MONITORING ASTHMA

LUNG BIOLOGY IN HEALTH AND DISEASE

Executive Editor

Claude Lenfant

Former Director, National Heart, Lung, and Blood Institute
National Institutes of Health
Bethesda, Maryland

The opinions expressed in these volumes do not necessarily represent the views of the National Institutes of Health.

MONITORING ASTHMA

Edited by

Peter G. Gibson
Hunter Medical Research Institute
New South Wales, Australia

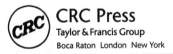

CRC Press
Taylor & Francis Group
Boca Raton London New York

CRC Press is an imprint of the
Taylor & Francis Group, an **informa** business

CRC Press
Taylor & Francis Group
6000 Broken Sound Parkway NW, Suite 300
Boca Raton, FL 33487-2742

First issued in paperback 2019

© 2010 by Taylor & Francis Group, LLC
CRC Press is an imprint of Taylor & Francis Group, an Informa business

No claim to original U.S. Government works

ISBN-13: 978-1-57444-855-9 (hbk)
ISBN-13: 978-0-367-39231-4 (pbk)

A CIP record for this book is available from the British Library.

Library of Congress Cataloging-in-Publication Data available on application

Visit the Taylor & Francis Web site at
http://www.taylorandfrancis.com

and the CRC Press Web site at
http://www.crcpress.com

Introduction

Half a century ago, infectious diseases were the major public health burden across the globe. Today, chronic diseases have emerged as the leading causes of death and disability worldwide, especially in developed countries but increasingly in the Third World as well. In the United States, asthma is said to affect up to 25 percent of children under 18 years of age and about 3–5 percent of adults. Fortunately, the U.S. death toll from asthma—less than 4,000 per year—is modest. In contrast, however, both morbidity and impaired quality of life from this disease are substantial and troubling.

Among the chronic diseases, asthma has characteristics that require specific and often individualized management approaches. During the past 20 years biomedical research has vastly increased our understanding of the pathogenesis of asthma, and this knowledge has provided physicians with pharmacologic tools to gain better control of the disease. Increasingly important is an emerging belief that approaches other than drugs can play an essential role in asthma management, sometimes reducing or even supplanting the need for medications. These non-pharmacological approaches are essentially dependent on effective "monitoring," the subject of this volume.

In his preface, editor Dr. Peter Gibson emphasizes the requirement for multifaceted monitoring. First, the patient—or the family, in the case of young children—must play a critical role in recognizing the symptoms that herald a need for therapeutic action. The techniques of self-monitoring are many, but the success of their application is dependent on the patient's knowledge about asthma and the available ways to control the disease's manifestations.

Also, critical components of successful monitoring are the physicians, nurses, and others involved in the care of the patient. These health-care professionals must have the tools to monitor the progression of the disease and its response to treatment, and to identify the environmental factors or activities that lead to exacerbations. In addition, recent research has shown the importance of empathy on the part of the health professional *vis á vis* the patient's reaction to his or her disease.

Over the years, the series of monographs Lung Biology in Health and Disease has addressed many aspects of asthma management, but only recently has it been recognized that careful monitoring can be an effective tool to control the physical and psychological consequences of the disease. This volume brings to the readership all the elements of monitoring that are required for the care of patients with asthma and evidence of the benefits that can accrue. Its authorship is multinational, thus adding the value of experiences tailored to cultural and health system differences. I am grateful to Dr. Gibson and to the authors for providing the opportunity to introduce this volume to our readership.

Claude Lenfant, MD
Gaithersburg, Maryland

Preface

Asthma is responsible for a vast and increasing level of illness in our society. Since asthma is a chronic illness, subject to periodic exacerbations and remissions, the monitoring of asthma is an essential component of asthma management. Not only is it necessary for physicians to monitor the management of the patient with asthma, there are also opportunities and benefits associated with self-monitoring of asthma by individuals with asthma, and for monitoring the quality and cost of care delivered to patients with asthma. Indeed, monitoring asthma outcomes is an essential step towards the successful implementation of the National Guidelines for the Management of Asthma.

This book deals with monitoring asthma from each of these perspectives. Self-monitoring by patients with asthma can involve measurements of symptoms or lung function using a variety of tools that can be recorded in a diary or via electronic means. This also involves the increasing and exciting possibilities of monitoring asthma using the Internet. Each of these parameters is considered, together with critical reviews of the individual's monitoring devices and their interpretation using familiar and innovational statistical techniques.

Health professionals also need to monitor patients with asthma. This not only involves monitoring control of asthma, but also management skills, adherence to treatment, and the investigation of significant asthma triggers, such as in occupational asthma. There are also some exciting developments from research that may be applicable to monitoring patients with asthma. These include the benefits of monitoring airway responsiveness in clinical practice together with markers of airway inflammation.

A crucial aspect of asthma care involves putting all the different pieces together. This means delivering the best quality asthma care at a variety of levels. In order to do this, it is important to monitor the quality and cost of asthma care. Some exciting developments have occurred in this area in a variety of disciplines. These are reviewed and examined in the context of monitoring asthma care. In addition, the important lessons learned from post-marketing surveillance and monitoring asthma mortality are examined and described in this book.

Monitoring of asthma is an important part of good asthma care. This book will be a valuable resource for health professionals involved in asthma care who are seeking to monitor patients in their practice or to help patients as they learn to monitor their illness. This book will also be of value to health system administrators and policy makers in outlining the successful approaches of monitoring the quality and cost of asthma care.

Peter G. Gibson

Contributors

R. J. Adams   The Queen Elizabeth Hospital Campus and Health Observatory, University of Adelaide, Woodville, South Australia, Australia

Sandra D. Anderson   Department of Respiratory Medicine, Royal Prince Alfred Hospital, Camperdown, Australia

C. L. Armour   Faculty of Pharmacy, University of Sydney, Sydney, Australia

Deborah F. Baker   Centre for Epidemiology and Research, NSW Health Department, North Sydney, Australia

M. A. Berry   Department of Respiratory Medicine and Thoracic Surgery, Institute for Lung Health, Glenfield Hospital, Leicester, U.K.

Peter B. Boggs   The Asthma 2000 Group, The Asthma-Allergy Clinic Center of Excellence, Shreveport, Louisiana, U.S.A.

S. Bosnic-Anticevich   Faculty of Pharmacy, University of Sydney, Sydney, Australia

John D. Brannan   Department of Respiratory Medicine, Royal Prince Alfred Hospital, Camperdown, Australia

André Cartier   Department of Chest Medicine, Hôpital du Sacré-Cœur de Montréal, Montréal, Québec, Canada

Anne B. Chang   Department of Respiratory Medicine, Royal Children's Hospital, Brisbane, Queensland and Department of Paediatrics and Child Health, University of Queensland, Queensland, Australia

Pierre Ernst Division of Clinical Epidemiology, Royal Victoria Hospital, McGill University Health Center, Montreal, Canada

Felicity S. Flack Telethon Institute for Child Health Research and Centre for Child Health Research, University of Western Australia, Perth, Western Australia

Denyse Gautrin Department of Chest Medicine, Hôpital du Sacré-Cœur de Montréal, Montréal, Québec, Canada

R. H. Green Department of Respiratory Medicine and Thoracic Surgery, Institute for Lung Health, Glenfield Hospital, Leicester, U.K.

Fazel Hayati Edgewood College, Madison, Wisconsin, U.S.A.

Ildiko Horvath Department of Pathophysiology, National Koranyi Institute for Pulmonology, Budapest, Hungary

Alan James West Australian Sleep Disorders Research Institute, Sir Charles Gairdner Hospital, and School of Medicine and Pharmacology, University of Western Australia, Nedlands, Western Australia, Australia

Elizabeth F. Juniper Department of Clinical Epidemiology and Biostatistics, McMaster University, Hamilton, Ontario, Canada

Heikki Koskela Department of Respiratory Medicine, Kuopio University Hospital, Kuopio, Finland

I. Krass Faculty of Pharmacy, University of Sydney, Sydney, Australia

Manon Labrecque Department of Chest Medicine, Hôpital du Sacré-Cœur de Montréal, Montréal, Québec, Canada

Catherine Lemiere Department of Chest Medicine, Hôpital du Sacré-Cœur de Montréal, Montréal, Québec, Canada

Jörg D. Leuppi Respiratory Medicine, University Hospital Basel, Basel, Switzerland

Jean-Luc Malo Department of Chest Medicine, Hôpital du Sacré-Cœur de Montréal, Montréal, Québec, Canada

Guy B. Marks Australian Centre for Asthma Monitoring, Woolcock Institute of Medical Research, Sydney, Australia

Tim O'Meara Woolcock Institute of Medical Research, University of Sydney, Sydney, Australia

I. D. Pavord Department of Respiratory Medicine and Thoracic Surgery, Institute for Lung Health, Glenfield Hospital, Leicester, U.K.

Neil Pearce Centre for Public Health Research, Massey University Wellington Campus, Wellington, New Zealand

Helen K. Reddel Woolcock Institute of Medical Research and University of Sydney, Camperdown, New South Wales, Australia

R. E. Ruffin The Queen Elizabeth Hospital Campus and Health Observatory, University of Adelaide, Woodville, South Australia, Australia

B. Saini Faculty of Pharmacy, University of Sydney, Sydney, Australia

Susan M. Sawyer Department of Respiratory Medicine, Centre for Adolescent Health, Royal Children's Hospital, and Department of Pediatrics, The University of Melbourne, South Australia, Australia

D. E. Shaw Department of Respiratory Medicine and Thoracic Surgery, Institute for Lung Health, Glenfield Hospital, Leicester, U.K.

Peter D. Sly Telethon Institute for Child Health Research and Centre for Child Health Research, University of Western Australia, Perth, Western Australia

Samy Suissa Division of Clinical Epidemiology, Royal Victoria Hospital, McGill University Health Centre, and the Departments of Epidemiology and Biostatistics and Medicine, McGill University, Montreal, Canada

Euan Tovey Woolcock Institute of Medical Research, University of Sydney, Sydney, Australia

Claire Wainwright Department of Respiratory Medicine, Royal Children's Hospital, Queensland, Australia

Donald J. Wheeler Statistical Process Controls, Inc. Knoxville, Tennessee, U.S.A.

Margaret Williamson Australian Centre for Asthma Monitoring, Woolcock Institute of Medical Research, Sydney, Australia

D. H. Wilson The Queen Elizabeth Hospital Campus and Health Observatory, University of Adelaide, Woodville, South Australia, Australia

Richard Wootton Centre for Online Health, University of Queensland, Queensland, Australia

Contents

1

Symptoms: Monitoring, Perceptions

R. J. ADAMS, D. H. WILSON, and R. E. RUFFIN

The Queen Elizabeth Hospital Campus and Health Observatory,
  University of Adelaide,
Woodville, South Australia, Australia

Symptom monitoring is not new. It has been occurring in one form or another from before the time asthma was recognized as an entity. Symptoms have resulted in people seeking help/diagnosis/treatment from health professionals before the era of lung function tests. Symptoms still play a major part in people presenting to health professionals which, in turn, may lead to the diagnosis of asthma.

In this chapter, we will focus on asthma in adults and explore the causes of symptoms, extend the symptom concept from "usual" asthma symptoms, look at the purpose of monitoring, examine influences that may affect the detection of asthma symptoms, describe some of the tools for asthma symptom monitoring, and suggest a framework which includes consideration of perception in asthma management.

Asthma Symptoms

It has been widely taught that one or more of the symptoms of cough, wheeze, shortness of breath, and chest tightness occurring in a variable or episodic time frame is/are the common or cardinal asthma symptoms

(1). These symptoms are not specific for asthma. They can occur individually or in combination with a range of other pulmonary diseases. These include airway diseases such as bronchitis and bronchiectasis, parenchymal lung disease such as emphysema or interstitial lung disease such as pulmonary fibrosis. The specificity of asthma symptoms is likely to be increased when details of triggering factors, seasonal variation, and response to treatment are explored (2). The mechanisms for asthma symptoms are:

1. Cough—via airway irritant receptor stimulation by chemicals from the inflammatory process in the airways, bronchoconstriction or the presence of mucous in the airways (3).
2. Wheezing—from bronchoconstriction or narrowing of the airway lumen by smooth muscle contraction, thickening of the airway wall and/or the presence of mucous in the lumen (4). This may be inspiratory or expiratory, with the latter being more frequent.
3. Chest tightness—due to narrowing of small airways resulting in airway closure causing gas trapping giving the sensation of chest tightness (5).
4. Shortness of breath—because of (a) the increased work ofbreathing due to a shift to a higher functional residual capacity for tidal breathing because of airway closure, and asa result of breathing against increased airway resistance and (b) as a result of ventilation–perfusion mismatch occurring from of variable airway narrowing affecting the distribution of ventilation. (The end result of severe mismatch being hypoxemia) (5).

However, we should probably extend our "conceptualization" of symptoms. It is usual to consider diurnal variation in taking an asthma history. Nocturnal symptoms are commonly used to measure asthma severity. However, it is also useful to delineate symptoms in relation to rest and exercise. Exercise is used as a stress test in other disease states e.g., coronary artery disease, and we should use "stress" as one of the associations for asthma symptoms.

Reduced exercise capacity also becomes an internal marker or a symptom when compared with (an individuals) best or usual exercise capacity and is commonly used by health professionals to assess asthma control during the review process.

Furthermore, the educated asthma patient self-monitors their status and responds to increases in the cardinal symptom (s) or reduction in exercise capacity by taking reliever or bronchodilator medication. So bronchodilator use in response to altered asthma status or the presence of asthma symptoms is an example of self-monitoring in every asthma patient using as required short-acting bronchodilator medication. We should consider bronchodilator use in two ways: (a) a symptom action, as increasing use will most often be a response to an increase in symptoms and may or may not trigger an appropriate event such as an Emergency Department visit or an unscheduled general practitioner visit as part of the patients asthma action plan, and (b) an integrated outcome of symptom monitoring which sums recognized symptoms. Other events such as courses of oral corticosteroids, unscheduled medical practitioner visits and Emergency Department visits may be considered as possible outcomes of symptom monitoring. Now is the time to elevate both exercise capacity compared with best or usual, and reliever medication use into the "cardinal symptom group" for asthma. Recognition of some of the limitations of symptom monitoring described later should be applied to bronchodilator use. Some people will use their bronchodilator through habit, or as a preventative strategy to reduce the risk of exercise-induced bronchoconstriction or continue to use bronchodilator unnecessarily before preventer medications because they have been told in the 1980s that it was necessary to "open up the airways" and let the preventer agent penetrate more deeply into the airways. Consequently, a more appropriate candidate for inclusion as an essential element of asthma assessment is frequency of bronchodilator use for symptom relief, or rescue use rather than routine use before preventer medication or exercise.

Purpose of Symptom Monitoring

Any discussion of symptom monitoring must consider the purpose of such an exercise. The reasons for assessing symptoms are to allow individual classification of asthma status, detect individual asthma exacerbations, and to measure community asthma burden, which may in turn reflect asthma management practice over time. The classification of asthma status whether this be labelled seventy or control is used as a basis for determining the intensity and direction of treatment, including doctor review, and subsequently for monitoring the effectiveness of individual treatment and whether further changes are needed. A number of national and international classification schemes have been developed (6–8). These guidelines generally propose that assessment of asthma status is based on symptomatic and functional assessments, including the frequency and severity of asthma symptoms, the frequency of rescue bronchodilator use, and measures of lung function or airway caliber. Functional assessments include how asthma affects the patient and family, with the goal that therapy should allow patients to have few symptoms and little interference with activities (8). Therefore, a more global concept of control would assess both the recent and chronic symptoms of asthma as well as a patients' functional status. It can therefore be argued that "symptom" monitoring requires measuring all these components in some way and classifying them to arrive at a sense of an individual's asthma status and management needs. This would then encompass the outcome of "asthma control" that has been defined as the composite goal of treatment identified in the GINA guidelines (7). It is relevant to note that a recent study reports low level of agreement amongst pediatric asthma specialists in classifying asthma severity in eight case summaries (9).

Asthma symptom burden can be conceptualized as three components: short-term symptom burden, long-term symptom burden, and functional status (10). Short-term symptom burden considers the recent time period, for example, over the past 4 weeks, and can be further categorized on the basis of reported recent daily/morning symptoms and nocturnal symptoms. Long-term symptoms include the frequency of asthma exacerbations, as well as the average frequency and severity or usual symptoms over a period, for example, 12 months. This formulation captures the intermittent or episodic nature of asthma symptoms for many people. Functional impact arises from the impact on activities of living from asthma. It can be a general measure ["limitation on daily activities" (11)] or broken down into at least three components: physical activities, social activities, and nocturnal impact (sleeping) (10). Included in this could be exercise limitation, as well as limitations such as avoiding certain places or activities that trigger symptoms.

People with asthma report varying patterns of timing of asthma symptoms. Fuhlbrigge et al. (10) using a survey of a representative U.S. population sample, found that only 58% of people with asthma were classified similarly on the basis of their report of both day- and night-time symptoms. Colice et al. (12), in a clinical trial population, also observed a similar lack of concordance between types of asthma symptoms. Both studies found that nocturnal symptoms occurred more commonly than day-time symptoms. However, when both day- and night-time symptoms were grouped into a combined measure of short-term symptoms, a much higher proportion of individuals were classified as having moderate-to-severe persistent symptoms than were found by either measure alone.

Juniper et al. (13) used a factor analysis to explore relationships within different aspects of asthma health status. These authors found that day-time asthma (including symptoms and day-time beta-agonist use) and night-time asthma were distinct components of asthma status. These results are consistent with the notion proposed by Kraft and Martin (14) that nocturnal asthma is distinct from day-time asthma although this notion has been challenged by others (15). Bai et al. (16) retrospectively analyzed 17 respiratory symptoms in a population sample of 1527 adults aged 18–55 years to determine whether some questions were better than others for predicting asthma. They found that questions which predicted asthma were those about asthma attack, chest tightness, shortness of breath at rest, and wheeze at rest or after exercise. They found that nocturnal cough did not help to differentiate a syndrome and suggested omitting it from adult asthma questionnaires. In contrast, Osman et al. (17) used scenarios to assess the relative importance of common symptoms in adults with asthma and found a different result. Day-time cough and breathlessness had greater influence on these adult asthmatics than wheeze or sleep disturbance. They also found that age influenced symptoms, with younger patients weighting breathlessness more than older patients. Regardless of whether one accepts a separation of day-time and nocturnal asthma, the literature can be interpreted to give support to the importance of the idea of a global composite measure of "asthma control," as the goal of management.

Functional Limitation

The other symptom group listed in guidelines as being important, but less commonly assessed in clinical studies, is functional activity limitation. In the study by Fuhlbrigge et al. (10) assessment of activity limitation showed that the impact of asthma on the daily activities of people with asthma was considerable. Two-thirds of individuals in this U.S. population survey reported that asthma had "some" or "a lot" of impact on physical activity. As the authors note, these results illustrate that evaluation of specific day- and night-time symptoms alone may underestimate the impact of asthma on patient's lives, and consequently over-estimate the degree of asthma control being achieved. This may then lead to recommendations for inadequate treatment and ongoing asthma burden to individuals.

Part of the difficulty in incorporating activity limitation into assessments of asthma control has been the lack of a clear methodology for measurement, or even agreement between health professionals and patients as to the significance of such limitations. Osborne et al. (18) compared patients' asthma severity as assessed by physicians with a severity score based on the NAEPP 2 guideline recommendations using the level of current asthma symptoms. They found no correlation between physician-assessed severity and symptom-based severity, and this lack of correlation persisted when asthma symptoms were separated into day-time and nocturnal symptoms. When patients have inadequate symptom control, lower physician estimates of symptom control have been associated with less use of inhaled corticosteroids than guidelines would recommend (19). This difficulty in recognizing what impact asthma is having with the consequence of under-treatment has been previously noted (20–22).

Symptom Monitoring and Exacerbations

An important use of symptom monitoring is the identification of exacerbations. Tattersfield et al. (23) found that during clinical asthma exacerbations that require treatment with oral corticosteroids, changes in peak expiratory flow (PEF), symptoms and rescue beta-agonist use occur in parallel prior to the exacerbation. This suggests none of these is superior in providing early warning of asthma exacerbations. Malo et al. (24) showed symptoms to be as effective as PEF in recognizing the onset of an exacerbation in people with moderate-to-severe asthma. Gibson et al. (25) demonstrated that symptoms usually precede changes in PEF in exacerbations induced by reduction of preventer medication. Similarly, peak-flow-based asthma action plans have not demonstrated superiority over symptom-based plans in managing exacerbations or reducing asthma morbidity (26–28). This may largely be because patients are more likely to initiate changes to therapy when more severe symptoms accompany falls in PEF than when symptoms are absent (29). Symptoms are also more closely linked to patients' global assessments of control and more likely to lead to seeking medical attention (30). Therefore, symptoms appear to be effective for monitoring and detecting exacerbations in patients with infrequent exacerbations or mild asthma (26), and in also people with moderate-to-severe asthma (28). To extrapolate findings from these publications into practice requires knowledge of the study group perception of their symptoms. This was not formally tested in these studies, although Adams et al. (28) excluded patients with known poor perception of symptoms from their study.

Respiratory infections, often viral, are associated with a high proportion of asthma exacerbations (31). Even people with well-controlled asthma remain vulnerable to infective asthma exacerbations (32). Reddel et al. (32) described a lack of responsiveness to beta-agonists as measured by PEF during presumed viral exacerbations in people with asthma. This is consistent with previous studies that reported patients describing diminished effectiveness of beta-agonists during infective exacerbations of asthma (33,34). In contrast, different mechanisms of inducing asthma exacerbations, such as reduction in inhaled corticosteroids or increased allergen exposure, as well as periods of poor asthma control, show airway lability as reflected by wide diurnal variability in PEF and bronchodilator responsiveness (25,35). Despite suggestions that use of long-acting beta-agonists could mask the symptoms of impending exacerbations (36), Tattersfield et al. (23) found that exacerbations "did not differ in severity or response to treatment" in people taking or not taking formoterol.

These findings have a number of implications for the use and interpretation of symptoms in monitoring for poor asthma control and asthma exacerbations. Symptoms of clinical respiratory infections, along with persistence of asthma symptoms despite rescue beta-agonist use, may need to be considered as a distinct form of asthma exacerbation. Whether these episodes should have a different specified treatment approach requires further research. Tattersfield et al. (23) examined whether certain types of changes in clinical state could identify exacerbations earlier. The occurrence of increased nocturnal symptoms may be relatively specific for prediction of an asthma exacerbation. However, these authors also found that the development of nocturnal symptoms was not sensitive, as most patients who went on to have an exacerbation did not have nocturnal symptoms 2 days prior to an attack. These findings suggest that in the education of patients regarding exacerbation identification, it may be beneficial to clarify that nocturnal symptoms are highly likely to indicate an impending attack that requires additional treatment. However, nocturnal symptoms cannot be solely used to identify an incipient exacerbation, as increased day-time symptoms and rescue beta-agonist use will be more common antecedents of an exacerbation.

We must exhibit caution in translating the data described above into clinical practice. These data are average data from controlled clinical settings in which the population has signed a form of contract i.e., a consent form after written information about what is required during the study. These studies often show disease status improvement during a run in period which possibly reflects improved adherence with medication regimens and a desire to satisfy the clinician. Also the data will not necessarily be transferable to an individual patient in an individual set of circumstances.

There may be differential effects in individuals. For example, wheezing may be present in some people and chest tightness may be more common in other individuals. The possible reasons for this may be variations between individuals but also variations in the type of stimulus. For example, small particle aerosols of histamine may cause more chest tightness than wheezing. In other words, it is possible that these different symptoms particularly in the same patient may indicate whether there is narrowing in the larger airways for wheezing or particularly narrowing in the peripheral airways for chest tightness. A common pattern is for adults with asthma to have more dyspnea and chest tightness rather than attacks of wheeze (37). However, the data from Bai et al. (16) and Osman et al. (17) show different schools of thought. Without training, individuals will presumably self-monitor symptoms on the basis of a range of factors including education and understanding of asthma and what it means.

There is no clear evidence to support whether a combination of symptoms is better than one symptom. The pattern is likely to vary amongst individual asthmatics. The challenge is to identify within an individual whether a combination of symptoms is better for that person.

The literature indicates that there is a need to coach patients to internally monitor symptoms against an absolute scale of good and poor control rather than in comparison to a "usual poorly controlled state." To facilitate this in practice, we will require a change in asthma management systems to allow time for patient "coaching." This may require an increase in time for the asthma review and/or a defined program of asthma review e.g., the Australian NAC 3+ Visit Plan, (38) and/or an increase or change in the type of health professional taking part in the asthma review process. Coaching has demonstrated effectiveness in other disease settings in improving self-assessment and self-management (39).

Symptom Perception

Within the asthma population there will be a range of awareness of symptoms reflecting the perception of the population. The perceptive ability of an individual patient will be influenced by psychosocial factors, genetic factors, situational and environmental circumstances, duration of asthma, the site of bronchoconstriction, and the type of any external stimulus.

Within the asthma population it may be a normal distribution, where at the bottom part of the normal distribution curve there are a group who have reduced awareness of symptoms and at the other end there will be a group who have increased awareness of symptoms (Fig. 1). The size of these populations is not known but they represent groups who have potentially opposing effects in terms of monitoring of asthma. The study of Salome et al. (40) supports a normal distribution with a wide confidence interval.

There are also likely to be abnormal populations of asthma who can have increased awareness. One may be a population who have a post-traumatic stress disorder following, for example, a near fatal or life-threatening episode of asthma and others with an anxiety disorder. There are likely to be other populations of asthmatic people who have apparently reduced

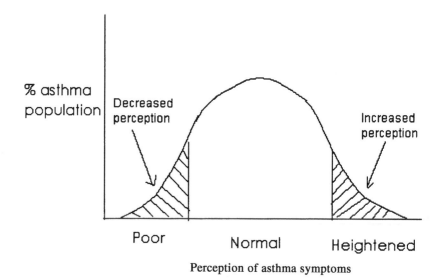

Figure 1   Perception of asthma symptoms.

awareness which may be related to denial, chronic poor control, or perhaps centrally acting medications including alcohol.

There are many factors which will influence perception and an individual's perception will not necessarily remain constant over time. Roisman et al. (41) reported interesting data on perception in asthma with several possible interpretations. They showed that in patients with asthma not exposed to corticosteroids, that there was good perception to methacholine-induced bronchoconstriction but poor perception with bradykinin induced bronchoconstriction. In asthmatics exposed to corticosteroids, the bronchoconstriction induced by both agents was well perceived. The data imply that perception may change with medication, but also that under particular circumstances different stimuli or trigger factors result in differently perceived bronchoconstriction. The authors proposed that eosinophilic inflammation and its magnitude were a determining factor for perception. Turcotte et al. (42) found no difference between bronchoconstrictors consisting of antigen, exercise and inhaled histamine, and the perception of acute bronchoconstriction. These authors proposed that it was the speed of the increase in airflow obstruction which caused variability in the perception of narrowing. Salome et al. (43) found that treatment with budesonide (1600 µg 3200 µg/day) for 8 weeks in 35 patients with poorly controlled asthma improved perception of bronchoconstriction induced by inhaled histamine. The improvement was not related to changes in FEV_1, airway responsiveness, nor blood eosinophils. Using a different model of resistive loads Jang and Choi (44) showed that an inhaled short-acting β_2-agonist improved the perception of dyspnoea in 20 patients with asthma of varying severity.

In a population sample, James et al. (45) showed that perception of mild and moderate degrees of airway narrowing from methacholine challenge varies widely between individuals, but is increased in subjects with mild asthma compared to nonasthmatics and this increase is independent of airway responsiveness.

Brand et al. (46) found supportive data in that asymptomatic hyperresponsive patients were less perceptive than symptomatic patients during a histamine challenge, but did find a relation with age, i.e., younger patients were more perceptive. Connolly et al. (47) showed that 34 elderly subjects were less aware of bronchoconstriction than young asthmatics. Boulet et al. (48) in contrast found that older patients were more perceptive and attributed this to high post-control saline inhalation scores. Of interest is that this study of 150 consecutive subjects did show a normal distribution pattern for perception of breathlessness during histamine challenge.

To summarize these studies: there are no simple demographic characteristics, blood eosinophil level, degree of airflow obstruction, or degree of airway hyper-responsiveness that allows the prediction of hypo- or hyperperceivers of bronchoconstriction. However, the necessity to identify these groups is emphasized by the findings of Rubinfeld and Pain (49) of the presence of a significant proportion of hypo-perceivers in the population with significant asthma.

In a review of symptom perception in asthma, Rietveld and Brosschot (50) propose that biomedical factors are more plausible in blunted perception and psychological factors in overperception. However, they emphasize that denial can account for blunted perception, and that emotional distress, panic, or selective perception can explain overperception. Hence, understanding the biomedical state of an individual and their psychological state will be paramount to understanding and interpreting an individuals symptoms.

The reporting of respiratory symptoms may also be influenced by psychological status (51). People with depression are more likely to report asthma symptoms (52,53). Psychological factors may influence asthma symptom monitoring in a number of possible ways. Depression is associated with decreased performance on problem solving (54), complex task performance (55), memory (56), and attention span (57). All of these cognitive processes can influence decision-making and perception of people with asthma. The effect of negative mood on symptom perception can also influence bronchodilator use. Main et al. (58) found that in the presence of negative mood, people seemed more likely to interpret non-specific symptoms as related to asthma and increased bronchodilator use. Bukstein (59) has noted that in asthma patients who had stable clinical markers such as lung function but who reported feeling that their asthma was "really bad and my energy is down," physicians learned to look for depression. It is clear that any method of assessing symptoms will need to allow for psychological status and physiological perception of changes in airway caliber. However, the effect of these factors on the symptom scoring systems outlined below is not well described. At present, clinical judgment remains the physician's best guide to integrating reported symptoms and the various factors that influence them.

Symptom Scoring Systems

The type of system will at least be partly dependent on the purpose. For clinical trials, both periodic questionnaires and daily diaries have been described as methods of recording the clinical asthma status. Few of these tools have undergone testing for validity and clinical responsiveness (24,25,60). Santanello et al. (11) have developed a daily asthma symptom diary and then averaged the daily score to come up with a weekly asthma symptom burden. In addition, they have validated diary scales constructed by experienced clinical asthma researchers based on unvalidated diary scales. The day-time symptom questions included 4 questions on: frequency of asthma symptoms in a day; how much bother the symptoms were; activity potential; and asthma affect on activities scored on a 0 (none) to 6 (all) scale. The nocturnal question was about waking with asthma symptoms scored on a 4-point scale from no to "awake all night." The day-time symptom scale showed good internal consistency (Cronbach's alpha coefficient 0.90–0.92). The test–retest reliability of the day- and night-scales was reasonably good (intraclass correlation coefficient 0.69–0.87). Both scales showed responsiveness to a change in asthma status produced by therapy. This tool is relatively simple and under copyright.

Other validated tools include those described by Gibson et al. (25), Malo et al. (60), and Steen et al. (61). Gibson et al. (25) used a daily asthma symptom diary (cough, chest tightness, breathlessness, and wheeze) and a weekly asthma symptom questionnaire to document loss of asthma control or not, in a steroid withdrawal study. Malo et al. (60) used a daily symptom diary (night-time asthma, symptoms on wakening, and school/work absence) to estimate asthma exacerbation in comparison to peak flow monitoring. Steen et al. (61) developed and validated a 10-item asthma symptom questionnaire which reflected the last month and were scaled on 5 points for frequency of symptoms and a 4-point scale for bother from symptoms. They also examined the responsiveness to change and found that the questionnaire was more sensitive to change in asthma status than a generic measure of general health perception.

A range of other symptom-scoring systems have been described. The Aas score (62) is derived from the frequency and severity of asthma episodes over the previous one year. The 5-point scale uses number and severity of episodes, lung function, hospitalization, and use of corticosteroids. The Hargreave score (63) uses symptoms, inhaled β_2-agonists, lung function, and PEF variability to generate four levels of severity assessed at one point in time. The Brooks Disease Severity Score (64) uses attack, day and night symptoms, cough, exertional dyspnea, and maintenance therapy to create a possible scoring range of 6–30. This assessment is based on what has occurred over the previous 6 months. Each of the scores exhibit a correlation with lung function i.e., FEV_1, measured at the time of assessment (65). These scores represent a combination of patient symptoms, events, and physiological measures and take time to apply.

Symptom scores are often used in clinical trials of respiratory medications to define benefit, and to determine loss of asthma control. The number of symptom free days has become a popular way of defining benefit of a preparation in a comparative study (66).

Because good or optimal asthma control is a target for all clinicians, there is a developing emphasis on measuring control rather than severity. Control is a concept which incorporates symptoms, functional ability, and ideally lung function. Several tools to measure asthma control utilize asthma symptoms and medication use only. One tool has been developed by Juniper et al. (67) by surveying clinicians internationally for the importance of individual symptoms developing a questionnaire and validating it.

The survey gave the 87 clinicians 10 options for selecting their five most important symptoms. These five were from greatest importance—woken at night by symptoms; limitation of normal daily activities; waking in the morning with symptoms; dyspnea and wheeze. Cough, chest discomfort, sputum, coloured sputum, and need to clear throat were symptoms not ranked highly by clinicians. It is interesting to note the discrepancy or mismatch between patient studies showing cough and dyspnoea were important.

The five most important symptoms over the previous 7 days are marked on a 7 point scale and average β_2-agonist use/day and bronchodilator FEV_1 included to give the Asthma Control Questionnaire. This relatively brief tool for assessing short-term control has been shown to have reasonable discriminative abilities in distinguishing stable from unstable groups.

Other tools to assess control have been developed and validated. Katz et al. (68) produced an 11-item perceived control of asthma questionnaire which addresses the domains of perceived responsibility for disease management, perceived ability to cope and control asthma, and any sense of futility or fatalism related to asthma.

Vollmer et al. (69) developed and validated the Asthma Therapy Assessment Questionnaire (ATAQ) which was intended to detect suboptimal management and barriers to management. ATAQ asks about: self-perception of asthma control; missed work, school or usual activities due to asthma; night-time wakening due to asthma and use of reliever medication. All categories were for the last 4 weeks and were graded as yes or no for a control problem and summed to give an index from 0 to 4.

Framework

In the ideal world, an individual asthma patient would have some form of assessment of perception made intermittently. The simplest method is measurement of bronchodilator response in an office review or prior to an office review. During this maneuver the patient is asked, "can you feel the difference from the bronchodilator?" If yes, is it small, moderate or large? and the clinician matches this with the FEV_1 bronchodilator response. (Note there is the opportunity to check device use at this time.) The clinician then will be able to arrive at an assessment of perception. If this is not possible, there are two other ways to assess perception — (i) a formal provocative test in the laboratory (histamine, methacholine, exercise, hypertonic saline, or mannitol) or (ii) a retrospective or prospective correlation between symptoms and PEF readings.

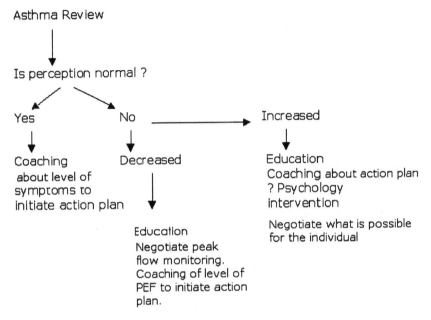

Figure 2   Future of symptom monitoring.

If the clinician makes the assessment of reasonable perception, the clinician can match their assessment of control (67) vs. patients perceived control (68). If there is no mismatch, then coach the patient with regard to symptoms, including bronchodilator use, which indicate the need for action in an asthma exacerbation (Fig. 2).

If perception is blunted, encourage the patient to undertake frequent PEF monitoring and provide a written action plan with the identification of PEF levels at which specific therapies or action are to take place.

If perception is heightened, encourage discussion as to possible reasons and if necessary refer for psychological intervention. Desensitization of heightened perception may be possible with PEF monitoring.

It is still possible to have a mismatch of control between patient and health professional in either direction in the latter circumstances. The exploration of the reasons for this mismatch, and strategies to remedy this mismatch, are important to implement. It will come as no surprise that we need further research to validate the above framework.

References

1. Woolcock AJ. Asthma. In: Murray JF, Nadel JA, eds. Textbook of Respiratory Medicine. 2nd ed. Philadelphia: WB Saunders, 1994:1288–1330.

2. Cogo A, Beghe B, Corbetta L, Fabbri L. Diagnosis in adults. In: O'Byrne PM, Thomson NC, eds. Manual of Asthma Management. 2nd ed. London: WB Saunders, 2001:63–80.
3. Fuller RW, Jackson DM. Physiology and treatment of cough. Thorax 1990; 45:425–430.
4. Wiggs B, Moreno R, James A, Hogg JC, Paré P. A model of the mechanics of airway narrowing in asthma. In: Kaliner MA, Barnes PJ, Persson CGA, Lenfant C, eds. Asthma. Its Pathology and Treatment. Lung Biology in Health and Disease Vol. 49. New York: Marcel Dekker, 1991:73–101.
5. Larsen GL, Cherniack RM, Irvin CG. Pulmonary physiology of severe asthma in children and adults. In: Szefler SJ, Leung DYM, Lenfant C, eds. Severe Asthma Pathogenesis and Clinical Management. Lung Biology in Health and Disease Vol. 86. New York: Marcel Dekker, 1996:77–101.
6. British Thoracic Society, National Asthma Campaign, Royal College of Physicians of London in association with the General Practitionerin Asthma Group et al. The British guidelines on asthma management: 1995 review and position statement. Thorax 1997; 52(suppl 1):S1–S21.
7. National Heart Lung and Blood Institute, Global initiative for asthma. Global strategy for asthma management and prevention.NHLB1/VHO workshop report. National Institutes of Health, Bethesda 1995: National Heart Lung and Blood Institute publication number 95–3659.
8. National Institutes of Health/National Heart, Lung, and Blood Institute. National Asthma Education and Prevention Program Expert Panel. Clinical Practice Guidelines. Expert Panel report 2: guidelines for the diagnosis and management of asthma, Vol. publication no. 97-4051. Bethesda, MD: National Institutes of Health/National Heart, Lung, and Blood Institute, 1997.
9. Baker KM, Brand DA, Hen J. Classifying asthma. Disagreement among specialists. Chest 2003; 124:2156–2163.
10. Fuhlbrigge AL, Adams RJ, GuilbertTW, Grant E, Lozano P, Janson SL, Martinez F, Weiss KB, Weiss ST. The burden of asthma in the United States: level and distribution are dependent on interpretation of the national asthma education and prevention program guidelines. Am J Respir Crit Med 2002; 166:1044–1049.
11. Santanello NC, Barber BL, Reiss TF, Friedman BS, Juniper EF, Zhang J. Measurement characteristics of two asthma symptom diary scales for use in clinical trials. Eur Resp J 1997; 10:646–651.
12. Colice GL, Vanden Burgt J, Song J, Stampore P, Thompson PJ. Categorizing asthma severity. Am J Respir Crit Care Med 1999; 160:1962–1967.
13. Juniper EF, Wisniewski ME, Cox FR, Emmett AH, Nielsen KE,O'Byrne PM. Relationship between quality of life and clinical status in asthma. A factor analysis. Eur Respir J 2004; 23:287–291.
14. Kraft M, Martin RJ. Nocturnal asthma. In: Barnes PJ, Grunstein MM, Leff AR, Woolcock AJ, eds. Asthma. Philadelphia, USA: Lippincott-Raven Publishers, 1997:2005–2024.
15. Weersink EJ, Postma DS. Nocturnal asthma: not a separate disease entity. Respir Med 1994; 88:483–491.

16. Bai J, Peat JK, Berry G, Marks GB, Woolcock AJ. Questionnaire items that predict asthma and other respiratory conditions in adults. Chest 1998; 114:1343–1348.

17. Osman LM, McKenzie L, Cairns J, Friend JAR, Godden DH, Legge JS, Douglas JG. Patient weighting of importance of asthma symptoms. Thorax 2001; 56:138–142.

18. Osborne ML, Vollmer WM, Pedula KL, Wilkins J, Buist AS, O'Halloran M. Lack of correlation of symptoms with specialist assessed long-term asthma severity. Chest 1999; 115:85–91.

19. Wolfenden LL, Diette GB, Krishnan JA, Skinner EA, Steinwachs DM, Wu AW. Lower physician estimates of underlying asthma severity leads to under treatment. Arch Intern Med 2003; 163:231–236.

20. Burdon JG, Juniper EF, Killian KJ, Hargreave FE, Campbell EJ. The perception of breathlessness in asthma. Am Rev Respir Dis 1982; 126:825–828.

21. McFadden ER Jr. Clinical physiologic correlates in asthma. J Allergy Clin Immunol 1986; 77:1-5.

22. Sears MR. Increasing asthma mortality: fact or artifact? J Allergy Clin Immunol 1998; 82:957–960.

23. Tattersfield AE, Postma DS, Barnes PJ, Svensson K, Bauer CA, O'Brien PM, Lofdahl CG, Pauels RA, Ullman A. Exacerbations of asthma: a descriptive study of 425 severe exacerbations. Am J Respir Crit Care Med 1998; 160:594–599.

24. Malo JL, Arch eweque JL, Trudeau C, d'Aquino C, Cartier A. Should we monitor peak expiratory flow rates or record symptoms with a simple diary in the management of asthma?. J Allergy Clin Immunol 1993; 91:702–709.

25. Gibson P, Wong B, Hepperle M. A research method to induce and examine a mild exacerbation of asthma by withdrawal of inhaled corticosteroid. Clin Exp Allergy 1992; 22:525–532.

26. Turner MO, Taylor D, Bennett R, Fitzgerald JM. A randomized trial comparing peak flow expiratory flow and symptom self-management plans for patients with asthma attending a primary care clinic. Am J Respir Crit Care Med 1998; 157:540–546.

27. Grampian Asthma Study of Integrated Care (GRASSIC). Effectiveness of routine self-monitoring of peak flows in patients with asthma. BMJ 1994; 308:564–567.

28. Adams RJ, Boath K, Homan S, Campbell DA, Ruffin RE. A randomized trial of peak flow and symptom based action plans in adults with moderate to severe asthma. Respirology 2001; 6:297–304.

29. Lahdensuo A, Haahtela T, Herrala J, Kava T, Kirivanta K, Kuusisto K, Pekurinen M, Perämäki E, Saarelainen S, Suahn T, Liljas B. Randomized comparison of cost effectiveness of guided self management and traditional treatment of asthma in Finland. BMJ 1998; 316:1138–1139.

30. Boulet LP, Boulet V, Milot J. How should we quantify asthma control? A proposal. Chest 2002; 122:2217–2223.

31. Nicholson KG, Kent J, Iceland DC. Respiratory viruses and exacerbations of asthma in adults. BMJ 1993; 307:982–986.

32. Reddel H, Ware S, Marks G, Salome C, Jenkins C, Woolcock A. Differences between asthma exacerbations and poor asthma control. Lancet 1999; 353:364–369.
33. Abisheganaden J, Sin Fai Lam KN, Lim TK. A profile of acute asthma patients presenting to the emergency room. Singapore MedJ 1996; 37:252–254.
34. Rebuck AS, Read J. Assessment and management of severe asthma. Am J Med 1971; 51:788–798.
35. Meijer GG, Postma DS, van der Heide S. Exogenous stimuli and circadian peak expiratory flow variation in allergic asthmatic children. Am J Respir Crit Care Med 1996; 153:237–242.
36. McIvor RA, Pizzichini E, Turner MO, Hussack P, Hargreave FE, Sears MR. Potential masking effects of salmeterol on airway inflammation in asthma. Am J Respir Crit Care Med 1998; 158:924–930.
37. Bronniman S, Burrows B. A prospective study of the natural history of asthma: relapse and remission rates. Chest 1986; 90:480–484.
38. National Asthma Council Australia. The asthma 3+ visit plan. http://www. National asthma.com.au.
39. Vale MJ, Jelinek MV, Best JD, Dart AM, Grigg LI, Hare DL, Ho BP, Newman RW, McNeil JJ. COACH study group. Coaching patients on achieving cardiovascular health ((COACH): a multicenter randomized trial in patients with coronary heart disease. Arch Intern Med 2003; 163:2775–2783.
40. Salome CM, Xuan W, Gray EJ, Belooussova E, Peat JK. Perception of airway narrowing in a general population sample. Eur Respir J 1997; 10:1052–1058.
41. Roisman GL, Peiffer Cl, Lacronique JB LeCae A, Dusser DJ. Perception of bronchial obstruction in asthmatic patients: relationship with bronchial eosinophilic inflammation and epithelial damage and effect of corticosteroid treatment. J Clin Invest 1995; 96:12–21.
42. Turcotte H, Corbeil F, Boulet LP. Perception of breathlessness during bronchoconstriction induced by antigen, exercise and histamine challenges. Thorax 1990; 45:914–189.
43. Salome CM, Reddel HK, Ware SI, Roberts AM, Jenkins CR, Marks. GB, Woolcock AJ. Effects of budesonide on the perception of induced airway narrowing in subjects with asthma. Am J Respir Crit Care Med 2002; 165:15–21.
44. Jang A, Choi I. Increased perception of dyspnoea by inhalation of short acting β_2 agonist in patients with asthma of varying severity. Ann Allergy Asthma Immunol 2000; 84:79–83.
45. James AL, Carroll N, DeKlerk N, Elliott J, Musk AW, Ryan G. Increased perception of airway narrowing in patients with mild asthma. Respirology 1998; 3:241–245.
46. Brand PLP, Rijcken B, Schouten JP, Koeter GH, Weiss ST Postma DS. Perception of airway obstruction in a random population sample. Relationship to airway hyperresponsiveness in the absence of respiratory symptoms. Am Rev Respir Dis 1992; 146:396–401.
47. Connolly MJ, Crowley JJ, Charan NB, Nielson CP, Vestal RE. Reduced subjective awareness of bronchoconstriction provoked by methacholine in elderly asthmatic and normal subjects measuredon a simple awareness scale. Thorax 1992; 47:410–413.

48. Boulet LP, Leblanc P, Turcotte H. Perception scoring of induced bronchoconstriction as an index of awareness of asthma symptoms. Chest 1994; 105:1430–1433.
49. Rubinfeld AR, Pain MCF. Perception of asthma. Lancet 1976; 24:882–884.
50. Rietveld S, Brosschot JF. Current perspectives on symptom perception in asthma: a biomedical and psychological review. Int J Behav Med 1999; 6:120–134.
51. Dale RE, Spitzer WO, Schechter MT, Suissa S. The influence of psychological status on respiratory symptom reporting. Am Rev Respir Dis 1989; 139:1459–1463.
52. Rimington LD, Davies DH, Lowe D, Pearson MG. Relationship between anxiety, depression and morbidity in adult asthma patients. Thorax 2001; 66: 226–271.
53. Goldney R, Ruffin R, Fisher L, Wilson D. Asthma severity symptoms and depression and the consequences for management. Med J Aust 2003; 178:437–441.
54. Silberman EK, Weingartner H, Post RM. Thinking disorder in depression. Arch Gen Psych 1983; 40:775–780.
55. Tarbuck AF, Paykel ES. Effects of depression on the cognitive function of young and older subjects. Psychol Med 1995; 25:285–295.
56. Paykel ES, Michael A, Sahakian BJ. Cognitive impairment in remission of bipolar affective disorders. Psychol Med 2000; 30:1025–1036.
57. Lemelin S, Baruch P, Vincent A, Laplante L, Everett J, Vincent P. Attention disturbance in clinical depression. Deficient distraction inhibition or processing resource deficit. J Nerv Ment Dis 1996; 184:114–121.
58. Main J, Moss-Morris R, Booth R, Kaptein AA, Kolbe J. The use of reliever medication in asthma: the role of negative mood symptom reports. J Asthma 2003; 40:357–365.
59. Bukstein DA. Practical approach to the use of outcomes in asthma. Immunol Allergy Clin North Am 1996; 16:859–891.
60. Malo JL, Cartier A, Merland N, Ghezzo H, Burek A, Morris J, Jennings BH. Four-time-a-day dosing frequency is better than a twice-a day regime in subjects requiring a high-dose inhaled steroid, budesonide, to control moderate to severe asthma. Am Rev Respir Dis 1989; 140:624–628.
61. Steen N, Hutchinson A, McColl E, Eccles MP, Hewison J, Meadows KA, Blades SM, Fowler P. Development of a symptom based outcome measure for asthma. BMJ 1994; 309:1065–1068.
62. Aas K. Heterogeneity of bronchial asthma. Allergy 1981; 36:3–14.
63. Hargreave FE, Dolovich J, Newhouse MT. The assessment and treatment of asthma: a conference report. J Allergy Clin Immunol 1990; 85:1098–1111.
64. Brooks SM, Bernstein L, Raghu Prasad PK, Maccia CA, MieczkowskiL L. Assessment of airway hyperresponsiveness in chronic stable asthma. J Allergy Clin Immunol 1990; 85:17–26.
65. Gautier V, Redier H, Pujol JL, Bousquet J, Proudhon H, Michel C, Daures JP, Michel FB, Godard PL. Comparison of an expert system with other clinical scores for the evaluation of severity of asthma. Eur Respir J 1996; 9:58–64.

66. Sculpher MJ, Buxton MJ. The episode free day as a composite measure of effectiveness. Pharmoeconomics 1993; 4:345–352.

67. Juniper EF, O'Byrne PM, Guyatt GH, Ferrie PJ, King DR. Development and validation of a questionnaire to measure asthma control. Eur Respir J 1999; 14:902–907.

68. Katz PP, Yelin EH, Smith S, Blanc PD. Perceived control of asthma: Development arid validation of a questionnaire. Am J Respir Crit Care Med 1997; 155:577–582.

69. Vollmer WM, Markson LE, O'Connor E, Sanocki LI, Fitterman L, Berger M, Buist AS. Association of asthma control with health care utilization and quality of life. Am J Respir Crit Care Med 1999; 160:1647–1652.

2

Quality of Life

ELIZABETH F. JUNIPER

Department of Clinical Epidemiology and Biostatistics, McMaster University, Hamilton, Ontario, Canada

Introduction

With a wide range of efficacious asthma medications and clear guidelines for their use now available (1–4), it is often low rates of patient compliance that poses the major challenge to effective asthma management (5–9). An important contributor to poor patient compliance may be a discrepancy between the goals of the clinician and those of the patient (10). Clinicians tend to focus on prevention of mortality and reduction of morbidity by good asthma control, whereas patients are usually more concerned with their ability to function normally in their day-to-day lives. Improved clinician awareness of patients' asthma-related quality of life goals and a willingness to address them may enhance patients' willingness to take medications and thus improve both their asthma control and their quality of life. Hence, there is a need for quick, valid, easy-to-use, self-administered, and clinic friendly quality of life questionnaires. The responses to these questionnaires can be used during the consultation to identify the patient's greatest needs, to ascertain how troublesome they are, and to ensure that they are included in the treatment plan. Questionnaires with strong measurement properties can also be used to monitor patient's progress over time.

Health-Related Quality of Life

The quality of a person's life may be considered in terms of its richness, completeness, and contentedness. A number of factors contribute to this sense of well-being and include good health, a secure social and occupational environment, financial security, spirituality, self-confidence, and strong, supportive family relationships. Each factor may be a determinant of a person's quality of life and may be closely inter-related with each of the others. For instance, a patient will often be able to deal with an illness better with good family support, a strong faith, and the financial ability to acquire nourishing food, shelter, and treatment.

Health-related quality of life can be considered as that part of a person's overall quality of life that is determined primarily by the person's health status and that can be influenced by clinical interventions. The definition by Schipper et al. (11) is both simple and focused: "the functional effects of an illness and its consequent therapy upon a patient, as perceived by the patient." The final phrase is important because it emphasizes that these are the impairments that patients themselves consider important. Schipper goes on to say that quality of life has four basic components: physical and occupational function, psychological state (emotional function), social interaction, and somatic sensation (the problems associated with symptoms).

This definition is used by many clinicians and academics and it has guided the development and validation of many disease-specific quality of life questionnaires (12). However, it is worth being aware that not everyone uses this definition, and in some quarters, the term has been discontinued. In the United States, and particularly within the U.S. pharmaceutical industry, "quality of life" has been replaced by "patient-reported outcomes." This has caused some confusion because clinicians tend to think that "patient-reported outcomes" are the ones, both subjective (e.g., symptoms) and objective (e.g., PEF), recorded by patients. Elsewhere, "quality of life" is referred to as "health status", but once again "health status" is often considered by clinicians to be any objective or subjective measure of patient's health. In recent years, there has been a growing public awareness of the concept of "quality of life" and so it seems sensible that the component of it that is associated with health should be called "health-related quality of life." For those of you who prefer "patient-reported outcomes" and "health status" when referring to the functional impairments that patients consider important, please forgive us for continuing to use "quality of life."

Why do We Need to Measure Quality of Life in Asthma?

There are three reasons for treating patients: to prevent mortality; to reduce the probability of future morbidity; and to improve patients' well-being (13). Most conventional clinical measures of asthma control and asthma severity assess the status of the airways and are primarily used to gauge whether the first two goals are being achieved. In the past, it was frequently assumed that these measures also provided insight into patients' well-being. Certainly, patients with very severe asthma tend to have a worse quality of life than patients with milder disease but a recent factor analysis has revealed that not only does quality of life not correlate closely with clinical status but is a very distinct component of asthma health status, and therefore, the impact that asthma has on a patient's quality of life cannot be inferred from the clinical indices and must be measured directly (Table 1) (14).

Table 1 Factor Analysis Showing That Quality of Life is a Distinct Component of Asthma Health Status (Varimax Rotated Factor Pattern)

	Factor 1	Factor 2	Factor 3	Factor 4
AQLQ[a] overall	93[b]	8	−24	−24
AQLQ activities	89[b]	11	−12	−17
AQLQ environment	83[b]	7	−3	−7
AQLQ symptoms	78[b]	6	−37	−30
AQLQ emotions	74[b]	5	−21	−24
FEV_1	0	92[b]	−8	−4
PEF (pm)	23	84[b]	−3	18
PEF (am)	15	83[b]	0	−11
FVC	15	80[b]	−2	8
FEF	−19	69[b]	−12	−16
Night-time waking	−24	−6	84[b]	15
Night-time rescue β_2-agonist	−10	−6	75[b]	18
Night-time symptoms	−25	−4	50[b]	47[b]
%Nights without β_2-agonist	13	6	−77[b]	−8
%Nights without waking	22	3	−84[b]	−7
Short of breath (daytime)	−30	−7	5	65[b]
Activity limitation	−37	−2	14	63[b]
PEF(pm–am)	17	5	−5	59[b]
Chest tightness (daytime)	−30	0	0	57[b]
Wheeze (daytime)	−23	6	16	50[b]
Rescue β_2-agonist (daytime)	−4	−10	18	46[b]
% days without β_2-agonist	4	0	−11	−44[b]

[a]Asthma Quality of Life Questionnaire.
[b]Statistically significant loading on factor (for clarity of reading, all values have been multiplied by 100).
Source: From Ref. 14.

Why should the relationship between clinical measures and quality of life be so weak? At the moment, there is no evidence as to whether the cause is purely extrinsic or a combination of intrinsic and extrinsic. An intrinsic component is suggested by the results of a pharmaceutical clinical trial that showed clinically important improvements in quality of life but no evidence of change in clinical asthma status in the intervention group compared with the control (15). The reason for this discrepancy has not yet been explained. However, extrinsic causes for the weak correlation between quality of life and clinical asthma are quite easy to understand. Let us take, as an example, two hypothetical patients with identical clinical asthma. Both women are 35 years of age with a moderate degree of bronchoconstriction (FEV$_1$: 65% predicted) and moderate airway hyper-responsiveness to methacholine (PC$_{20}$: 1 mg/mL). The first patient has very poor perception of airway narrowing. She works at home and can regulate her life style according to how she feels. She lives a very sedentary life and is generally a very relaxed person. The second patient is very different. She has very good perception of airway narrowing. She works in a high-pressure job and has to attend meetings where people smoke. She is an athlete and is a very "uptight" person. In the past, she has had a life-threatening asthma episode. Although both these patients present with similar degrees of airway narrowing and hyper-responsiveness, the second patient is likely to have much greater impairment of quality of life than the former as a result of her asthma. Similar scenarios can easily be imagined for children with asthma where additional factors, such as family support and desire to keep up with peers, will also affect the child's quality of life.

Quality of Life Impairments in Asthma

Adults

Extensive research has highlighted the functional impairments that are most troublesome to adults with asthma (Table 2) (16–20). They are certainly bothered by the symptoms themselves. The most troublesome are usually shortness of breath, chest tightness, wheeze, and cough. Many patients have problems with physical activities such as sports, hurrying, going upstairs, and shopping. Allergens may cause difficulties with daily occupational and social activities. Environmental stimuli, such as cigarette smoke, strong smells, and troublesome weather conditions, may limit family and social activities. Asthma patients are bothered by not being able to get a good night's sleep and often feel tired. In addition, they experience fears and concerns about having asthma and the need for medications and they become frustrated by their limitations. The functional impairments (physical, social, emotional, and occupational) that are important to patients are remarkably consistent in both sexes and across a wide range of ages,

Table 2 Functional Impairments Most Important to Adults with Asthma

Symptoms	Emotions	Activities	Environment
Short of breath	Afraid of not having medications available	Exercise/sports	Cigarettes
Chest tightness	Afraid of getting out of breath	Hurrying	Dust
Wheeze	Concerned about the need to use medications	Social activities	Air pollution
Cough		Pets	Cold air
Tired	Frustrated	Work/housework	Pollen

Source: From Ref. 16.

cultures, and severity of asthma (16,21). However, women tend to experience greater impairment in these problems than men (16,22); inner city African-Americans have poorer scores than other Americans (23); patients with low socioeconomic status are worse than higher groups (24); and patients with occupational asthma are worse than patients whose asthma is not of occupational origin (25). All of these observations have been made after correcting for clinical asthma severity.

Children

The burden of illness and functional impairments experienced by children with asthma are similar to those experienced by adults (Table 3) (26–29). In addition, children are troubled because they cannot integrate fully with their peers; they feel isolated and left out and this often causes them to feel frustrated, irritable, and angry. There is growing evidence that parents often have a poor perception of the problems and emotions that are troubling the

Table 3 Functional Impairments Most Important to Children with Asthma

Symptoms	Activities	Emotions
Short of breath	Sports and games	Feel different and left out
Chest tightness	Activities with friends	Frustrated
Cough	Playing with pets	Angry
Wheeze	School activities	Sad
Tired	Sleeping	Frightened /anxious

Source: From Ref. 26.

child and so it is essential to obtain quality of life information directly from the child (30–32). Children as young as 6 years have little difficulty understanding quality of life questionnaires and they are able to provide reliable and valid responses (33,34).

Selecting the Right Questionnaire for the Task

This section describes the types of questionnaires available, discusses their strengths and weaknesses, and then reviews the measurement properties that an instrument must have for specific types of use.

Questionnaires

Generic Health Profiles

There are two types of quality of life questionnaires: generic and specific. Generic health profiles are designed to be applicable to patients with all medical conditions (35–38). In adults, the most commonly used and the best validated is the Medical Outcomes Survey Short Form 36 (SF-36) (35). For children, probably the most widely used is the Child Health Questionnaire (39). These questionnaires measure impairment over a broad spectrum of functions, and the great advantage of generic instruments is that burden of illness can be compared across different medical conditions. For instance, one can compare the burden of illness experienced by patients with asthma, COPD, rhinitis, inflammatory bowel disease, rheumatoid arthritis, etc. (40,41). However, because they are required to be broad in their comprehensiveness, they have very little depth, and therefore impairments that are important to patients with a specific condition may not be included. Consequently, in many conditions, including asthma, generic instruments are not only unable to identify specific problems in individual patients, but also unresponsive to small but important changes in quality of life (42,43). Therefore, the use of generic instruments in both clinical practice and clinical trials is limited.

Disease-Specific Questionnaires

The inadequate depth of focus of generic health profiles leads to the development of disease-specific questionnaires. These instruments include all the functional impairments (physical, emotional, social, and occupational) that are most important to patients with a specific disease and are therefore ideal for identifying specific problems that are bothering individual patients (17–20,44). In addition, a number of studies have shown that disease-specific questionnaires are very much more sensitive to change in patients' quality of life than generic health profiles (33,42–44). These questionnaires are not only used extensively in clinical trials, but also in clinical practice to help identify patients' asthma goals and to evaluate the effect of interventions.

Measurement Properties

Face and Content Validity

When selecting an instrument, one needs first to ensure that it has face and content validity, that is to say, the instrument appears, on reading the items, to measure what it purports to measure (face validity) and the items in a questionnaire have been selected using recognized procedures that ensure that they capture all the areas of function that are considered important by patients (content validity) (12,45,46). Questionnaires in which items have been selected by clinicians rarely have content validity because there is no evidence that the impairments that they have selected are important to patients. Neither is there evidence that the questionnaires include the problems that patients consider most troublesome.

Evaluative vs. Discriminative Properties

Instruments that are to be used in cross-sectional studies (e.g., screening and surveys) must have good discriminative properties (47) because they are required to *discriminate* between patients and groups of patients of different levels of impairment. Instruments that are to be used in longitudinal studies (clinical trials and clinical practice) need good evaluative properties (47) because they are required to *evaluate* change in impairment over time.

Discriminative Properties

An instrument that is to be used to distinguish between individuals or groups of patients at a single point in time, for example, between individuals who do or do not have impaired quality of life or, within asthma patients, between those who have mild, moderate, or severe impairment require reliability and cross-sectional validity (47).

Reliability is the ability of the instrument to measure differences between patients at a single point in time (signal is between-subject variance, noise is within-subject variance). The test statistic usually used to express reliability is the intraclass correlation coefficient that relates the between-subject variance to the total variance. (Cronbach's alpha, which measures the internal consistency, i.e., similarity of the questions, does not give an indication of this property).

Occasionally, it is possible to evaluate whether a questionnaire is measuring what it purports to measure (validity) by comparing it with a gold-standard (criterion validity). This may occur when a shorter or simpler version of a well-established, validated questionnaire has been developed to measure the same construct (concept) as the original. For instance, the standardized and mini versions of the Asthma Quality of Life Questionnaire (48,49) were validated against the original version (44). When there is no gold standard, the developer puts forward hypotheses or constructs that, if they are met, provide evidence that the instrument is valid (construct validity). The approach frequently used is the demonstration that the various domains of a new quality of life instrument correlate in a predicted manner with other indices of asthma severity and with other quality of life instruments (21,22,26,44,50).

Evaluative Properties

An instrument that is to be used to measure longitudinal change within an individual or group of patients must have good responsiveness and longitudinal validity (47). Responsiveness is the ability of the instrument to respond to small but clinically important changes that occur either spontaneously or as the result of an intervention. The signal is the true within-subject change over time, and the noise is the within-subject variance unrelated to the true within-subject change; the relationship between the two is known as the responsiveness index (51). If a formal estimate of the responsiveness index is not available, an instrument that has already performed well in a clinical trial will probably have acceptable responsiveness.

Evaluative instruments also require longitudinal validity. Longitudinal validity is usually demonstrated by showing that changes in the various domains of the new quality of life instrument correlate in a predicted manner with changes in other outcome measures, such as clinical asthma severity and generic quality of life.

Most developers publish reliability and cross-sectional validity data and, good as these may be, they are no guarantee that the instrument will be capable of performing well in a clinical trial. There are now a number of studies in which patients experienced clinically important changes in quality of life, but which instruments, with good reliability and cross-sectional validity, failed to detect.

Interpretation of Quality of Life Data

For many disease-specific quality of life questionnaires, we now have estimates of what difference or change in score can be considered clinically meaningful. This value is usually referred to as the minimal important difference (MID). It has been defined as "the smallest difference in score that patients perceive as beneficial and would mandate, in the absence of troublesome side effects and excessive cost, a change in the patient's management" (52).

Clinical Trials

Using the MID to interpret clinical trial data is not as simple as might first appear. Just comparing the mean differences between treatment groups with the MID is very inadequate, may lead to erroneous conclusions and a lot of valuable information is lost. Patients are very heterogeneous in their responses to interventions, and by only looking at the mean, one ignores the distribution about the mean. We have developed a method, using the proportions of patients who improve and deteriorate by the MID on the trial interventions to calculate the number-needed-to-treat (53). This is the number of patients who need to be treated with the new intervention for one to have a clinically important improvement in their quality of life over and above that which they would have had on the control treatment. Statisticians have been warning for years about the limitations of only looking at mean data and ignoring distributions, but terms like "confidence intervals" and "standard deviations" usually draw a veiled glaze over the eyes of non-statisticians. We believe that this method of presenting quality of life results not only addresses the concerns of statisticians, but also provides clinicians with a conceptually easy and clinically meaningful way of understanding the results of clinical studies.

Clinical Practice

The MID are determined by examining change in the questionnaire score relative to patients' perception of change (global rating of change) (52) or linking the change scores to other clinical indices whose MID is well established (54). Whichever method is used, clinicians should recognize that although MIDs may be accurate for group data, there may be quite large differences between individual patients. Therefore, the MID should only be used as a rough guide, and discussion with the patient about whether they consider any change that have experienced as important should also be included in any decision-making. However, it is also important to remember that both patients and clinicians may be very inaccurate in their ability to estimate change in status over time (55,56). For estimating whether changes in quality of life scores are clinically important, it is probably wisest to use all sources of information recognizing their strengths and weaknesses.

Quality of Life in Clinical Trials

The recognition of the importance of quality of life, the poor correlation between the conventional clinical indices of airway impairment, and quality of life and the advent quality of life instruments with strong measurement properties has ensured that most asthma clinical trials now include quality of life as one of the primary end-points (57). These instruments are short, easily understood, and usually in self-administered format making completion very little burden either to the investigator or to the patient. In fact, we have found that patients enjoy completing quality of life questionnaires because they can relate to the questions and know that the things that are important to them are being taken into consideration. In addition, national pharmaceutical regulatory agencies often require quality of life data for new product submissions.

Quality of Life in Clinical Practice

As we have already identified, patients are treated for three reasons: to bhprevent mortality, to reduce the probability of future morbidity, and to improve patient's well-being (quality of life) (13). Clinicians treating asthma tend to focus on the first two goals, prevention of mortality and reduction of morbidity, and they use the conventional clinical measures of asthma control to assess the status of the airways and to gauge whether these two goals are being achieved. This behavior is in accordance with international guidelines (1–4) for the treatment of asthma that identify that clinicians should endeavor to minimize asthma symptoms, airway narrowing, short-acting β_2-agonist use and activity limitation (i.e., achieve good asthma control).

However, patients' own goals may be very different from those of clinicians and that although patients are concerned about mortality, their primary goals are usually concerned with their quality of life (10). Most patients seek help from their clinicians in order to feel better and to function better in their every-day activities. They want to be able to enjoy their sports, function well at work, participate social activities with their friends and family, and cope easily with day-to-day activities of living. In addition, they want to have their fears and concerns addressed. These fears and concerns often include anxiety about the use of medications.

Shared-Decision Making

Shared-decision making (58) is an approach to patient management in which the clinician and the patient decide together on the patient's management plan (Table 4). In asthma, the clinician brings to the encounter expertise in diagnosis, the goals of clinical asthma control, and asthma treatment options. The patients bring to the encounter their own goals for improving asthma-related quality of life, concerns about medications, and likes/dislikes of various forms of treatment regimens. Together, the clinician and patient negotiate an asthma management plan that works towards both their goals and which, most importantly, the patient is willing to follow.

Inadequate asthma control frequently occurs when patients take the decision-making role away from clinicians and make their own choices

Table 4 Shared Decision-Making Model in Asthma

Decision maker	Clinician alone	Clinician and patient	Patient alone
Model	Paternalistic	Shared decision-making	"Informed" decision-making
Primary goals	Asthma control	Asthma control Asthma-related quality of life Acceptable treatment regimen	Asthma-related quality of life Acceptable treatment regimen
Information	Clinician knows about diagnosis, guidelines for asthma control, and treatment options	Exchange of facts and treatment preferences	In the model, the patient is provided with all the facts in order to make the decision.
Decision-maker	Clinician alone	Clinician and patient	Patient alone
Reality	Majority of treatment strategies are decided by clinicians on their own	Clinician's and patient's goals achieved	Patients, without the facts, reject the clinician's directions and decide for themselves how to take their medication Non-compliance

about their management (usually a conscious or sub-conscious decision not to take their medication as prescribed). Most patients do not have an adequate understanding of asthma and the mechanisms of action of the interventions to make such decisions and usually fail to meet both their own goals and those of the clinician. Although patients usually do not want to be the prime decision maker (59,60), they take over that role when they are unhappy with a treatment regimen paternalistically prescribed for them by their clinician. With the Internet and other modern technologies providing patients with a plethora of information, often inaccurate or misleading, they need a supportive environment in which they can discuss treatment options. Shared-decision making requires clinicians to move out of their conventional role as the sole decision-maker and engage with the patient in a discussion of the clinical goals, the patient's personal goals, and the management options. Already, there is evidence that willingness of physicians to discuss management is strongly related to asthma outcomes and patient's satisfaction (61). Initial studies have suggested that quality of life questionnaires may have an important role by facilitating the identification of patients' goals and concerns. After the patient has completed the questionnaire in the waiting room, a quick scan of the responses allows the clinician to focus on problems that are most troublesome and this quickly leads to the identification of the patient's treatment goals. Initial studies in primary care have suggested that when clinicians are provided with Mini Asthma Quality of Life Questionnaire (49) data during a consultation, prescribing practices are altered (62,63) and similar experiences have been reported in children. Feedback from patients has been positive. They report that they like the questionnaires because their own concerns are being addressed and they have identified that the questionnaires give them permission to discuss asthma-related concerns, other than symptoms, with their clinician. However, the real test of whether there is a place for quality of life questionnaires in this model of clinical practice will be whether both asthma control and quality of life are enhanced by the use of the questionnaires. There are currently international studies, both in primary and secondary care, addressing this question.

Practical Considerations

Methods of Administration

Self-Report vs. Interviewer Administered

Paper versions of questionnaires completed by patients themselves in the clinic remain the most popular method for collecting quality of life data. The strengths and weaknesses of the various methods are shown in Table 5. Although there are many studies showing very little difference in overall scores when questionnaires are completed by patients and when

Table 5 Methods of Administration

Method of administration	Advantages	Disadvantages
Self-completed in clinic (paper)	Most popular method because of accurate, easy, and cheap Honest responses (no embarrassment or wanting to please the interviewer) Clinic staff available if get confused No missing responses Time for patients to think about responses	Need some literacy and numeracy skills Must attend the clinic
Self-completed in clinic (computer)	Honest responses No missing responses (if permitted by ethics) Time for patients to think about responses No transcription errors	Very difficult to program High "screw-up" rate (none are "idiot proof") Clinic/patient requires a computer Train clinic staff in computer use Patients need basic computer skills Expensive
Interviewer administered in clinic	No missing responses Correct misunderstood questions or response options Patient requires minimal numeracy skills (ideal for young children and adults with low literacy skills)	Employ and train interviewers Risk of interpretation and/or response guidance by interviewer Embarrassment or desire to please may affect responses Poor interviewing can be a source of error

(Continued)

Table 5 Methods of Administration (*Continued*)

Method of administration	Advantages	Disadvantages
Telephone	No missing responses Patients do not have to attend clinic More honest responses than postal (minimal family input)	Patients must have a phone Employ and train interviewers Provide patients with response options before the phone call Cannot be sure that patient is the respondent
Post	Patients do not have to attend clinic Time for patients to think about responses	Missing data and questionnaires not returned Patient must have literacy and numeracy skills Nobody to ask if patient has understanding problems Family may influence patient's responses Questionnaires lost in post
Surrogate	Better than nothing	Inaccurate—response may not reflect patient's experiences (especially emotional)

administered by a trained interviewer, it is usually considered wise to stick to one method when the patient is being followed over time. In clinical trials, a minority of patients may not have adequate reading or numeracy skills. There is minimal risk of bias if these patients consistently have the questionnaire administered by an interviewer while the rest of the patients complete it on their own.

Telephone vs. Clinic

Studies comparing telephone vs. clinic interviews are far less consistent, and so it is sensible to check whether the questionnaire that you are using has been evaluated for telephone administration. Some questionnaires score consistently higher by telephone, whereas others score lower (64,65). It is important not to mix telephone interviews with clinic ones in a clinical trial or when following individual patients.

Electronic vs. Paper

Scores from electronic and paper versions are usually very similar (66). However, although programmers have been trying for over a decade, there are still very few successful systems for electronic data collection. Programming can be quite complicated in order to overcome both practical and ethical problems. On the practical side, it is important for patients to be able to check and change responses they have already given. Programming flexible movement around questionnaires and providing change options can be quite difficult. In addition, the screen on hand-held devices is often not large enough to include a complete question plus response options. On the ethical side, many countries now require patients to be able to skip questions they do not want to answer. Questionnaires that have been successfully programmed then tend to run into practical problems because they cannot be made totally "idiot proof." Apart from problems caused by people who are not computer literate, some patients and clinic staff love to "find out how it works," and manage to get into incredibly secure software, and then the whole system crashes. It then takes a programmer to get it back into action.

Postal vs. Clinic

It is always best if patients are on their own when they complete questionnaires and there is only one way to ensure that this happens and that is in the clinic. There is a risk when questionnaires are completed outside the clinic that you get a family consensus. In addition, some patients do not want their families to know what they are really experiencing, whereas others seek their family's guidance on both interpretation of questions and choice of responses. Although postal completion runs the risk of missing data, a recent study comparing postal and clinic completion suggested that failure to attend the clinic might be comparable to the missing postal data (67).

Children

A large number of studies in a wide range of childhood illnesses have shown that parents have a very poor perception of the problems that bother the child (30–32). There have been a number of hypotheses as to why this happens such as the parent imagining how they would feel if they had the illness, not knowing about the child's experiences at school and at night, the child not wanting the parent to know about their true experiences because of over/under protection, etc. Whatever the reason, the message is the same, "ask the child." There is strong evidence that children as young as 6 years can respond to quality of life questionnaires accurately and reliably (33,34). The problem with going any younger is that the concept of time does not develop until about 6 years of age and if you ask children how they have been "over the last week," for instance, they cannot understand. They know how they are "now" but with functional impairments varying during the day and from day to day. It is necessary to include several days in an assessment of quality of life so as to get an average and not accidentally catch a peak or trough. Children over about 11 years can usually self-complete questionnaires with no help. The limiting factor in going any lower does not appear to be reading skills but a willingness to concentrate. Little boys tend to scatter responses like confetti, so that they can get on with more interesting activities!

Cultural Adaptations

Adapting quality of life questionnaires for another language and culture is a great deal more complicated than doing a simple translation (68). Although the problems that are important to asthma patients are fairly consistent across continents and cultures, there are occasionally minor differences that need to be taken into consideration. For instance, although "feeling frustrated" is important to patients in most countries, Portuguese patients say they do not experience this emotion and accept asthma and its effects on their day-to-day lives as something with which they have to live. Parents in North America feel "anger" that their child has asthma, whereas in rest of the world "sadness" is a more commonly identified emotion (69). Part of the adaptation process must ensure that the problems that are important to local patients are included in the new language ("content validity").

The process usually involves a team of translators working closely with the developer because it is important that the team accurately understands the meaning of each question. Members of the team should not only be medical linguists, but also skilled in clinical measurement and scaling. There are usually two forward translations by independent translators whose primary language is the one into which the questionnaire is being translated. There is then a reconciliation of the two forward translations followed by two backward translations, ideally by people whose primary language is English (or the original language of the questionnaire). Probably, the most important part of the whole process is the testing in patients (cognitive debriefing). The purpose of this phase is to ensure that the words chosen by the translators are easily and accurately understood by patients and that all the important problems have been included. It is very important to use the words that patients themselves use to describe their symptoms and limitations, not the terms used by clinicians.

Ideally, every new cultural adaptation should undergo a complete validation. However, this is expensive and time consuming. There is now good evidence that if the cultural adaptation is done to a high standard, the resulting questionnaire will have measurement properties very similar to those of the original. When a quality of life questionnaire is used in a multinational clinical trial (70), data from the various languages can be used to confirm the consistency of some of the measurement properties (usually responsiveness and construct validity). In addition, Cronbach's alpha will provide evidence of the internal consistency of the items across the different languages. However, such analyses make the assumption that similar patients were enrolled in each country and that they have all responded in a similar manner to the intervention.

Copyright

Most of the quality of life questionnaires are copyrighted by the developer. This is to ensure that they are not modified, translated, or sold (paper and electronic) without the developer's permission. The most important reason for copyrighting is to ensure that nobody changes the questions, response options, or time specification each of which can invalidate the instrument. Rogue versions that get into general circulation can cause enormous problems because users often do not know that they are not using the original instrument. Entire studies have been lost by investigators not getting an original from the developer. As mentioned earlier, cultural adaptation is specialized work and most developers like to ensure that it is done to the highest standard and that there is only one authorized version available in each language.

Conclusion

Apart from achieving good asthma control, an important aim of asthma management should also be to ensure that the patients' own goals are identified and addressed. These goals cannot be inferred from the conventional clinical measures of asthma control, as quality of life correlates poorly with these indices. The inclusion of simple quality of life questionnaires in the routine clinical management of asthma patients may help to identify patients' goals and ensure that they are included in a negotiated treatment plan. Willingness to follow a negotiated plan should lead to both improved quality of life and asthma control.

References

1. National Institutes of Health (National Heart, Lung and Blood Institute). Global strategy for asthma management and prevention. Global initiative for asthma. Bethesda, MD: National Institutes of Health, April 2002. Publication No. 02-3659.
2. British Thoracic Society, Research Unit of the Royal College of Physicians of London, King's Fund Centre, National Asthma Campaign. Guidelines for management of asthma in adults I: chronic persistent asthma. Br Med J 1990; 301:651–653.
3. Thoracic Society of Australia and New Zealand. Woolcock A, Rubinfeld AR, Seatle JP, Landau LL, Antic R, Mitchell C, Rea HH, Zimmerman P. Asthma management plan 1989. Med J Aust 1989; 151:650–653.
4. Ernst P, Fitzgerald JM, Spier S. Canadian asthma consensus conference: summary of recommendations. Can Respir J 1996; 3:89–100.
5. Cerveri I, Locatelli F, Zoia M, et al. International variations in asthma treatment compliance: the results of the European Community Respiratory Health Survey (ECRHS). Eur Respir J 1999; 14:288–294.
6. Chambers C, Markson L, Diamond J, et al. Health beliefs and compliance with inhaled corticosteroids by asthmatic patients in primary care practices. Respir Med 1999; 93:88–94.
7. Apter A, Reisine S, Affleck G, et al. Adherence with twice-daily dosing of inhaled steroids. Socioeconomic health belief differences. Am J Respir Crit Care Med 1998; 157:1810–1817.
8. Spector S. Non-compliance with asthma therapy—are there solutions? J Asthma 2000; 37:381–388.
9. Buston K, Wood S. Non-compliance amongst adolescents with asthma: listening to what they tell us about self-management. Fam Pract 2000; 17:134–138.
10. Stahl E, Hyland ME. Unmet needs of asthma patients, and how these are reflected in attitudes to the disease and its treatment. Eur Resp J 2002; 20:410s.
11. Schipper H, Clinch J, Powell V. Definitions and conceptual issues. In: Spilker B, ed. Quality of Life and Pharmacoeconomics in Clinical Trials. Philadelphia: Lippincott-Raven Publishers, 1996:11–23.

12. Juniper EF, Guyatt GH, Jaeschke R. How to develop and validate a new quality of life instrument. In: Spilker B, ed. Quality of Life and Pharmacoeconomics in Clinical Trials. 2nd ed. New York: Raven Press Ltd, 1995:49–56.

13. Guyatt GH, Naylor D, Juniper EF, Heyland D, Cook D and the Evidence-Based Medicine Working Group. Users' guides to the medical literature. IX. How to use an article-about health-related quality of life. JAMA 1997; 277: 1232–1237.

14. Juniper EF, Wisniewski ME, Cox FM, Emmett AH, Nielsen KE, O'Byrne PM. Relationship between quality of life and measures of clinical status in asthma: a factor analysis. Eur Respir J 2004; 23:287–291.

15. Juniper EF, Price DB, Stampone P, Creemers JPHM, Mol SJM, Fireman P. Improvements in asthma quality of life but maintenance of conventional clinical indices in patients changed from CFC-BDP to approximately half the dose of HFA-BDP. Chest 2002; 121:1824–1832.

16. Juniper EF, Guyatt GH, Epstein RS, Ferrie PJ, Jaeschke R, Hiller TK. Evaluation of impairment of health-related quality of life in asthma: development of a questionnaire for use in clinical trials. Thorax 1992; 47:76–83.

17. Marks GB, Dunn SM, Woolcock AJ. A scale for the measurement of quality of life in adults with asthma. J Clin Epidemiol 1992; 45:461–472.

18. Hyland ME, Finnis S, Irvine SH. A scale for assessing quality of life in adult asthma sufferers. J Psychomat Res 1991; 35:99–110.

19. Maille AR, Kaptein AA, Koning CJM, Zwinderman AH. Developing a quality of life questionnaire for patients with respiratory illness. Monaldi Arch Chest Dis 1994; 49:76–78.

20. Creer TL, Wigal JK, Kotses H, McConnaughy K, Winder JA. A life activities questionnaire for adult asthma. J Asthma 1992; 29:393–399.

21. Sanjuas C, Alonso J, Sanchis J, Casan P, Broquetas JM, Ferrie PJ, Juniper EF, Anto JM. The quality of life questionnaire with asthma patients; the Spanish version of the Asthma Quality of Life Questionnaire. Arch Bronconeumol 1995; 31:219–226.

22. Leidy NK, Coughlin C. Psychometric performance of the Asthma Quality of Life Questionnaire in a US sample. Qual Life Res 1998; 7:127–134.

23. Blixen CE, Tilley B, Havstad, Zoratti E. Quality of life, medication use, and health care utilization or urban African Americans with asthma treated in emergency departments. Nursing Res 1997; 46:338–341.

24. Apter AJ, Reisine ST, Affleck G, Barrows E, ZuWallack RL. The influence of demographic and socioeconomic factors on health-related quality of life in asthma. J Allergy Clin Immunol 1999; 103:72–78.

25. Malo JL, Boulet LP, Dewitte JD, Cartier A, L'Archeveque J, Cote J, Bedard G, Boucher S, Champagne F, Tessier G, Contandriopoulos AP, Juniper EF, Guyatt GH. Quality of life of subjects with occupational asthma. J Allergy Clin Immunol 1993; 91:1121–1127.

26. Juniper EF, Guyatt GH, Feeny DH, Ferrie PJ, Griffith LE, Townsend M. Measuring quality of life in children with asthma. Qual Life Res 1996; 5:35–46.

27. Creer TL, Wigal JE, Kotses H, Hatala JC, McConnaughty K, Winder JA. A life activities questionnaire for childhood asthma. J Asthma 1993; 30:467–473.

28. Christie MJ, French D, Sowden A, West A. Development of child-centred disease-specific questionnaires for living with asthma. Psychosomat Med 1993; 55:541–548.
29. Osman L, Silverman M. Measuring quality of life for young children with asthma and their families. Eur Respir J 1996; 9(suppl 21):S35–S41.
30. Guyatt GH, Juniper EF, Feeny DH, Griffith LE. Children and adult perceptions of childhood asthma. Pediatrics 1997; 99:165–168.
31. Wood PR, Hidalgo HA, Prihoda TJ, Kromer ME. Comparison of hispanic children's and parents' responses to questions about the child's asthma. Arch Pediatr Adolesc Med 1994; 148:43.
32. Theunissen NCM, Vogels TGC, Koopman HM, Verrips GHW, Zwinderman KAH, Verloove-Vanhorick SP, Wit JM. The proxy problem: child report versus parent report in health-related quality of life research. Qual Life Res 1998; 7:387–397.
33. Juniper EF, Guyatt GH, Feeny DH, Griffith LE, Feme PJ. Minimum skills required by children to complete health-related quality of life instruments: comparison of instruments for measuring asthma-specific quality of life. Eur Respir J 1997; 10:2285–2294.
34. Juniper EF, Howland WC, Roberts NB, Thompson AK, King DR. Measuring quality of life in children with rhinoconjunctivitis. J Allergy Clin Immunol 1998; 101:163–170.
35. Stewart AL, Hays R, Ware JE. The MOS short-form general health survey. Reliability and validity in a patient population. Med Care 1988; 26:724–732.
36. Bergner M, Bobbitt RA, Carter WB, Gilson BS. The sickness impact profile: development and final revision of a health status measure. Med Care 1981; 19:787–805.
37. Hunt SM, McKenna SP, McEwen J, et al. A quantitative approach to perceived health status: a validation study. J Epidemiol Community Health 1980; 34: 281–286.
38. Nelson E, Wasson J, Kirk J, Keller A, Clark D, Dietrich A, Stewart A, Zubkoff M. Assessment of function in routine clinical practice: description of the COOP chart method and preliminary findings. J Chron Dis 1987; 40(suppl 1):S55.
39. Landgraf JM, Maunsell E, Nixon Speechley K, Bullinger M, Campbell S, Abetz L, Ware JE. Canadian-French, German and UK versions of the Child Health Questionnaire: methodology and preliminary item scaling results. Qual Life Res 1998; 7:433–445.
40. Bousquet J, Knani J, Dhivert H, Richard A, Chicoye A, Ware JE, Michel FB. Quality of life in asthma. 1. Internal consistency and validity of the SF-36 questionnaire. Am J Respir Crit Care Med 1994; 149:371–375.
41. Bousquet J, Bullinger M, Fayol C, Marquis P, Valentin B, Burtin B. Assessment of quality of life in patients with perennial rhinitis with the French version of the SF-36 health status questionnaire. J Allergy Clin Immunol 1994; 94: 182–188.
42. Rutten-van Molken MPMH, Clusters F, Van Doorslaer EKA, Jansen CCM, Heurman L, Maesen FPV, Smeets JJ, Bommer AM, Raaijmakers JAM.

Comparison of performance of four instruments in evaluating the effects of salmeterol on asthma quality of life. Eur Respir J 1995; 8:888–898.

43. Juniper EF, Norman GR, Cox FM, Roberts JN. Comparison of the standard gamble, rating scale, AQLQ and SF-36 for measuring quality of life in asthma. Eur Respir J 2001; 18:38–44.
44. Juniper EF, Guyatt GH, Ferrie PJ, Griffith LE. Measuring quality of life in asthma. Am Rev Respir Dis 1993; 147:832–838.
45. Feinstein AR. The theory and evaluation of sensibility. Feinstein AR, ed. Clinimetricso. Westford, MA: Murray Printing Co., 1987:141–166.
46. Juniper EF, Guyatt GH, Streiner DL, King DR. Clinical impact versus factor analysis for quality of life questionnaire construction. J Clin Epidemiol 1997; 50:233–238.
47. Guyatt GH, Kirshner B, Jaeschke R. Measuring health status: what are the necessary measurement properties. J Clin Epidemiol 1992; 45:1341–1345.
48. Juniper EF, Buist AS, Cox FM, Feme PJ, King DR. Validation of a standardized version of the Asthma Quality of Life Questionnaire. Chest 1999; 115:1265–1270.
49. Juniper EF, Guyatt GH, Cox FM, Ferrie PJ, King DR. Development and validation of the Mini Asthma Quality of Life Questionnaire. Eur Respir J 1999; 14:32–38.
50. Rowe BH, Oxman AD. Performance of an asthma quality of life questionnaire in an outpatient setting. Am Rev Respir Dis 1993; 148:675–681.
51. Guyatt GH, Walter S, Norman G. Measuring change over time: assessing the usefulness of evaluative instruments. J Chron Dis 1987; 40:171–178.
52. Juniper EF, Guyatt GH, Willan A, Griffith LE. Determining a minimal important change in a disease-specific quality of life questionnaire. J Clin Epidemiol 1994; 47:81–87.
53. Guyatt GH, Juniper EF, Walter SD, Griffith LE, Goldstein RS. Interpreting treatment effects in randomised trials. Br Med J 1998; 101:163–170.
54. Lydick E, Epstein RS. Interpretation of quality of life changes. Qual Life Res 1993; 2:221–226.
55. Guyatt GH, Norman GR, Juniper EF, Griffith LE. A critical look at transition ratings. J Clin Epidemiol 2002; 55:900–908.
56. Juniper EF, Chauhan A, Neville E, Chatterjee A, Svensson K, Mörk A-C, Stähl E. Clinicians tend to overestimate improvements in asthma control: an unexpected observation. Primary Care Respir J 2004; 13:181–184.
57. Juniper EF, Johnston PR, Borkhoff CM, Guyatt GH, Boulet LP, Haukioja A. Quality of life in asthma clinical trials: comparison of salmeterol and salbutamol. Am J Respir Crit Care Med 1995; 151:66–70.
58. Mazur DJ. In: Shared Decision Making in the Patient–Physician Relationship. Tampa: Hillsboro Printing Company, 2001.
59. Gibson PG, Talbot PI, Toneguzzi RC. Self-management, autonomy and quality of life in asthma. Chest 1995; 107:1003–1008.
60. Adams RJ, Smith BJ, Ruffin RE. Patient preferences for autonomy in decision making in asthma management. Thorax 2001; 56:126–132.

61. Adams R, Smith B, Ruffin R. Impact of the physician's participatory style in asthma outcomes and patient satisfaction. Ann Allergy Asthma Immunol 2001; 86:263–271.

62. Bawden R. Impact of having a patient's quality of life scores on nurse management of patients with chronic asthma . IPCRG Conference, Amsterdam, 2002.

63. Jacobs JE, van de Lisdonk EH, Smeele I, van Weel C, Grol RPTM. Management of patients with asthma and COPD: monitoring quality of life and the relationship to subsequent GP interventions. Fam Pract 2001; 18:574–580.

64. McHorney C, Kosinski M, Ware JE. Comparison of costs and quality of norms for the SF-36 Health Survey collected by mail versus telephone interview: results from national survey. Med Care 1994; 34:551–567.

65. Fowler FJ, Roman AM, Zhu XD. Mode effects in the survey of medicare prostate surgery patients. Proc Surv Meth Sec, Am Sociol Assoc 1993:730–735.

66. Caro JJ, Caro I, Caro J, Wouters F, Juniper EF. Does electronic implementation of questionnaires used in asthma alter responses compared to paper implementation. Qual Life Res 2001; 10:683–691.

67. Pinnock H, Sheikh A, Juniper EF. Evaluation of an intervention to improve successful completion of the Mini-AQLQ: comparison of postal and supervised completion. Primary Care Respir J 2004; 13:36–41.

68. Acquadro C, Jambon B, Ellis D, Marquis P. Language and translations issues. In: Spilker B, ed. Quality of Life and Pharmacoeconomics in Clinical Trials. Philadelphia: Lippincott-Raven Publishers, 1996:575–585.

69. Juniper EF, Guyatt GH, Feeny DH, Ferrie PJ, Griffith LE, Townsend M. Measuring quality of life in the parents of children with asthma. Qual Life Res 1996; 5:27–34.

70. Stahl E, Postma DS, Juniper EF, Svensson K, Mear I, Lofdahl C-G. Health-related quality of life in asthma studies. Can we combine data from different countries? Pulm Pharmacol Ther 2003; 16:53–59.

3

Monitoring Cough: Diary, Electronic Monitoring and Significance in Asthma

ANNE B. CHANG

Department of Respiratory Medicine, Royal Children's Hospital,
    Brisbane, Queensland and Department of Paediatrics and
    Child Health, University of Queensland,
Queensland, Australia

Introduction

The frequency and/or severity of the common asthma symptoms of wheeze, chest tightness, and cough are main components of the classification of asthma severity in adults (1) and children (2). Each symptom is however not diagnostic for asthma and the recent British Asthma guidelines caution against the use of any symptom in isolation (3). As cough is the most common symptom presenting to general practitioners (4) and asthma a common chronic disorder, there is high potential for a chance overlap between cough and asthma, without there being a clear causal link between the two conditions. Nevertheless cough is a prominent symptom in many people with asthma and good control of asthma symptoms is a component of effective asthma management. This chapter reviews current evidence on the use of the symptom of cough and objective cough indices as an indicator of asthma control. Whether isolated cough represents asthma is beyond the scope of this chapter and reviews are available elsewhere (5–7).

General Issues on Cough as a Symptom and Outcome Measure

Cough, like other subjective symptoms in clinical medicine, has limitations as an outcome measure (8). Studies based in London have shown that parents of children with other respiratory noises (wheeze, snoring, stridor) often use the wrong label (9,10). Cough is a distinct audible sound and unlike wheeze can be easily distinguished by non-medical personnel. However, this has not been tested in a research setting. In the last decade, the need for objective markers for cough as a marker of asthma has been highlighted (8,11). The importance of objectively measuring cough in clinical research is reflected in the several documented limitations of symptom questionnaires. Firstly, questions on isolated cough are largely poorly reproducible (12). The kappa value relating the chance-corrected agreement between answers to questions on cough ranges from 0.14 to 0.57 (12,13). In contrast, questions on isolated wheeze and asthma attacks are highly reproducible with kappa values of 0.7–1.0 (12). However, when cough is combined with another positive symptom such as "cough with phelgm" (12) and "cough with colds" (14) the repeatability of the questions is enhanced (Cohen's kappa of 0.63 and 0.53, respectively). Secondly, nocturnal cough is unreliably and inconsistently reported when compared to objective measurements in both adults (15) and children (16,17). Using overnight tape recording of 56 nights Archer and Simpson (16) showed the unreliability of nocturnal cough reporting in children with asthma. Falconer et al later confirmed the poor agreement between subjective and objective assessment of nocturnal cough (Cohen's kappa of 0.3). However, when the ability to detect change rather than whether cough was present or absent (agreement) was measured, two groups have reported that parents were able to detect change (18,19). Although the change in cough frequency measured objectively significantly correlated to changes in cough scores (18), the relationship is only moderate and better in children with a history of troublesome recurrent cough (Spearman $r=0.52$) than in children without ($r=0.38$) (18).

Thirdly, cough is subject to period-effects (spontaneous resolution of cough) (20). Thus non-randomized placebo controlled intervention studies have to be interpreted with caution (21). The therapeutic benefit of placebo treatment for cough has been reported to be as high as 85% (21). Fourthly, as cough is cortically modulated (5) it is subjected to psychological influences (22–24). In adults with cough, subjective scoring of cough does not correlate with cough frequency over a 20-min period but correlates with mood scores (25). Rietveld et al. (22) showed that children were more likely to cough under certain psychological settings. Fifthly, subjective perception of cough severity is dependent on the population studied (26). In children without a history of recurrent cough, the correlation of daytime to nighttime cough is higher than those with recurrent cough, and they have a lower ratio of daytime to nighttime cough (26). This study suggests that nighttime cough, although less reliably reported, is perceived as more troublesome. Sixthly, "normal" children cough occasionally as described by two studies that objectively measured cough frequency (26,27). Normal children without a preceding upper respiratory tract infection in the last 4 weeks have up to 34 cough epochs per 24 hr. In another study where controls were children (with or without recent upper respiratory tract infection) considered well by parents and attending school and were age, gender and season matched, 0–141 cough epochs per 24 hr (median 10) were recorded in these children (26). Finally, the data on isolated cough in children significantly differs from adults. In community settings, epidemiological studies have shown that isolated cough is rarely asthma (28,29). Recent work on airway inflammatory markers in community children with isolated persistent cough show that unlike the adult literature, most children with persistent isolated cough do not have asthma as their airway inflammatory markers are significantly different to children with asthma (30,31). Gibson et al. (31) concluded from their community-based survey of children with chronic respiratory symptoms that "persistent cough and recurrent chest colds without wheeze should not be considered a variant of asthma" (31). In contrast to paediatric data, a high percentage (40–43%) of adults with chronic cough have asthma (32,33) and there is little doubt that the aetiology of cough would depend on the setting and population studied (31,34).

Measurements of Cough Severity

The symptom of cough is widely used in research as an outcome measure in clinical studies on asthma in both children (35–37) and adults (38,39). However validated cough measurements/systems have only recently existed (18,40). In addition to the considerations described above when measuring cough severity specifically for asthma, one has to be cognisant that like the many available objective markers for asthma severity, objective tests for cough severity also measure different aspects of cough and these indices are not interchangeable. The choice of the cough index depends on the reason for performing the measurement (41). Broadly, indices of cough severity can be divided into subjective and objective indices.

Subjective Scores, Cough Diaries and Assessment Scores

Gulsvik and Refvem (42) have shown that respiratory symptoms recorded as discrete variables are far less reliable that rating scores or respiratory disability. Whilst previous clinical studies on asthma utilised isolated cough as an indicator of asthma control (35) (all largely unvalidated systems), more recent validated asthma diary cards (43,44) and asthma specific quality of life systems for both children (45) and adults (46) have removed isolated cough as an indicator of asthma severity or exacerbation. Cough diaries like other symptoms and quality of life scores in children's diary-cards can be parent-completed or child-completed (18). This factor is an additional variable in diary-cards of children's symptoms. There is an increasing trend for older children to complete their own questionnaires (47) as child-completed responses have been shown to be significantly different to those completed by parents (48). Although cough-specific diary cards completed by children had a higher correlation with objectively measured cough frequency than diary cards completed by parents, the difference was not significant (18,26).

Cough-specific diary cards can be related to general severity scales (eg., Likert scale, visual analog scale) or categorically based on limitation or effect on activity (verbal category descriptive score) (Fig. 1a and b)

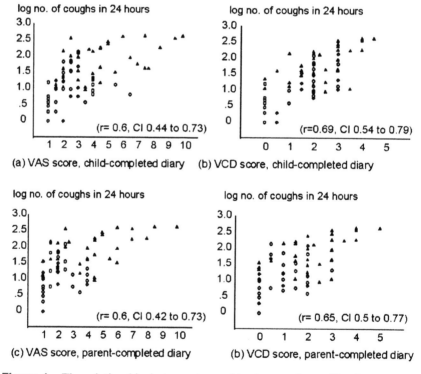

Figure 1   The relationship between two subjective cough specific diary cards vs cough frequency (reproduced with permission from Ref. 18). Figure shows correlation (Spearman) between the log frequency of cough measured by the cough meter (number of coughs in 24 hr) vs. the visual analog score (VAS) and the verbal category descriptive scale (VCD) as recorded by the child and parent(s) of the subjects (*triangles*) and controls (*circles*).

(18). In a study that compared these scores to objective monitoring, the most valid subjective method of scoring cough in children over 6 years old is the verbal category descriptive score completed by children with parental assistance (Fig. 2). Nocturnal cough diary cards have been repeatedly shown to be inaccurate and are hence invalid (16,18). Indeed despite the wide use of cough as an outcome measure there is only one validated cough-specific diary card for children (18) and adults (15). However, this study and other studies (15,16) comparing objective and subjective scores for cough assume that subjects and parents judge the severity of cough on the frequency of cough. It is possible that subjects assess the severity of cough on other aspects of cough such as the length of the paroxysms, loudness of the cough, effects of cough (post tussive vomiting, incontinence) which would not necessarily correlate to the frequency of cough. Validated cough-specific quality of life measures now exist for adults (49,50) but none are yet available for children.

Cough Monitoring Devices

Non-Ambulatory Systems: Cough Analysers and Tape-Recorder Systems

Physical characteristics of cough have been analysed in different ways: electromyogram (EMG) or activity of muscles used to generate cough (the expiratory muscles of respiration) (51), cough sounds analysis (52,53), airflow that results from the cough (51), cough frequency/counts (16,54). Cox's group (51) showed that abdominal EMG activity as a measurement of cough intensity correlated well with the airflow and volume produced by coughing. Piirila and Sovijarvi (55) analysed spectrographically the acoustic and dynamic characteristics of cough in asthma, bronchitis, tracheobronchial collapse syndrome, and fibrotic pulmonary disease. They found that during a cough, there is an average of 2.6 ± 0.8 expiratory flow phases and that the sound always occurred simultaneously with the expiratory flow phase. The counting of cough using audio tape recorder systems has been used for almost 40 years (16,54). An automated system of quantifying cough using a static charged sensitive bed with a microphone was later described (56). In the system described by Salmi et al. (56) the acoustic signal was high pass filtered and rectified, and for the first time allowed electronic discrimination of single cough events. Ambulatory tracheal sound recording for 72 hr has been used by Rietveld et al (57) in children. This system is dependent on detection of cough and wheeze sounds recorded from a microphone placed over the suprasternal notch and recorded on tape.

(a)   Day 1   Day 2

Date   ———————   ———————

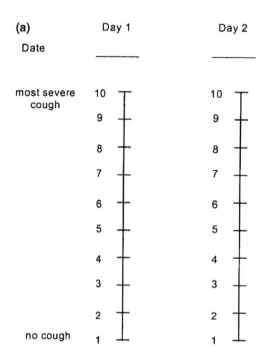

most severe   10   10
    cough
            9   9

            8   8

            7   7

            6   6

            5   5

            4   4

            3   3

            2   2

no cough   1   1

(b)

(reproduced from Cough: Mechanisms, Causes and Therapy. Blackwell Science 2003:in press)

Day of month	1st	2nd	3rd	4th	5th	6th	7th
Score **day**-time (0-5)							

Day-time score

0 = No cough during the day

1 = Cough for one-two short periods only

2 = Cough for more than two short periods

3 = frequent coughing but does <u>not</u> interfere with school or other day time activities

4 = frequent coughing which <u>does</u> interfere with schoolwork or some day time activities

5 = cannot perform most usual daytime activity due to severe coughing

Figure 2   Cough-specific diary cards. (a) The Visual Analog Scale (VAS). (b) The validated verbal category descriptive score. *Source*: Ref. 18.

Electronic Cough Meters

The systems described previously were forerunners to the development of the first ambulatory cough meter described by the Brompton group (15). The cough meter which objectively defines cough frequency is based on the recognition of cough signals from the simultaneous activity of muscles of expiration and generation of sound when coughing occurs (15). The Brompton cough meter allowed continuous recording of up to 4 hr and episodic recording for up to 48 hr and utilised a digital logger. The EMG and audio signals were preprocessed using high pass and low pass filters; which were 1.3 kHz and 5 kHz, respectively for the audio signal and 120 Hz and 5 kHz for the EMG. Sampling rates of 50 Hz were used and the τ_c (time constant) was 30μs. The Brompton cough meter was indeed elegant but the authors did not validate the cough meter using a previous standard i.e., an audio tape recorder system. The "validation of the cough meter" was performed using experimental induction of cough and differentiating the cough signal from signals of other events (sighing, loud speech, throat clearing, forced expiratory manoeuvres, sneezing) (15). Using a cough processor adapted onto a Holter monitor, we described and validated a 24-hr continuous recording system for cough frequency (58). The Australian cough meter developed specifically for children utilised different filter cut-offs and time constant from the Brompton cough-meter. The filters for the audio signal consisted of a 4-pole high pass Butterworth filter with a −3dB point at 1200 Hz and a roll off of 24 dB/octave and a 2-pole low pass filter, with the −3dB point at 5000 Hz and the roll of 12dB/octave. For the EMG signal, the low pass filter was the same as the audio system but the high pass filter had a −3dB point at 200 Hz. Amplification of the signal gains were 11 for the audio signal and 981 for the EMG signal. Both the EMG and the audio signals were then full wave rectified and further filtered with a low pass Butterworth filter 55Hz to give a τ_c of 3μs. Audio (from the sound of cough) and EMG signals (from the muscles involved in the generation of cough: diaphragm, intercostal, and abdomen muscles) (59) are different (e.g., different peak frequencies, amplitude and intensity) in children to that in adults. It is thus not surprising that the optimum filters and time constant in the paediatric system are different to that for the adult system. Placement of leads for the paediatric system (58) is also different to that for adults (Fig. 3) (15). The paediatric system described above was not tested in infants who will undoubtedly also have different EMG and audio thresholds which may not be recorded by a cough meter that does not allow adjustment of EMG and audio signals. A recent system adapted for use in infants only had a sensitivity of 81% when compared to a gold standard (video monitoring) (60). There was also a systemic error in the adapted cough meter described as it consistently recorded higher cough epochs in infants who had > 4 coughs/hr (60). Cough-meters are currently the only

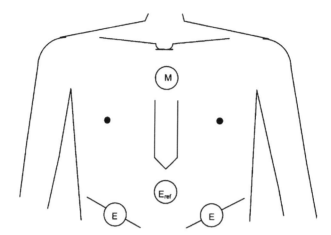

Figure 3 Placement of microphone and electrodes for the cough meter in children (58). Electronic cough monitoring is based on pattern recognition of simultaneous audio signal (picked up by microphone) and EMG signals generated from respiratory muscles of expiration (see section on cough monitoring devices) *Abbreviations:* M, microphone; E, EMG electrodes; E_{ref}, reference electrode.

ambulatory objective monitoring tool for cough and have been suggested as a monitoring tool in asthma (11). Although the cough-meter has been used in clinical studies to determine response of cough to asthma medications (61), currently its expense and technical requirements limit its use to research settings.

Other Objective Cough Measurements

The many other objective ways of defining cough severity in children and adults are beyond the scope of this chapter and have recently been reviewed elsewhere (41,62). The concept of cough sensitivity measures will however be briefly discussed as it is increasingly used in research on cough in both adults and children (63–65).

Cough can be chemically stimulated by a variety of tussive agents (acetic acid, capsaicin, nebulised fog etc) (5). Capsaicin is the most commonly used tussive agent in clinical research and its utility for clinical research purposes have been documented (63,65,66). As cough receptors are unevenly distributed in the airways (5), standardisation of airway deposition is important for test validity in both adults and children (40,67). This is arguably more important in children who have smaller airways and who are less likely to comply with complex respiratory manoeuvres like maintaining an open glottis throughout actuation of the dosimeter (delivery of nebulising solution). For measurements to be interpretable, measures of repeatability within the laboratory are important. Inspiratory flow has been shown to influence repeatability measurements of cough sensitivity (40,67) and hence should be regulated. Gender is known to influence cough sensitivity in adults but not in children (63). Other influences on cough sensitivity are airway calibre and age (63). A full description of a standardised reliable method of measuring cough sensitivity to capsaicin is available elsewhere (40). The commonly used outcomes measures for cough sensitivity are C2 (the lowest concentration that stimulates 2 or more coughs) and C5 (the lowest concentration that stimulates 5 or more coughs). Other outcome measures that have been described are number of coughs within a specific time period (eg.,10′sec) and cough latency. Unlike the C2 and C5 measurements, no repeatability studies have been performed on these other outcome measurements.

Significance of Cough in Asthma

The interpretation of cough as a symptom as asthma was previously thought to be a key factor in the under-diagnosis of asthma. In the past as cough was under-recognised as a symptom of asthma as first described by McFadden (68). However, the trend has swung and the use of the symptom of isolated cough as representative of asthma has partly contributed to the reported increased prevalence of asthma (69–71). In a paper that provided a breakdown of the method of how asthma was diagnosed, the symptom of cough alone accounted for the largest rise in asthma prevalence (72). Between 1990 and 1993, the change in the cumulative prevalence of wheeze was 0.6% and that of troublesome cough was 3%. This group accounted for the biggest increase in the "frequency of asthma and its symptoms" (72). In the UK Kelly et al. (69) showed that in 1993 doctors were twice as likely to diagnose asthma on the basis of isolated cough when compared to 1991. Although the prevalence of respiratory symptoms was unchanged between the two studies, the number of children who were diagnosed with asthma, as well as the number of children who were receiving medications for asthma, significantly increased (69). Another community based study (28) has also reported the over-diagnosis of asthma in children when isolated cough is used as the diagnostic criterion. In a hospital outpatient setting, the over-diagnosis of cough as asthma has also been documented (34).

Children and adults with asthma can present with cough and cough dominant asthma phenotypes in adults and children have been described (7,73). Increasingly asthma subtypes have been described such as eosinophil dominant and neutrophil dominant asthma that require different treatment strategies (74). Cough variant asthma (isolated cough i.e., without wheeze, dyspnoea, or spirometric evidence of airway obstruction) may yet represent a different phenotype or spectrum as the physiology of cough is different to that of asthma. Adults with "cough variant asthma" that did not respond to bronchodilators and corticosteroids responded to leukotriene receptor antagonist (75). Adults and children with cough-dominant asthma have transient increase in cough sensitivity when compared to those without cough-dominant asthma (63,66,73).

Is cough a feature in all with asthma? Because of the variability of diagnostic methods in asthma (29,76), determinations of how often people with classical asthma (as opposed to isolated cough diagnosed as asthma) cough are not readily available. Current data suggest that most but not all asthmatics cough (5,57,77). In a South African study (excluding children diagnosed with asthma based on isolated cough) only 8 of the 362 children with wheeze did not have cough at presentation (78). Using objective monitoring only 50% of children with asthma exacerbation had cough (57).

Nocturnal cough is often used as a hallmark of asthma as children with asthma are often reported to have troublesome nocturnal cough (79). However Ninan et al. (80) found that only a third children with isolated nocturnal cough (absence of wheeze, shortness of breath or chest tightness) had asthma in a large cross sectional epidemiological study. To date there are no studies that have objectively documented that nocturnal cough is worse than daytime cough in children and adults with asthma. In children with recurrent cough the correlation between day-time and night-time cough frequency, although significant, is only modest (Spearman r of 0.5) (26). In a group of children with asthma reported to have troublesome cough, only a median of 6 cough epochs per night was recorded (81). In comparison, 46 children considered well by parents and attending school and were age, gender and season matched to children with recurrent cough had 0–57 cough epochs per night (median 0) (26). In a cross sectional study of 796 children nocturnal cough, which mostly occurred in conjunction with other symptoms, was the most common nocturnal symptom in children with apparently otherwise stable asthma (79). Nocturnal cough in children with wheeze tends to occur throughout the night with a peak between 8–10pm whereas children without wheeze tend to cough in the morning between 5–7am (82). In Thompson et al. (81) study however, children with asthma had peak coughing times 2 hr after going to bed and two hours before rising. In adults, nocturnal cough is related to asthma as well as female gender, increased body mass index, rhinitis, smoking and environmental smoke exposure. The female gender had the highest odds ratio in the multivariate analysis for association with nocturnal cough (83).

Anecdotally, clinicians sometimes refer cough associated with asthma as a "tight" cough. However the validity, sensitivity, and specificity of this has not been defined. Cough associated with asthma in children (without other diseases and respiratory tract infections) is dry (3). In adults, cough with asthma can be dry (7) or productive (83) but other confounding factors such as gender and anxiety are highly significant in adults (84). Moreover these aspects have not been rigorously examined and given the wide overlap of asthma with cough from other diseases especially in adults (see section on cough, asthma and other associated conditions), the quality of cough associated with pure asthma can be difficult to ascertain. The quality of cough associated with asthma has been reported on digital assessment to be less intense (via tussiphonogram) (85), longer with a lower upper limit frequency on spectrogram (55) and have different bursts or peaks on spectral analysis with fast Fourier transformation (53). Although the characteristics of an asthmatic cough have significantly different digital parameters to non-asthmatic cough, there is a considerable overlap (53). To date none of these techniques are clinically used. Using ambulatory tracheal sounds monitoring for 72 hr in 90 children, Rietveld et al. (77) described that the diagnostic sensitivity of cough for wheeze was 34% and specificity was 35%.

Cough, Bronchocontriction and Airway Responsiveness-Clinical Laboratory Studies

The physiology of cough (86,87) and bronchoconstriction are both complex and beyond the scope of this chapter. There are however several studies that have looked at cough and bronchoconstriction in clinical laboratory studies, where by many groups have described that physiologically cough and bronchoconstriction can be separately stimulated and inhibited. Medications (lignocaine, oral codeine) that inhibit cough have no effect on bronchoconstriction and conversely, medications (cromoglygate, atropine) that inhibit the pharmacologically induced bronchoconstriction have no effect on the cough response of adults (88–93). Using non-isotonic water as a bronchoconstrictor agent and cough stimulant, Sheppard et al. (89) found that atropine and cromoglygate inhibited bronchoconstriction but had no effect on the cough response. When lignocaine was inhaled, the cough response was abolished but there was no effect on bronchoconstriction (89,91). Recently Wardlaw et al. (94) proposed a model involving micro-localisation as the organising principle in airway inflammation response (hence determining phenotypes) whereby inflammation localised to the epithelium and lamina propria results in symptoms of bronchitis (cough and mucus hypersecretion) and only if the airway smooth muscle is involved does asthma occur (94). Using induced sputum, Zimmerman et al. (95) described that although airway hyper-responseivess (AHR) can be found in some children with post infectious cough, these children do not have airway markers representative of asthma.

Cough, Asthma and Other Associated Conditions

When relating asthma severity to cough, important confounders such as socioeconomic deprivation (96) and obesity (97) have been found. Cough is the respiratory symptom that is most strongly related to socioeconomic deprivation (96) and poverty has also been shown to influence asthma severity (98). People with asthma have increased prevalence of other diseases (e.g., chronic obstructive airway disease, gastroesophageal reflux, atopy, allergic rhinitis, obstructive sleep disorders, obesity) that are also associated with chronic cough. Cough is a key feature in adults with chronic obstructive airway disease which may or may not co-exist with an "asthma component" (94,99). Obstructive sleep disorders and gastroesophageal reflux are more common in children and adults with asthma (100,101) and increased cough problems are associated with these disorders (84,102,103). Appropriate management of these disorders reduces comorbidities without additional asthma therapy (104–106). Gastroesophageal reflux alone accounts for 10–20% of adults with chronic cough (106). In Chinn's recent review of the literature on obesity and asthma, Chinn concluded that the association between obesity and asthma is strong, possibly through several mechanisms including gastroesophageal reflux (97). The prevalence of atopy in people with asthma is higher than non-asthmatics and in adults the concept of "atopic cough" is accepted (107). When exposed to airborne pollutants people with asthma are more likely to have a coughing illness, without necessarily affecting their asthma control, in comparison to non asthmatics (108,109). Different pollutants can also cause independent effects on cough and asthma. Just et al. (110) described that black smoke and nitrogen dioxide were associated with increases in the occurrence of nocturnal cough whereas ozone was associated with an increase in the occurrence of asthma attacks with changes in lung function (increase in PEF variability and a decrease in PEF) (110). Asthma-like diseases are also increased in respiratory diseases such as bronchiectasis (111), cystic fibrosis (112) and bronchiolitis obliterans (113) all of which has cough as a major feature of the underlying illness.

Cough as a Marker of Asthma Control

Cough is the most common symptom presenting to general practitioners (4,114) and viral respiratory infections, which also cause cough, has been reported as the aetiological reason in 80% of childhood asthma exacerbations (115). When a person with asthma coughs, determining if the cough is related to asthma or other aetiology can be a challenge when other symptoms of asthma are absent and/or when objective measurements such as exhaled nitric oxide or spirometry are unavailable. Misdiagnosis of isolated cough as asthma is common in children (34,116) and anecdotally children have become Cushingoid when increasing doses of corticosteroids are used to treat cough in children with asthma. Also, asthma severity of can be categorised using several methods such as assessment of serum, airway and urine inflammatory markers, clinical symptoms, pulmonary function indices, degree of AHR, quality of life. Airway inflammation has recently been recognised as a determinant of asthma symptoms and physiology, and some have advocated sputum rather than clinical indices as the outcome measure (17,118). Current knowledge of neutrophilic and eosinophilic airway inflammation in adult and childhood asthma (94,119) would render the "best" universal measure of asthma severity unknown, and the most sensitive measurement may not necessarily reflect clinical relevance. Relating the also many indices of cough severity such as cough sensitivity thresholds (capsaicin, citric, acetic acid), frequency (day or night), diary cards (parent or child-reported), cough amplitude etc to asthma severity indices is thus difficult. Arguably individual or isolated symptom reporting in asthma is inappropriate (8,42). Nevertheless, relevant questions that arise in relating cough to asthma monitoring summarised in Table 1 is discussed in the following section.

Table 1 Questions on the Relationship Between Cough with Monitoring Asthma

	Pathophysiology question	Clinical relevance
1	Does the onset of cough herald an exacerbation of asthma?	Should asthmatics initiate acute asthma management plan at the onset of cough?
2	What is the relationship between cough indices and asthma severity in acute asthma?	Should severity of cough be used as a marker of severity in acute asthma?
3	How does cough severity indices relate to asthma severity in the resolution phase of asthma? And How soon should cough resolve if cough is related to asthma?	Should acute asthma therapy be continued until cough totally resolves?
4	Does the presence of cough in otherwise clinically stable asthma indicate persistent inflammation?	Should anti-inflammatory medications be increased if cough is present?
5	Does the presence of isolated nocturnal cough indicate more severe/unstable asthma?	Should anti-inflammatory medications be increased if isolated nocturnal cough is present?
6	Does coughing with exercise indicate asthma instability?	Should anti-inflammatory medications be increased if isolated cough is present with exercise?

Studies Relating Cough Indices to Asthma Severity

Most studies in asthma have used increased cough in conjunction with other asthma symptoms of wheeze and dyspnoea as a marker of asthma stability in both hospitalised acute exacerbations (74) and epidemiological studies (120). Despite the difficulties described above in evaluating the relationship between cough severity and asthma severity, studies that have examined this relationship using objective measurement(s) will be presented in this section. There are few studies that have directly studied the questions posed in Table 1 and some data are thus indirect inferred. Data relating cough with asthma severity indices are summarised in Table 2(a) children and (b) adults.

The two studies that have directly examined whether the onset of cough heralded the onset of an asthma exacerbation have found that cough is only modestly predictive of the onset of an asthma exacerbation and the relationship is lost early (57,121). In the Rietveld et al. study (57) where 30 controls and 60 children with asthma were objectively monitored with tracheal sound monitoring for 24–72 hr respectively, cough occurred at the onset of the asthma exacerbation only in 2 of the 6 children. The 2nd study utilised subjective reporting in children with cough-dominant asthma found that the onset of cough did herald the onset of an asthma exacerbation as cough scores related to asthma diary scores (121). However, this relationship was no longer present by day 3 of the mild exacerbation (121). In the former study (57), children with asthma did cough more than controls but cough frequency in the remission phase of asthma was no different to that of controls. Cough severity defined by subjective scores did not relate to asthma severity defined subjectively or objectively by sputum eosinophils, IL8, ECP and FEV_1 variability in the later study (Table 3) (121). In hospitalised children recovering from a severe asthma attack oximetry recordings (widely accepted marker of acute asthma severity (1,3) in both adults and childhood asthma) correlated better to daytime tests of lung function ($r=0.711$) than nocturnal cough frequency ($r=0.56$) (122). These children recorded 1–156 cough epochs (median 39.5) per night. Nocturnal cough frequency correlated with the mean overnight oxygen saturation (SpO_2) but the lower mean SpO_2 may be related to a technical artefact as an apparent brief fall in SpO_2 may occur during coughing and the associated movement artefact. Cough frequency did not correlate with peak expiratory flows, morning or evening clinical scores (122). Following presentation for asthma to an emergency department, Stevens et al. (123) described that 46% of the 388 children had persistent cough at 1 week and 23% at 2 weeks. However, cough severity was not measured and cough was only verbally reported in the study (123).

Many scoring systems for assessing acute asthma exist (11,124) and the problems associated with them have been summarized (11). Cough

Table 2 Studies Relating Markers of Cough Severity to Asthma Severity in Children and Adults with Asthma

Refs	Asthma severity measures	Cough severity	Study setting	Relationship between cough and asthma variables
(a) Studies relating markers of cough severity to asthma severity in children with asthma (see section on studies relating cough indicate asthma severity for details)				
Brooke et al. (82)	Diary, night SpO$_2$, lung volumes, PEF & variability, spirometry	Nocturnal cough frequency (tape recorder)	Community, no respiratory infection in last 4-weeks, room temperature & humidity measured ($n = 100$)	Cough frequency associated with lower overnight room temperature ($p = 0.016$) in those with wheeze. No relationship between cough and any other variable
Chang et al. (73)	Spirometry, clinical	CRS to capsaicin	Hospitalised, acute asthma (DI), post discharge (D7-10, week 4–6) ($n = 31$)	No relationship between CRS thresholds and FEV$_1$
Chang et al. (121)	Sputum ECP, eosinophils, asthma diary score, IL8, MPO, FEV$_1$ and variability, AHR to HS	Verbal category cough scores, CRS to capsaicin	Serial measurements (baseline, D1,D3,D7, D28) in cohort of children with mild asthlima exacerbation ($n = 21$)	No relationship bewteen CRS to sputum eosinophils, IL8, ECP or MPO
Hoskyns et al. (122)	Clinical score, day and night SpO$_2$, lung volumes, R_{aw}, PEF & variability, spirometry	Nocturnal cough frequency (tape recorder)	Hospitalised, acute asthma, pre discharge ($n = 22$)	Negative correlation between log$_e$ cough and mean night SpO$_2$ ($r = -0.564$), RV:TLC ($r = -0.45$). No correlation between log$_e$ cough

(Continued)

Table 2 Studies Relating Markers of Cough Severity to Asthma Severity in Children and Adults with Asthma (*Continued*)

Refs	Asthma severity measures	Cough severity	Study setting	Relationship between cough and asthma variables
Hoskyns et al. (135)	Clinical score, day and night SpO$_2$, lung volumes, R_{aw}, PEF & variability, spirometry	Nocturnal cough frequency (tape recorder)	Community, stable asthma (n = 21)	and any expiratory flow, clinical score, airway resistance No relationship between night cough and any measure
Rietveld et al. (57)	PEF, clinical symptoms	Cough and wheeze frequency (tape recorder)	Community & residents of asthma centre (asthma n = 60, no asthma n = 30)	Presence and frequency of cough independent of PEF, wheeze and self-reported dyspnoea.
Rietveld et al. (77)	Spirometry, clinical symptoms	Cough frequency (tape recorder)	Community, stable asthma, histamine challenge (asthma n = 30, no asthma n = 30)	Cough frequency independent of FEV$_1$, wheezing, dyspnoea, and severity of asthma
Shimuzu et al. (140)	Spirometry, AHR to histamine	CRS to acetic acid	Community, stable asthma, histamine induced FEV$_1$ change (n = 19)	No relationship between CRS thresholds and FEV$_1$, PC$_{20}$
(b) Studies relating markers of cough severity to asthma severity in adults with asthma				
Hsu et al. (15)	FEV$_1$ and peak flow diurnal variation	Cough frequency (cough meter)	Ambulatory Asthma (n = 21) Others (n = 26)	No relationship between cough frequency and diurnal peak flow or FEV$_1$
Fujimura et al. (93)	Spirometry	CRS to capsaicin and tartaric acid	Laboratory using methacholine and	FEV$_1$ decrease (from methacholine) and increase (from procterol) had

Study				Results
Minoguchi et al. (64)	Sputum eosinophils, AHR to histamine	CRS to capsaicin	procaterol (n = 22) Randomised parallel group study, using allergen inhalation (HDM) (n = 8)	no relationship to CRS No relationship between CRS to eosinophilie inflammation or to AHR to histamine
Niimi et al. (130)	Clinical severity of classic asthma, bronchial eosinophils, and serum ECP	Subjective asthma cough score (unvalidated)	Outpatients (asthma n = 21, CVA n = 14, controls n = 7)	Clinical severity correlated to serum ECP and bronchial
Rundell et al. (137)	Spirometry, airway hyperresponsiveness to exercise	Symptom reporting	Elite athletes with AHR to exercise challenge (n = 158)	Proportion of AHR positive and AHR negative athletes reporting two or more symptoms was not different. Sensitivity and specificity of 0.61 and 0.69 respectively.
Ware et al. (134)	QOL activities scale, Marks scales, SF-36-scales, Sleep problem scale, Physician assessed changes: cough, chest tightness, wheezing, shortness of breath, overall condition.	Physician assessed cough severity	Assessments during phases of a randomised controlled trial using beclomethasone (n = 142)	Related best to "physical symptoms" derived from mark's scale (relative validity of 1), poorest relation amongst all physician assessed changes to the best subjective score (breathlessness from Mark's scale), no relationship to sleep disturbance, variable statistically significant relationship to other scales with relative validity ranging from 0.25–0.71)

AHR airway hyper-responsiveness; CRS, cough receptor sensitivity; CVA, cough variant asthma; D, day; ECP, eosinophil cationic protein; HDM, house dust mite; MPO, myeloperoxidase; PEF, peak expiratory flow; QOL, quality of life; R_{aw} = airway resistance.
Source: Adapted from 1694/id.

severity does not feature in any of these scores of acute asthma and clinicians do not utilise cough as a marker of acute asthma severity. In laboratory studies, there was no relationship between cough sensitivity and airway calibre measured by FEV_I in both the acute and interval phase of asthma (73). In contrast, improvements in FEV_I correlated with the reduction in sputum eosinophils and eosinophil cationic protein (ECP) in the recovery phase of acute severe asthma (125).

In the treatment of cough associated with asthma, many early studies in adults and children reported that cough *completely resolved* by 3–7 days (68,126–128) with medications such as non steroidal drugs such as theophylline (126), terbutaline and major tranquillisers (68). Creticos, in his summary of data on the therapeutic effects of nedocromil on inflammation and symptoms reported that cough symptom scores improved by 30% by day 2 (39). In the study by Cherniack et al. (38) nedocromil had a greater effect in the subgroup of adults who had cough-dominant asthma, when compared to those who did not have cough at baseline (pretreatment).

Most studies have evaluated the relationship between cough frequency and asthma severity and have found no relationship. Childhood asthma differs from adult asthma in several distinctive ways, but they also share some common features (129). Studies relating cough severity to asthma in children however, are concordant with studies on adults with asthma. Using an ambulatory cough meter, Hsu et al. (15) showed that cough frequency did not relate to asthma severity measured by FEV, and diurnal variation of peak flow. Experimentally studies have shown that cough receptor sensitivity thresholds do not relate to airway calibre and AHR in adults with asthma as summarized (5). During stable asthma but not during exacerbations, one study has described that child recorded asthma and cough scores and parent recorded cough scores were significantly higher in ETS exposed children when compared to ETS non-exposed children (121).

Using allergen airway challenge in adults with known allergen sensitivity, Minogushi et al. (64) described that cough sensitivity to capsaicin was not associated with eosinophilic inflammation of the airways. Despite the significant increase in sputum eosinophils, there was no change in cough sensitivity in these patients with allergic asthma whose main symptoms are wheezing and dyspnoea but not cough (64). In children with cough-dominant asthma, we had earlier reported no relationship between eosinophilic inflammation (sputum eosinophils and sputum ECP) and cough sensitivity or subjective cough scores (121). Niimi el al. however reported that in their group of adults with cough variant asthma (CVA), bronchial eosinophils and serum ECP correlated to clinical cough scores (range 1–3 and based on response to theophylline and inhaled beta$_2$-agonist used). This cohort clearly had spirometric evidence of airway obstruction (mean FEV_1 was 79.7% predicted, range 51.9–116.6%; mean $MMEF_25\%$ 44.3% predicted, range 11.8–76.6%) (130). Diette et al. (131) reported that

Table 3 Relationship Between a Validated Cough Scoring System and Several Indices of Asthma at Day 1 and Day 3 of a Mild Asthma Exacerbation in Children

Spearman correlation (2 tailed p)	Asthma score (parent rec[a])	Cough score (child rec[a])	Cough score (parent rec[a])	Child's QOL[b]	Parents QOL[b]	IL-8	Sputum ECP
Day 1							
Asthma score (child rec[a])	0.75 (0.008)	0.88 (0.001)	0.84 (0.001)	-0.014 (0.97)	0.24 (0.48)	-0.76 (0.031)	-0.83 (0.04)
Asthma score (parent rec[a])		0.75 (0.013)	0.78 (0.004)	-0.27 (0.43)	-0.22 (0.51)	-0.79 (0.02)	-0.76 (0.03)
Cough score (child rec[a])			0.97 (0.0001)	0.11 (0.76)	0.19 (0.6)	-0.43 (0.29)	-0.58 (0.13)
Cough score (parent rec[a])				-0.27 (0.43)	0.2 (0.56)	0.55 (0.16)	-0.58 (0.14)
Child's QOL[b]					0.51 (0.11)	0.29 (0.49)	-0.17 (0.69)
Parents QOL[b]						0.12 (0.48)	-0.14 (0.74)
IL-8							0.43 (0.34)
Day 3							
Asthma score (child rec[a])	0.86 (0.001)	0.62 (0.06)	0.64 (0.03)	0.33 (0.39)	-0.25 (0.57)	-0.58 (0.13)	-0.25 (0.55)
Asthma score (parent rec[a])		0.41 (0.23)	0.55 (0.08)	0.3 (0.43)	-0.14 (0.74)	-0.69 (0.06)	-0.24 (0.57)
Cough score (child rec[a])			0.89 (0.001)	0.07 (0.39)	-0.26 (0.57)	0.03 (0.95)	-0.42 (0.3)
Cough score (parent rec[a])				0.24 (0.53)	-0.26 (0.53)	-0.06 (0.9)	-0.07 (0.87)
Child's QOL[b]					0.24 (0.57)	-0.43 (0.4)	-0.37 (0.47)
Parents QOL[b]						-0.8 (0.1)	-0.7 (0.19)
IL-8							0.41 (0.32)

[a]rec = recorded.
[b]QOL = Quality of life.
Source: From Ref. 121.

in older patients with asthma the presence of chronic cough, amongst other factors, was a risk factor for hospitalisation. However Satoh et al. outlined that the study omitted influence of important details such as the effect of cardiac disease on respiratory symptoms (132).

Does the presence of nocturnal cough represent more severe or unstable asthma? In Meijer et al. (79) cross sectional study of 796 children with asthma attending routine clinics (79), nocturnal wheezing and dyspnoea on waking discriminated between mild vs. moderate and severe asthma (parental reports), but no data was given for nocturnal cough. As odds ratio for all significant associations were given except for nocturnal cough, it is inferred that nocturnal cough was non-discriminatory for the severity of asthma. Mitra et al. (133) however argues that symptoms are more important than objective markers in childhood asthma and showed a difference primarily in morning and nocturnal cough but not in other symptoms (nocturnal wheeze, morning dyspnoea, nocturnal dyspnoea). This study (133) however has to be interpreted in the context of the problems in interpreting isolated cough and other studies showing cough especially nocturnal cough as a poorer marker when compared to other subjective symptoms (134). Other groups that have measured nocturnal cough objectively have shown no difference between treated and untreated children with asthma (82). Brooke et al. (82) specifically examined the relationship between nocturnal cough and asthma severity in a population-based cohort of children with asthma. In children aged 4–7 years who were free from a viral respiratory infection in the previous 4 weeks, they concluded that although nocturnal cough was more common in children with asthma, there was little agreement between recorded and reported night cough and that it could not be used to predict objective measurements of asthma severity (82). Two groups have thus questioned the importance of the sleeping environment (e.g., temperature, dampness, pollutants, and smoke exposure) rather than asthma severity per se as the major contributor to nocturnal cough in children (82,135). Hoskyn et al. (135) studied children with clinically stable asthma and persistent nocturnal cough and found no relationship between nocturnal cough and all measured indices of asthma everity (daytime lung function, airway resistance, mean SpO_2, morning and evening peak expiratory flow, overnight peak expiratory flow variability and diary card score). Nocturnal cough in association with asthma related to decreased temperature and humidity rather than asthma severity defined by peak flow variability, AHR, ventilatory function and oximetry (82,135).

Although cough with exercise may indicate asthma, the symptom of cough in isolation is also nonspecific. Exercise-induced asthma is common in children with asthma who do not receive anti-inflammatory treatment (136) but, like the difficulty in relating cough in isolation as a symptom of asthma, that of cough and exercise has an additional difficulty as any person with a coughing illness, will cough more when exercising. Post exercise

cough was the most common symptom reported in elite athletes but self-reported symptoms of cough lacked sensitivity and specificity (0.61 and 0.69, respectively) for exercise induced asthma determined by AHR to exercise (137), arguably the most accepted definition of exercise induced asthma (136). Specificity for wheeze, dyspnoea and excessive mucus formation was 0.82, 0.83 and 0.85, respectively. In adult athletes, the sensitivity and specificity of exercise related cough in detecting AHR to methacholine was 43% and 77%, respectively whilst that for breathlessness, chest tightness and wheeze was higher at 45% and 83%, respectively (138). Sixty-four (72.7%) of the 88 children who presented to cardiologist with chest pain and had ventilatory evidence of exercise induced asthma, only 6 (7%) had cough on exertion and the commonest respiratory symptom in the group was dyspnoea (139).

Application (Case Study)

An 8-year old Caucasian girl had been managed with asthma medications since aged 4 years based on symptoms of cough and intermittent wheeze and exertional dyspnoea. She had a variable response to beta$_2$-agonists and had been increasingly troubled with recurrent cough, which is a mixture of dry and productive cough. Following her asthma action plan, each coughing exacerbation was managed with increased inhaled and oral corticosteroids. As the interval phase between episodes were short, a physician then placed her on daily oral steroids in addition to an increasing dose of inhaled corticosteroids (fluticasone 1500 μg/day, salmeterol and leukotriene receptor antagonist) with an equivocal effect on the frequency and severity of her coughing exacerbations. Further history during respiratory consultation revealed that the child's recurrent cough was usually an isolated symptom without wheeze, chest tightness or wheeze. By then she had been on daily oral prednisolone for 12 months. High resolution CT scan showed radiological bronchiectasis which is presumed post-infectious as all investigations (sweat test, neutrophil and lymphocyte function, immunoglobulins, cilia biopsy) were negative. Her spirometry was repeatedly normal and despite prior use of oral corticosteroid therapy she had been growing normally. After effective management of her bronchiectasis (chest physiotherapy and antibiotics), she was weaned off oral steroids over a period of several months, inhaled corticosteroids reduced to 250 μg/day and her parents reeducated on the management of her mild asthma. Her spirometry remained normal and growth significantly improved (growth velocity changed from 2.4cm/year to 7.7cm/year) since weaning of oral corticosteroids.

Key points in case history:

- The child's troublesome recurrent isolated cough was representative of acute bronchitis or an infective exacerbation of underlying bronchiectasis rather than asthma exacerbations. The indication for this child's erroneous escalating doses of corticosteroids was solely based on cough. Although cough features prominently in most asthma action plans (1), isolated cough if used as a marker of asthma stability, should be carefully and recurrently evaluated. Cough if related to asthma should substantially improved in 1–2 weeks and if not, the diagnosis should be reevaluated (5,6).

- Using a paediatric asthma scoring system (2), this child would be erroneously placed in the second most severe group of children with asthma and increase use of anti-inflammatory treatment for asthma would then be indicated. This case study illustrates a pitfall in the utilisation of isolated cough as a marker of asthma stability.
- The use of electronic cough monitoring in this child would not have been clinically useful. The utility of separate asthma diary card (43) (with cough removed as a symptom) and cough diary card (18) would have shown the discordance between the symptoms of dyspnoea and wheeze to that of cough.

Summary

As our understanding of the pathophysiology of asthma improves, different phenotypic manifestations of asthma are increasingly appreciated. It is likely that as with the difference between eosinophilic dominant asthma and neutrophil-dominant asthma, those with cough dominant asthma, cough variant asthma differ from classical asthma. The use of isolated cough as a symptom for control of asthma is problematic because of its low specificity for asthma and also because of the many limitations intrinsically related to the assessment of cough. There is little doubt that children and adults with asthma can present with cough and cough heralds the onset of instability in some but not all with asthma. Caution must be exercised when cough in isolation is utilised as a marker of asthma control. An asthmatic with isolated cough should be carefully evaluated for other causes of the cough and overlapping disorders. In the absence of other symptoms and markers of asthma control, a cough that does not respond to asthma therapy (inhaled corticosteroids and bronchodilators) within 1–2 weeks is rarely related to classical asthma. Perhaps Wardlaw's model of asthma in conjunction with a model relating cough sensitivity and AHR (5) explain the variability of the symptom of cough in people with asthma (94).

References

1. Asthma management Handbook. Melbourne: National Asthma Council Australia Ltd, 2000.

2. Rosier MJ, Bishop J, Nolan T, Robertson CF, Carlin J, Phelan PD. Measurement of functional severity of asthma in children. Am J Respir Crit Care Med 1994; 149:1434–1441.
3. British Guideline on the Management of Asthma. Thorax 2003; 58:il–i94i.
4. Britt H, Miller GC, Knox S, Charles J, Valenti L, Henderson J et al. Bettering the Evaluation and Care of Health—A Study of General Practice Activity. 2002; AIHW Cat. No. GEP-10.
5. Chang AB. State of the Art: cough, cough receptors, and asthma in children. Pediatr Pulmonol 1999; 28:59–70.
6. Chang AB, Asher MI. A review of cough in children. J Asthma 2001; 38: 299–309.
7. Chung KF, Lalloo UG. Diagnosis and management of chronic persistent dry cough. Postgrad Med J 1996; 72:594–598.
8. O'Connor GT, Weiss ST. Clinical and Symptom Measures. Am J Respir Crit Care Med 1994; 149:S21–S28.
9. Cane RS, Ranganathan SC, McKenzie SA. What do parents of wheezy children understand by "wheeze? Arch Dis Child 2000; 82:327–332.
10. Cane RS, McKenzie SA. Parents' interpretations of children's respiratory symptoms on video. Arch Dis Child 2001; 84:31–34.
11. de Blic J, Thomson A. Short-term clinical measurement: acute severe episodes. Eur Respir J Suppl 1996; 21:4s–7s.
12. Brunekreef B, Groot B, Rijcken B, Hoek G, Steenbekkers A, de Boer A. Reproducibility of childhood respiratory symptom questions. Eur Respir J 1992; 5:930–935.
13. Clifford RD, Radford M, Howell JB, Holgate ST. Prevalence of respiratory symptoms among 7 and 11 year old schoolchildren and association with asthma. Arch Dis Child 1989; 64:1118–1125.
14. Luyt DK, Burton PR, Simpson H. Epidemiological study of wheeze, doctor diagnosed asthma, and cough in preschool children in Leicestershire. Br Med J 1993; 306:1386–1390.
15. Hsu JY, Stone RA, Logan-Sinclair RB, Worsdell M, Busst CM, Chung KF. Coughing frequency in patients with persistent cough: assessment using a 24 hour ambulatory recorder. Eur Respir J 1994; 7:1246–1253.
16. Archer LNJ, Simpson H. Night cough counts and diary card scores in asthma. Arch Dis Child 1985; 60:473–474.
17. Falconer A, Oldman C, Helms P. Poor agreement between reported and recorded nocturnal cough in asthma. Pediarr Pulmonol 1993; 15:209–211.
18. Chang AB, Newman RG, Carlin J, Phelan PD, Robertson CF. Subjective scoring of cough in children: parent-completed vs. child-completed diary cards vs. an objective method. Eur Respir J 1998; 11:462–466.
19. Davies MJ, Fuller P, Picciotto A, McKenzie SA. Persistent nocturnal cough: randomised controlled trial of high dose inhaled corticosteroid. Arch Dis Child 1999; 81:38–44.
20. Evald T, Munch EP, Kok-Jensen A. Chronic non-asthmatic cough is not affected by inhaled beclomethasone dipropionate. A controlled double blind clinical trial. Allergy 1989; 44:510–514.

21. Eccles R. The powerful placebo in cough studies? Pulm Pharmacol Ther 2002; 15:303–308.
22. Rietveld S, Van BI, Everaerd W. Psychological confounds in medical research: the example of excessive cough in asthma. Behav Res Ther 2000; 38:791–800.
23. Dales RE, Spitzer WO, Schechter MT, Suissa S. The influence of psychological status on respiratory symptom reporting. Am Rev Respir Dis 1989; 139:1459–1463.
24. Butani L, O'Connell EJ. Functional respiratory disorders. Ann Allergy Asthma Immunol 1997; 79:91–99.
25. Hutchings HA, Eccles R, Smith AP, Jawad MSM. Voluntary cough suppression as an indication of symptom severity in upper respiratory tract infections. Eur Respir J 1993; 6:1449–1454.
26. Chang AB, Phelan PD, Robertson CF, Newman RG, Sawyer SM. Frequency and perception of cough severity. J Paediatr Child Health 2001; 37:142–145.
27. Munyard P, Bush A. How much coughing is normal? Arch Dis Child 1996; 74:531–534.
28. Faniran AO, Peat JK, Woolcock AJ. Persistent cough: is it asthma? Arch Dis Child 1998; 79:411–414.
29. McKenzie S. Cough–but is it asthma? Arch Dis Child 1994; 70:1–2.
30. Fitch PS, Brown V, Schock BC, Taylor R, Ennis M, Shields MD. Chronic cough in children: bronchoalveolar lavage findings. Eur Respir J 2000; 16:1109–1114.
31. Gibson PG, Simpson JL, Chalmers AC, Toneguzzi RC, Wark PAB, Wilson A, et al. Airway eosinophilia is associated with wheeze but is uncommon in children with persistent cough and frequent chest colds. Am J Respir Crit Care Med 2001; 164:977–981.
32. McGarvey LP, Heaney LG, MacMahon J. A retrospective survey of diagnosis and management of patients presenting with chronic cough to a general chest clinic. Int J Clin Pract 1998; 52:158–161.
33. McGarvey LP, Heaney LG, Lawson JT, Johnston BT, Scally CM, Ennis M, et al. Evaluation and outcome of patients with chronic non-productive cough using a comprehensive diagnostic protocol. Thorax 1998; 53:738–743.
34. Thomson F, Masters IB, Chang AB. Persistent cough in children—overuse of medications. J Paediatr Child Health 2002; 38:578–581.
35. Ilangovan P, Pederson S, Godfrey S, Nikander K, Noviski N, Warner JO. Treatment of severe steroid dependent preschool asthma with nebulised budesonide suspension. Arch Dis Child 1993; 68:356–359.
36. van Essen-Zandvliet EE, Hughes MD, Waalkens HJ, Duiverman EJ, Kerrebijn KF, and the Dutch CNSLD Study Group. Remission of childhood asthma after long-term treatment with an inhaled corticosteroid (budesonide): can it be achieved? Eur Respir J 1994; 7:63–68.
37. Konig P, Eigen H, Ellis MH, Ellis E, Blake K, Geller D, et al. The effect of nedocromil sodium on childhood asthma during the viral season. Am J Respir Crit Care Med 1995; 152:1879–1886.
38. North American Tilade Study Group. A double-blind multicenter group comparative study of the efficacy and safety of nedocrmil sodium in the management of asthma. Chest 1990; 97:1299–1306.

39. Creticos PS. Effects of nedocromil sodium on inflammation and symptoms in therapeutic studies. J Allergy Clin Immunol 1996; 98:S143–S149.

40. Chang AB, Phelan PD, Roberts RGD, Robertson CF. Capsaicin cough receptor sensitivity test in children. Eur Respir J 1996; 9:2220–2223.

41. Chang AB, Phelan PD, Robertson CF, Roberts RDG, Sawyer SM. Relationship between measurements of cough severity. Arch Dis Child 2003; 88:57–60.

42. Gulsvik A, Refvem OK. A scoring system on respiratory symptoms. Eur Respir J 1988; 1:428–432.

43. Santanello NC, Barber BL, Reiss TF, Friedman BS, Juniper EF, Zhang J. Measurement characteristics of two asthma symptom diary scales for use in clinical trials. Eur Respir J 1997; 10:646–651.

44. Santanello NC, Demuro-Mercon C, Davies G, Ostrom N, Noonan M, Rooklin A, et al. Validation of a pediatric asthma caregiver diary. J Allergy Clin Immunol 2000; 106:861–866.

45. Juniper EF, Guyatt GH, Feeny DH, Feme PJ, Griffith LE, Townsend M. Measuring quality of life in children with asthma. Qual Life Res 1996; 5:35–46.

46. Juniper EF, Guyatt GH, Epstein RS, Ferrie PJ, Jaeschke R, Hiller TK. Evaluation of impairment of health related quality of life in asthma: development of a questionnaire for use in clinical trials. Thorax 1992; 47:76.

47. Richards JM Jr, Hemstreet MP. Measures of life quality, role performance and functional status in asthma research. Am J Respir Crit Care Med 1994; 149:S31–S39.

48. Juniper EF, Guyatt GH, Dolovich J. Assessment of quality of life in adolescents with allergic rhinoconjunctivitis: Development and testing of a questionnaire for clinical trials. J Allergy Clin Immunol 1994; 93:413–423.

49. Birring SS, Prudon B, Carr AJ, Singh SJ, Morgan MD, Pavord ID. Development of a symptom specific health status measure for patients with chronic cough: Leicester Cough Questionnaire (LCQ). Thorax 2003; 58:339–343.

50. Irwin RS, French CT, Fletcher KE. Quality of life in coughers. Pulm Pharmacol Ther 2002; 15:283–286.

51. Cox ID, Wallis PJW, Apps CP, Hughes DTD, Empey DW, Osman RCA. An electromyographic method of objectively assessing cough intensity and use of the method to assess effects of codeine on the dose-response curve to citric acid. Br J Clin Pharmac 1984; 18:377–382.

52. Piirila P, Sovijarvi ARA. Objective assessment of cough. Eur Respir J 1995; 8:1949–1956.

53. Thorpe CW, Toop LJ, Dawson KP. Towards a quantitative description of asthmatic cough sounds. Eur Respir J 1992; 5:685–692.

54. Woolf CR. Objective assessment of cough suppressants under clinical conditions using a tape recorded. Thorax 1964; 19:125–130.

55. Piirila P, Sovijarvi ARA. Differences in acoustic and dynamic characteristics of spontaneous cough in pulmonary diseases. Chest 1989; 96:46–53.

56. Salmi T, Sovijarvi ARA, Brander P, Piirila P. Long-term recording and automatic analysis of cough using filtered acoustic signals and movements on static charge sensitive bed. Chest 1988; 94:970–975.

57. Rietveld S, Rijssenbeek-Nouwens LH. Diagnostics of spontaneous cough in childhood asthma: results of continuous tracheal sound recording in the homes of children. Chest 1998; 113:50–54.

58. Chang AB, Newman RG, Phelan PD, Robertson CF. A new use for an old Holter monitor: an ambulatory cough meter. Eur Respir J 1997; 10: 1637–1639.

59. Scarpelli EM. Pulmonary Mechanics and Ventilation. In: Scarpelli EM, ed. Pulmonary Physiology. Philadelphia: Lea & Febiger, 1989:33–54.

60. Corrigan DL, Paton JY. Pilot study of objective cough monitoring in infants. Pediatr Pulmonol 2003; 35:350–357.

61. Chang AB, Phelan PD, Carlin J, Sawyer SM, Robertson CF. Randomised controlled trial of inhaled salbutamol and beclomethasone for recurrent cough. Arch Dis Child 1998; 79:6–11.

62. Chung KF. Assessment and measurement of cough: the value of new tools. Pulm Pharmacol Ther 2002; 15:267–272.

63. Chang AB, Phelan PD, Sawyer SM, Del Brocco S, Robertson CF. Cough sensitivity in children with asthma, recurrent cough, and cystic fibrosis. Arch Dis Child 1997; 77:331–334.

64. Minoguchi H, Minoguchi K, Tanaka A, Matsuo H, Kihara N, Adachi M. Cough receptor sensitivity to capsaicin does not change after allergen bronchoprovocation in allergic asthma. Thorax 2003; 58:19–22.

65. Choudry NB, Fuller RW. Sensitivity of the cough reflex in patients with chronic cough. Eur Respir J 1992; 5:296–300.

66. O'Connell F, Thomas VE, Pride NB, Fuller RW. Capsaicin cough sensitivity decreases with successful treatment of chronic cough. Am J Respir Crit Care Med 1994; 150:374–380.

67. Hansson L, Wollmer P, Dahlback M, Karlsson J-A. Regional sensitivity of human airways to capsaicin-induced cough. Am Rev Respir Dis 1992; 145:1191–1195.

68. McFadden ER. Exertional dyspnea and cough as preludes to acute attacks of bronchial asthma. N Engl J Med 1975; 292:555–558.

69. Kelly YJ, Brabin BJ, Milligan PJM, Reid JA, Heaf D, Pearson MG. Clinical significance of cough and wheeze in the diagnosis of asthma. Arch Dis Child 1996; 75:489–493.

70. Chang AB, Newson TP. Trend in occurrence of asthma among children and young adults Labelling of cough alone as asthma may partially explain increase. Br Med J 1997; 315:1015–1015.

71. Chang AB, Powell CV. Non-specific cough in children: diagnosis and treatment. Hosp Med 1998; 59:680–684.

72. Comino E, Mitchell CA, Bauman A, Henry RL, Robertson CF, Abramson MJ et al. Asthma management in eastern Australia, 1990 and 1993. Med J Aust 1996; 164:403–406.

73. Chang AB, Phelan PD, Robertson CF. Cough receptor sensitivity in children with acute and non-acute asthma. Thorax 1997; 52:770–774.

74. Gibson PG, Norzila MZ, Fakes K, Simpson J, Henry RL. Pattern of airway inflammation and its determinants in children with acute severe asthma. Pediatr Pulmonol 1999; 28:261–270.

75. Dicpinigaitis PV, Dobkin JB, Reichel J. Antitussive effect of the leukotriene receptor antagonist zafirlukast in subjects with cough-variant asthma. J Asthma 2002; 39:291–297.

76. Pearce N, Beasley R, Pekkanen J. Role of bronchial responsiveness testing in asthma prevalence surveys. Thorax 2000; 55:352–354.

77. Rietveld S, Rijssenbeek-Nouwens LH, Prins PJ. Cough as the ambiguous indicator of airway obstruction in asthma. J Asthma 1999; 36:177–186.

78. Green R, Luyt D. Clinical characteristics of childhood asthmatics in Johannesburg. S Afr Med J 1997; 87:878–882.

79. Meijer GG, Postma DS, Wempe JB, Gerritsen J, Knol K, van Aalderen WM. Frequency of nocturnal symptoms in asthmatic children attending a hospital out-patient clinic. Eur Respir J 1995; 8:2076–2080.

80. Ninan TK, Macdonald L, Russel G. Persistent nocturnal cough in childhood: a population based study. Arch Dis Child 1995; 73:403–407.

81. Thomson AH, Pratt C, Simpson H. Nocturnal cough in asthma. Arch Dis Child 1987; 62:1001–1004.

82. Brooke AM, Lambert PC, Burton PR, Clarke C, Luyt DK, Simpson H. Night cough in a population-based sample of children: characteristics, relation to symptoms and associations with measures of asthma severity. Eur Respir J 1996; 9:65–71.

83. Janson C, Chinn S, Jarvis D, Burney P. Determinants of cough in young adults participating in the European Community Respiratory Health Survey. Eur Respir J 2001; 18:647–654.

84. Ludviksdottir D, Bjornsson E, Janson C, Boman G. Habitual coughing and its associations with asthma, anxiety, and gastroesophageal reflux. Chest 1996; 109:1262–1268.

85. Korpas J, Kelemen S. Tussiphonographic analysis of cough sound recordings performed by Schmidt-Voigt and Hirschberg and Szende. Acta Physiol Hung 1987; 70:167–170.

86. Canning BJ. Interactions between Vagal Afferent Nerve Subtypes Mediating Cough. Pulm Pharmacol Ther 2002; 15:187–192.

87. Undem BJ, Carr MJ, Kollarik M. Physiology and plasticity of putative cough fibres in the Guinea pig. Pulm Pharmacol Ther 2002; 15:193–198.

88. Eschenbacher WL, Boushey HA, Sheppard D. Alteration in osmolarity of inhaled aerosols cause bronchoconstriction and cough, but absence of a permeant anion causes cough alone. Am Rev Respir Dis 1984; 129:211–215.

89. Sheppard D, Rizk NW, Boushey HA, Bethel RA. Mechanism of cough and bronchoconstriction induced by distilled water aerosol. Am Rev Respir Dis 1983; 127:691–694.

90. Fuller RW, Karlsson J-A, Choudry NB, Pride NB. Effect of inhaled and systemic opiates on responses to inhaled capsaicin in humans. J Appl Physiol 1988; 65:1125–1130.

91. Choudry NB, Fuller RW, Anderson N, Karlsson J-A. Separation of cough and reflex bronchoconstriction by inhaled local anaesthetics. Eur Respir J 1990; 3:579–583.

92. Fahy JV, Wong HH, Geppetti P, Reis JM, Harris SC, Maclean DB, et al. Effect of an NK1 receptor antagonist (CP-99,994) on hypertonic saline-

induced bronchoconstriction and cough in male asthmatic subjects. Am J Respir Crit Care Med 1995; 152:879–884.

93. Fujimura M, Sakamoto S, Kamio Y, Matsuda T. Effects of methacholine induced bronchoconstriction and procaterol induced bronchodilation on cough receptor sensitivity to inhaled capsaicin and tartaric acid. Thorax 1992; 47:441–445.

94. Wardlaw AJ, Brightling CE, Green R, Woltmann G, Bradding P, Pavord ID. New insights into the relationship between airway inflammation and asthma. Clin Sci (Lond) 2002; 103:201–211.

95. Zimmerman B, Silverman FS, Tarlo SM, Chapman KR, Kubay JM, Urch B. Induced sputum: comparison of postinfectious cough with allergic asthma in children. J Allergy Clin Immunol 2000; 105:495–499.

96. SIDRIA. Asthma and respiratory symptoms in 6–7 yr old Italian children: gender, latitude, urbanization and socioeconomic factors. Eur Respir J 1997; 10:1780–1786.

97. Chinn S. Obesity and asthma: evidence for and against a causal relation. J Asthma 2003; 40:1–16.

98. Partridge MR. In what way may race, ethicity or culture influence asthma outcomes? Throax 2000; 55:175–176.

99. Jeffery PK. Differences and similarities between chronic obstructive pulmonary disease and asthma. Clin Exp Allergy 1999; 29(suppl 2):14–26.

100. Redline S, Tishler PV, Schluchter M, Aylor J, Clark K, Graham G. Risk factors for sleep-disordered breathing in children. Associations with obesity, race, and respiratory problems. Am J Respir Crit Care Med 1999; 159: 1527–1532.

101. Taniguchi MH, Moyer RS. Assessment of risk factors for pneumonia in dysphagic children: significance of videofluoroscopic swallowing evaluation. Dev Med Child Neurol 1994; 36:495–502.

102. Field SK, Sutherland LR. Gastroesophageal reflux and asthma: are they related? J Asthma 1999; 36:631–644.

103. Irwin RS, Madison JM, Fraire AE. The cough reflex and its relation to gastroesophageal reflux. Am J Med 2000; 108:73–78.

104. Teramoto S, Ohga E, Matsui H, Ishii T, Matsuse T, Ouchi Y. Obstructive sleep apnea syndrome may be a significant cause of gastroesophageal reflux disease in older people. J Am Geriatr Soc 1999; 47:1273–1274.

105. Kerr P, Shoenut JP, Millar T, Buckle P, Kryger MH. Nasal CPAP reduces gastroesophageal reflux in obstructive sleep apnea syndrome. Chest 1992; 101:1539–1544.

106. Johnston BT, Gideon RM, Castell DO. Excluding gastroesophageal reflux disease as the clause of chronic cough. J Clin Gastroenterol 1996; 22: 168–169.

107. Fujimura M, Sakamoto S, Matsuda T. Bronchodilator-restrictive cough in atopic patients: bronchial reversability and hyperresponsiveness. Int Med 1992; 31:447–452.

108. Andriessen JW, Brunekreef B, Roemer W. Home dampness and respiratory health status in european children. Clin Exp Allergy 1998; 28:1191–1200.

109. Ostro B, Lipsett M, Mann J, Braxton-Owens H, White M. Air pollution and exacerbation of asthma in African-American children in Los Angeles. Epidemiology 2001; 12:200–208.

110. Just J, Segala C, Sahraoui F, Priol G, Grimfeld A, Neukirch F. Short-term health effects of particulate and photochemical air pollution in asthmatic children. Eur Respir J 2002; 20:899–906.

111. Field CE. Bronchiectasis: a long term follow-up of medical and surgical cases from childhood. Arch Dis Child 1961; 36:587.

112. Balfour-Lynn IM, Elborn JS. "CF asthma": what is it and what do we do about it? Thorax 2002; 57:742–748.

113. Chang AB, Masel JP, Masters B. Post-infectious bronchiolitis obliterans: clinical, radiological and pulmonary function sequelae. Pediatr Radiol 1998; 28:23–29.

114. Morice AH. Epidemiology of cough. Pulm Pharmacol Ther 2002; 15: 253–259.

115. Johnston SL, Pattemore PK, Sanderson G, Smith S, Lampe F, Josephs L. Community study of role of viral infections in exacerbations of asthma in 9–11 year old children. Br Med J 1995; 310:1225–1229.

116. Lokshin B, Lindgren S, Weinberger M, Koviach J. Outcome of habit cough in children treated with a brief session of suggestion therapy. Ann Allergy 1991; 67:579–582.

117. Parameswaran K, Pizzichini E, Pizzichini MM, Hussack P, Efthimiadis A, Hargreave FE. Clinical judgement of airway inflammation versus sputum cell counts in patients with asthma. Eur Respir J 2000; 15:486–490.

118. Green RH, Brightling CE, McKenna S, Hargadon B, Parker D, Bradding P, et al. Asthma exacerbations and sputum eosinophil counts: a randomised controlled trial. Lancet 2002; 360:1715–1721.

119. Gibson PG, Simpson JL, Saltos N. Heterogeneity of airway inflammation in persistent asthma: evidence of neutrophilic inflammation and increased sputum interleukin-8. Chest 2001; 119:1329–1336.

120. Gibson PG, Wlodarczyk JW, Hensley MJ, Gleeson M, Henry RL, Cripps AW, et al. Epidemiological association of airway inflammation with asthma symptoms and airway hyperresponsiveness in childhood. Am J Respir Crit Care Med 1998; 158:36–41.

121. Chang AB, Harrhy VA, Simpson JL, Masters IB, Gibson PG. Cough, airway inflammation and mild asthma exacerbation. Arch Dis Child 2002; 86: 270–275.

122. Hoskyns EW, Heaton DM, Beardsmore CS, Simpson H. Asthma severity at night during recovery from an acute asthmatic attack. Arch Dis Child 1991; 66:1204–1208.

123. Stevens MW, Gorelick MH. Short-term outcomes after acute treatment of pediatric asthma. Pediatrics 2001; 107:1357–1362.

124. Bishop J, Carlin J, Nolan T. Evaluation of the properties and reliability of a clinical severity scale for acute asthma in children. J Clin Epidemiol 1992; 45:71–76.

125. Pizzichini MMM, Pizzichini E, Clelland L, Efthimiadis A, Mahony J, Dolovich J, et al. Sputum in severe exacerbations of asthma. Am J Respir Crit Care Med 1997; 155:1501–1508.
126. Cloutier MM, Loughlin GM. Chronic cough in children: a manifestation of airway hyperreactivity. Pediatrics 1981; 67:6–12.
127. Hannaway PJ, Hopper GDK. Cough Variant Asthma in Children. JAMA 1982; 247:206–208.
128. Konig P. Hidden asthma in children. Am J Dis Child 1981; 135:1053–1055.
129. Busse W, Banks-Schlegel SP, Larsen GL. Childhood- vs. adult-onset asthma. Am J Respir Crit Care Med 1995; 151:1635–1639.
130. Niimi A, Amitani R, Suzuki K, Tanaka E, Murayama T, Kuze F. Eosinophilic inflammation in cough variant asthma. Eur Respir J 1998; 11:1064–1069.
131. Diette GB, Krishnan JA, Dominici F, Haponik E, Skinner EA, Steinwachs D, et al. Asthma in older patients: factors associated with hospitalization. Arch Intern Med 2002; 162:1123–1132.
132. Satoh H, Sekizawa K. Elderly asthmatic patients. Arch Intern Med 2003; 163:122.
133. Mitra AD, Ogston S, Crighton A, Mukhopadhyay S. Lung function and asthma symptoms in children: relationships and response to treatment. Acta Paediatr 2002; 91:789–792.
134. Ware JE Jr, Kemp JP, Buchner DA, Singer AE, Nolop KB, Goss TF. The responsiveness of disease-specific and generic health measures to changes in the severity of asthma among adults. Qual Life Res 1998; 7:235–244.
135. Hoskyns EW, Beardsmore CS, Simpson H. Chronic night cough and asthma severity in children with stable asthma. Eur J Pediatr 1995; 154:320–325.
136. Carlsen KH, Carlsen KC. Exercise-induced asthma. Paediatr Respir Rev 2002; 3:154–160.
137. Rundell KW, Im J, Mayers LB, Wilber RL, Szmedra L, Schmitz HR. Self-reported symptoms and exercise-induced asthma in the elite athlete. Med Sci Sports Exerc 2001; 33:208–213.
138. Turcotte H, Langdeau JB, Bowie DM, Boulet LP. Are questionnaires on respiratory symptoms reliable predictors of airway hyper-responsiveness in athletes and sedentary subjects?. J Asthma 2003; 40:71–80.
139. Wiens L, Sabath R, Ewing L, Gowdamarajan R, Portnoy J, Scagliotti D. Chest pain in otherwise healthy children and adolescents is frequently caused by exercise-induced asthma. Pediatrics 1992; 90:350–353.
140. Shimuzu T, Mochizuki H, Tokuyama K, Morikawa A. Relationship between the acid-induced cough response and airway responsiveness and obstruction in children with asthma. Thorax 1996; 51:284–287.

4

Electronic Monitoring of Lung Function in Asthma: Technical Aspects, Clinical Applications

HELEN K. REDDEL

Woolcock Institute of Medical Research and University of Sydney, Camperdown, New South Wales, Australia

Context of Electronic Spirometric and Peak Flow Monitoring

Electronic spirometers and peak flow meters, with their capabilities in recording, storing, processing, and displaying large data sets, have an obvious and increasing role in the monitoring of asthma. The first such devices suitable for home monitoring were described in the early 1980s, and more sophisticated devices have subsequently been developed. However, at least partly because of cost, electronic monitoring devices are not yet in widespread use.

The two most relevant settings for electronic monitoring are in clinical asthma management and in clinical trials. In both of these settings, electronic devices can usually provide two basic functions: first, to inform the patient about their current lung function, and second, to store accumulated data for later display, review, and analysis. One of the most striking features of the literature about electronic monitoring devices is the wide range of device capability and of study methodology. The following information is therefore largely empirical.

Types of Electronic Monitoring Devices

Modified Mini-Wright. The Mini-Wright peak flow meter (Clement Clarke International, Harlow, U.K.) has a long history of use as a mechanical monitoring device in asthma. With certain modifications, including a pressure port at the mouthpiece, the Mini-Wright has been adapted to provide several models of electronic monitors. With the VM1 (1), which does not store data, peak expiratory flow (PEF) and forced expiratory volume in one second (FEV_1) are displayed on-screen, and a PEF value can also be read from the Mini-Wright scale. Later models have included VMX Mini-Log (PEF only) (2) and VM Plus (PEF and FEV_1) (3).

Turbine Spirometers. These were originally developed as compact laboratory spirometers (4), using photoelectronics to detect rotation of a low-inertia vane. The Micro Medical DiaryCard, which could display four lines of questionnaire text, was used for two long-term studies: a 2 year emphysema study in Denmark (5) and an 18 month asthma study in Australia (6). Several other portable turbine spirometers have been developed, for example, AM1 (7), AM2, and AM2+(Viasys Healthcare GmbH, Hoechberg, Germany), which feature sophisticated questionnaire functions, Micro DiaryCard (Micro Medical, Rochester, U.K.), which displays scrolling questionnaire text, Spirotel (MIR, Rome, Italy), and the small Airwatch meter (8).

Pneumotachograph. Several portable devices, such as the Vitalograph Data Storage Spirometer (no longer available) (9) and the PEF/FEV_1 Diary (Vitalograph, Maids Moreton, U.K.) (10), were developed using Fleisch-type pneumotachographs to measure pressure drop across a linear resistance. OneFlow devices (Clement Clarke International, Harlow, U.K.) (11) utilize the Venturi effect to measure pressure drop across a constriction.

Other measurement methods include a *hot wire anenometer* system in the PeakLog (Medtrac Technologies Inc, Denver, Colorado, U.S.A.) (12), which measures flow by calculating the drop in temperature of heated wires; a *variable orifice* system in the KoKoPeak Pro (PDS Inc, Louisville, Colorado, U.S.A.); and *digital ultrasonic* flow measurement in the EasyOne spirometer (ndd Medical Technologies, Andover, Massachusetts, U.S.A.) (13).

The available devices vary considerably in size and weight, and portability may be a particular issue if measurements are required during working hours.

Validation of Electronic Monitoring Devices

Quality control issues relating to home monitoring have been able to be studied much more rigorously and accurately with electronic devices than with mechanical peak flow meters.

Guidelines Relating to Monitoring Devices

The new category of "monitoring devices" was added in the 1994 update of the American Thoracic Society (ATS) guidelines for Standardization of Spirometry (14). These guidelines are summarized in Table 1. It was recognized that, during monitoring, repeatability (precision) was of greater priority than accuracy, in order to ensure that trends could be detected above signal noise. The guidelines, therefore, specified the same level of repeatability for both monitoring and diagnostic devices (3% or 50 mL for FEV_1 and FVC). The accuracy criterion for FEV_1 and FVC was less stringent for monitoring devices, although accuracy becomes an issue particularly for clinical trials if a device needs to be replaced during monitoring. The accuracy and repeatability requirements for PEF were almost identical with those for diagnostic devices. For monitoring devices, resolution was set at 50 mL For FEV_1 and FVC and at 10 L/min for PEF, with constant graduations across the entire range. Although adherence with the earlier-mentioned guidelines should be regarded as the minimal acceptable standard, electronic monitoring devices are obviously capable of considerably greater accuracy and precision than mechanical devices, and it is hoped that the guidelines will be updated to reflect this. In the meantime, it would be preferable for devices to report spirometric results in a format that reflects the accuracy of the device, for example, not reporting PEF to three digits if accuracy is only $\pm 10\%$ at the high end of the range.

Procedures for selection of FEV_1 and FVC from supervised maneuvers are specified in the ATS guidelines (14), but there are no such instructions for monitoring devices, reflecting the lack of such capability at the time. For PEF, the ATS guidelines specify that the highest of at least three readings should be used, with no reproducibility criterion (14). A within-session reproducibility criterion of 10% is, however, recommended by the NAEP/NHLBI guidelines (15) and of 40 L/min by the European Respiratory Society (16).

Regulations Relating to Electronic Monitoring Devices

In 1997, detailed regulations (21 CFR Part 11) relating to electronic records were issued by the United States Food and Drug Administration (FDA). These regulations were directly relevant to electronic monitoring in pharmaceutical studies conducted for regulatory purposes and included technical requirements such as password protection, procedural controls such as audit trails, and administrative controls. However, following widespread concern that these regulations would be unduly restrictive of the appropriate use of electronic technology, it was announced in September 2003 that the Part 11 document was under review. The advice given in the present chapter is not intended for regulatory studies. However, it would

Table 1 ATS Guidelines for Monitoring Devices (BTPS) (14)

Requirement	Monitoring device		Diagnostic device	
	FEV$_1$ and FVC	PEF	FEV$_1$ and FVC	PEF
Range	0.50–8 L	100 to ≥750 L/min, ≤850 L/min	0.50–8 L	Not specified
Accuracy	±5% or ±0.100 L, whichever is greater	±10% or ±20 L/min, whichever is greater	±3% or ±0.050 L, whichever is greater	±10% or ±0.400 L/sec (24 L/min), whichever is greater
Precision (reproducibility)	±3% or ±0.050 L, whichever is greater	Intradevice: ≤5% or ≤10 L/min, whichever is greater Interdevice: ≤10% or ≤20 L/min, whichever is greater	±3% or ±0.050 L, whichever is greater	±5% or ±0.200 L/sec (12 L/min), whichever is greater
Linearity	Within 3% over range	Within 5% over range	Not applicable	Not applicable
Graduations	Constant over entire range: 0.100 L	Constant over entire range: 20 L/min	Not applicable	Not applicable
Resolution	0.050 L	10 L/min	Not specified	Not specified
Resistance	< 2.5 cm H$_2$O/L/sec from 0 to 14 L/sec	< 2.5 cm H$_2$O/ L/sec from 0 to 14 L/sec	< 1.5 cm H$_2$O/ L/sec	< 1.5 cm H$_2$O/ L/sec

Minimum recommendations of ATS for full range monitoring and diagnostic devices (14). Additional recommendations are specified for low-range devices.

be appropriate to maintain an audit trail of changes to device or software configuration during any clinical trial.

Validation of Electronic Devices in Laboratory Studies

Early studies used a variety of methods for testing the accuracy of electronic spirometers (4,17,18). In 1992, it was recommended that volume–time waveform no. 24 (ATS-24) should be used for testing PEF meters (19). This was superseded in 1994 when the ATS adopted 26 standardized flow-time waveforms, recorded from actual subjects, for testing of portable PEF meters and spirometers (14). However, computerized waveform generators are not usually available for routine checking of calibration during the course of long-term monitoring. Irvin and colleagues (8,20) described a system for evaluating the performance of PEF meters (mechanical and electronic) during multicenter clinical trials, by placing the device inside a testing chamber, connected in series between a calibration syringe and a spirometer. Dirksen et al. (18) have drawn attention to the limitations of mechanical calibration systems.

Validation of Electronic Devices with Supervised Maneuvers

Several authors have examined the accuracy of electronic monitoring devices by having patients or normal volunteers perform maneuvers under supervision on the electronic device and a reference spirometer or PEF meter (3,7,21–24). In general, these studies have shown acceptable agreement between the electronic device and the reference device. However, there are several methodological issues relating to such testing (3), depending on whether the two devices are tested separately or in series. For example, with separate testing, there may be real differences between test sessions, whereas with testing in series, the two devices may require different maneuvers, for example, some pneumotachographs need an inspiratory effort to signal end of expiration, or may store different maneuvers from the same test session, or one device may have an impact on the airflow reaching the downstream device. Richter et al. (7) found a reduction in FEV_1 by about 4% when the AM1 was used in series with a pneumotachograph by human subjects but not when the same test rig was used with a waveform generator.

Validation of Electronic Devices in Home Testing

For each device, testing in a wide range of patients is essential because of the potential for unusual maneuvers or external factors in the home environment. Absolute values for PEF, FEV_1, and FVC from unsupervised home monitoring cannot be directly compared with those recorded in conventional laboratory spirometry because of the impact of factors such as time of day and prior β_2-agonist use. Results may be expected to be lower without the usual vigorous verbal encouragement from laboratory personnel. In lung transplant recipients, FEV_1 and FVC were 120 and 150 mL lower respectively, from home monitoring compared with at clinic visits on the same day (25). In patients with poorly controlled asthma, we found that FVC recorded at clinic visits was slightly higher than average evening FVC recorded at home on Micro Medical DiaryCard spirometers in the following week [mean difference 57 mL, Standard deviation (SD) 40 mL, unpublished data].

Within-session reproducibility with Micro Medical DiaryCards (Fig. 1) was reported for 33 subjects with poorly controlled asthma in the long-term budesonide study (26). The ATS reproducibility criterion for supervised maneuvers of 200 mL was satisfied for FEV_1 in 90% of these unsupervised sessions. For PEF, the upper 95% confidence limit for reproducibility was 21.4 L/min (5.8%) during study run-in, suggesting that a reproducibility target of 20 L/min should be achievable by most patients. Absolute reproducibility for FEV_1 and PEF did not correlate with baseline lung function and did not change significantly despite large improvements in lung function after 8 weeks of budesonide (26). Children, not surprisingly, are less able to perform reproducible spirometric maneuvers during home monitoring. In a group of 110 children aged 5–10 years who used Vitalograph Data Storage spirometers, reproducibility declined with decreasing age, with an overall mean of 77% of test sessions meeting the ATS reproducibility criterion (SD 17, range 21–100%) (9).

Functions of Electronic Spirometers/Peak Flow Meters

Electronic monitoring devices have a wide range of capabilities, and the choice of device may depend on the requirements of the setting, whether it is for clinical practice or for a clinical trial. However, the most basic initial requirement is compatibility with the operating system with which the software is to be used. Table 2 summarizes some of the other features that may need to be considered.

Date and Time Stamp

Most electronic monitoring devices record the date and time of each test session, and some can be configured to automatically update for daylight saving. The internal clock is usually set from the central computer during configuration, so it is important to ensure that the date and time on the central computer remain correct, in order to avoid possible overwriting of data. It may be necessary to alter the computer's regional date/time configurations to ensure that date and time data are exported correctly.

Alarms

Some devices can be configured with audible alarms as a reminder to the patient. Although this may be useful to enhance adherence with monitoring in COPD studies or for multiple daily measurements in occupational asthma, alarms are not as appropriate for general asthma studies in that it may be desirable to record spirometry on waking.

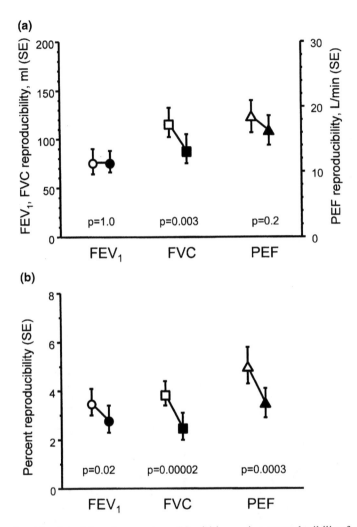

Figure 1 Absolute (**a**) and percentage (**b**) within-session reproducibility for FEV$_1$, FVC, and PEF from electronic monitoring in asthma. Reproducibility = (best value−second best value of each electronic monitoring session) expressed (**a**) in mL (FEV$_1$ and FVC) and L/min (PEF) and (**b**) as a percentage of the best value, in week 0 (*open symbols*) and week 9 of budesonide treatment (*closed symbols*). Chart shows median ± IQR; *p*-values are for comparison of week 0 and week 9. Absolute within-session reproducibility for FEV$_1$ and PEF did not change significantly, despite large improvements in FEV$_1$ and PEF. From Ref. 26.

Table 2 Choosing an Electronic Spirometer/Peak Flow Meter

Feature	Comments	Chapter Section
Method of measurement	Check that device type has been validated in the relevant disease stage/age group	Types of Electronic Monitoring Devices
Size, weight	Portability important if measurements are required during working hours. Protective case useful, but as device is used daily, it needs to be able to be removed easily	
Compliance with ATS waveforms	Check for compliance report	Guidelines Relating to Monitoring Devices
Operating system	Check that the device software is compatible with the operating system of the computer(s) on which it will be used	Functions of Electronic Spirometers/Peak Flow Meters
Date and time stamp	Are date and time set from base computer? Is there provision for adjustment for daylight saving?	Date and Time Stamp
Alarm function to remind patients to carry out measurement	Good for multiple daily measurements, for example, occupational asthma. Not necessarily appropriate for normal asthma monitoring—measurement on waking more appropriate	Alarms
Prompt to perform spirometry	If prompt is an icon, is it unambiguous? If text, is wording appropriate and unambiguous?	Prompt to Perform Spirometry

	Questions	
	Is the patient prompted for three maneuvers? Is it easy to record data on the device without instructions?	Non-Volatile Memory
Non-volatile memory	Will data be lost if batteries are removed or go flat? After how many days?	Resolution
Resolution	Is resolution uniform across the measurement range?	Storage Capacity
Storage capacity	Does device store results? What is minimum interval between uploading? Does it depend on selected configuration? If storage capacity is exceeded, does device stop recording or overwrite existing data?	Recording Options
Recording options	Does the device store all maneuvers or only the best? If only the best maneuver or best individual results are stored, what selection process? Can these be customized? Are flow-volume loops stored?	Quality Control Processes
Quality control checks	Are real time quality control checks available/configurable? Is feedback given to the patient to correct their technique?	End-of-test Display
End-of-test display	Is the best PEF displayed to the patient at the end of the session? Can the PEF be concealed from the patient if necessary?	Studies of Perception of Asthma

(Continued)

Table 2 Choosing an Electronic Spirometer/Peak Flow Meter (*Continued*)

Feature	Comments	Chapter Section
Warning about low lung function	Can "action points" be set? Are they applied to individual maneuvers or to the best result? Can an alert message be customized?	Link with Asthma Action Plans
Questionnaire functions	Are the questionnaire functions easy to use and unambiguous? How many text characters for questions? Is a branching questionnaire structure available? What format is available for answers (numeric, binary, visual analog, text); if text, how many characters?	Questionnaire Functions
Communication	Can the spirometer be linked to another device, for example, portable digital assistant (PDA)? How are data uploaded to the central computer (cable/infrared/modem/telephone, etc.)? Is the method of communication compatible with facilities at the site of use?	Communication
Durability	Has the device been used in any long-term studies? Are there any potentially flimsy connections (e.g., modular plugs)? (For turbine devices) Are the vanes protected by a screen?	Durability
Maintenance	What solution is needed to sterilize the device between patients? Is it readily available?	Maintenance

Ease of use	Try using the device yourself with minimal instructions	Ease of Use and Acceptability
	Are the buttons clearly labeled? Are the screen icons unambiguous? Are there any complex or tedious steps? Are there any critical steps in configuring the device or performing a test session?	
	How are after-midnight "evening" results handled? Does this affect any derived values?	After Midnight Recordings
Derived values	Are the equations for predicted values appropriate and correct? Is an adjustment for race available?	Derived values
	How is PEF variability calculated? (Amplitude percentage mean, amplitude percentage maximum, etc.)	
	How is personal best PEF calculated?	
Exported data	Are exported questionnaire and spirometry files directly linked?	Link with Asthma Action plans
	Is each line of exported data identified by subject ID, study site, date and time?	Exporting Data
	Are exported data in a format that can be imported into a clinical trial database?	
	Is date/time format compatible with local system (U.S./European)?	
Trend displays	Is the trend display in a user-friendly format? (e.g., showing only the best result from each session)	Trend Displays

(Continued)

Table 2 Choosing an Electronic Spirometer/Peak Flow Meter (*Continued*)

Feature	Comments	Chapter Section
Security	Is an audit trail maintained for any changes to the configuration of devices during a clinical trial?	Preparing Data Sets for Analyses
Centralized data handling	Is this available, where needed?	Centralized Data Handling
Technical support	How quickly is technical support available to practitioners and patients?	Priorities in Use of Electronic Monitoring Devices
Cost	For routine clinical use, is cost warranted by benefits in convenience and display? For clinical trial use, can the cost be spread over several studies or can the devices be leased?	

Prompt to Perform Spirometry

Many devices have a visual prompt for spirometry, ranging from a simple cartoon-style icon, to a single word such as "Go," to several words of text. The patient should be prompted for a minimum of three maneuvers in a test session. The clarity of prompts on each device should be checked within the setting of their use, for example, the AM2 prompt is "Exhale fully and deeply", but Australian usage of "exhale" suggests a relaxed rather than a forceful expiration.

Non-volatile Memory

Loss of data was reported in some early electronic monitoring studies when device batteries became flat or were removed by patients (17,27). Most devices now store data in non-volatile memory, although in one study in which we participated, data were lost from multiple Airwatch devices because of battery failure.

Storage Capacity

Some electronic devices (OneFlow Tester, VM1) do not store lung function results, so a paper diary is still needed. However, most electronic devices store data from a month to a year of monitoring, with the capacity sometimes depending on how many variables or flow-volume loops are stored. When the storage capacity is exceeded, some devices overwrite the earliest recorded results, for example, KoKoPeak Pro (one month capacity). Other devices, for example, AM2, display a warning when the memory is almost full, and cannot record further data if data transfer does not occur within a few days. In a clinical trial, the device storage capacity may determine the interval between visits unless remote uploading is available.

Resolution

The ATS specification for PEF resolution (10 L/min) is very generous in the context of electronic devices. Resolution for PEF on the AM1 rises from 1 L/min at low flow rates to 10 L/min at high flow rates (7), but this may not be obvious as high-range results are still reported to the nearest single digit.

Recording Options

A minimum of three maneuvers should be performed in a test session. The majority of devices record PEF and FEV_1, and some also store FEV_6 or FVC. Some devices store the results for all maneuvers but others, to increase storage capacity, store only selected "best" results. The ATS guidelines specify only that PEF should be the highest recorded value (14). Some devices, for example, OneFlow FVC, store the highest individual result for each variable. The VM-Plus meter stores the highest FEV_1 and its associated PEF (3); this approach results in lower PEF results than if the highest PEF is stored (26). If the PEF value stored by a device is different from the highest value displayed to the patient, there may be some confusion for asthma action plans or for covert adherence studies (10,28). The Vitalograph Data Storage spirometer stores the maneuver with largest $FEV_1 + FVC$ (29). However, this does not appear advisable as FEV_1 and FVC from unsupervised maneuvers may be lower than from supervised maneuvers (25). Some devices, for example, Micro DiaryCard, allow customization of the maneuver selection criteria. Storage of flow-volume loops may facilitate screening of outlying data (26).

Quality Control Processes

Real-time quality control checks may be useful during home spirometry, to avoid delays in detecting technique problems. The Micro DiaryCard, for example, incorporates a range of configurable quality control processes with text alerts, such as a prompt to blow faster if time to PEF is > 120 msec. Some devices record quality control data, for example, the Vitalograph Data Storage spirometer applies a 5% reproducibility criterion to the two maneuvers with highest $FEV_1 + FVC$ and records the percentage difference if this is not achieved (29).

End-of-test Display

In most settings, it is appropriate to display at least the PEF result to the patient at the end of each maneuver, to encourage good effort. If the patient is using a PEF-based asthma action plan, it is advisable for the highest PEF (or the stored value) to be retained on screen for at least 60 sec, so that the patient has adequate time for comparison with the trigger point. Most devices automatically switch off after 90 sec to avoid battery drain.

Link with Asthma Action Plans

Some electronic spirometers can be configured with one or more customized trigger (action) points for use with an asthma action plan. The device may display PEF against colored "traffic light" zones (e.g., KoKoPeak Pro) or may display a configurable message if the PEF falls below a specified trigger point (e.g., Micro DiaryCard). The calculation of trigger points may be based on predicted PEF, a clinic measurement of post-bronchodilator PEF, or the patient's personal best PEF calculated from previous recordings. Personal best PEF is defined in asthma guidelines as the highest PEF from 2 to 3 weeks of twice daily monitoring during good asthma control and has been found to reach maximal levels after only 3 weeks of inhaled corticosteroid treatment (30). Electronic monitoring devices offer the opportunity for application of electronic algorithms, based on quality control analysis of the patient's previous PEF data, with more sensitive and specific detection of exacerbations than can be achieved with simple percentage trigger points (31). The software algorithm by which current PEF is compared with the trigger point should be applied *after* the determination of the "best" result for the test session in order to avoid inappropriate alerts. It should be noted that the guidelines definition of "personal best" PEF is different from the lifetime "best-ever" calculation that is used by sports persons to refer to their "PB" for speed, distance, etc., and is calculated by some electronic spirometers (30). Calculations based on best-ever PEF may result in inappropriate alerts if the device is used even once by someone other than the patient. For example, if the patient's PEF is around 350 L/min with a trigger point of 70% best and the device is used even once by someone with a PEF of 600 L/min, then an alert may be displayed on every subsequent use by the patient until the device is reconfigured.

Questionnaire Functions

Clinical asthma trials almost invariably include monitoring of symptoms and β_2-agonist use, and like paper PEF diaries, paper questionnaire diaries are subject to high levels of data falsification (32). Several electronic monitoring devices incorporate some type of questionnaire function, but there is a wide range of capabilities. Some devices (e.g., KoKoPeak Pro, PEF/FEV$_1$ Diary) display an icon or number on the screen for each "question," but the patient needs to refer to printed material for the precise meaning. This system is not appropriate for clinical trials, given the paramount requirement for both intra- and inter-patient consistency in interpretation of questionnaire wording throughout a study. For example, the screen may show an icon of an inhaler, but the patient may forget mid-study whether it refers to β_2-agonist or inhaled corticosteroid use. Some monitoring devices can display text questions, for example, Spirotel—two lines each of 16 characters. Questions on the Micro DiaryCard device can be up to 70 characters, giving much greater flexibility; however, each question scrolls slowly across the screen, and we find that after a few weeks of monitoring, patients often key in their answer without reading the entire question. The AM2 and AM2+have a flexible questionnaire design, with three lines of text for each question, multiple possible text or numeric answers, and the option of a branching questionnaire structure. Answers on electronic monitoring devices may be numeric, binary (yes/no), visual analog, or text. Once again, it is important to ensure that available responses are unambiguous. With the DiaryCards used in the long-term budesonide study (6), only numeric answers were possible, so we incorporated the answer code into the question text (e.g., "Was Ventolin used in last 4 hr? 1=No, 3=Yes").

Given the importance of symptom diary data in the outcomes for clinical asthma trials, it may prove more cost-effective to develop personal digital assistant programs that can be linked with electronic spirometers than to try to combine both functions in one device. This strategy is already being used in some studies (33), and allows a user-friendly interactive interface with essentially unlimited flexibility in the design of questions and answers.

Communication

For most monitoring devices, data are uploaded to a personal computer by cable (infrared for KoKoPeak Pro), and some can directly link to a printer (e.g., PEF/FEV$_1$ meter). For clinical trials, it is helpful to have the option for printing of data recorded since the previous visit. Some devices have the capacity for remote uploading by modem (e.g., AM2), acoustic coupler (e.g., Spirotel) or telephone jack (e.g., Airwatch). Other innovative methods of communication are being tested, for example, Vitalograph PEF/FEV$_1$ Diary linked to a PDA with inbuilt mobile phone. It is important to check the compatibility of the device with communication systems in the country of use. For example, we found in 2000 that Airwatch meters required seven-digit telephone numbers for uploading, but Australia, like many other countries, has eight-digit telephone numbers.

Durability

Few studies have examined the durability of electronic monitoring devices. Dirksen et al. (18) reported consistency of calibration of 30 Micro Medical DiaryCards over 2 years, with an unexplained decline in calibration in only one device. We reported durability of 61 Micro Medical DiaryCards that were used twice daily for 18 months (26). The main mechanical problem was with the cable (not used in the current MicroDiary model) that had approximately a 10% failure rate. This was manifested by cessation of recording preceded by a brief decrease (or, rarely, a marked increase) in PEF. Breakage of the lugs on the modular connections was common after about 12 months but did not affect data recording. On four occasions, a decrease in PEF, FEV$_1$, and FVC with no change in symptoms was found to be due to tangling of a hair around the turbine spindle, and was corrected by its removal (26); the subsequent model has an intervening screen that should prevent this occurring. Airwatch meters appeared to have substantial durability problems in the 10-week study by Martin et al. (8). Of 101 devices issued, 17 were recalled prior to use because of possible electronic problems; of the remainder, 18 (21%) demonstrated failure of the rotor/housing component, with a further nine (11%) experiencing electronic failure. Mechanical peak flow meters, of course, are also vulnerable to equipment failure (20), although this may be less noticeable as the problem is more likely to be a gradual drift in recordings with time rather than abrupt failure.

Maintenance

Patients should be advised not to perform spirometry immediately after meals, to avoid deposition of food particles within the device. Electronic spirometers should be checked and washed at regular intervals or if there is an unexplained change in lung function; turbine devices can be moved rapidly through the air to check for free movement of the vane. The manufacturers' instructions for sterilization of devices between patients should be followed carefully, as use of an inappropriate solvent may damage components.

Ease of Use and Acceptability

When choosing an electronic monitoring device, it is particularly important to check that the device has a user-friendly design and configuration, in order to enhance adherence with monitoring and minimize data errors. It may be helpful to initially try the device oneself with only minimal instructions, as this is the way consumers often approach a new household device such as a television remote control. Are the buttons clearly labeled? Are the screen icons unambiguous? Is the PEF easy to read? Are there any complex or tedious steps involved in a test session? Using a single button for spirometry and questionnaire functions, for example, KoKoPeak Pro, may cause confusion for patients. Are there any critical steps, either in configuring the device or in performing a test session? For example, Redline et al. (34) noted that unless the "ON" switch on the VMX was pressed, electronic recording would not occur, although the Mini-Wright component would still display a PEF result; in the same study, incorrect configuration led to loss of data from 8% of the devices (34).

Surprisingly, few studies have examined the acceptability of electronic spirometers to patients. Lefkowitz et al. (35) reported that when patients who had used both an Assess peak flow meter and an Airwatch meter (including its telephone transmission function) were given a free choice, 27/29 selected the electronic device. The 10 subjects studied by Godschalk et al. (23) carried out 2 weeks of monitoring on each of a Micro Medical DiaryCard and a Mini-Wright peak flow meter plus paper diary. Figure 2 shows that the electronic device was preferred by most of the patients for recording of symptoms, the alarm function, readability and for overall preference, with portability the only feature for which the Mini-Wright was preferred over this early electronic device.

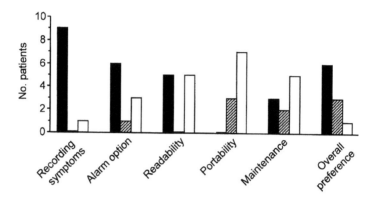

Figure 2 Patient preference for electronic vs. conventional monitoring in a study of 10 patients who used a Micro Medical DiaryCard and a Mini-Wright peak flow meter plus paper diary each for 2 weeks (23). Figure shows the number of patients who preferred the electronic device (*black*) or conventional monitoring (*hatched*) or who expressed no preference (*white*) for each feature. *Source*: Derived from Ref. 23.

Performance Issues

Standardization of Conditions for Monitoring

Some clinical asthma trial protocols have applied time windows or restrictions on β_2-agonist use to home monitoring. Spirometric monitoring may be used to provide the equivalent of repeated daily clinic spirometry, such as after lung transplant (36). However, in asthma, home monitoring is also intended to assess the characteristic within-day and between-day variability of lung function within the patient's usual environment. Conditions for monitoring should therefore not be artificially manipulated on a long-term basis, except in order to exclude equipment and performance error. A good analogy is with blood pressure assessment; at a clinic visit, patients rest supine for 15 min before blood pressure is measured, whereas ambulatory blood pressure recordings, either in clinical trials or in clinical practice, are carried out with the patient performing their usual daily activities.

Time Windows

In clinical trials, laboratory spirometry is often performed within strict time windows, and some studies have applied similar requirements to home monitoring. However, a circadian pattern is present in only about 50% of days (1), and the acrophase (time of maximum value) for FEV_1 can range between 0800 and 1600 hr in individual subjects (1). The acrophase is determined more by waking time than by time of day (37), and waking time may vary from day to day. Delaying spirometry for even 15 min after waking can significantly increase PEF and FEV_1 (38). A pragmatic approach, which allows sampling of a range of daily lung function and facilitates adherence, is to ask patients to record spirometry immediately upon waking and then 12 hr later (after return from work, if applicable).

Prior β_2-Agonist Use

Clinical trials usually specify that, before clinic spirometry, short-acting β_2-agonist should be withheld for 6–8 hr and long-acting β_2-agonist for 12–15 hr. Some studies have similarly required patients to withhold salbutamol for 4 or even 6 hr prior to every home PEF session. This requirement would be neither feasible nor desirable in severe asthma or during long-term monitoring, as it would impose an unacceptable burden on the patient, could cause significant bias in symptom and bronchodilator reporting, and could reduce monitoring adherence. When β_2-agonist is used more than 2.2 occasions/day (4.4 puffs/day), almost one-third of twice-daily PEF data is likely to be performed within 4 hr after bronchodilator (39). We examined the effect of such "post-bronchodilator" data on standard PEF indices (Fig. 3). During poorly controlled asthma, a median of 29% of test sessions was "post-bronchodilator", falling to 0% after eight weeks of budesonide. This systematic change in reliever use resulted in an underestimation of improvement in average morning and evening PEF and unpredictable changes in diurnal variability (amplitude percent mean). Exclusion of "post-bronchodilator" data from analysis would introduce selection bias by omission of "sick days". Calculation of PEF variability as the lowest morning PEF percentage highest (40) ("Min%Max") was unaffected by inclusion of post-bronchodilator data (39).

Spirometric Technique

In order to avoid non-asthma-related variation in lung function variables, patients must be thoroughly trained on the device prior to commencing home monitoring, with repeat training at subsequent visits (41). When a spirometric maneuver is used, PEF is slightly lower than from a short sharp "peak flow" maneuver (21,42). This is possibly due to a slightly longer incidental breath-hold before the full maneuver (42) or to elimination of artifactually high values from a "spitting" technique (16). During training, it is important to highlight the need for consistent posture (sitting or standing), full inspiration, a close seal between lips and mouthpiece, fast start to expiration, and prolonged expiration. In the long-term budesonide study, four of 33 subjects recorded short maneuvers ($FEV_1 = FVC$) on more than 10% occasions during the first 2 weeks of monitoring. Two of these subjects recovered correct technique following instruction at the second visit (29). A quality control message, or an audible prompt after 1 sec (e.g., VMPlus), can be helpful in ensuring that maneuvers are not truncated.

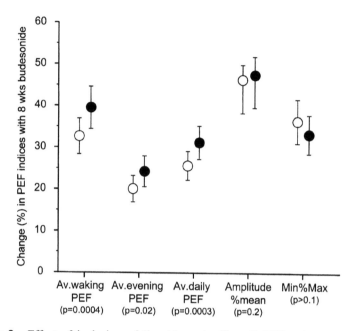

Figure 3 Effect of inclusion of "post-bronchodilator" PEF values on improvement in PEF indices after 8 weeks of budesonide treatment ($n = 43$). Unfilled circles show PEF indices based on all PEF data including within 4 hr after bronchodilator, filled circles show PEF indices based only on pre-bronchodilator PEF. Error bars show 95% confidence intervals. *p*-values: paired *t*-tests comparing the two methods of analysis. *Source*: Adapted from Ref. 39.

Influence of Non-asthma Events

During long-term monitoring, lung function may be influenced by non-asthma events, although this is not likely to be unique to electronic devices. However, no adjustment would usually be made in clinical trial data for variations in lung function due to non-asthma events reported by patients, apart from excluding obviously artifactual data. In the long-term budesonide study, we examined the effect of reported non-asthma events on lung function data (26). Some painful conditions, such as migraine, resulted in a 20–50 L/min reduction in PEF due to impaired effort. Coughing during spirometry led to a reduction in all variables. Some effects were specific to turbine-style spirometers, for example, all variables were reduced when spirometry was performed outside in windy weather or near a fan, and some, obviously artifactual data (FEV_1 0.3 L, FVC 0.3 L, and PEF 1 L/min), were due to laughing or coughing near the turbine. We also observed *increased* PEF and FEV_1 data for one subject when the subject phonated during spirometry for several weeks; this was confirmed during supervised maneuvers but was not found on simultaneous pneumotachograph readings (26). The increase in recorded PEF and FEV_1 was presumably due to inertial spinning of the turbine during the repetitive momentary closure of the vocal cords during phonation. As phonation during spirometry is not unusual, its effect with other types of monitoring devices should be established.

Maneuver-Induced Bronchoconstriction

A successive fall in FEV_1 or PEF through a test session would be expected to occur by chance in up to 1/6 session (17%), but may indicate maneuver-induced bronchoconstriction (43), sometimes found in severe asthma. In poorly controlled asthma, we found sequential reductions for FEV_1 in 15.3% (SD 12.8) and for PEF in 16.2% (SD 11.8) of test sessions, i.e., no more often than expected by chance (26). There was no association with baseline lung function and no significant change in maneuver-induced bronchospasm after 8 weeks of budesonide treatment ($p > 0.4$).

Processing Issues

After-Midnight Recordings

During the long-term budesonide study, over 11% of evening sessions were performed after midnight (range 0–39%) (26). Such data carry the date stamp of the following day. However, most electronic spirometers assume a midnight-to-midnight "day," which results in misclassification of such test sessions to the "morning" of the next day. This can result in errors in calculations based on morning results, for example, average morning PEF, or in calculations that require two readings per day, for example, diurnal variability or assessment of adherence. In occupational asthma, when PEF is performed every 2–3 hr, computerized division of the date/time record is possible (44). For twice daily monitoring with diary spirometers, we include a specific question to distinguish "morning" and "evening" sessions; this also facilitates division of test sessions for shift workers. If linked questionnaires are not available, an alternative is to adopt a cut-point of 3 A.M. for the end of a "day", as we found that non-shift workers performed only 0.4% of evening sessions after this time (26). After-midnight readings should also be considered when selecting time periods for analysis of data in a clinical trial. This can be done using a cut-point of 3 A.M., for example, by selecting data from first test session after 3 A.M. on "Start Date" up to and including last test session before 3 A.M. on "End Date+1." Alternatively, one can base time period selection on "Effective Date" rather than true date, with post-midnight sessions assigned an effective date of "True Date −1."

Time Zone Changes

During monitoring in the 18-month budesonide study, 15% of subjects undertook travel across time zones. The circadian rhythm of lung function changes rapidly after a time zone shift (37); so, it is most appropriate after upload of data to allocate test sessions to morning or evening according to local time rather than time in the place of origin; i.e., the "effective" date and time of testing should be calculated from the patient's record of their time-zone changes.

Derived Values

Some monitoring devices provide calculations of standard derived variables, such as percentage-predicted lung function or diurnal variability. It cannot be assumed that these calculations will be based on correct assumptions. For example, programs calculating predicted values from European Community for Steel and Coal equations sometimes omit the footnoted adjustment for subjects 20–25 years old (45). Pre-programed calculations of diurnal variability or adherence often treat post-midnight sessions as the morning session of the following day.

Extraneous Data

It is not unusual for patients, despite instructions, to allow another person such as a family member to use their peak flow meter, and such data must be excluded from analysis. With diary spirometers, we include a specific question for this purpose. Some studies exclude data that lie more than two SDs outside the mean (34), but this approach would censor data from asthma exacerbations (31). A requirement for entry of a personal identification number (PIN) before each session, to comply with FDA regulations, would not in fact prevent the device being used with the patient's permission and could reduce adherence with monitoring because of the daily inconvenience (46). For clinical trial applications, device manufacturers must develop systems by which extraneous data can be flagged.

Exporting Data

Standard operating procedures for handling of other clinical trial data would indicate that each line of electronically collected data should be uniquely identified by study code, site code, and patient code, date and time. To avoid complex data handling, questionnaire and spirometry data should be exported in the same file or should be linked together. If not, the time stamp for a particular test session may not be the same on the two files, making linkage difficult. Exporting procedures should facilitate routine archiving of datasets. Prior to any data analysis, the format of exported date/time records should be checked for compatibility with local date/time formats (U.S./European).

Trend Displays

Electronically collected data are particularly suitable for rapid transformation into graphical displays, and most electronic monitoring devices are packaged with display software for use by patients or medical staff. If all maneuvers are being stored by the device, it is less confusing for the display to show only the best PEF or FEV_1 from each session, so that patterns of airflow obstruction can be identified (47). The format in which PEF charts are displayed, particularly the vertical:horizontal scale, can have a major impact on the visual appearance of the data, with horizontally compressed charts improving ease of recognition of exacerbations and of long-term trends (48). Use of a consistent chart scale will allow development of expertise in pattern recognition, as has occurred in occupational asthma.

Preparing Data Sets for Analysis

When processing electronically recorded spirometry and questionnaire datasets from Micro Medical DiaryCard, Micro DiaryCard, and Jaeger AM2 devices in clinical trials, we have adopted the following quality control procedures (26): (a) make corrections to questionnaire data if needed, provided the date and time are identified in writing; (b) exclude sessions identified as "Extra Sessions" or "Other Person"; (c) adjust date/time record to local time for travel across time zones or daylight saving; (d) allocate each session to "morning" or "evening", from a specific question or by using default 3 A.M. cutpoint (See section on After–Midnight Recordimgs); (e) calculate "Effective Date" (See section After-Midnight Recording) to allow for sessions recorded after midnight; (f) for any maneuver with $FEV_1 = FVC$, exclude FEV_1 and FVC; (g) identify outlying values from data plots and SD calculation and screen the stored flow-volume loops for these maneuvers; (h) for DiaryCard and AM2, add study code and patient code to each line of data; (i) for AM2, identify the spirometry data that match each session of questionnaire data. We initially excluded the first 2 days' data for learning effect (49), but other investigators have not found this to be necessary (29). For clinical trial settings, it is important to maintain an audit trail for any data corrections or processing.

Centralized Data Handling

Many of the earlier-mentioned data handling procedures could be facilitated or avoided by better design of monitoring devices. However, for large clinical trials, there may be an advantage in utilizing a centralized data management system. This facility is currently provided by some of the larger manufacturers of electronic monitoring devices (e.g., Viasys, Vitalograph) and by some independent biomedical data management companies. If such a system is used, it is important for the relevant operating procedures to be incorporated at the stage of protocol development.

Uses of Electronic Monitoring Devices

Following are some examples of clinical asthma studies that demonstrate the specific capabilities of electronic monitoring devices.

Assessment of Adherence with Conventional Monitoring

One of the most striking uses of electronic monitoring in asthma has been to covertly investigate adherence with *conventional* pen-and-paper PEF monitoring. This followed suspicion about the accuracy of paper diaries, particularly in occupational asthma (50). In covert adherence studies, patients are asked to write down the PEF results displayed by the device but are not informed that these are being recorded. Many such studies, in widely varying settings, have now provided unequivocal evidence for poor adherence with paper PEF diaries, with high rates of data fabrication (2,4,10,12,22,27,29,34,51–53). The equivalent of clinical trial medication "dumping" may occur; for example, Chowienczyk et al. (54) described a patient who performed 54 forced expirations over 3 hr and entered these data retrospectively on the paper diary. In occupational asthma studies, with short periods of monitoring 6–8 times per day, approximately one-quarter of paper diary data are falsified (2,22). In a general asthma study with twice daily monitoring for 3 months, Verschelden et al. (51) found apparent adherence of 54% but with 22% of results fabricated, true adherence was 44%. Côté et al. (53) subsequently measured adherence over 12 months when PEF monitoring was incorporated into the patients' asthma management. This included a PEF-based action plan and PEF-based adjustment of medication. Despite this, true adherence with monitoring was low even in the first month (mean 63%) and declined to 33% at 12 months, with most of the paper diaries maintained with fabricated results. Several covert studies have demonstrated that poor adherence with monitoring is also a problem in the management of asthma in children, even when the families are given extended information about the planned use of the PEF data (10), when contingency management strategies are used in an attempt to enhance adherence with monitoring (12), or when the carer rather than the child makes the diary entry (34). In each of these short (3–5 weeks) studies, adherence declined with time, and there were no obvious predictive factors for poor adherence.

Poor adherence and data falsification in paper PEF monitoring may have major implications in clinical asthma management, for example, inappropriate changes in medication. In clinical trials, the power of the study to detect a therapeutic response is likely to be reduced, and this may impact on the required sample size. In both of these settings, there may be systematic bias as patients may be more likely to remember to use their conventional PEF meter when symptomatic.

Enhancement of Adherence with Monitoring

Although there is ample evidence of unacceptably poor adherence with conventional monitoring, these studies do not provide any information about adherence with electronic monitoring itself, without the requirement for a paper diary. This was examined in one of the earliest electronic monitoring studies (54), with Micro Medical DiaryCards. One group knew that the device was recording their lung function; the remaining subjects were not informed of this and were required to transcribe the PEF results into paper diaries. There was a dramatic difference in adherence over 8 weeks between the two groups (median 94% for electronic monitoring alone, 61% for paper diaries). There was thus early evidence that reduction in the burden of PEF monitoring, by removing the need to write down the results, might actually enhance adherence. In the long-term budesonide study, in which patients were fully aware of the DiaryCard's recording capabilities, and which incorporated regular visual feedback of results, and PEF-based action plans and medication down-titration, median adherence with twice daily monitoring declined only from 96% to 89% over 18 months (55). In contrast, there were no entries at all on 39% of 8-week paper diaries used by the same patients for a simple study task (unpublished data). It is taken for granted in consumer marketing that non-user friendly features will decrease the likelihood of use of a product. Inconvenience and practical difficulties have been found to be significant contributors to poor adherence with medical instructions (46). Conventional paper PEF monitoring places a substantial burden on patients, which may be reduced by use of well-designed electronic devices.

Studies of Perception of Asthma

Some monitoring devices can be configured to conceal PEF from the patient, in order to avoid potential confounding of symptom assessment. For example, Higgs et al. (56) used the Codaflow device to demonstrate the impact of knowledge of PEF on the perception of asthma symptoms. Affleck et al. (33) assessed the relationship between changes in mood and asthma symptoms, by modifying the PeakLog device to conceal its output.

Relationship of Changes in FEV$_1$ to Changes in PEF

Discussions about PEF monitoring have often been qualified with comments about the unreliability and effort dependence of PEF measurements, particularly when unsupervised. There was therefore much anticipation that FEV_1 meters would result in an improvement in the reliability of home-monitored data. However, studies with electronic devices have provided some reassurance about the validity of PEF monitoring in asthma. For example, PEF was as satisfactory as FEV_1 for describing circadian variations in lung function in normals and asthmatics (1) and had better sensitivity and specificity than FEV_1 for diagnosis of occupational asthma, using specific occupational challenges as the gold standard (57). In the long-term budesonide study (6), electronic monitoring demonstrated symmetrical, although smaller, improvements in FEV_1 compared with PEF, with a similar time course following initiation of budesonide treatment (Fig. 4) (6). Similarly, symmetrical falls were seen in both FEV_1 and PEF during viral infections, although the fall in FEV_1 was smaller in magnitude than the fall in PEF (58). Previous suspicions about the validity of PEF monitoring may have had a solid foundation in poor adherence and data falsification with paper diaries and may have been affected by use of a PEF rather than a spirometric maneuver.

Identification of Variable Lung Function

Clinical trials often require documentation of current or previous bronchodilator reversibility, to confirm the diagnosis of asthma. Electronic monitoring has been used to document increased variability in subjects who did not meet a reversibility criterion at their first visit (6,59). Home monitoring has also been used to identify improvement in PEF variability with corticosteroids (60), and to demonstrate a significant decrease in lung function after experimental rhinovirus infection (61), when there were no significant changes in clinic lung function.

Assessment of Outcomes in Clinical Trials

The long-term budesonide study (6) was designed to assess, in patients with poorly controlled asthma, whether a very high starting dose of budesonide would lead to greater improvement in asthma outcomes, or permit lower long-term budesonide doses, than a lower starting dose. Sixty-one subjects used Micro Medical DiaryCards twice daily for 18 months, with 8-weekly visits. The study design incorporated a 14 month period of budesonide dose down-titration determined by a clinical algorithm (symptoms, β_2-agonist use, PEF variation) that was calculated from the electronic diary data. Quality control checks and processing of diary card data were carried out during each visit, and the data were available for immediate visual feedback to the patient and for determination of eligibility for dose reduction. Because of the reliability of the electronic diary data, as well as high levels of adherence with monitoring (55), detailed information was available about the time course of changes in asthma outcomes (Fig 5). Night waking

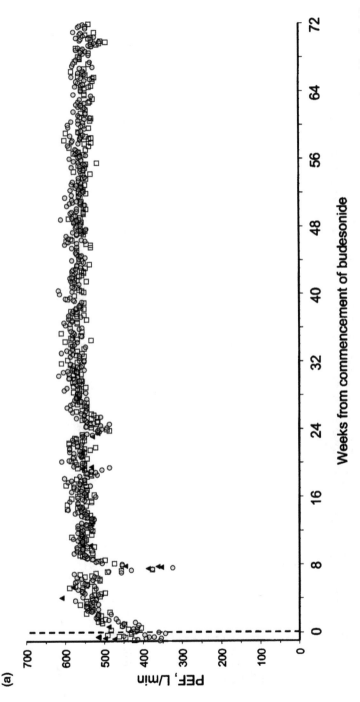

Figure 4 Typical cumulative PEF and FEV1 chart used for patient feedback during the long-term (18 months) budesonide study (6). Panel **a** shows PEF data, and Figure **b** (see p. 98) shows FEV1 data. Grey circles show morning pre-bronchodilator values, open squares show evening pre-bronchodilator values, and black triangles show "post-bronchodilator" data (recorded less than 4 hr after bronchodilator).

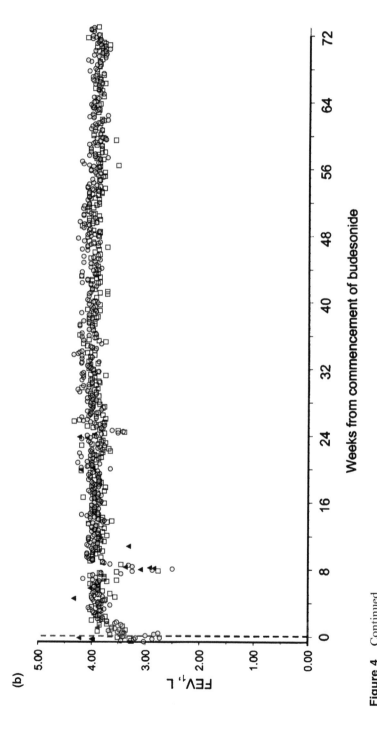

Figure 4   Continued

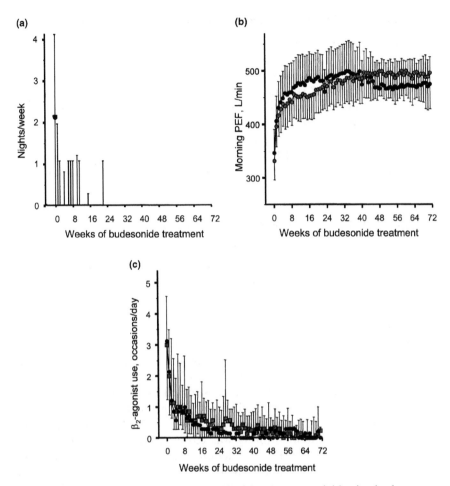

Figure 5 Time course of change in asthma outcome variables in the long-term budesonide study (6). Spirometric and questionnaire data from electronic monitoring were averaged for each week. Data for the 3200 μg/day starting dose group are shown in black, and for the 1600 μg/day group in gray. (a) Night waking due to asthma, nights/week (median, IQR), (b) Morning pre-bronchodilator PEF. (L/min) (mean, 95% CI); (c) Rescue β_2-agonist use (median, IQR). *Source*: Adapted from Ref. 6.

resolved within < week in the majority of subjects. Morning pre-bronchodilator PEF demonstrated a first dose effect of 35 L/min compared with run-in, with an overall improvement of 135 L/min, reaching a statistical plateau by week 14 (30). In contrast, as-needed β_2-agonist use continued to improve to week 30 and by study completion/withdrawal averaged less than once a week, despite reduction in budesonide dose to a median of 800 μcg/day by study completion (6).

Differences Between Asthma Exacerbations and Poor Control

Routine generation of horizontally compressed cumulative charts of morning, evening, and "post-bronchodilator" PEF and FEV_1 data at each visit in the long-term budesonide study also facilitated the identification of distinctive characteristics of spontaneously occurring viral exacerbations compared with poorly controlled asthma. Both of these states were characterized by frequent asthma symptoms, night waking, increased β_2-agonist use, and reduced lung function, but during poor asthma control, there was high within-day PEF variability and good bronchodilator reversibility, whereas during viral exacerbations, there was low within-day PEF variability and no evidence of response to β_2-agonist (58).

Implementation of Asthma Management Programs

A small number of uncontrolled studies have used electronic monitoring devices in asthma management programs. In one study, 22 adults with stable asthma monitored PEF daily for 2 weeks, and for 4 weeks after implementation of an asthma management plan, monitored PEF on 1 day per week or with increased symptoms. The electronic spirometer was used to identify low PEF days on which subjects should have changed their medication use, which was monitored covertly by Nebulizer Chronolog. The study demonstrated that most patients were willing to increase, but not to double, their inhaled corticosteroid when PEF fell below the assigned trigger point (52). In a 6-month study of 99 children selected for willingness to use the Airwatch monitoring system, self-reported medication use improved although adherence with monitoring declined (62). In the long-term budesonide study, electronic monitoring was closely incorporated into asthma management (6), with a PEF-based action plan for detection and management of exacerbations, a clinical algorithm based on electronic diary and PEF data for sequential down-titration of inhaled corticosteroid dose, and visual feedback of cumulative PEF and FEV_1 charts to patients at each visit. It is interesting to note that previous studies of the utility of asthma action plans have been based on written PEF diaries, and there is an obvious need, given the known poor adherence and data falsification with such systems, for further studies to assess action plans with a more user-friendly interface as can be obtained with electronic monitoring.

Occupational Asthma

There is an extensive literature on the role of peak flow monitoring in work-related respiratory disease, and expert visual recognition of characteristic PEF changes, originally developed by Burge and colleagues, is well-established in the diagnosis of occupational asthma (64). The same investigators went on to develop a computerized system of analysis of occupational PEF records (OASYS) (64), which has subsequently been adapted for use with the PEF/FEV$_1$ Diary. Other studies of occupational asthma are currently underway using the EasyOne spirometer, with customized software providing real time coaching in spirometry technique, an algorithm of questions about work-related factors, and an incentive system of points to encourage adherence. Because of the potential economic implications of confirmation or exclusion of a diagnosis of occupational asthma, the device was configured to conceal PEF from the patient for these studies (13).

Priorities in Use of Electronic Monitoring Devices

In *general clinical practice*, the primary expectation from using electronic monitoring in preference to conventional monitoring may be facilitation of better asthma management, from both the patient's and the doctor's perspective. In order to achieve this, the device would need to have the following characteristics: (a) easy to use, easy to teach; (b) integrated with an asthma action plan; (c) reproducible results; (d) technical support for patient and physician; (e) user-friendly trend displays; (f) small size; (g) durable, with an expected lifetime of several years; and (h) compatible with multiple operating systems. If a device had these features, and if there was a clear message from health-care professionals about how to interpret and act upon the recorded data, consumers could be prepared to pay somewhat more than for a mechanical meter. However, the cost benefit comparison may be difficult, as mechanical peak flow meters tend not to fail catastrophically (20); so, there is little perception in the community or by health-care professionals of their limited lifespan. None of the currently available electronic monitoring devices appear to be completely appropriate for routine clinical use at present, largely because of cost and user-unfriendly features.

For *clinical trials*, the primary expectation from an electronic monitoring device may be improved data reliability, with the expectation of cost savings for future studies. In order to achieve this, the device system would need to be considerably more sophisticated than for general clinical practice: (a) easy to use, easy to teach; (b) accurate and reproducible spirometric data; (c) symptom diary with unambiguous text (same device or linked device); (d) rapid objective identification of exacerbations; (e) ready accessibility of training and technical support for staff and patients; (f) export of data files in a format suitable for company databases; (g) validation to FDA standards of the device and any associated software; (h) an audit trail of any changes in device, configuration, or software during setup or use; and (i) compatibility with multiple different operating systems. Before electronic monitoring becomes widely adopted, there is a need for industry-wide discussion about quality control processes for the devices themselves and for processing of electronically recorded data. For a pharmaceutical company, the cost of conventional peak flow monitoring may be perceived as minimal and predictable (purchase of cheap single-patient peak flow meters, double data entry, data clarification for transcription errors), whereas the initial cost of setting up electronic monitoring may be greater because of the higher purchase cost (unless the devices are leased) and the need to set up new standard operating procedures. However, because of the compelling evidence of widespread data falsification with conventional pen-and-paper diaries, there is little justification for continuing to use such monitoring for either lung function or symptoms in clinical asthma trials. As electronic devices become more suitable for clinical trial requirements and as more clinical trials utilize electronic monitoring, the cost effectiveness of obtaining reliable data may become more obvious.

References

1. Troyanov S, Ghezzo H, Cartier A, Malo J-L. Comparison of circadian variations using FEV_1 and peak expiratory flow rates among normal and asthmatic subjects. Thorax 1994; 49:775–780.
2. Quirce S, Contreras G, Dybuncio A, Chan-Yeung M. Peak expiratory flow monitoring is not a reliable method for establishing the diagnosis of occupational asthma. Am J Respir Crit Care Med 1995; 152:1100–1102.
3. Bastian-Lee Y, Chavasse R, Richter H, Seddon P. Assessment of a low-cost home monitoring spirometer for children. Pediatr Pulmonol 2002; 33:388–394.
4. Chowienczyk PJ, Lawson CP. Pocket-sized device for measuring forced expiratory volume in one second and forced vital capacity. Br Med J (Clin Res Ed) 1982; 285:15–17.
5. Dirksen A, Holstein-Rathlou NH, Madsen F, Skovgaard LT, Ulrik CS, Heckscher T, Kok-Jensen A. Long-range correlations of serial FEV_1 measurements in emphysematous patients and normal subjects. J Appl Physiol 1998; 85:259–265.
6. Reddel HK, Jenkins CR, Marks GB, Ware SI, Xuan W, Salome CM, Badcock CA, Woolcock AJ. Optimal asthma control, starting with high doses of inhaled budesonide [erratum in Eur Respir J 2000; 16:579]. Eur Respir J 2000; 16:226–235.
7. Richter K, Kanniess F, Mark B, Jorres RA, Magnussen H. Assessment of accuracy and applicability of a new electronic peak flow meter and asthma monitor. Eur Respir J 1998; 12:457–462.
8. Martin RJ, Pak J, Kunselman SJ, Cherniack RM. Assessment of the AirWatch lung function monitoring system. Asthma Clinical Research Network (ACRN). J Allergy Clin Immunol 1999; 103:535–536.
9. Pelkonen AS, Nikander K, Turpeinen M. Reproducibility of home spirometry in children with newly diagnosed asthma. Pediatr Pulmonol 2000; 29:34–38.
10. Kamps AW, Roorda RJ, Brand PL. Peak flow diaries in childhood asthma are unreliable. Thorax 2001; 56:180–182.

11. Barrabe P, Choudat D, Dessanges J.-F. Electronic pocket spirometer with memorization of peak expiratory flow (PEF) and forced expiratory volume in one second (FEV₁). Rev Mal Respir 1999; 16:402–403.

12. Burkhart PV, Dunbar-Jacob JM, Fireman P, Rohay J. Children's adherence to recommended asthma self-management. Pediatr Nurs 2002; 28:409–414.

13. Mortimer KM, Fallot A, Balmes JR, Tager IB. Evaluating the use of a portable spirometer in a study of pediatric asthma. Chest 2003; 123:1899–1907.

14. American Thoracic Society. Standardization of spirometry, 1994 Update. Am J Respir Crit Care Med 1995; 152:1107–1136.

15. Cherniak R, Hurd S, for the NAEP and NHLBI. Statement on Technical Standards for Peak Flow Meters. NIH Publication No. 92–2113a. US Department of Health and Human Services, 1992.

16. Quanjer PH, Lebowitz MD, Gregg I, Miller MR, Pedersen OF. Peak expiratory flow: conclusions and recommendations of a working party of the European Respiratory Society. Eur Respir J 1997; 10(Suppl 24):2s–8s.

17. Hitchings DJ, Dickinson SA, Miller MR, Fairfax AJ. Development of an accurate portable recording peak-flow meter for the diagnosis of asthma. J Biomed Eng 1993; 15:188–192.

18. Dirksen A, Madsen F, Petersen OF, Vedel AM, Kok-Jensen A. Long term performance of a hand held spirometer. Thorax 1996; 51:973–976.

19. National Asthma Education Program. Expert Panel Report on Diagnosis and Management of Asthma. NIH Publication No. 92-2113a. US Government Printing Office, Washington, DC, 1992.

20. Irvin CG, Martin RJ, Chinchilli VM, Kunselman SJ, Cherniack RM. Quality control of peak flow meters for multicenter clinical trials. The Asthma Clinical Research Network (ACRN). Am J Respir Crit Care Med 1997; 156:396–402.

21. Gunawardena KA, Houston K, Smith AP. Evaluation of the turbine pocket spirometer. Thorax 1987; 42:689–693.

22. Malo JL, Trudeau C, Ghezzo H, L'Archevêque J, Cartier A. Do subjects investigated for occupational asthma through serial peak expiratory flow measurements falsify their results? J Allergy Clin Immunol 1995; 96:601–607.

23. Godschalk I, Brackel HJ, Peters JC, Bogaard JM. Assessment of accuracy and applicability of a portable electronic diary card spirometer for asthma treatment. Respir Med 1996; 90:619–622.

24. Quirce S, Contreras G, Moran O, Abboud R, Kennedy S, Dimich-Ward H, Chan-Yeung M. Laboratory and clinical evaluation of a portable computerized peak flow meter. J Asthma 1997; 34:305–312.

25. Lindgren BR, Finkelstein SM, Prasad B, Dutta P, Killoren T, Scherber J, Stibbe CL, Snyder M, Hertz MI. Determination of reliability and validity in home monitoring data of pulmonary function tests following lung transplantation. Res Nurs Health 1997; 20:539–550.

26. Reddel HK, Ware SI, Salome CM, Jenkins CR, Woolcock AJ. Pitfalls in processing home electronic spirometric data in asthma. Eur Respir J 1998; 12:853–858.

27. Chowienczyk PJ, Lawson CP, Morris J, Kermani A, Cochrane GM. Electronic diary to record physiological measurements. Lancet 1992; 339:251.

28. Anees W, Huggins V, Burge PS. Reliability of PEF diaries. Thorax 2001; 56:742.
29. Wensley DC, Silverman M. The quality of home spirometry in school children with asthma. Thorax 2001; 56:183–185.
30. Reddel HK, Marks GB, Jenkins CR. When can personal best peak flow be determined for asthma action plans? Thorax 2004; 59:922–924.
31. Gibson PG, Wlodarczyk J, Hensley MJ, Murree-Allen K, Olson LG, Saltos N. Using quality-control analysis of peak expiratory flow recordings to guide therapy for asthma. Ann Intern Med 1995; 123:488–492.
32. Stone AA, Shiffman S, Schwartz JE, Broderick JE, Hufford MR. Patient non-compliance with paper diaries. Br Med J 2002; 324:1193–1194.
33. Affleck G, Apter A, Tennen H, Reisine S, Barrows E, Willard A, Unger J, ZuWallack R. Mood states associated with transitory changes in asthma symptoms and peak expiratory flow. Psychosom Med 2000; 62:61–68.
34. Redline S, Wright EC, Kattan M, Kercsmar C, Weiss K. Short-term compliance with peak flow monitoring: results from a study of inner city children with asthma. Pediatr Pulmonol 1996; 21:203–210.
35. Lefkowitz D, Klimas JT, Ross RN. Comparison of a new hand-held interactive airway monitoring system and a conventional peak expiratory flow meter in the management of asthma. Am J Manag Care 1996; 2:1227–1235.
36. Finkelstein S, Lindgren B, Prasad B, Snyder M, Edin C, Wielinski C, Hertz M. Reliability and validity of spirometry measurements in a paperless home monitoring diary program for lung transplantation. Heart Lung 1993; 22:523–533.
37. Cinkotai F, Sharpe T, Gibbs A. Circadian rhythms in peak expiratory flow rate in workers exposed to cotton dust. Thorax 1984; 39:759–765.
38. Eckert B, Mitchell C, Brennan T, Huxham G. Diurnal variation in airway calibre: influence of time of measurement. Aust N Z J Med 1995; 25:A453.
39. Reddel HK, Ware SI, Salome CM, Marks GB, Jenkins CR, Woolcock AJ. Standardization of ambulatory peak flow monitoring: the importance of recent beta2-agonist inhalation. Eur Respir J 1998; 12:309–314.
40. Reddel HK, Salome CM, Peat JK, Woolcock AJ. Which index of peak expiratory flow is most useful in the management of stable asthma? Am J Respir Crit Care Med 1995; 151:1320–1325.
41. Gannon PF, Belcher J, Pantin CF, Burge PS. The effect of patient technique and training on the accuracy of self-recorded peak expiratory flow. Eur Respir J 1999; 14:28–31.
42. Wensley D, Pickering D, Silverman M. Can peak expiratory flow be measured accurately during a forced vital capacity manoeuvre? Eur Respir J 2000; 16: 673–676.
43. Enright PL, Sherrill DL, Lebowitz MD. Ambulatory monitoring of peak expiratory flow. Reproducibility and quality control. Chest 1995; 107:657–661.
44. Newton D, Gannon P, Burge P, Pantin C, Middleton J. An evaluation of a computer based system to divide peak expiratory flow records. Eur Respir J 1992; 5(suppl 15):403s.
45. Quanjer PH, Dalhuijsen A, Van Zomeren B. Summary equations of reference values. Bull Europ Physiopathol Respir 1983; 19(suppl 5):45–51.

46. DiMatteo M. Enhancing patient adherence to medical recommendations. JAMA 1994; 271:79–83.
47. Turner-Warwick M. On observing patterns of airflow obstruction in chronic asthma. Br J Dis Chest 1977; 71:73–86.
48. Reddel HK, Vincent SD, Civitico J. The need for standardisation of peak flow charts. Thorax 2005; 60:164–167.
49. Quackenboss JJ, Liebowitz MD, Krzyzanowski M. The normal range of diurnal changes in peak expiratory flow rates. Relationship to symptoms and respiratory disease. Am Rev Respir Dis 1991; 143:323–330.
50. Burge P. Use of serial measurements of peak flow in the diagnosis of occupational asthma. Occup Med 1993; 8:279–294.
51. Verschelden P, Cartier A, L'Archeveque J, Trudeau C, Malo JL. Compliance with and accuracy of daily self-assessment of peak expiratory flows (PEF) in asthmatic subjects over a three month period. Eur Respir J 1996; 9:880–885.
52. van der Palen J, Klein JJ, Rovers MM. Compliance with inhaled medication and self-treatment guidelines following a self-management programme in adult asthmatics. Eur Respir J 1997; 10:652–657.
53. Côté J, Cartier A, Malo JL, Rouleau M, Boulet LP. Compliance with peak expiratory flow monitoring in home management of asthma. Chest 1998; 113:968–972.
54. Chowienczyk PJ, Parkin DH, Lawson CP, Cochrane GM. Do asthmatic patients correctly record home spirometry measurements? Br Med J 1994; 309:1618.
55. Reddel HK, Toelle BG, Marks GB, Ware SI, Jenkins CR, Woolcock AJ. Analysis of adherence to peak flow monitoring when recording of data is electronic. Br Med J 2002; 324:146–147.
56. Higgs CMB, Richardson RB, Lea DA, Lewis GTR, Laszlo G. Influence of knowledge of peak flow on self-assessment of asthma: studies with a coded peak flow meter. Thorax 1986; 41:671–675.
57. Leroyer C, Perfetti L, Trudeau C, L'Archeveque J, Chan-Yeung M, Malo JL. Comparison of serial monitoring of peak expiratory flow and FEV$_1$ in the diagnosis of occupational asthma. Am J Respir Crit Care Med 1998; 158:827–832.
58. Reddel H, Ware S, Marks G, Salome C, Jenkins C, Woolcock A. Differences between asthma exacerbations and poor asthma control [erratum in Lancet 1999; 353:758]. Lancet 1999; 353:364–369.
59. Pelkonen AS, Hakulinen AL, Turpeinen M. Bronchial lability and responsiveness in school children born very preterm. Am J Respir Crit Care Med 1997; 156:1178–1184.
60. Pelkonen AS, Hakulinen AL, Hallman M, Turpeinen M. Effect of inhaled budesonide therapy on lung function in school children born preterm. Respir Med 2001; 95:565–570.
61. Grunberg K, Timmers MC, de Klerk EP, Dick EC, Sterk PJ. Experimental rhinovirus 16 infection causes variable airway obstruction in subjects with atopic asthma. Am J Respir Crit Care Med 1999; 160:1375–1380.
62. Marosi A, Stiesmeyer J. Improving pediatric asthma patient outcomes by incorporation of effective interventions. J Asthma 2001; 38:681–690.

63. Gannon PFG, Burge PS. Serial peak expiratory flow measurement in the diagnosis of occupational asthma. Eur Respir J 1997; 10(suppl 24):57s–63s.
64. Burge PS, Pantin CF, Newton DT, Gannon PF, Bright P, Belcher J, McCoach J, Baldwin DR, Burge CB. Development of an expert system for the interpretation of serial peak expiratory flow measurements in the diagnosis of occupational asthma. Midlands Thoracic Society Research Group. Occup Environ Med 1999; 56:758–764.

5

Asthma and Telemedicine

CLAIRE WAINWRIGHT

Department of Respiratory Medicine,
Royal Children's Hospital,
Queensland, Australia

RICHARD WOOTTON

Centre for Online Health,
University of Queensland,
Queensland, Australia

Abstract

Although the literature contains a number of reports of early work involving telemedicine and chronic disease, there have been comparatively few studies in asthma. Most of the work in asthma has concerned remote monitoring of patients in the home, for example, transmitting spirometry data via a telephone modem to a central server. The object is to improve management. A secondary benefit is that patient adherence to prescribed treatment is likely to be improved. Early results are encouraging. Other studies have described the cost-benefits of a specialist asthma nurse who can manage patients by telephone contact, as well as deliver asthma education. Many web-based resources are available for the general public or health-care professionals to improve education in asthma, although their quality is highly variable. The work on telemedicine in asthma clearly shows that the technique holds promise in a number of areas. Unfortunately—as in telemedicine generally—most of the literature refers to pilot trials and feasibility studies, with short-term outcomes. Large-scale, formal research trials are required to establish the cost-effectiveness of telemedicine in asthma.

Introduction

Asthma represents a significant burden of ill health in society and affects approximately 10% of adults and up to 20% of children in the USA, Australia, and the UK. The annual cost of asthma in the United States was estimated as 12.7 billion US dollars in 1998 (1). The management of asthma includes managing the acute exacerbations, as well as chronic management aimed at reducing the severity and frequency of acute exacerbations and maintaining optimum health and lung function. Health outcomes for children and adults with asthma may be optimized through education, adherence to appropriate therapy, regular review, and in the case of young people and adults with asthma, by promotion of self-management. Many of these activities might be enhanced or supported by utilization of telemedicine where appropriate.

The widespread availability of the PC and of relatively low-cost, digital telecommunications led to an upsurge of interest in telemedicine in the 1990s. Much of this work has concerned acute patients in hospitals (2). However, in the last few years there has been increasing interest in the possible use of telemedicine for managing chronic disease, and the literature contains a number of reports of early work. The majority of the work is in diabetes, and there are comparatively few studies in asthma. For example, a search of the Medline database (December 2003) for papers containing the keyword "telemedicine" returned a total of 5741, of which 121 (2.1%) concerned diabetes, and only 25 (0.4%) concerned asthma.

What Is Telemedicine?

Telemedicine is a general term used to define health-care activities carried out at a distance (3). It therefore encompasses all aspects of health care, from diagnosis and management to the continuing education of health-care professionals, whenever distance is involved. Other synonyms for telemedicine include the terms telehealth, online health, and e-health. The use of the term telehealth is due to the perception that "health" implies broader societal aims than the narrower focus of "medicine." The use of the term e-health is more recent and implies telemedicine activities that take place via the Internet, especially those with a commercial focus. Nonetheless, the term telemedicine remains firmly embedded in the literature. In the interests of simplicity, telemedicine is used here as a generic term encompassing all distance medicine delivery techniques.

There are essentially two types of telemedicine techniques—those that occur in real-time and those that are pre-recorded. Real-time telemedicine is interactive, requiring the presence of the specialist and the non-specialist at the same time, albeit in different locations. A well-accepted example of real-time telemedicine is giving health-care advice over the telephone, something that most health professionals hardly think twice about. More advanced techniques include real-time teleconsulting when one party consults with another using videoconferencing equipment (Fig. 1). The point is that both parties are in live communication via whatever medium is in use. Thus, either party can ask a question and receive an immediate reply.

In contrast, pre-recorded or store-and-forward telemedicine does not require the simultaneous presence of the parties concerned at each location, i.e., the health-care provider and the recipient of that care do not have to be available at the same time. Information can be transmitted to a specialist health-care provider, by e-mail for instance, and then viewed later at a more convenient time by the specialist. An increasingly common form of pre-recorded telemedicine is teleradiology, in which an electronic image of the x-ray examination is transmitted to a radiologist, often in another hospital, for reporting.

The common ground between real-time and pre-recorded telemedicine is the increased accessibility to medical and health-care expertise when distance is involved. Telemedicine is not therefore a technology as such, but rather a *technique* for delivering care when the individuals concerned are located in different places. The technique involves modifying normal clinical practice to adapt to the novel circumstances of communicating at a distance, rather than in person. In using telemedicine, clinicians and other health-care workers owe the same duty of care as with the conventional forms of delivery.

Why Telemedicine in Asthma?

What components of asthma management are likely to be enhanced by telemedicine? In chronic diseases generally, experience shows that prevention, early detection, and management may all be improved by suitable interventions(4). For asthma, it should be possible to deliver the necessary interventions by an appropriate telemedicine technique. For example, patient education can be delivered by videoconference (5), and home monitoring in various forms can be used for early detection of exacerbations (6), for better management of exacerbations (7), and to improve adherence (8). The following aspects are discussed in more detail below:

- patient education;
- remote monitoring;
- adherence;
- telephone follow-up;
- screening.

As well as support for the patients, successful chronic disease management involves support for health-care professionals. This may

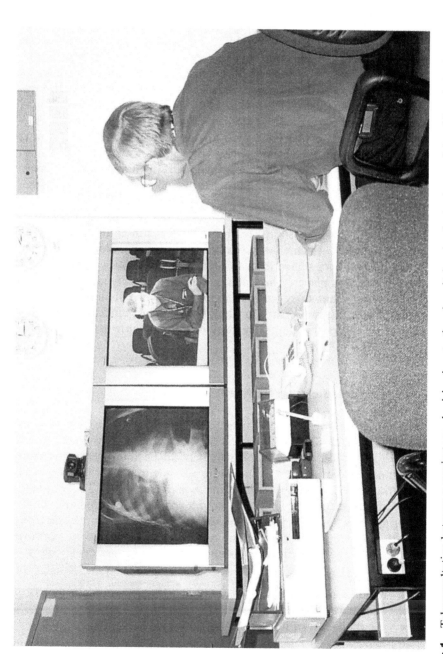

Figure 1 Teleconsultation between a respiratory physician in a tertiary hospital and a doctor in a peripheral hospital using videoconferencing.

include the provision of guidelines, decision support tools, and clinical information systems. Again, telemedicine techniques can be used to provide such support, and successful outcomes have been demonstrated in other chronic diseases, such as diabetes.

Successful chronic disease management involves communication between health-care professionals, and between health-care professionals and the patient. Again the techniques of telemedicine are likely to have an increasing role in chronic disease management including asthma, particularly in situations where communication is difficult, such as in rural and remote communities.

Patient Education

Education and support for the patient involve the provision of information and access to self-help tools. Asthma education is a cornerstone of management but there are surprisingly few studies examining the role of telemedicine in asthma education. Some patient education in metered-dose inhaler (MDI) technique has taken place by videoconferencing (using equipment located in health-care facilities), Table 1 (5,9). For subjects who have access to facilities where suitable videoconferencing equipment is available, this approach seems likely to be useful. Many web-based systems are available for the general public or health-care professionals to improve education in asthma, although their content and quality are highly variable (10). While definitive trials have yet to be carried out, early results suggest that a computer-assisted education program promoting change in knowledge and self-management in children aged 9–13 years can improve self efficacy and self-management behaviors at least in the short-term management of asthma (11).

Unfortunately, while many studies have looked at the benefits of asthma education in adults or in children, there is little evidence about which components of asthma education are beneficial and this may make the role of telemedicine in asthma education more difficult to define. The components of asthma education include specific education about the disease, medication, and self-management, the use of specific devices to administer medication and a written management plan. A Cochrane review has shown that asthma education programs using a written management plan are more likely to decrease the utilization of health services compared with programs that do not use such a plan (12). However, the contribution of the written asthma plan to the education program is not known since trials have so far been too small and the results too inconsistent to allow firm conclusions to be drawn (13). One study has examined the benefit of a specific educational component of asthma education in adults. Côte et al. (14) showed that a structured educational intervention emphasizing self-management with a written management plan improved peak expira-

Table 1 Educational Studies. The Study Shown in Italics was a Randomized Trial

Study	Participants per group	Intervention	Results	Implications
Bynum et al. 2001 (5)	36 subjects randomly assigned to control (21) or intervention group (15)	Metered-dose inhaler technique taught by videoconferencing	The video group significantly improved their technique	Videoconferencing is an effective teaching medium
Chan et al. 2001 (9)	12 elderly subjects in a residential home!	Metered-dose inhaler technique taught by videoconferencing	Half of the subjects improved their technique after 3 months in comparison with baseline performance	Videoconferencing is an effective teaching medium

tory flow rates, reduced the number of urgent medical visits for asthma, improved quality of life scores and improved patients' knowledge of asthma during 12 months follow-up. The study group was compared with a control group given no education other than education on use of an inhaler device and a group who were given limited education with an asthma management plan and education on use of an inhaler device. Unfortunately, no studies have comprehensively compared methods of delivering education and the design of most studies has not enabled the identification of the specific component or components of the educational package that was key in the improvement in clinical outcomes found.

Remote Monitoring

Most studies involving telemedicine and asthma have involved remote monitoring of patients in the home, for example, transmitting spirometry data via a telephone modem to a central server, Table 2 (6,7,15–17), although videoconferencing and telephone calls have been used as well. Kokubu et al. (6) carried out a formal randomized controlled study of an intervention that combined many of these aspects. In their trial, patients were equipped with a portable device (the "Air Watch") to record PEF and FEV_1. The data could subsequently be transmitted via an ordinary telephone line to a central server, from which the telemedicine nurse could fax a summary to the patient's physician. The telemedicine nurse also carried out regular follow-up by telephone. In a six-month study of 66 patients, medication adherence was higher in the telemedicine group (though not significantly), but there was a substantial reduction in the hospitalization rate in the intervention group ($P < 0.001$), as well as reduced numbers of visits to the emergency department. The lower rates of hospitalization and fewer hospital visits appear likely to make the telemedicine intervention cost-effective.

Adherence

The object of the remote monitoring studies is to improve management. A secondary benefit is that patient adherence to prescribed treatment is likely to be improved through the use of telemedicine although this has not been systematically examined. Morbidity from asthma in both children and adults is related to their adherence to therapy (18,19). Adherence to therapy for chronic conditions is difficult. Adherence to regular preventative therapy in asthma has been examined using self-report, caregiver's report, weight of metered dose inhaler and by electronic monitoring of inhaler actuation (20). Even in studies where patients know they are being monitored adherence tends to wane with time and averages about 50%. Simplifying medication regimes, regular review with appointment reminders, and promotion of self-management are all associated with improved adherence

Table 2 Clinical Studies. The Study Shown in Italics was a Randomized Trial

Study	Participants per group	Intervention	Length of study	Results	Implications
Bruderman and Abboud, 1997 (15)	39 asthma patients	Home monitoring, portable spirometer. Data transmission by telephone modem	—	In 19 patients, analysis of the spirometry data detected early signs of deterioration	Home monitoring may improve management
Finkelstein et al. 1998 (16)	10 subjects	Home monitoring—portable spirometer and palmtop computer. Data transmission by telephone modem	2–21 days	Average data transmission time was about 1 min by PSTN and 6 min by mobile phone	Feasibility study
Kokubu et al. 1999 (6)	High-risk patients randomly assigned to control or intervention group	Home monitoring—nurse provided instructions by telephone	6 months	Significant decrease in emergency room visits; improved PEF values in telemedicine group	Effective system for poorly controlled asthma
Romano et al. 2001 (17)	17 patients with persistent asthma	Telemedicine (video conferencing) follow-up visits at a school clinic	6 months	Symptom scores improved	Feasibility study
Steel et al. 2002 (7)	33 patients	Remote monitoring from home. Data transmission via telephone modem	2 weeks	80% compliance with monitoring; 52% compliance with transmission of results	Feasibility study

(21), although this has not been examined with-electronic monitoring of adherence. Concerns that adherence might be reduced in elderly people because of potential technophobia have not been borne out by surveys that show that the elderly have positive attitudes to technology generally, and to telemedicine and telecare specifically (22,23). Videophones have been used successfully to improve treatment adherence in other conditions. For example, DeMaio et al. (24) used low-cost analog videophones for video communication between patients' homes and a chest clinic. Patients undergoing treatment for tuberculosis were called at pre-arranged times, displayed the daily dosage of medication and swallowed the pills in view of the camera. Patient adherence was excellent (95%) and similar to adherence in face-to-face therapy. There were substantial time and travel savings through the use of telemedicine. A similar effect could be expected in asthma.

Telephone Follow-up

There are studies describing the cost benefit advantages of a specialist asthma nurse who can manage patients by telephone contact, as well as deliver asthma education (25–28). Most of these studies have compared cost benefits before and after a specialist asthma nurse program was established and the separate components of the intervention have not been examined. Some of these studies have used telephone monitoring in addition to face-to-face education sessions, thus adding a telemedicine component to the education/health management package (25,26,28). However, the design of these studies has not allowed an assessment of the benefit derived from the different components of the interventions used. A recent randomized controlled study by Pinnock et al. (29) reported that routine review of asthma care by telephone consultation with an asthma nurse enabled more adults with asthma to be reviewed without apparent clinical disadvantage. In addition, they felt that the shorter duration of the telephone consultations meant that the telephone consultation was likely to be an efficient option for general practices with a specialist asthma nurse. There are some significant concerns about this study discussed in letters by Huynh and Lavars (30) and by McKinstry et al. (31), which should be considered in the design of future telemedicine interventions. They felt that the study sample was not representative of the target population and most patients approached to take part either did not reply or did not consent. The clinical outcomes focused on patient satisfaction rather than more objective clinical measures such as lung function or objective assessment of medication delivery. In addition, while telephone reviews might be regarded as efficient because they were shorter and more focussed on asthma, it is possible that face-to-face reviews might integrate opportunistic preventative health screening, such as blood pressure measurement, and thus provide a more cost-effective service.

Screening

Telemedicine has been used for screening in many chronic conditions. The object is to improve early detection of complications in chronic disease or early diagnosis of a disease process. The majority of the work to date has concerned the transmission of image data, such as retinal photographs. However, some small studies have investigated the use of daily spirometry data in adults with asthma with a view to the early detection and treatment of exacerbations. This approach is of great interest in reducing the use of acute medical services, and preventing the loss of school and workdays for the community by the identification of asthma exacerbations. Portable spirometers have been found to be accurate and reliable (32); however, a screening tool needs to be sensitive and specific enough for this type of approach in order to be cost effective in practice. Unfortunately, while this may be the case for retinal photographs, the trends have not been systematically studied for home spirometry and lung function, Large-scale trials are now required to prove the cost-effectiveness of this approach to screening. In addition, long-term adherence to this type of monitoring in the home is unlikely to be sustained and cost benefits need to be carefully examined.

Clinical Guidelines, Decision Support Tools and Clinical Information Systems

National guidelines have been widely available both electronically and in paper form for many years in most industrialized nations and have been designed to provide a consistent appropriate standard of care for patients with asthma although adherence to guidelines is notoriously poor. The use of computerized evidence-based guidelines on asthma management in adults in a well-designed large primary care study was examined by Eccles et al. (33) and rather disappointingly no effect was found on adherence to guidelines or patient reported clinical outcomes. Further work is obviously required.

Telemonitoring systems and clinical information systems are often designed for one type of chronic disease or to operate with one or two specific monitoring devices. The data generated are usually transferred to a central database and the software components are usually specific to the data produced by particular devices. This can lead to multiple different systems being required for different diseases and monitoring equipment. Generic data modelling tools for telemonitoring have now been developed and may in the future facilitate the use of telemedicine for diverse health-care requirements (34).

Promising Developments

As described above, much of the use of telemedicine in chronic disease management concerns diabetes. In the latter condition, it is encouraging to note that formal RCTs are beginning to obtain evidence for the cost-effectiveness of telemedicine. For example, Biermann et al. (35) carried out a trial on patients on insulin therapy who were randomly assigned to control ($n = 16$) or telecare ($n = 27$). The latter group used blood glucose meters which could store and then transmit their data over an ordinary telephone line. Data were transmitted every 1–3 weeks and a telephone consultation was carried out once per month. The telemedicine intervention was equally effective as conventional care in reducing HbA_{1c}. Because of the savings in patient travel, there were substantial societal gains in using telemedicine, amounting to Euro 650 per patient per year.

One potential barrier to the use of telemedicine in chronic disease management is reimbursement, since in many countries health-care providers must deal with patients face to face if they are to be paid for the work. In the United States, a national managed care company has recently established reimbursement for web-based Internet consultations between patients and their physicians (36). Privacy issues have been addressed by utilizing secure network procedures. The scheme is limited to chronic conditions such as diabetes, asthma, and congestive heart failure, and will reimburse up to 24 consultations per year at a rate of $25 each. Reimbursement, when it was permitted in other areas, did not lead to a dramatic increase in telemedicine, so the effect in chronic disease management remains to be seen.

Unanswered Research Questions

The work to date demonstrates that telemedicine is feasible in asthma, and in certain areas, it appears effectual. The fundamental research question at present is whether telemedicine is cost effective. The conventional method of assessing the strength of the evidence would be a systematic review, in which each piece of work was classified according to the study design, from a meta-analysis of randomized controlled trials (strongest) to simple anecdotes or case reports (weakest). Unfortunately, in the work related to asthma—as in telemedicine generally—most of the literature refers to pilot trials and feasibility studies, with short-term outcomes.

There are few studies to date examining the use of telemedicine in asthma care and formal studies of cost effectiveness are awaited. It is worth noting that formal studies of cost effectiveness in telemedicine are difficult to carry out, which may be one reason why so few have yet been attempted.

In the trials of home monitoring so far conducted it has not always been easy to discern the effect of telemedicine itself vs. the effect of increased contact with health-care professionals or even the novelty effect of the technology. As always in telemedicine research, careful study design will be required.

Other Issues

Common concerns that are often raised in discussions about the use of telemedicine include:

- the medicolegal implications of practising in a "new" way;
- the acceptability to users of the technique (i.e., acceptability to patients and carers, and to health-care staff);
- reimbursement.

Broadly speaking, the medicolegal position of doctors involved in telemedicine is similar to that in which the telephone, fax, email, or letter are used instead. It has been suggested that provided the staff involved behave in a prudent manner, the medicolegal risks of telemedicine are acceptable (37–40). Furthermore, there may be occasions on which it is inappropriate *not* to use telemedicine if that is considered to be best practice in the circumstances.

There is now a considerable literature on aspects of the acceptability of telemedicine to users. Generally speaking, this body of work shows that telemedicine is acceptable to patients and to doctors, although recent reviews have shown that some of the studies have been methodologically weak (41,42). Nonetheless, it would be hard to conclude that dissatisfaction with telemedicine is a significant problem.

Few countries have systems in place by which doctors can be reimbursed for participating in telemedicine. This is often cited as a barrier to the general adoption of telemedicine into routine practice. In the United States, there has been some recent relaxation in the rules regarding reimbursement for episodes of telehealth (43), and it remains to be seen whether this will lead to a dramatic rise in activity.

Conclusion

Telemedicine appears to be a promising technique for the management of asthma but good quality studies are scarce and the generalizability of most findings is rather limited. Telemedicine can provide convenient rapid communication between health-care workers and patients that could lead to better monitoring of quantitative variables and may improve adherence to therapy thereby reducing the need for acute health-care visits and the workdays and school days lost to the community because of acute exacerbations. Formal cost-effectiveness studies will be required to prove this. In addition, education appears to be a promising area for telemedicine and asthma, but is at an earlier stage of examination.

References

1. Redd CR. Asthma in the United States: burden and current theories. Environ Health Perspect 2002; 110(suppl 4):557–560.
2. Jaatinen PT, Forsstrom J, Loula P. Teleconsultations: who uses them and how? J Telemed Telecare 2002; 8(6):319–324.
3. Wootton R. Telemedicine: a cautious welcome. Br Med J 1996; 313:1375–1377.
4. Weingarten SR, Henning JM, Badamgarav E, Knight K, Hasselblad V, Gano A, Ofman JJ. Interventions used in disease management programmes for patients with chronic illness—which ones work? Meta-analysis of published reports. Br Med J 2002; 325:925–928.
5. Bynum A, Hopkins D, Thomas A, Copeland N, Irwin C. The effect of telepharmacy counseling on metered-dose inhaler technique among adolescents with asthma in rural Arkansas. Telemed JE Health 2001; 7(3):207–217.
6. Kokubu F, Suzuki H, Sano Y, Kihara N, Adachi M. [Article in Japanese—Telemedicine system for high-risk asthmatic patients]. Arerugi 1999; 48(7): 700–712.
7. Steel S, Lock S, Johnson N, Martinez Y, Marquilles E, Bayford R. A feasibility study of remote monitoring of asthmatic patients. J Telemed Telecare 2002; 8(5):290–296.
8. Finkelstein J, O'Connor G, Friedmann RH. Development and implementation of the home asthma telemonitoring (HAT) system to facilitate asthma self-care. Medinfo 2001; 10(Pt 1):810–814.
9. Chan WM, Woo J, Hui E, Hjelm NM. The role of telenursing in the provision of geriatric outreach services to residential homes in Hong Kong. J Telemed Telecare 2001; 7(1):38–46.
10. Croft DR, Peterson MW. An evaluation of the quality and contents of asthma education on the World Wide Web. Chest 2002; 121(4):1301–1307.
11. Shegog R, Bartholomew LK, Parcel GS, Sockrider MM, Masse L, Abramson SL. Impact of a computer-assisted education program on factors related to asthma self-management behavior. J Am Med Inform Assoc 2001; 8(1):49–61.
12. Gibson PG, Coughlan J, Wilson AJ, Abramson M, Bauman A, Hensley MJ, Walters EH. Self-management education and regular practitioner review for adults with asthma (Cochrane Review). Cochrane Database Syst Rev 2003(1):CD001117.
13. Toelle BG, Ram FS. Written individualised management plans for asthma in children and adults. Cochrane Database Syst Rev 2002(3):CD002171.
14. Côté J, Bowie DM, Robichaud P, Parent J-G, Battisti L, Boulet L-P. Evaluation of two different educational interventions for adult patients consulting with an

acute asthma exacerbation. Am J Respir Crit Care Med 2001; 163(6):1415–1419.

15. Bruderman I, Abboud S. Telespirometry: novel system for home monitoring of asthmatic patients. Telemed J 1997; 3(2):127–133.

16. Finkelstein J, Hripcsak G, Cabrera M. Telematic system for monitoring of asthma severity in patients' homes. Medinfo 1998; 9(Pt 1):272–276.

17. Romano MJ, Hernandez J, Gaylor A, Howard S, Knox R. Improvement in asthma symptoms and quality of life in pediatric patients through specialty — care delivered via telemedicine. Telemed J E Health 2001; 7(4):281–286.

18. Bauman LJ, Wright E, Leickly FE, Crain E, Kruszon-Moran D, Wade SL, Visness CM. Relationship of adherence to pediatric asthma morbidity among inner-city children. Pediatrics 2002; 110(1 Pt l):e6.

19. Schmier JK, Leidy NK. The complexity of treatment adherence in adults with asthma: challenges and opportunities. J Asthma 1998; 35(6):451–454.

20. Bender B, Wamboldt FS, O'Connor SL, Rand C, Szefler S, Milgrom H, Wamboldt MZ. Measurement of children's asthma medication adherence by self report, canister weight, and Doser CT. Ann Allergy Asthma Immunol 2000; 85(5):416–421.

21. Sawyer SM. Action plans, self monitoring and adherence: changing behaviour to promote better self-management. Med J Aust 2002; 177(suppl):S72–S74.

22. Bratton RL, Short TM. Patient satisfaction with telemedicine: a comparison study of geriatric patients. J Telemed Telecare 2001; 72(suppl):85–86.

23. Levy S, Bradley DA, Morison MJ, Swanston MT, Harvey S. Future patient care tele-empowerment. J Telemed Telecare 2002; 82(suppl):52–54.

24. DeMaio J, Schwartz L, Cooley P, Tice A. The application of telemedicine technology to a directly observed therapy program for tuberculosis: a pilot project. Clin Infect Dis 2001; 33(12):2082–2084.

25. Greineder DK, Loane KC, Parks P. A randomised controlled trial of a pediatric asthma outreach program. J Allergy Clin Immunol 1999; 103:436–440.

26. Greineder DK, Loane KC, Parks P. Reduction in resource utilization by an asthma outreach program. Arch Pediatr Adolesc Med 1995; 149(4):415–420.

27. Forshee JD, Whalen EB, Hackel R, Butt LT, Smeltzer PA, Martin J, Lavin PT, Buchner DA. The effectiveness of a one-on-one nurse education on the outcomes of high-risk adult and pediatric patients with asthma. Manag Care Interface 1998; 11(12):77–78.

28. Kelly CS, Morrow AL, Schults J, Nakas N, Strope GL, Adelman RD. Outcomes evaluation of a comprehensive intervention program for asthmatic children enrolled in Medicaid. Pediatrics 2000; 105:1029–1035.

29. Pinnock H, Bawden R, Proctor S, Wolfe S, Scullion J, Price D, Sheikh A. Accessibility, acceptability, and effectiveness in primary care of routine review of asthma: pragmatic, randomised controlled trial. Br Med J 2003; 326:477–479.

30. Huynh T, Lavars C. Routine telephone review of asthma. Br Med J 2003; 326(7401):1267;author reply 1268.

31. McKinstry B, Heaney D, Walker J, Wyke S. Routine telephone review of asthma: further investigation is required. Br Med J 2003; 326(7401):1267;author reply 1268.

32. Abboud S, Bruderman I. Assessment of a new transtelephonic portable spirometer. Thorax 1996; 51(4):407–410.
33. Eccles M, McColl E, Steen N, Rousseau N, Grimshaw J, Parkin D, Purves I. Effect of computerised evidence based guidelines on management of asthma and angina in adults in primary care: cluster randomised controlled trial. Br Med J 2002; 325:941–948.
34. Cai J, Johnson S, Hripcsak G. Generic data modeling for home telemonitoring of chronically ill patients. Proc AMIA Symp 2000:116–120.
35. Biermann E, Dietrich W, Rihl J, Standl E. Are there time and cost savings by using telemanagement for patients on intensified insulin therapy?. A randomised, controlled trial. Comput Methods Programs Biomed 2002; 69(2): 137–146.
36. Smith SP. Internet visits: a new approach to chronic disease management. J Med Pract Manage 2002; 17(6):330–332.
37. Stanberry B. The legal and ethical aspects of telemedicine. 1: Confidentiality and the patient's rights of access. J Telemed Telecare 1997; 3(4):179–187.
38. Stanberry B. The legal and ethical aspects of telemedicine. 2: Data protection, security and European law. J Telemed Telecare 1998; 4(1):18–24.
39. Stanberry B. The legal and ethical aspects of telemedicine. 3: Telemedicine and malpractice. J Telemed Telecare 1998; 4(2):72–79.
40. Stanberry B. The legal and ethical aspects of telemedicine. 4: Product liability and jurisdictional problems. J Telemed Telecare 1998; 4(3):132–139.
41. Mair F, Whitten P. Systematic review of studies of patient satisfaction with telemedicine. Br Med J 2000; 320(7248):1517–1520.
42. Miller EA. Telemedicine and doctor-patient communication: an analytical survey of the literature. J Telemed Telecare 2001; 7(1):1–17.
43. Puskin DS. Telemedicine: follow the money modalities. Online J Issues Nurs 2001; 6(3):2.

6

At-Home Monitoring of Serial Lung Function Using Statistical Process Control Theory and Charts[*]

PETER B. BOGGS

The Asthma 2000 Group, The Asthma-
Allergy Clinic Center of Excellence,
Shreveport, Louisiana, U.S.A.

FAZEL HAYATI

Edgewood College,
Madison, Wisconsin, U.S.A.

DONALD J. WHEELER

Statistical Process Controls, Inc.
Knoxville, Tennessee, U.S.A.

Summary

Background: Over the past 6 years we have adapted the techniques of statistical process control (SPC) to the daily monitoring of peak expiratory flow rate (PEFR) and/or FEV_1 in the care of patients with asthma. The primary statistical tool is the Individual Value and Moving Range Chart (XmR chart), which integrates knowledge of the serial AM PEFR pre-bronchodilator values and their day-to-day variation together in a manner that enables the physician and the patient to make more informed decisions. This article introduces our adaptation of this statistical technique: the Functional Behavior Chart, so named because each chart provides insights into the function over time the system of care being monitored is capable of delivering. Case examples are provided.

Objective: Introduce the use of a simple and proven statistical technique to the monitoring of lung function in the care of patients with asthma.

---

[*]Software used to generate the charts in this chapter: SPC-PC IV Starter Kit. Version 3.21. Quality America, Inc. Tuscon, Arizona, U.S.A.

Methods: Discussion of methodology of using Functional Behavior Charts in asthma care and provide case examples.

Conclusion: The statistical analysis of serial lung function provided by the Functional Behavior Chart provides a perspective of asthma care not otherwise available to either patient or clinician through traditional run charting methods.

Introduction

Home Monitoring of Serial Lung Function

The home monitoring of serial lung function has been suggested as a clinical tool for several decades. Until recently, because of a combination of technical limitations and costs, it was only possible to measure peak expiratory flow rate (PEFR). However, several instruments are now available that make it possible to measure both PEFR and the 1-sec forced vital capacity (FEV_1) using inexpensive equipment that captures and retains data electronically (1,2).

Expectations of At-Home Monitoring

With the ability to monitor serial PEFR at-home came expectations that this would (i) permit patients to be full participants in their care; (ii) improve communication between patient and physician; (iii) help in the identification of inflammation-inducing and bronchospasm-producing triggers; (iv) link lung function measurements and specific treatment actions; (v) enable the prediction/early detection of exacerbations; (vi) provide a rational means by which to assess the effect of medication changes on lung function/asthma; (vii) permit the measurement of daily variation in serial PEFR; and (viii) assist in the diagnosis of asthma. Although the monitoring of PEFR has met some of these past promises to varying degrees, it has not been able to do so at the level of congruity needed to invite commitment on the part of either physicians or patients and is underutilized in patient assessment and care (3–23).

Why Lung Function Monitoring is Underutilized

There are several reasons for the underutilization of serial lung function monitoring in asthma care. (i) The current run charting paradigm (green, yellow, red zone concept) is incapable of predicting either an exacerbation or the risk of an exacerbation of asthma. (ii) This system has no rules governing what constitutes a statistical signal of change (*improved* or *reduced* function), leaving such to subjective interpretation. (iii) Confounding literature suggests that the monitoring of symptoms may be as effective as monitoring serial PEFR in predicting exacerbations of asthma. (iv) Patients do not regularly commit to the at-home monitoring of lung function. (v) There is a lack of enthusiastic acceptance of home monitoring by physicians. (vi) Confusion generated by a lack of agreement between published PEFR-driven treatment plans regarding the PEFR levels at which specific actions should take place. (vii) Many training programs do not emphasize home monitoring of lung function, and hence, send the message to physicians in training and their patients that such monitoring is not important. (viii) Because the traffic light charting methodology has become a *paradigm*, it is difficult to see beyond the boundaries and limitations it imposes (23,24).

A New Way of Monitoring and Interpreting Serial Lung Function

This chapter describes our adaptation (Functional Behavior Chart) of the techniques of statistical process control (SPC) to the at-home monitoring and interpretation of serial lung function (PEFR). SPC was developed in the context of interpreting serial data in an industrial setting (25–31). It is a thoroughly proven methodology that is easy to understand and apply. By examining serial data for statistical evidence of systematic process changes, this approach provides a way of separating the routine variation, which encumbers the straightforward interpretation of traditional serial data in run chart format, from the exceptional variation, which deserves special attention. As a bonus, this approach provides a reasonable approximation of the range within which future lung function values will fall given the continuation of the current system of care: the range of functional capability of the system. This enables risk assessment and invites anticipatory care rather than reactive care. Thus, by providing a framework for the analysis and interpretation of serial data, the use of SPC techniques makes explicit the potential of serial monitoring as an important part of the overall system of asthma care (23).

Because PEFR is the lung function test most accessible for at-home monitoring at this time, it is the focus of this chapter. However, our method can be used to serially monitor any lung function measurement (PEFR, FEV_1, etc.). We anticipate increased accessibility to simple, relatively inexpensive, and accurate FEV_1 monitoring in the very near future. Because the purpose of an XmR chart is to examine and characterize the behavior of the underlying process or system and because the behavior of interest here is lung function, we call our adaptation of SPC charts, Functional Behavior Charts.

The Functional Behavior Chart provides a framework for making sense of serial data. By means of a structured approach to analysis, this chart allows both the physician and the patient to identify changes in the patient's functional capability. Changes for the better can easily be identified with interventions or changes in environment, and causes of changes for the worse can be identified and dealt with in a timely manner. It is of note that an unintended consequence of the patient's involvement in collecting and applying the data has a powerful impact upon their commitment to the data collection process. We prefer the term *commitment* to compliance. By providing constant, instantaneous feedback in an easily understood format, the patient can see the effects of non-compliance in a graphic and dramatic manner.

Basic Theory and Terminology

The theoretical and empirical basis of SPC was introduced by Dr. Walter A. Shewhart, a physicist at Bell Laboratories, in a seminal book *Economic Control of Quality of Manufactured Product* in 1931 (25). His colleague, another physicist, Dr. W. Edwards Deming actively promoted the use of Shewhart's techniques for over 55 years (26). Primarily because of Dr. Deming's efforts, SPC has become one of the core tools of the quality improvement movement. It is interesting that although the theory and tools developed by Shewhart have been used worldwide in the context of improving the quality and outcomes of manufacturing processes for over 70 years, they have only recently been adapted to medicine and to patient care (26,28,31).

Concepts

Asthma Care as a System

A *system* is a set of inter-related dependencies that together produce an outcome. All systems are capable of producing exactly what they are designed to produce but no better (32,33). Each person's asthma care system is composed of many elements: causal agents, trigger agents, genetic abilities, environmental exposures, medications used, skills employed, avoidance measures needed and followed, need for and implementation of immunotherapy, etc., all of which interact to enable that person to achieve a given range of function. This range of function can be defined using a Functional Behavior Chart.

A typical Functional Behavior Chart (normal person, no asthma) is shown in Fig. 1. It has two parts: the X chart and the moving range (mR) chart, hence the generic label of XmR chart.

X Chart

The X chart contains the original data and is usually shown as the upper chart. It is the graph of the serial AM PEFRs measured during the observation period. The X chart can have up to seven lines: a central line and three pairs of lines placed symmetrically around the central line at distances of one-, two-, and three-sigma units. The three-sigma lines are the boundaries

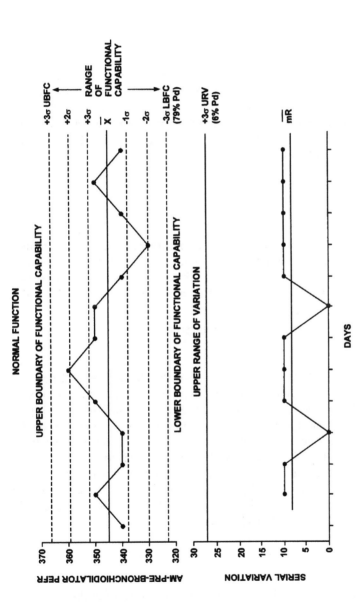

Figure 1 General structure of the XmR-type of SPC chart of serial AM-prebronchodilator PEFRs. In the context of asthma care, we call this a Functional Behavior Chart.

of functional capability [upper boundary of functional capability (UBFC) and lower boundary of functional capability (LBFC)]. The method of computing the values for these lines from the patient's data is provided in what follows.

mR Chart

The (mR) chart is the lower chart. It is a graph of the serial differences (variation) between successive pairs of AM-to-AM PEFRs. This chart has two lines: a central line that represents the average variation between serial PEFRs and an upper boundary for routine variation known as the upper range of variation (URV) limit. As the serial differences are, by definition, non-negative, the mR chart has a lower boundary of 0.

Baseline

To establish a baseline, the patient is asked to record serial AM pre-bronchodilator PEFRs for at least 14 days. These values are then used to compute the values for the reference lines described earlier. The formulas for these computations are simple, involving two averages and some multiplication, addition, and subtraction. While not absolutely necessary, software is available that will produce the charts and reference lines.

Terminology, Construction, and Interpretation of Charts

Sigma

The term sigma, used earlier, refers to a specialized measure of dispersion. This measure is computed in such a way that it will capture the routine variation without being unduly inflated by any exceptional variation that is present. For an XmR chart, this measure of dispersion *must* be based upon the mRs. It cannot be based on any other measure of dispersion. Specifically, it cannot be based upon the traditional descriptive standard deviation statistic. For Functional Behavior Charts, the appropriate way to compute sigma is to divide the average mR by the constant 1.128. This computation captures the routine variation in the serial PEFRs without being unduly inflated by changes in the clinical status of the patient.

Central Lines

The central line for the X chart is the average of the serial PEFRs during the observation period of the chart. The formula for calculating this is

$$\overline{X} = \frac{\sum X}{n}$$

where n is the number of observations.

The central line for the mR chart will be the average of the mRs. This is the average of the serial AM-to-AM differences between the measured PEFRs during the observation period. The formula for calculating this is

$$\overline{mR} = \frac{\sum mR}{n-1}$$

As n serial PEFRs will yield $n-1$ serial differences, the sum mentioned earlier is divided by $n-1$.

Upper Boundary of Functional Capability

This is the upper limit of the X chart. It is the upper limit of functional capability under current asthma care system. The UBFC value is three-sigma units above the central line of the X chart. It is calculated as follows:

$$UBFC = \overline{X} + 3\left(\frac{\overline{mR}}{1.128}\right)$$
$$UBFC = \overline{X} + 2.66\,\overline{mR}$$

Lower Boundary of Functional Capability

Of greater interest is the lower bound of functional capability (LBFC). This is the lower limit of the X chart. It is the lower limit of functional capability under current asthma-care system. The LBFC value is three-sigma units below the central line of the X chart. It is calculated as follows:

$$LBFC = \overline{X} - 3\left(\frac{\overline{mR}}{1.128}\right)$$
$$LBFC = \overline{X} - 2.66\,\overline{mR}$$

Upper Range of Variation

This is the upper boundary for routine variation in the serial PEFR values. It characterizes volatility in the functional values of the patient in the context of the current system of care. This limit is found by multiplying the average mR by 3.268.

$$URV = 3.268\,\overline{mR}$$

The reader is urged to consult the text references for a more detailed explanation and for the construction of process behavior charts (23,25–31).

The Range of Functional Capability

The *range of functional capability* is the difference between the UBFC and LBFC. This range serves as a guide to the range of function the current system of care each patient is following is capable of delivering. As long as there is no change in the system of care (internally or externally), the patient is not likely to perform outside this range: for better or worse.

Normal Population

We recruited 100 normal subjects who monitored PEFR every Morning, mid-afternoon, and bedtime daily for 14 days for the purpose of understanding the range of normal function for the various PEFR chart indices we were charting. Analysis of their 14-day serial AM PEFR data revealed the following:

1. Ninety-five of these normal subjects had an LBFC that exceeded 69% of their predicted and 70% of their personal best PEFR score. Thus, the 95th percentile of this normal panel had an LBFC at 69% predicted/ 70% personal best.
2. The average mR for these 100 normal subjects was 4.8% of predicted and 4.3% of personal best. As the mR characterizes the day-to-day variation, this value is important in determining when a patient's clinical status is stable (23).

Contrasting Functional Control and Chronic Predictability

The XmR chart characterizes the variation present in a sequence of values as being either routine or exceptional. *Routine* variation is characteristic of a steady-state process and is said to be due to many common causes (no one of which is dominant). *Exceptional* variation is characteristic of a system that is being affected by one or more dominant causal factors (also known as special causes or assignable causes) (23,25–31). As we will outline in what follows, the distinction between these two types of variation is useful in determining how to proceed in improving the system of care. The limits of Functional Behavior Chart allow characterization of the variation present in the serial measures of lung function. When a patient's PEFR scores display only routine variation that patient can be said to have a predictable range of functionality and the outer, three-sigma limits will define the range of functional capability for that patient. (Because that range of functionality may not be desirable, we must make a distinction between predictable functionality and clinical control of asthma.) When a patient's PEFR scores display predictable functionality, we can say that unless the patient's asthma system of care is altered (internally or externally), the current system of care will deliver measures of lung functionality that will continue to fall within the range of functional capability (the three-sigma limits), and the only way to achieve improved lung functionality will be for the patient and physician to change the system of care. Predictable functionality is characteristic of a steady-state system of care that has achieved all that it is going to achieve.

Exceptional variation in a patient's PEFR scores may be taken as an indication of both a change in functionality and a change in clinical status. Commonly accepted, statistically valid signals of exceptional variation are (i) a single point outside one of the three-sigma limits on the X chart or a single mR above the upper range of variation (ii) at least two out of three successive values beyond one of the two-sigma lines on the X chart; (iii) at least four out of five successive values beyond one of the one-sigma lines on the X chart; and (iv) at least eight successive values on one side of the central line on the X chart (Fig. 2).

Regardless of how exceptional variation manifests, it is always an indication of a change in patient status. This awareness of changes in status provides valuable information regarding events external to the care system or changes in the care system itseif. Signals on the high side of the X chart are signals of improved functionality. If this improved functionality is due to a change in the system of care, then we have evidence of its effectiveness, if this improved functionality is unexpected, then finding the assignable cause can be helpful in modifying the system of care. Signals on the low side of the X chart are signals of decreased functionality. The assignable causes of such detrimental changes will help the physician and the patient learn what to avoid. mRs that exceed the upper-range limit will indicate sudden changes in status that can be either favorable or detrimental. Either way, the Functional Capability Chart and its detection rules offer opportunities

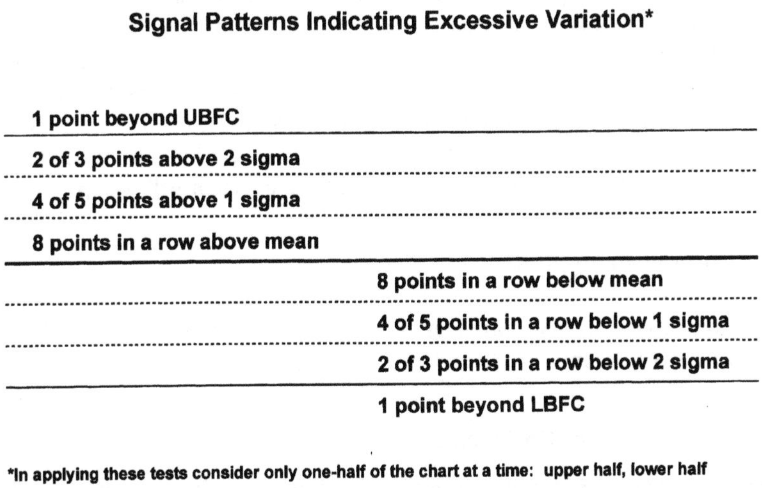

Signal Patterns Indicating Excessive Variation*

1 point beyond UBFC	
2 of 3 points above 2 sigma	
4 of 5 points above 1 sigma	
8 points in a row above mean	
	8 points in a row below mean
	4 of 5 points in a row below 1 sigma
	2 of 3 points in a row below 2 sigma
	1 point beyond LBFC

*In applying these tests consider only one-half of the chart at a time: upper half, lower half

Figure 2 Signals of excessive variation. *Source*: From Ref. 27.

for improvement, which can be easily missed using the traditional run chart display.

Functional Control of Asthma

When interpreting a Functional Capability Chart, we use the baseline of the normal subjects as minimal criteria by which to judge when a patient has achieved functional control:

1. No signals of exceptional variation should be present.
2. The LBFC must exceed or equal 70% predicted (PEFR) or 69% predicted for FEV_1.
3. It is preferable that the URV of the mR chart be <10% of predicted (PEFR of FEV_1). However, this may not be possible with some patients due to the increased variation that is characteristic of asthma.

We acknowledge that a larger sample of normal people must be studied to improve our interpretation and we are in the process of developing such study for both PEFR and FEV_1.

Acquiring Serial PEFR Data

Peak Expiratory Flow Rates

PEFR is measured as follows: the patient breathes normally and then executes a maximal inspiration followed immediately by a maximal, forced expiration. Breath-holding at total lung capacity prior to executing the forced expiratory effort from which the PEFR is generated, is considered unacceptable technique in our center (21,22). Each of the patients reported here consistently demonstrated correct technique for the PEFR maneuver.

PEFRs are measured every morning (within 15 min of arising) and *before* bronchodilator throughout the observation period. The best of three efforts is chosen and recorded. In this report, patients used the MiniWright Flowmeter (Clement Clarke). Patients were instructed on the proper use of the device and their techniques were checked on each follow-up.

Clinical Examples

Examples of how we use Functional Behavior Charts in the day-to-day care of people with asthma are found in Fig. 1–6.

Normal Person: No Asthma

Figure 1 displays predictable functional variation as there are no signals on the chart. The LBFC (79% Pd) and the URV (6% Pd) are at a level one

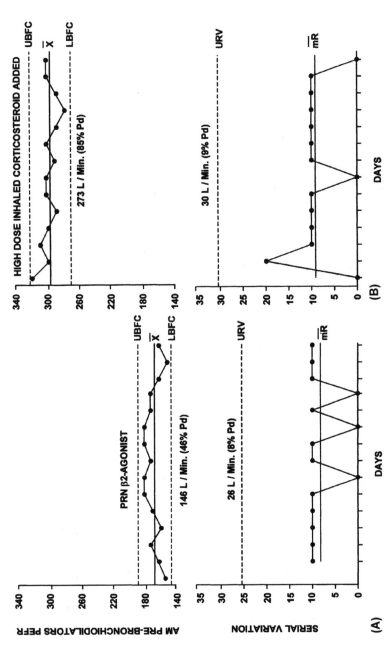

Figure 3 First intervention: (A) using prn β₂-agonist and (B) high-dose inhaled corticosteroid added with reduction in use of prn β_2 agonist.

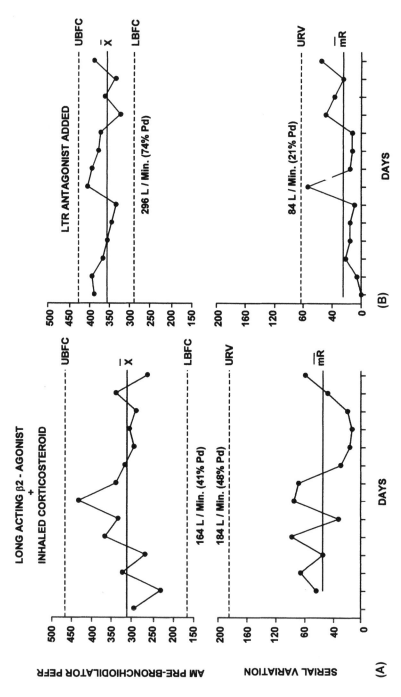

Figure 4　Assessing the addition of a third medication: (A) combination agent of long-acting β_2-agonist and inhaled corticosteroid and (B) addition of Leukotriene receptor antagonist.

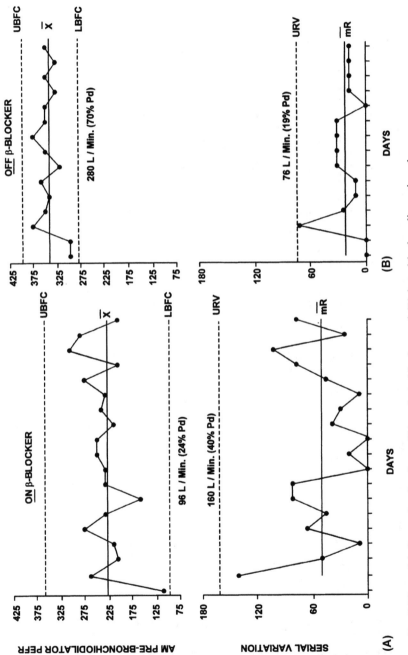

Figure 5 Differential diagnosis of asthma: (A) on beta-blocker and (B) beta-blocker discontinued.

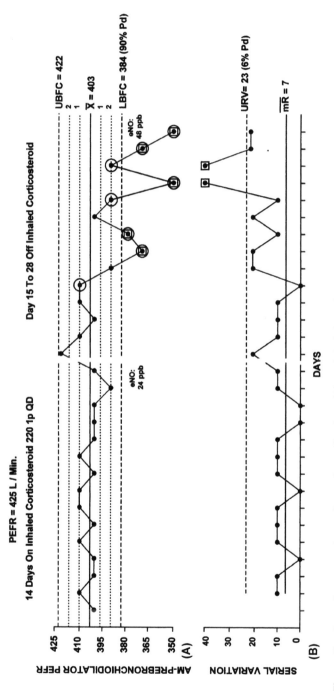

Figure 6 Assessing a step-down change in medication: (A) on-inhaled corticosteroid and (B) Off-inhaled corticosteroid. *Note:* Expired nitric oxide (eNO) measurements were made at the end of each phase.

expects to see in a group of normal people. The serial morning PEFRs charted suggest that this patient is functionally normal and not at functional risk due to the system of care being followed. Because no signals of excessive variation are present, the focus of improvement efforts should be on improving the general system of care.

Monitoring First Interventions

The functional behavior chart (Fig. 3) shows two periods of time: the baseline (A) and (B) a period following a change in the system of care the patient was following. During baseline (Fig. 3A) using only prn β_2-agonists, the patient was functioning far below normal (LBFC is 46% Pd). The variation between the patient's serial observations was not excessive (8% Pd). However, on follow-up (Fig. 3B) after the addition of a high-dose inhaled corticosteroid, the patient's function normalizes and the LBFC increases to 85% Pd and the patient's URV changes slightly to 9% Pd. As no signals of excessive variation are present, the focus of further improvement efforts should be the general system of care.

Assessing the Addition of a Third Medication

A patient after using a combination medication (long-acting β_2 agent and high-dose inhaled corticosteroid) remains dysfunctional at a level that is of concern (Fig. 4). A leukotriene receptor antagonist (LTRA) was added and the patient was monitored. During the period when only the combination medication was used (Fig. 4A), the LBFC was low (41% Pd) and the URV was excessive (48% Pd). Following the introduction of an LTRA (Fig. 4B), the LBFC improved to 74% Pd and the URV improved to 21% Pd. As no signals of excessive variation are present, the focus of further improvement efforts should be on the general system of care.

Help in the Differential Diagnosis of Asthma

A middle-aged female presented with cough and intermittent wheezing of relatively recent onset (Fig. 5). Her history indicated that a beta-blocker had been started 3 months before symptoms began. She was asked to monitor serial AM PEFRs for 2 weeks, then stop the beta-blocker. She was instructed to continue to monitor PEFRs until her revisit 2 weeks after discontinuation of the beta-blocker. During the time on the beta-blocker (Fig. 5A), her LBFC was low (24%) and her URV was quite high (40%). During the 15-days off the beta-blocker (Fig. 5B), she became asymptomatic, her LBFC improved to 70% Pd, and her URV began to normalize (19% Pd). The beta-blocker was discontinued and her cough and wheeze did not return.

Assessing a Step-Down Change in Medication

A gentleman had been asymptomatic on a low dose of inhaled corticosteroids for over 1 year. Because of this he was asked to discontinue the inhaled corticosteroid and revisit in 1 month, recording serial AM PEFRs for the 14 days preceding the revisit (Fig. 6). Here, we did something slightly different: we imposed the baseline limits (Fig. 6A) onto the follow-up data to see if a significant change from baseline occurred. As you can see (Fig. 6B), multiple signals occurred between day 15 and day 28. Do not be confused by the improvement signal on day 19: it is an artifact produced by displaying all the numbers from day 15 to day 28 on a single chart and the fall in function from day 20 thru day 28. The important information is in the multiple signals of deterioration seen between day 21 and day 28. Clearly, there has been a functional change in association with the discontinuation of the inhaled corticosteroid. In addition, his expired nitric oxide (eNO) was measured on day 15 of baseline (24 ppb) and showed a 100% increase on day 28 following discontinuation of the inhaled corticosteroid. The only reason we could identify for the change in function during days 15–28 was discontinuation of the inhaled corticosteroid. The focus of improvement was to eliminate the cause of the signals of deterioration by reintroducing the medication. It is of note that in spite of the strong signals of deterioration and the rise in eNO, he was *asymptomatic* when seen on day 28. This is an example of the charting information providing a clinical perspective not available from the assessment of symptoms.

Discussion

What Functional Behavior Charts can do for Asthma Care

Traditional PEFR serial run charting provides *nothing* that is not also provided by the Functional Behavior Chart. Both types of chart show the serial lung function (PEFR or FEV_1) values and the between-point variation. Moreover, both charts can be constructed to accommodate the simultaneous recording of symptom scores and medications used, if desired. However, the Functional Behavior Chart provides a perspective of asthma care not available to either patient or clinician using the traditional run charting methods:

- The limits on the Functional Behavior Chart incorporate and combine the information contained in *both* the serial lung function measurements and the serial variation into a useful characterization of the variation inherent in the system of care prescribed by the physician and practiced by the patient. Knowledge of the actual and potential variation inherent in the system of care followed is fundamental to the clinical management of asthma.

By making this characterization visible, the Functional Behavior Chart replaces a subjective evaluation with a picture that both physician and patient can use to make intelligent decisions regarding the system of care.

- The Functional Behavior Chart filters out the routine variation that always complicates the interpretation of raw PEFR scores and provides *patient specific, statistically valid signals* of any change in clinical status. Each such signal provides information about the direction of the change, the time when the change occurred, and the magnitude of the change in status—all of which are relevant to clinical decision-making.

- By allowing a patient's functionality to be characterized as being either predictable within limits or unpredictable, the Functional Behavior Chart provides the physician with a guide to how to manage the system of care. When a patient displays predictable functionality, but is not yet clinically up to the status of normal functionality, the clinical focus should be directed toward a review of the current system of care to look for opportunities to further improve care. When a patient displays unpredictable functionality, the focus is upon the identification of the reason for the changes in status, with the emphasis upon incorporating causes of improved functionality and removing causes of deteriorating functionality.

- The Functional Behavior Chart provides the ability to "see" the potential range of lung function that the current system of care is capable of delivering. This benefit, which is of immense clinical value, is not available with traditional asthma run charting. In particular, the Functional Behavior Chart provides warnings of potential exacerbations in two ways. One of these occurs when the LBFC falls below the level needed to effectively remove carbondioxide. The other occurs when the upper range of variation stays high even though the average PEFR scores are fairly good.

Thus, the Functional Behavior Chart facilitates asthma care in four specific ways: (i) It provides a visual characterization of the range of functionality that can be anticipated from the current system of care; (ii) it provides a way to know when the patient's clinical status has changed and provides information that will help to identify the reason for that change; (iii) it provides a way to characterize functionality as predictable or unpredictable, which is a guide on how to proceed with developing and improving the system of care; and (iv) it provides a warning of potential exacerbations in clinical status when the limits of functionality fall into danger zones. Each of these aspects of the Functional Behavior Chart enhances both patient's and physician's ability to meaningfully work together to improve the system of care. We call this general application as anticipatory asthma care.

What Functional Behavior Charts Cannot Do

- The Functional Behavior Chart cannot tell you what caused a change in clinical status, but when a change does occur, it can tell you when, in what direction, and by how much the functionality has changed. This enables more focused questioning and facilitates causal identification.
- The Functional Behavior Chart cannot anticipate a *change* in clinical status, but it can help you to anticipate clinical problems associated with poor or volatile functionality. Therefore, although the Functional Behavior Chart cannot tell you in advance when an exacerbation will occur, it can warn you that the potential for an exacerbation is present.

Unanswered Questions

Unanswered questions concerning the use of Functional Behavior Charts in asthma care include the following:

- Normal values: Functional Behavior Charts need to be developed on a sufficiently large sample of normal people to further refine the definition of normal functionality. Of particular interest in this regard are the LBFC and the URV for both PEFR and FEV_1.
- Formal clarification of information provided by Functional Behavior Charts in relation to that provided by other tools, such as quality of life questionnaires, symptom scores, spirometry, sputum cytology, eNO, etc., is needed.
- Do "which is best" comparisons detract from the larger question of how to get the most from each tool we use, as well as from the perspective they offer when integrated?
- Clarification of which signals are clinically most helpful and which least helpful.
- Diffusion of knowledge: how best to disseminate knowledge and skill in the use of Functional Behavior Charts to physicians and healthcare workers, as well as how to simplify the process for patients.
- How might Functional Behavior Charts facilitate commitment to long-term treatment programs by all involved in the care of people with asthma?

Conclusion

Good asthma care is about helping a patient achieve and sustain a system of care that is capable of delivering a range of functionality over time that is as near to normal as possible. To accomplish this, one endeavors to optimize function, to minimize the variation between serial functional measurements, to avoid taking action when action in not required, to take action when action is required, to focus actions more appropriately, and to anticipate the limits within that future function will fall given no internal or external alteration of the system of care. Although these clinical perspectives are not consistently available to either physician or patient using the traditional run-chart perspective, they are all available using Functional Behavior Charts. Good asthma care should not happen by accident.

Acknowledgment

Appreciations to Mr. Jim Wilson, Wilson Medical Illustrations, Shreveport, Louisiana for producing the graphics in this chapter.

References

1. Guidelines for the Diagnosis and Management of Asthma. Expert Panel Report. National Institutes of Health. Publication No. 92-3091, 1992.
2. Global Initiative For Asthma. Global Strategy for Asthma Management and Prevention. National Heart, Lung, and Blood Institute/WHO Workshop Report. National Institutes of Health. Publication No. 95-3659, 1995.
3. Redline S, Wright EC, Kattan M, et al. Short-term compliance with peak flow monitoring: results from a study of inner city children with asthma. Pediatr Pulmonol 1996; 21:203–210.
4. Melzer AA, Smolensky MH, D'Alonzo GE, et al. An assessment of peak expiratory flow as a surrogate measurement of FEV_1 in stable asthmatic children. Chest 1989; 96:329–333.
5. Malo J, L'Archeveque JL, Trudeau RT, et al. Should we monitor peak expiratory flow rates or record symptoms with a simple diary in the management of asthma? J Allergy Clin Immunol 1993; 91:702–709.
6. Clark NM, Evans D, Mellins RB. Patient use of peak flow monitoring. Am Rev Respir Dis 1992; 145:722–725.
7. Charlton I, Charlton G, Broomfield J, Mullee MA. Evaluation of peak flow and symptoms only self-management plans for control of asthma in general practice. Br Med J 1990:1355–1359.
8. Effectiveness of routine self-monitoring of peak flow in patients with asthma. Grampian Asthma Study of Integrated Care (GRASSIC). Br Med J 1994; 308:564–567.

9. Kliaustermeyer WB, Kurohara M, Guerra GA. Predictive value of monitoring expiratory peak flow rates in hospitalized adult asthma patients. Ann Allergy Asthma Immunol 1990; 64:281–284.

10. Li JT. Home peak expiratory flow rate monitoring in patients with asthma. Mayo Clin Proc 1995; 70:649–656.

11. Lebowitz MD. The use of peak expiratory flow rate measurements in respiratory disease. Pediat Pulmonol 1991; 11:166–174.

12. Beasley R, Cushley M, Holgate ST. A self-managment plan in the treatment of adult asthma. Thorax 1989; 44:200–204.

13. Neuhauser D, Headrick L, Miller DM. The best asthma care: a case problem in continuous quality improvement. Am J Med Qual 1992; 7:76–80.

14. Woolcock A, Rubinfeld AR, Seale JP, et al. Asthma management plan. Med J Austr 1989; 151:650–653.

15. Hargreave FE, Dolovich J, Newhouse MT. The assessment and treatment of asthma: a conference report. J Allergy Clin Immunol 1990; 82:1098–1111.

16. Chemlick F, Doughty A. Objective measurements of compliance in asthma treatment. Ann Allergy Asthma Immunol 1994; 73:527–532.

17. Garrett J, Fenwick JM, Taylor G, et al. Peak expiratory flow meters: who uses them and how does education affect the pattern of utilization? Aust N Z J Med 1994; 24:521–529.

18. Verschelden P, Cartier A, L'Archeveque J, Trudeau C, Malo JL. Compliance with and accuracy of peak expiratory flow (PEF) in asthmatic subjects over a three month period. Eur Respir J 1996; 9:880–885.

19. Malo JL, Cartier A, Ghezzo H, Chan-Yeung M. Compliance with peak expiratory flow readings affects the within- and between-reader reproducibility of interpretation of graphs in subjects investigated for occupational asthma. J Allergy Clin Immunol 1996; 98:1132–1134.

20. Mendoza GR. Peak flow monitoring. J Asthma 1991; 28:161–177.

21. Sly PD. Peak expiratory flow monitoring in pediatric asthma: is there a role? J Asthma 1996; 33:277–287.

22. Matsumoto I, Walker S, Sly PD. The influence of breathhold on peak expiratory flow in normal and asthmatic children. Eur Respir J 1996; 9:1363–1367.

23. Boggs P. Peak expiratory flow rate control chart: a breakthrough in asthma care. Ann Allergy Asthma Immunol 1996; 77:429–432.

24. Barker JA. Paradigms: the business of discovering the future. "The Paradigm Question". New York: Harper-Collins 1993; 147.

25. Shewhart WA. Economic Control of Quality of Manufactured Product. D. Van Norstrand Co, Inc., 1931.

26. Deming WE. Out of Crisis. MIT, CAES, 1994.

27. AT&T. Statistical Quality Control Handbook. Indianapolis, Indiana: AT&T, 1956.

28. Wheeler DJ, Chambers DS. In: Understanding Statistical Process Control. SPC Press, Inc., 1986.

29. Wheeler DJ. Advanced Topics In Statistical Process Control. SPC Press, Inc., 1995.

30. Wheeler DJ. Understanding Variation: The Key To Managing Chaos. SPC Press, Inc., 1993.

31. Wheeler DJ, Poling SR. Building Continual Improvement, A Guide For Business. SPC Press, Inc., 1998.
32. Senge P. The fifth discipline. The art and practice of the learning organization. Currency. 1990.
33. Forrester JW. Principle of Systems. Productivity Press, Inc. 1961.

7

Monitoring Adherence

SUSAN M. SAWYER

Department of Respiratory Medicine, Centre for Adolescent Health, Royal Children's
  Hospital, and Department of Pediatrics, The University of Melbourne,
  South Australia, Australia

It is often simply assumed that people with chronic illnesses such as asthma are adherent with their treatments. However, poor adherence has been repeatedly demonstrated across all disease types, treatment regimens, and population groups. A review of adherence of long-term treatments for life-threatening disorders reveals mean adherence rates of approximately 50% (1). It should therefore be no surprise that between 30% and 70% of people with asthma have been shown to be poorly adherent (2).

Poor adherence is more likely when the illness is chronic, when it is asymptomatic or characterized by episodic or recurrent symptoms, or when the medication regime is complex, such as requiring multiple medications or time-intensive behavioral interventions. As these features characterize persistent asthma, attention to adherence is strongly recommended as an integral component of clinical care.

There are major differences between the effects of prescribed treatments in controlled experimental environments when compared with their use and their effectiveness in the community, where a range of complex barriers commonly reduces adherence with the treatment regimen. There are multiple reasons, both inadvertent and more intentional, for this discrepancy between what is recommended and what actually happens. For example, the most frequently cited reason for inconsistent (or no) use of inhaled corticosteroids in one asthma study related to the belief that inhaled corticosteroids were unnecessary during asymptomatic periods: 62% of those who used inhaled corticosteroids inconsistently reported only using them when needed (3). Other major concerns relate to side effects, especially in children (4).

While changes made to the treatment regimen by patients may have little effect on asthma outcomes much of the time, impressive effects can be seen at other times. For example, an elderly person might inappropriately stop their twice daily preventer, thinking it is no longer necessary following resolution of their symptoms, only to find their symptoms recur over time. The parent of a child with asthma, fearful of potential side effects of inhaled corticosteroids on growth, administers a once daily dose instead of the recommended twice daily administration, even though it fails to sufficiently control their child's symptoms. A young adult with asthma may continue to smoke despite knowing that asthma is significantly worse with smoking. A young professional with asthma is "too busy" to see his or her general practitioner regularly for asthma review and continues to use a much higher dose of preventer than what has long been truly indicated, exposing them to unnecessary side effects. A single parent with severe asthma cannot afford the asthma preventer recommended by her doctor, and relies instead on cheaper reliever medication that achieves less than ideal asthma control. Another young man with asthma does not seek timely medical assessment of his deteriorating asthma and is hospitalized in ICU with an acute, severe episode requiring ventilation.

Poor adherence can thus have significant repercussions in terms of reduced quality of life to the individual and unnecessary costs to the health system. Progression of disease, exacerbation of disability, unnecessary prescriptions of more potent drugs with greater side effects, more frequent medical emergencies, and ultimately, failure of treatments can all result from poor adherence. Conversely, better adherence with an evidence-based asthma regimen, such as more timely medical assessment of acute asthma, more regular medical review of persistent asthma, more consistent preventer use or greater rates of smoking cessation will result in better asthma outcomes at less cost to the health system.

However, patients have complex lives and the potential benefits of adherence with the recommended asthma treatment regimen must be balanced by patients (not doctors!) against a range of factors, such as the financial costs of medication, less tangible fears of side effects, or even unconscious concerns about what it means to have to rely on medication. While poorly adherent patients are commonly blamed by health professionals for their poor asthma outcomes, understanding the patient's perspective and the extent to which they do or do not follow recommended treatments is central to understanding how adherence, and thus health outcomes, can be improved.

What Is Meant by Adherence?

The terms "adherence" and "compliance" are generally used interchangeably in the medical literature to refer to the extent to which a patient follows the prescribed health-care regimen. The association of compliance with blind obedience makes some people dislike the term, preferring to use the term "adherence" instead, which is defined as an "active, voluntary, collaborative involvement of the patient in a mutually acceptable course of behavior to produce a desired preventative or therapeutic result." (5) According to this definition, adherence in its fullest sense implies that the recommended treatment has been fully explained by the health professional and that there has been understanding, agreement and follow through by the patient.

Adherence as a term is most commonly applied to prescribed medications, however, it refers equally to the breadth of behaviors required for illness management. In asthma, while various asthma management guidelines have been introduced to guide health professionals' delivery of evidence-based care, the implementation of these guidelines requires a complex set of adherence behaviors by patients and doctors alike. For example, implementation of most Asthma Management Plans requires doctors to work with patients to use reliever and preventer medication where appropriate, avoid asthma triggers, arrange for regular monitoring of asthma, and to seek health care in an appropriate and timely manner (6,7).

Patterns of Adherence

Adherence is a dynamic phenomenon. People may be highly adherent with one element of the treatment regimen but less adherent with another. For example, an adult with asthma may be poorly adherent with his or her preventer medication, using it very irregularly, yet may consistently seek regular medical review. Alternatively, a teenager may see his or her doctor infrequently, yet remain adherent with the treatment regimen. The same person may be adherent with a particular medication or intervention at one time, but less adherent at another time.

Adherence has been shown to vary with the type of therapy, the severity of illness, the relationship with the health professional, competing life events, and the patient's own internal cost/benefit analysis. For example, the diagnosis of asthma may be associated with significant anxiety. As a result, there may be excellent adherence with preventer medication when it is first introduced. However, as the patient becomes less concerned about the diagnosis, or its symptoms, adherence commonly lessens with time.

There are many different reasons why people do not adhere to recommended asthma treatments (3,4). People may be unwittingly poorly or non-adherent because of misunderstanding the regimen, forgetting instructions, or simply forgetting their medication. On the other hand, people may actively decide not to take the prescribed medication because they feel better and believe it is no longer required, because of concern of side effects, fear of addiction, a lack of belief in the medication, or because of cultural beliefs about medication such as "less is best." Lask (8) describes three types of non-adherent patients: "refusers" who say they do not want or need a particular treatment; "procrastinators" who say they will adhere more in time, but just do not seem to get around to it; and "deniers" who will not admit to poor adherence even when it is obvious they are non-adherent. Commonly, however, people are simply busy and without regular treatment routines, find it hard to remember to do what has been recommended. This is particularly the case with medical appointments, where the use of appointment reminders has been shown to powerfully improve clinic attendance (9), even in high-risk populations (10). In these settings, "forgetting" is the most common reason reported for failure to attend (10,11), rather than more deep-seated resistance to prescribed treatments. However, the term "forgetting" is also an easy shorthand for a range of other more complex explanations.

How do we describe these variable patterns of adherence? Adherence is commonly referred to by clinicians and by the medical literature as a dichotomous construct—patients are either adherent or not (12,13). Clinicians most commonly use this construct negatively in referring to patients as non-compliant (13). In contrast, the medical literature commonly uses the term non-adherence or non-compliance to refer to any behavior that deviates from what has been prescribed. "Poor adherence" or "partial adherence" better describes the common patterns of variable adherence than "non-adherence", a term better restricted to those patients who are truly non-adherent with their treatment regimen.

Monitoring Adherence

There are a number of ways that adherence to medication can be monitored, both indirectly and directly.

Response to Treatment

Improvement following the introduction of a new treatment can generally be assumed to reflect reasonable adherence with the treatment regimen. However, as outlined in Table 1, poor adherence is not the only explanation

Table 1   Reasons for Lack of Treatment Response

An 8-year-old girl was prescribed inhaled corticosteroids twice daily using a MDI and spacer because of a long history of nocturnal cough, shortness of breath on exertion, and the frequent need of reliever medication. She was reviewed 2 months later, at which time there has been no improvement in her symptoms.

Reasons for the lack of response to treatment include:

1. Incorrect diagnosis.
2. Incorrect aerosol device use
3. Insufficient dose of inhaled corticosteroid prescribed
4. Poor adherence with the prescribed inhaled corticosteroid

   a. Non-adherence (e.g., prescription was not filled because of lack of confidence that medication was indicated, concerns about side effects of medication, etc.)
   b. Non-adherence (e.g., prescription was filled but medication was not taken at all because of lack of confidence that medication was really needed, concerns about side effects of medication, cost of medication, etc.)
   c. Poor adherence due to genuine confusion about dose (e.g., once daily was administered regularly instead of twice daily as prescribed)
   d. Variably poor adherence (e.g., due to lack of treatment routines, family holidays, improved symptoms with less commitment to treatment regimen, etc.)
   e. Poor adherence due to confusion about duration of treatment (e.g., parents thought it was alright to cease medication when symptoms resolved)

---

of lack of response. Clarification of whether the medication has actually been taken, in what dose, and with which device is always indicated when a patient is reviewed.

Health Professional Assessment

Health professionals commonly believe they can identify patients who are adherent and who are not, despite adherence behaviors not being specifically questioned in most consultations. Presumably, many health professionals are basing their assumptions on the response to treatment. However, our clinical assessments are also likely to reflect our beliefs that adherence is worse in particular groups, such as adolescents, or better in other groups, such as the well educated. This is despite the lack of evidence that adherence is determined by income, education, personality, age, sex, or disease severity. There is, however, evidence that aspects of denial, such as denial of illness severity, disruption to routines from personal or family crises, and depression are associated with poorer adherence. Health professionals generally overestimate patient adherence. In so doing, they fail to identify large numbers of poorly adherent patients. Indeed, it appears that health professionals identify less than half of poorly adherent patients (14).

Self-report

While patients and their families are experts about their own behavior, monitoring adherence by asking the patient how well they have been following recommended treatment is not as straightforward as it sounds. Patients may feel comfortable informing their health professional about the extent of adherence when it is reliable, but for a range of reasons, are less able to admit to poor adherence. Indeed, studies demonstrate that, like doctors, patients consistently over-estimate their adherence. For example, a study of adults compared self-reported MDI use with electronic measurement (15). One in five subjects who reported high adherence did not have this confirmed electronically. However, that 100% of those reporting low adherence could be believed is a very valuable fact in relationship to how we interpret what patients tell us what they do (or do not do). Self-reported adherence can be useful in particular contexts, such as when comparing the relative adherence of different treatments by a single patient. However, it is unreliable if detailed or accurate information about adherence behaviors is sought, such as in clinical trials.

Prescription Refill Rates

Primary non-adherence, the failure to fill an initial therapy prescription, is estimated to occur in 20% of all prescriptions written. This can reflect patient illness beliefs or problems of doctor–patient communication, such as lack of agreement with the explained rationale for the medication, or more straightforward factors such as symptom resolution and the belief, rightly or wrongly, that medication is no longer necessary. An Australian study of community prescriptions for inhaled corticosteroids demonstrated that only 72% of prescriptions were filled in those with mild persistent asthma, in comparison to 78% in those with moderate asthma and 89% in those with severe disease (16).

How long a puffer lasts can be a useful indirect indicator of medication usage. Clinically, this is particularly helpful in relationship to assessment of asthma control, where very infrequent replacement of reliever medication may be a sign of good asthma control. It can also be a helpful indicator of preventer adherence. For example, a 60-dose puffer should last for 30 days if one puff twice daily is actually taken. This approach is less helpful when people use more than one puffer of the same medication (to keep at work or school in addition to at home) as commonly occurs.

Biochemical Measurement

Biochemical analysis of blood or urine levels of a particular drug or its metabolites provides a direct measure of adherence with medication. However, these assays generally only provide an accurate picture of medication used within the past 24 hr, thus greatly limiting the practicality of biological monitoring over a longer period. The invasiveness of these tests, as well as the cost, further limit the applicability of these tests. Other issues to consider are pharmacokinetic variation and confounding effects, such as the effect of smoking on theophylline levels. Serum assays are available for theophylline, but minimal systemic absorption of inhaled asthma medications currently limits the usefulness of biochemical assays in most patients with asthma.

Medication Measurement

Medication measurement, such as pill counting or weighing residual medication within aerosol devices or puffers, is a direct measure of adherence. An advantage of weighing is that it can assess adherence over a longer time period. Another advantage is that it is relatively cheap. However, device or puffer weighing is not particularly reliable when patients know that adherence is being monitored, as in a clinical trial. For example, the study reported earlier by Rand et al. (15) compared self-report to both device weights and electronic monitoring. Device weighing was reliable in only 39% cases when compared with electronic monitoring. One reason for poor reliability is due to patients "dumping" their medication in an effort to make their adherence appear better than it really is. For example, in the above study, 14% of patients dumped medication by activating their MDI on multiple occasions in the 24 hr prior to the known return of their MDIs at their next clinic visit.

Counting Devices

Many of the newer aerosol devices, such as the Turbuhaler® and the Accuhaler®, have counters to count down the remaining available puffs within the device. This can be very helpful, especially for parents or carers, in identifying when a new inhaler is required. Parent monitoring of aerosol device counters is also useful to check how often medication is used. However, a limitation of counters to assess adherence is the common practice of individuals having more than one puffer of the same medication, or when children share puffers.

Electronic Monitoring

The advent of microchip technology has enabled small electronic monitoring devices to be attached to various aerosol devices to record very detailed information about their use. The most precise electronic devices record both the date and time of actuations, while others record only the number of actuations within a 24-hr period. Devices generally have a "rolling memory," continually recording adherence but only retaining data from the most recent period, such as 30 days, for downloading and analysis.

While these devices record actuations rather than patient use per se, the detailed data provided about patterns of medication use enable experienced researchers to confidently interpret these data (15,17). Major benefits of electronic monitoring include the capacity to monitor adherence over a period of time, the detailed data they provide, and the lack of requirement for active patient cooperation. These devices are not without limitations, particularly in cost, which currently restricts their use to research settings. Battery failure has been a problem with certain devices, although researchers generally report high levels of accuracy and reliability (15,17). While the main benefit of electronic monitoring is the detailed adherence information obtained, they do not identify whether the device is used correctly.

Why Monitor Adherence?

Understanding adherence with the health-care regimen is highly relevant to clinical practice in asthma, as well as having important implications for clinical research.

Why Monitor Adherence in Clinical Settings?

Knowledge of adherence behaviors in asthma can greatly influence clinical decision-making, whether in terms of the diagnosis or the ongoing management. Given the lack of strict diagnostic criteria for asthma, response to treatment can significantly contribute to the confidence about a new diagnosis of asthma. There can be many reasons for an apparent lack of response to medication, including an incorrect diagnosis (Table 1). Knowledge of whether a patient has actually taken the medication can help explain a lack of response to treatment, rather than question the underlying diagnosis itself.

It is less common for health professionals to reflect on the range of reasons for improved symptoms, as we generally assume that symptomatic improvement is due to an appropriate response to treatment. However, as outlined in Table 2, response to treatment is only one possible explanation for improvement. Checking with patients whose symptoms have improved whether they have actually taken the medication can be instructive! Understanding that symptoms have improved without medication can help get the diagnosis right as well as prevent the continued prescription of unnecessary medications.

Knowledge of adherence behaviors can similarly be used to influence ongoing asthma management. For example, a patient with good asthma control despite poor adherence could be expected to maintain reasonable control with a reduced dose of preventer, especially if better adherence could be achieved. In contrast, one would reduce the preventer dose more carefully in someone with good asthma control and good adherence. While

Table 2 Possible Explanations for Treatment Response

A 16-year-old young man was recently prescribed inhaled corticosteroids twice daily using a dry powder inhaler because of a short history of nocturnal cough, shortness of breath on exertion, and frequent requirement for reliever medication. He was reviewed 2 months later at which time there has been a marked improvement in his symptoms.

Possible explanations for the improvement in symptoms include:

1. Correct diagnosis of asthma, with improvement due to correct dose of inhaled corticosteroids, appropriately used aerosol device, and reasonable adherence with prescribed treatment
2. Correct diagnosis of asthma, but a larger than necessary dose of inhaled corticosteroid resulted in clinical improvement despite poor device use or variable adherence
3. Incorrect diagnosis of asthma, with correct device use and good adherence. Symptoms improved naturally (following resolution of post viral cough), rather than as a result of adherence with the prescribed treatment.

in this situation, good asthma control is likely to result from reasonable adherence, it may not. Reducing the dose of preventer medication will provide clarification.

Why Monitor Adherence in Research Settings?

Just as it is widely assumed that patients with asthma are more or less adherent, it is commonly assumed that subjects who volunteer for clinical research studies are particularly adherent. The foolishness of this assumption is immediately apparent when one reflects that the various studies that have detailed the extent of poor adherence have all been performed in research subjects!

Measuring adherence should be an integral element of both drug development and clinical research studies. Phase 1 and 2 studies of new drug development that aim to determine dose toxicity profiles and dose–response must be absolutely certain that any clinical effect accurately reflects the dose that was thought to have been administered.

It could be argued that monitoring adherence is less relevant for Phase 3 studies, especially double-blind studies, as these more closely represent the way in which medication is taken in the "real" world. However, research subjects are not necessarily representative of the clinical population in terms of adherence, albeit that they may be representative in terms of age and gender. Thus, adherence within these populations, and as a result, the potential effect size of the intervention cannot be assumed to be the same as in clinical populations.

How Much Is Enough?

How much adherence is enough depends on the disease or disorder, the medication or treatment, and the setting. Within research settings, 100% adherence is desirable in Phase 1 and 2 drug development studies where precise knowledge of effectiveness and toxicity profiles is required. Less than 100% adherence is better tolerated in Phase 3 studies, although how much less adherence is tolerable will depend on the particular drug and the disorder in question. Ensuring that adherence is approximately the same in both arms of a Phase 3 controlled study is especially important, especially if the study is not double blind.

The question of how much adherence is enough is more vexed within clinical settings. Do we expect patients to be adherent 100% of the time? Presumably, that depends on the severity and nature of the disease and the effectiveness and toxicity of the treatment in question. We might wish that transplanted patients were 100% adherent with immunosuppressive medications, however, poor adherence is also seen in these populations. Adherence rates rarely exceed 80%, even in clinical research studies that include life threatening and severe disorders (5). While most health professionals would not expect 100% adherence with asthma preventer medications, what level might we tolerate?

Most asthma studies describe good adherence to lie between 80% and 110% of the recommended regimen. However, what might this really mean? For example, an electronic monitoring study that reports 50% adherence with a twice daily preventer over the last month might mean that a patient has taken one puff a day regularly over this time. Or it might mean they took 1 puff twice a day for 2 weeks and no medication at all during the other 2 weeks. If group rather than individual data is presented, it could also mean that 50% of patients were adherent with twice daily medication and 50% were completely non-adherent. Both individual and group adherence data should therefore be interpreted carefully.

It might be argued that, regardless of the extent of adherence, that it is sufficient if the patient is responding appropriately or is stable. Thus, in people with asthma, the issue of adherence with the treatment regimen might be considered irrelevant unless patients have unstable or severe asthma. Certainly, there should be less concern of poor adherence in patients whose asthma is readily managed. Yet, this means we might not be concerned by the patient who in reality has mild-to-moderate asthma but, because of erratic adherence, requires a high dose of preventer to achieve reasonable control. Knowledge of erratic adherence would presumably be clinically important: more regular adherence of a lesser dose could result in equally stable asthma with less risk of side effects and at reduced cost to the health system.

Whose Problem Is Poor Adherence?

Attending to adherence in children is primarily the parents' responsibility. Adolescents gradually become more responsible for their own health behaviors as they mature through their teenage years. For young people, the line between parent reminders about medication and "nagging" can be especially tricky and warrants particular attention (18). However, regardless of age, the support of family and carers is an important component of good adherence.

What of health professionals? If we believe that poor adherence affects only a minority of people with asthma and that there is little health professionals can do to improve patient adherence, then we effectively construct poor adherence as the patient's problem (13). In doing so, it becomes easy to conceptualize people with poor adherence as irresponsible or irrational. In contrast, when we acknowledge that over half of the population is less than fully adherent with their health-care regimen, and that these people are in all likelihood just like us, it becomes easier to understand the different roles that health professionals can play in promoting better adherence with asthma treatment.

As adherence with asthma management guidelines improves health outcomes (19), it is clearly the health professional's responsibility to engage in adherence-promoting strategies. In this regard, understanding the extent of health professionals' poor adherence in relationship to evidence-based asthma management guidelines is highly pertinent (20), although beyond the scope of this chapter.

Monitoring Adherence Universally

The dynamic nature of poor adherence and our failure to identify those who are more or less adherent clinically suggests that strategies to improve adherence in people with asthma should be applied universally, rather than restricting these approaches to those who we believe have a problem.

An important starting point is to ask about adherence at every consultation. Simple questioning about what medication is or is not being taken is recommended as the first step, especially given the lack of consistency between what medications patients with asthma are taking and what their health professionals think they are taking. A non-judgmental manner using an information-rich approach is suggested, as described in the following scenario. Focusing on barriers to adherence, especially in relationship to medication routines, directs the orientation of the consultation from identifying problems to building solutions. Rather than the health professional jumping in to "fix the problem," working with the patient to help them identify their own solutions is the challenge.

Scenario. Non-judgmental questioning using an information-rich approach

You recently prescribed a twice daily asthma preventer for a middle-aged woman who has redeveloped symptoms of asthma in adult life, having had asthma as a child. She has been reliably adherent with her morning dose but very erratic with her evening dose of medication, despite her commitment to the treatment regimen. While her symptoms are much better than previously, her asthma is still not ideally controlled.

Example 1

Doctor: So, how are things with your asthma? Everything going OK? Any problems with your medication?

Patient: It seems to be OK. My asthma is much better than before.

Doctor: Good. Don't hesitate to see me in the future if you have any further problems.

This approach does not specifically question adherence behaviors. It does not encourage the patient to admit any difficulties with adhering to the treatment regimen. It fails to use an information-rich approach: her poor adherence with the evening dose has not been identified, neither have the reasons why she is adherent with the morning dose been explored. It is thus a missed opportunity to reinforce positive behaviors and to help develop more effective routines. The doctor made no firm commitment for regular asthma review.

Example 2

Doctor: So, how are things with your asthma? Last time we discussed how your recent symptoms were consistent with asthma and I suggested you recommence the same type of medication you used as a child, 2 puffs twice a day. Tell me, how have things been with the medication? Have you been taking any?

Patient: Oh yes, it seems to be OK. My asthma is much better than before.

Doctor: Good. But I know how easy it is to forget medication, especially when your symptoms start to improve. Tell me, which dose are you more likely to forget, the morning or evening dose?

Patient: The evening dose! It's a disaster! (laughs).

Doctor: What about the morning dose? How often are you forgetting that one?

Patient: I don't seem to have a problem there. I might forget now and again, but not much at all.

Doctor: Why is that?

Patient: I have a really good routine in the morning. I get out of bed, clean my teeth and take my puffer ...

Doctor: And at night? Do you have any routines with your medication at night?

Patient: (Reflects briefly) I've been working really late recently and I just collapse into bed exhausted. You're right, I don't really have a routine with the evening dose.

Doctor: Do you do anything regularly in the evenings. Would that make it easier to remember?

Patient: I clean my teeth in the evening as well. I suppose I should just take it then, like in the morning.

Doctor: Sounds like a good idea. I'd like to see you in 1 months time to see how things go, as your asthma is still not ideally controlled at the moment. I expect that taking the evening dose more regularly will make all the difference.

Notice that the non-judgmental and information-rich approach helped the patient admit less than ideal adherence. The doctor reinforced the positive routines around the morning dose and identified the poor evening adherence. The doctor helped the patient to come up with her own ideas about an evening routine. The doctor committed to future asthma review, providing a reason why. An information-rich strategy results in a slightly longer consultation which feels far more effective.

Other strategies focus on good doctor–patient communication, simplification of the treatment regimen, and regular medical review, as outlined in Table 3. While a detailed discussion of how to improve adherence with

Table 3 Universal Strategies to Improve Adherence

Focus on adherence at each consultation
    Clarify patient understanding and use of all medications
    Probe for poor adherence using a non-judgmental and information-rich approach
    Identify (or help develop) medication routines
Practice good communication skills (20)
    Listen to the patient's perspective
    Maintain interactive conversation
    Identify underlying worries or concerns
    Give specific reassuring information
    Reach agreement on short-term goals
    Help patients use specific criteria for decision-making.
Simplify the treatment regimen
    Minimize the number of medications
    Minimize the dose frequency
    Use the same type of aerosol inhaler as much as possible
Review regularly
    Use appointment reminders
    Review written asthma action plan

---

the health-care regimen is beyond the scope of this chapter, the range of adherence-promoting strategies should be conceptualized to extend well beyond the four walls of the health consultation to include school and community settings and the public policy arena (13). School-based strategies to improve the management of asthma in primary and secondary schools, community strategies to reduce the social stigma associated with asthma, government priorities in health care and research funding, and government policy in relationship to reducing environmental tobacco smoke exposure exemplify the breadth of approaches that will, over time, improve individual adherence with asthma treatments and result in improved health outcomes for those with asthma, both now and in the future.

References

1. Sackett DL, Snow JC. The magnitude of compliance and non-compliance. In: Haynes RB, Taylor DW, Sackett DL, eds. Compliance in Health Care. Baltimore: The Johns Hopkins University Press, 1979:11–22.
2. Rand CS, Wise RA. Monitoring adherence to asthma medication regimens. Am J Respir Crit Care Med 1994; 149:S69–S76.
3. Chambers CV, Markson L, Diamond JJ, Lasch L, Berger M. Health beliefs and compliance with inhaled corticosteroids by asthmatic patients in primary care practices. Respir Med 1999; 93:88–94.
4. Sawyer SM, Fardy J. Bridging the gap between doctors' and patients' expectations of asthma management. J Asthma 2003; 40(2):131–138.
5. Meichenbaum D, Turk DC. Treatment adherence: terminology, incidence and conceptualization. In: Facilitating Treatment Adherence. Plenum Press, 1987; 19–39.
6. Woolcock A, Rubinfeld AR, Seale JP, Landau LL, Antic R, Mitchell C, Rea HH, Zimmerman P. Asthma management plan. Med J Aust 1989; 151: 650–653.
7. National Asthma Campaign. Asthma Management Handbook. Melbourne: National Asthma Campaign, 1998.
8. Lask B. Non-adherence to treatment in cystic fibrosis. J R Soc Med 1994; 87(suppl 21):25–27.
9. Macharia WM, Leon G, Rowe BH, Stephenson BJ, Haynes B. An overview of interventions to improve compliance with appointment keeping for medical services. JAMA 1992; 267:1813–1817.
10. Sawyer SM, Zalan A, Bond LM. Improving clinic attendance in adolescents: a randomised controlled trial of telephone reminders. J Paediatr Child Health 2002; 38:79–83.
11. Conway SP, Pond MN, Hamnett T, et al. Compliance with treatment in adult patients with cystic fibrosis. Thorax 1996; 51:29–33.
12. Kettler LJ, Sawyer SM, Winefield HR, Greville HW. Determinants of adherence in adults with cystic fibrosis. Thorax 2002; 57:459–464.
13. Sawyer SM, Aroni R. The sticky issue of adherence. J Paediatr Child Health 2003; 39:2–5.

14. Steele DJ, Jackson TC, Gutman MC. Have you been taking your pill? The adherence-monitoring sequence in the medical interview. J Fam Pract 1990; 30:294–299.
15. Rand CS, Wise RA, Nides M, et al. Metered-dose inhaler adherence in a clinical trial. Am Rev Respir Dis 1992; 146:1559–1564.
16. Watts RW, McLennan G, Bassham I, el-Saadi O. Do patients with asthma fill their prescriptions? A primary compliance study. Aust Fam Physician 1997; 26(suppl 1):s4–s6.
17. Spector SL, Kinsman R, Mawhinney H, et al. Compliance of patients with asthma with an experimental aerosolized medication: implications for controlled clinical trials. J Allergy Clin Immunol 1986; 77:65–70.
18. Sawyer SM. Management of asthma in adolescents. In: Walls RS, Jenkins CM, eds. Understanding Asthma: A Management Companion. : MacLennan and Petty, 2000:262–270.
19. Gibson PG, Coughlan J, Wilson AJ, et al. Self-management education and regular practitioner review for adults with asthma. In: Cochrane Collaboration, ed. Cochrane Library. Issue 2. Oxford: Update Software, 2000.
20. Cabana MD, Rand CS, Power NR, Wu AW, Wilson MH, Abboud PC, Rubin HR. Why don't physicians follow clinical practice guidelines? A framework for improvement. JAMA 1999; 282:1458–1465.
21. Clark NM, Gong M, Schork MA, et al. Impact of education for physicians on patient outcomes. Pediatrics 1998; 101:831–836.

8

Monitoring Asthma Triggers-Allergens

EUAN TOVEY and TIM O'MEARA

Woolcock Institute of Medical Research, University of Sydney,
Sydney, Australia

Introduction

In 1873, Dr Charles Blackley published his classic observations that linked the aerobiology of pollens and fungi with the diseases of asthma and rhinitis. These studies had been initiated by observation that his hayfever could be caused during winter by inhaling pollen from dried grass (1). Such allergic diseases were uncommon at that time; now they are of epidemic proportions, with a prevalence of up to 40% in some populations (2).

To better understand the role that allergen exposures play in allergic diseases, it is necessary to define and measure that exposure. While an acute episode of rhinitis is an example of a simple dose–response relationship, these relationships become more complex in the real world of acute and chronic exposures to a range of different sized particles, allergens, and modulating agents. In addition, mapping these relationships to clinical outcomes involves exploring both gene/environment interactions and the acquired and innate immune systems. Central to all this research are the simple questions "what exposure is occurring, and what role is it playing in the disease process?" This leads to: "how can the agents be identified, characterized and measured in ways that are relevant to understanding the disease?" This process is iterative; only by testing ideas about exposure against disease models can the most appropriate ways be discovered. Although genomics and proteomics are revolutionizing our molecular understanding of many pathogenic processes, the important drivers and modulators of allergic diseases are the environmental determinants. Thus, defining and understanding exposure is essential for the development of better strategies for disease therapy, prevention and management. Some other recent reviews of monitoring allergens include Refs (3–5).

A Primer on Allergens

The Nature of Allergens

Most of the allergens associated with asthma and rhinitis are glycosylated proteins of molecular weight 5–100 kDa that are abundant in, and readily extracted from, inhaled airborne particles. Susceptible people generally become allergic following natural exposure to exquisitely small doses, repeated over months or years. At present, no unifying biochemical features of allergens are recognized and the allergic proteins include those that function normally as enzymes, recognition molecules and transport molecules. Some allergens have independent immune functions, while for others no function is yet recognized, for example the Group 2 mite allergens. While an allergen is generally defined by its induction of, and binding to, immunoglobulin class E (IgE), allergens stimulate a much broader immune response including via receptors on T–cells and to other antibody isotypes (IgG 1–4, IgA, etc.) (6). In some cases, the carrier particles are also recognized via innate mechanisms (7). All of the latter occur whether people are allergic or not, and are probably important in modulating the overall immune response to exposure. Finally, extracts from natural allergen sources, such as mite feces, may contain other additional, non-allergenic, components which will stimulate IgG but not IgE (8), or possess potent independent immune functions (9).

Common Allergens

Overall, allergens can be sourced from almost every corner of the biosystem plus a few synthetic molecules. For allergy diagnosis, although clinical history is helpful, objective confirmation of allergy by in vivo challenge or in vitro testing is required. Such allergy may be induced through inhalation, ingestion, injection, dermal exposure and even indirectly via breast milk and possibly the placenta. For reasons probably and partly associated with exposure factors such as timing and particle size, as well as disease pathology, allergens differ somewhat in their likelihood of being associated with asthma and rhinitis. As a broad (and dangerous) generality, indoor allergens that provide perennial exposure to smaller airborne particles tend to be associated with asthma, whereas large-sized carriers of allergens, such as seasonal pollens, are more likely to be associated with rhinitis (10). There are many variations and overlaps, and asthma and rhinitis can each occur without the other in some subjects or both can occur within the same subject, or may fluctuate.

Which allergies are common in a population is determined by what molecules are common in the environment, so the determinants include geography, season, type of dwellings, occupation, lifestyle, and social settings. Within a community, the majority of allergies will be to a few common allergen sources (e.g., mites, cat dander, birch, ragweed or ryegrass pollens), and for each of these sources there are some allergenic molecules that are frequently recognized: for mites, for example, Der p 1, Der p 2, and Der p 3, and other molecules that are infrequently recognized. Indeed, at a finer level, most people are allergic to a slightly different pattern of these individual allergenic molecules. This even extends to allergic identical twins, who do not show complete concordance for specificity of responses to individual allergens. This suggests that the major influence of genetics on allergy concerns the propensity to regulate total IgE production, and not the response to individual allergens (11,12).

The accepted nomenclature system for individual allergens (13) uses the first three letters of the genus, a space, followed by the first letter of the species, a space, followed by an Arabic number. The number usually indicates the order in which they were identified, but can be changed by consent to reflect homologies between similar allergens of different species. For example, the allergens Der p 1 and Der f 1 are the homologous Group 1 allergens from *Dermatophagoides pteronyssinus* and *D. farinae*, respectively.

Mites and Cockroaches

Globally, the single most common group of allergens that people are allergic to, are those derived from a few species of mites found in the dust of houses. This is a function of the ability of such mites to use our detritus as a food source and that our domestic microclimates often achieve a comfort zone which suits mite proliferation. In terms of inducing allergen, mite allergens are also extraordinarily potent, with up to 25% of a person's total IgE directed against a single mite allergen (14). This focusing of the IgE response is staggering considering that in a hyper-immunized animal, only ~3% of total IgG is directed against a group of different antigens. The main determinants of the size of mite populations, and therefore allergen level at a domestic site, are the proportion of the year that the site provides an "ideal" microclimate (~25°C and 75% relative humidity). Sites of colonization typically occur within a fibrous matrix such as a mattress, clothing, bedding, etc. and where the mite's diet of shed human dander accumulates.

Reviews on the ecology, international distribution, and different allergens of mites are found elsewhere (15–19).

Several species of mites are included under the commonly used term "House Dust Mites"; (16) however, this term does not always include some domestic species common in tropical regions (20,21). Globally, the most common are *D. pteronyssinus* and *D. farinae,* which occupy niches that differ slightly in diet and microclimate tolerance. Either species may be dominant, or share different geographical locations and it is necessary to know their occurrence to select the appropriate immunoassay for allergen quantification. At least 19 mite allergens have been characterized so far (22), and these generally share a high level of homology between species. The most commonly used assays for mite allergens are for Der p 1, Der f 1, and Group 2 (combined Der f 2 and Der p 2) allergens. Several polymorphs of Der p 1 and Der f 1 are known to occur (23), and one is known to include an epitope bound by one of the monoclonal antibodies commonly used in assays, and thus existence of this polymorph potentially confounds accurate allergen measurement of this allergen in environmental samples (24). IgE staining of thin sections confirm that several allergens originate in the mite gut (25) and have enzymic functions consistent with a role in digestion (26). The main carriers of mite allergens, to which exposure occurs, were originally described as the mite feces (27), although more recently it has been appreciated that numerous amorphous flakes, of a range of sizes, also carry some Der p I (28). The particles carrying Der p 2 may be smaller (29). Although mites colonize various sites, the allergens become ubiquitously distributed throughout houses. We have modeled that about 60% of total daily mite aeroallergen exposure occurs while in beds (30).

Cockroach allergens are important in some urban, domestic environments, and in tropical countries (see review (31)). At least three species are important allergen sources; these differ in habitat and ecological niche, and only share some allergens. Although the reported presence of the cockroaches, or their collection on sticky traps can be used as a proxy for exposure, measurement of individual allergens in reservoir dust is more reliable. The extent that these allergens become airborne remains controversial; while some studies have collected aeroallergens only after aggressive dust disturbance (32), another study, using the very sensitive "Halogen^{TM}" assay, was able to detect aeroallergen even when rooms were unoccupied (33). In heavily infested houses, the allergens become ubiquitously distributed, with the highest concentrations in the kitchen. Recent allergen avoidance studies with cockroach allergens have produced encouraging clinical results (34).

Pets

Furred animals, including cats, dogs, rabbits, and mice, are widely owned pets or feral companions that share urban dwellings and can be important sources of several allergens. In some countries, more than 50% of households report owning cats (35). While the major cat allergen, Fel d 1, and the major dog allergen, Can f 1, appear to be common to all breeds, it is less clear whether different breeds differ in the diversity and novelty of their allergens; certainly there are numerous additional cat and dog allergens. Allergen-specific immunoassays are available for Can f 1 (dog) and Fel d 1 (cat) allergens. Although the biochemistry and origins of cat and dog allergens differ, in both cases the aeroallergens are mainly associated with amorphous, dander-like particles. Because of their size and shape, the particles carrying pet allergens remain airborne much longer than those of mite allergens (36–38) and the airborne levels can be > 100-fold higher than those for mites (39). As a result of the airborne persistence of cat allergen, cat-allergic subjects can experience almost immediate symptoms on entering a house where a cat is resident without any deliberate dust disturbance. Not surprisingly, the main determinant of pet allergen levels is possession of the animal, but the allergen is readily transported from cat owners, whose house dust may exceed 3 mg allergen/g of dust, to non-owners through public routes. As a consequence, virtually all houses, independent of cat residency, have detectable cat allergens (>1 ng/g dust), as do schools and other indoor public places (40). As the majority of cat-allergic people do not own a cat, the level of incidental, private, and public exposure must be sufficient for sensitization to occur. We have shown that most aeroallergen exposure to cat allergen occurs in the living areas of houses and not in bed (30). In some U.S. inner city environments, particularly where exposure to mites and cat allergens is low, allergy to mice may be common, with sensitization in the population occurring even in the absence of observed mice (41).

The distinctive feature about cat and perhaps dog allergen exposure, that has only recently become apparent, is the complexity of any dose–response relationship. Several studies have shown that high personal and community cat exposure is associated with less cat allergy. The proposed mechanisms include "high-dose tolerance" (42) with accompanying deviation of TH2 responses to IgG4 (43) or possibly from accompanying high co-exposure to endotoxin. While children born into a cat owning family may have some protection from developing allergy and asthma, exposure of cat-allergic people to cats increases symptoms (44–48).

Pollens

Pollens are the male gametophyte stage of a plant's life cycle. Plants that disseminate pollen via the atmosphere (termed anemophylous) often produce large amounts of pollen, whereas those that pollinate via insects do not. Pollen grains are generally roughly spherical in shape, and vary in diameter from 10 to 70 μm depending on the species. The grains often have distinctive surface ornamentation (pores, channels, spikes) visible on microscopy, which aid their identification. Pollen grains will liberate allergens starting within seconds of contact with moisture and continuing for hours (49). During selected meteorological conditions, including thunderstorms (50), some pollen grains will rupture and liberate smaller allergenic fragments (51,52). On inhalation, these fragments may produce profound clinical consequences. In one such event (53), 215 of a local population of 55,000 attended the local hospital with asthma within 12 hr; of these, 31% had no prior history of asthma, only rhinitis. Thus, the clinical consequence of exposure to pollen allergens is not only the total quantity of exposure, but also the size of the carrier particle, which determines its site of deposition within the respiratory tract. During the pollen season, there may be independently fluctuating exposure to both pollen grains and smaller non-pollen carriers of the same allergens. The monitoring of such particles and the clinical consequences of such exposure over time has not been adequately explored.

Exposure to pollen is usually assessed by collecting and counting the grains; a technique that dates from the 1870s. The spatial distribution of airborne pollen changes with place and time (hours, days, and months), and there are now detailed pollen maps and calendars available for many geographic regions (54,55). These provide a generalized view of population exposure, whereas individual exposure may be highly determined by local sources and vary markedly between people in a similar location. Challenge studies have provided associations between doses, allergic sensitivity, and symptoms (56,57). While pollen exposure is associated with the outdoors, pollens do penetrate indoors and can seasonally peak in house dust (58).

Pollens elute numerous proteins, some of which function as allergens. These allergens differ between species and share homologies that loosely mimic their phylogenic relationships. What pollens are clinically important depends on the geographic location, and pollens that dominate as allergen sources include some grasses (ryegrass, timothy), ragweed, birch, olive, pine, and Parietaria. These may not necessarily be the most numerous pollens in an environment. At the level of simple microscopy, grass pollens all appear similar and are counted together, although their allergen content varies widely.

Where airborne pollen allergens, as quantified by immunoassays, have been compared to counts of pollen grains performed by microscopy, there is a surprising lack of concordance (59,60). This emphasizes the importance of non-pollen airborne carriers of these allergens and the confounding introduced by assuming all grains contain equal allergen. Measuring pollen allergens, however, requires that suitable specific assays are available, which may not be the case, and this approach is made more difficult by the diversity of pollens encountered in a single sample. One approach to overcome this has been to use pollen-specific IgE as the primary probe of "blotted" pollen allergens collected onto a solid phase (61). These techniques allow visualization of all personally relevant allergenic pollens.

Fungi

Fungi are the most enigmatic of the major allergen sources. While there is an extraordinary diversity of fungi, both indoors and outdoors, the majority of exposures are usually summarized with fewer than 10–30 species, see reviews (62–64). Sometimes, the larger sized spores (10–100 μm) have distinct physical appearances aiding their identification by microscopy, while smaller spores (2–5 μm) cannot be distinguished in this way. Here, identification relies on inspection of conidial structures (the shape of a group of spores in relationship to branching of hyphae) and/or culture and other techniques. These more recently include PCR (65) (see http://www2.ebi.ac.uk/ fasta3/ for sequences used to identify species). The sharing of common allergens within the diversity of species is dependant on phylogenic relationships.

The major distinctions of fungi from most other allergen sources are that the fungal allergens are largely the active products of the spores and hyphae (66) and thus allergen release varies with time nutritional and germination state and other factors. Secondly, fungi potentially contribute additional non-allergen components (1–3 beta glucan, mycotoxins, etc.) that stimulate innate immune responses and have a variety of immunological and biological effects.

Based on observations of the importance of germination in the production of allergens, we have hypothesized that "exposure" to a fungal allergen may be more a function of the extent of their germination occurring in the airways following inhalation, than simply the number of spores inhaled. Consistent with this is the observation that subjects with cystic fibrosis, who have impaired mucociliary clearance, are disproportionately allergic to fungi compared to other domestic allergens (67).

Almost all studies of exposure to fungal allergens have quantified the numbers and types of spores as a proxy for allergen exposure. Where measurement of both allergens and spores has been compared, a low correlation had been observed (68). However, the assessment of exposure to fungal allergens is confounded by the large number of allergens and fungal species that occur (which would require many different assays), and the relationships between the method of extraction of allergen and the quantity of allergen recovered. This area needs much more research. In addition, the quantity of fungal allergens collected in air and even in domestic dust samples has often been too low to measure by immunoassay (69). The domestic pattern of exposure to fungi has not been well studied. We performed one small study that showed that simultaneous personal exposure within houses was highly variable between individuals and was dependant on activity and dust disturbance (70). Whether greater exposure occurs indoors or outdoors, depends on the individual circumstances. As spores can be generated from both local indoor sources and penetrate into buildings from outdoors (more frequently with small than large spores), explaining high counts of small spores indoors requires parallel monitoring of outdoor spores.

The extent that observed mould growth is a reliable indicator of exposure is uncertain, see reviews (71,72). Certainly, questionnaires have been the basis of most clinical associations of fungi and asthma (73,74). Without confidence in the precision of single air samples, it is difficult to know the reliability of questionnaires. Recently, Chew et al.(75) found only a low association between the fungi present in the air and those recovered from domestic surfaces. A detailed study assessing the culture of fungi in dust concluded that measurement depended greatly on the method used and no single measure was reliable (76).

Occupational Allergens

Although allergic sensitization generally has its genesis during infancy, it may occur for the first time in adulthood, particularly in association with exposure to sensitizing occupational allergens. While IgE-based mechanisms are probably not involved for most low molecular weight occupational sensitizing agents, e.g., isocyanates, IgE-mechanisms are involved in responses to several high molecular weight proteins. This process may occur in combination with additional responses on co-exposure to non-allergens also causing respiratory symptoms, such as endotoxin (77,78), making identification of the role of allergens more complex. The common occupational allergens include latex (79,80), rodents and livestock (81,82), flour (83,84), and proteases such as amylase used in bakery and laundry products (85). Numerous more esoteric allergies associated with processing of plant or animal materials also occur; e.g., garlic, crab-processing factories, or types of agricultural mites used in biofriendly pest control. Not only is occupational asthma important from the perspective of occupational health and safety, it also demonstrates that becoming allergic is not restricted by the events of infancy, and that it may occur within the context of high coexposure to endotoxin (considered in some models to enhance "protection"). Occupational asthma, which involves more opportunities to study the time and dose of exposure, allows novel opportunities for the observation of the etiology of asthma. In occupational situations, the importance of measuring exposure is to define causal mechanisms and to develop and implement safer work practices, including primary avoidance.

Exposure and Clinical Outcomes

The role of Allergens in Generating Symptoms

The term "the allergic march" is commonly used to refer to the step-wise progressive effects of allergen exposure occurring over a period ranging from months to years leading to sensitization and clinical outcomes. (Others, noting the complexity of such gene environment interactions, have quipped that it is more a "long and winding road"). This march involves the production of allergen-specific -IgE, followed in a subset of these people by the occurrence of symptomatic allergic disease in the skin, nose and / or airways (see Ref. (86)). On allergen exposure, symptoms may be "immediate," that is within minutes, and or occur hours later—the so-called "late" responses. Cumulative, persistent, and subclinical exposure or acute high exposure may result in increases in nonspecific hyper–responsiveness or nasal "priming" lasting for days or weeks. Indeed, the different clinical events following a single and profound exposure to allergen occur over a timeframe ranging from seconds to weeks. Thus, at any time, it can be difficult to isolate the overlapping and cumulative effects of different individual events of allergen exposure, resulting in current symptoms. Much depends on the dose and particle size of the exposure and their immediate and long-term effects and the organs affected.

Defining Exposure

Much of the technical methodology, terminology, and thinking about allergen "exposure" has been borrowed from the well-established science of measuring occupational exposures. This evolved for measuring exposure to aerosolized particulates from coal, asbestos, metal oxides, heavy metal dust, etc. to establish disease risk and enforce occupational safety standards. While this forms a useful background, the technical requirements for occupational sampling and those for allergens differ. In developing occupational systems, much attention has been paid to the size fractions of the airborne dust, particularly the smaller particulates, and to overcoming the effects of the ambient airflows of between 0.5 and 5 m/sec found in occupational situations such as mines. Indeed, the proxy occupational "gold standard" has been a human dummy that, 20 times per minute, inhales 1 L of air through its mouth (equivalent of moderate work) while rotating on its axis in a wind tunnel with unidirectional and horizontal airflow. This is of limited relevance to domestic aeroallergen sampling.

Occupational concepts include the *inhalable* fraction, later termed the *inspired* fraction, representing the fraction that is removed from the ambient air, and the *respirable* fraction, which refers to those smaller particles that penetrate to the alveoli in the periphery of the lung. Samplers are compared to the *inhalability convention*, which describes an idealized convention for human harvesting of particles from the air. Other occupational concepts include *risk-relevant exposure measure* (the theoretical measure having a defined clinical effect), *the internal dose* (the amount that enters the body), and the *biologically effective dose* (the amount that interacts with a target site).

While occupational concepts are highly relevant to our thinking about the relationship of allergen exposure to disease outcomes, they have not been widely adopted in developing allergic disease models. This is due to the complexity and multiplicity of the clinical effects of allergens previously referred to, and their variability in size and allergen content, as well as host factors that modulate responsiveness. Indeed, in allergy, even the term "exposure" is often broadly and variably used to describe some weak and poorly validated proxy of what is actually inhaled. For example, the use in recent studies of allergen concentration in bed dust as a proxy for "exposure" to judge the clinical effectiveness of an intervention (87) would have been better served by using measures of aeroallergen. By better understanding the concepts of exposure, it should be possible to build more relevant models of their clinical effects.

The Morphology of Particles that Carry Aeroallergens and Their Clinical Effect

As described in the section on a primer on allergens, the airborne fraction of particles carrying the allergens of mites, cats, and cockroaches occur in a range of differently sized particles of different origins. What is present in the air at any time is the dynamic result of the generation and removal of such airborne particles. The majority of mite allergen settles over ~15 min, indicating that most is associated with relatively large particles, whereas a greater proportion of cat allergen remains airborne longer after disturbance, indicating more is associated with smaller, more buoyant, particles. Mechanisms in addition to gravitational settling affect the net loss of particles from the air. These include indoor air velocity, electrostatic charge, surface roughness, Brownian motion, and resuspension from multiple interior surfaces, as well as the additional generation of new aerosols. This phenomenon is complex and poorly understood. This is illustrated by the theoretical terminal settling velocities of particles of diameter 1, 5, and 20 µm being calculated as 0.072, 0.47, and 5.4 m/hr, respectively, while their observed deposition velocities (defined as the estimated net removal from the air), as derived from empirical data, are 0.13, 2.8, and 43 m/hr, respectively (88,89).

Information on apparent particle sizes of carriers of different allergens is contained in the following papers: mite (90–93) cat (30,38,91,94–96) dog (96,98) cockroach (32,99) and rodent (92,100). Pollen grains and fungal spores vary with the species.

Allergen-bearing particles may not exhibit "ideal" behavior, even including the concept of "effective aerodynamic diameter". Using cascade impaction sampling (which sorts particles according to aerodynamic size) combined with Halogen assay (which enables the visualization of particles carrying allergens on the cascade stages), we found that particles carrying mite and cat allergens are often associated with amorphous and flake–like particles that were distributed over a range of stages of a size selective impaction sampler—and not as predicted from their apparent diameter (96). How such nonideal particles behave in turbulent airflow in an airway during inhalation is unknown.

The aerodynamic size of the particles carrying allergen dictates their probable site of deposition in either the nose or lungs, which may in turn determine the clinical outcomes of acute and chronic exposure. Although there is no unified interpretation, numerous observations suggest that it is important. These include:

- The occurrence of "thunderstorm asthma" demonstrates marked, adverse, and both acute and persistent clinical consequences of "small particle" natural pollen allergen exposure, including in people with no prior history of asthma (53). While this generally is observed during springtime meteorological outflows that burst pollen grains, it may also occur on a smaller scale at other times under less dramatic conditions (52).
- The dose-dependent induction of asthma in cat-allergic subjects soon after entering a house where a cat is resident is attributable to small particles carrying cat allergen remaining airborne (101,102). Anecdotally, this does not occur when mite-allergic subjects enter a house with high mite allergen levels. The latter may, however, recall symptoms following major dust raising activity, such as handling stored clothing, emptying vacuum cleaners, etc.
- Clinical challenge with differently sized aerosols shows ~20-fold greater asthmatic response to challenge with same quantity of allergen when carried by 10.3 μm droplets compared to 1.4 μm droplets (103). This suggests that high concentrations at a few sites in the upper airways may be more important in inducing immediate symptoms than the same amount of allergen being more widely and deeply distributed.

Repeated laboratory challenge with sub-clinical doses of aerosolized allergen, too low to generate immediate symptoms, may increase airways hyper–responsiveness (104). This underscores the difficulty of measuring the immediate clinical outcomes of chronic exposure to small particles carrying allergens. It is unclear whether the increase in airways hyper-responsiveness that occurs following chronic natural exposure to allergens

(105), (or the decreases in airways hyperresponsiveness (AHR) following reduction in exposure (106), is a consequence of a high proportion of small particles or a low proportion of large particles entering the lung (90).

In summary, the size of particles carrying natural aeroallergens is likely to have a profound impact on the subsequent clinical effects, but this had not yet been incorporated into models of allergen exposure.

Thresholds of Exposure and Occupational Exposure Limits

The term "threshold" is used to describe an amount of exposure at which a biologically relevant event is detected, and below which there is no observed effect. Thresholds for mite allergens as originally proposed, were a concentration of 2 µg of Der p 1 / g of bed dust being associated with an increased prevalence of sensitization, and 10µg of Der p 1 / g of dust was associated with an increased risk of symptoms of acute asthma. These were calculated as the equivalent to an earlier proposition of 100 and 500 mites / g of dust (107). These levels became widely popular and are still cited, despite the Third International Workshop on Indoor Allergens, held in 1995, no longer supporting them (19). Although numerous studies supported these thresholds, it also became apparent that numerous others did not, e.g., (108,109). An interesting analysis relating cumulative exposure (mg/g × years) vs. community prevalence of sensitization has also been developed (110). Within a population, if there was a relationship, it was more likely sigmoidal in shape, than a threshold "step", and additionally was modulated by genetic susceptibility (111). It was even more difficult to demonstrate an association between asthma symptoms and mite allergen concentration (112).

Equivalent threshold values for cat (8 µg Fel d 1/g) (113), dog (10 µg/g) (114), and cockroach (Bla g 2 µg/g) (113) allergens have also been proposed, as well as occupational thresholds (115). However, while the values serve as useful markers of what constitutes a lower boundary of high exposure on a global scale, they are not explicit clinical predictors for individuals. More recently the proposed levels have been usefully applied to define the cutoff between exposure and nonexposure when examining synergistic effects of allergens, sensitization, and viruses for an association with risks for hospital admissions (116) or with exposure and sensitization, for asthma severity (117).

More recently, in some quarters, the pendulum of etiological interest has swung away from the concept that allergens play a major role in asthma causation, and has pointed instead to possible roles for neutrophils and innate mechanisms (as opposed to eosinophils and T-cell-IgE-based mechanisms) in both promoting and modulating the expression of asthma (118,119). While profound asthma can occur in the absence of any detectable allergy; such, allergy is also a frequent and associated feature of asthma in many people, particularly children. Only refinement of our understanding of both exposure and the molecular mechanisms of asthma will progress this.

Dose–Response Relationships

The pathways involved in both asthma and rhinitis that involve exposure to aeroallergens are presumed, at least in part, to be dose–dependent. These include:

1. The specificity of this response is defined by allergen–specific IgE, and allergen exposure is a prerequisite for sensitisation to a specific allergen.
2. As well as quantity, the timing of this exposure influences the likelihood of sensitization.
3. Subsequent allergen exposure of a sensitized person may have a variety of effects, including the generation of acute symptoms and chronic inflammatory changes or no apparent symptoms but chronic inflammatory changes.
4. The effects of accumulated chronic exposure over extended periods are even less well characterized, but may include irreversible changes to airway modeling (120,121) or expression of genes (120,122,123).

Although the currently recognized factors that influence an individual's risk of becoming allergic, or expressing asthma, focus on genes, early exposure and lifestyle, even identical twins, who share both genes and environment, are only moderately concordant for these outcomes and presumably other influences occur (124).

Issues that remain and confound include the following:

- Only subset of the population is likely to be affected by allergen exposure and their predisposition is a complex function of genetic susceptibility to sensitization and asthma phenotype, the involvement of multiple genes as well as environmental, timing, disease-history and lifestyle factors that modulate the focus of the immune system, and lung development, particularly during infancy.
- There is a variety of clinical outcomes and each may differ in the nature of chronic and acute aeroallergen exposure required. These outcomes include: sensitisation, development of hyper-responsive airways, maintenance of hyper-responsive airways, and acute symptoms of asthma.
- Much data on the relationship of allergen exposure to asthma outcomes has been developed with measurements of allergen concentrations in dust collected from a single site at a single time. This provides only a weak estimate for the actual total and

inhaled exposure of individuals and does not include any recognition of the size of the particles carrying allergens, the effects of timing, of non-allergen co-exposures and other variables.

- The relationship of exposure to outcomes probably differs between allergens: early exposure to high amounts of cat and perhaps dog may exert a protective effect on the development of sensitization and perhaps asthma, whereas late exposure does not. No such effects have been shown for mite or cockroach allergens. High fungal exposure may exert a nonspecific effect, increasing other allergies (125).
- There is a lack of quantitative human data examining dose–response relationships in sensitized subjects. This is in contrast to the surfeit of studies of human exposure to irritants and gases, or of mice to allergens. With the exception of a few isolated challenges with natural allergen sources (mainly with cat, pollen, and fungi), there has been little attempt to understand the pathological basis for variation between the responses to increases or decreases in allergen exposure of individuals.
- While asthma has close associations with atopy, the disorder comprises a spectrum of phenotypes involving different pathophysiological process. Many exacerbations may be triggered by non-allergens, e.g., viruses, although these may be dramatically increased by concurrent atopy and allergen exposure (116).

With occupational allergens, the difficulties of defining dose–response relationships become acute, as such sensitization can affect careers and defining standards for exposure may incur legal liabilities. Although limits have been proposed (115,126,127), they have not been widely adopted. Despite the aforementioned technical shortcomings (lack of standardization of sampling methods, protocols and assays, data expression, paucity of information linking "relevant" exposure to outcomes, individual susceptibility, etc.), the identification of standards to enforce protection of workers remains a priority.

Other Non–Allergen Airborne Components Involved in Respiratory Diseases

It needs to be recognized that airborne exposure to allergens usually occurs in parallel to exposure to numerous other gaseous and particulate materials, particularly micro-organisms, which may have independent or synergistic effects with allergens. Douwes et al. (128) have provided a comprehensive and recent overview. These components include, but are not limited to:

1. *Endotoxin*: These are a group of lipopolysacchrides (LPS) derived from the cell walls of all Gram–negative bacteria. Such exposure

is also considered as a proxy for more general microbial exposure, including CpG motifs (129), which are more generally associated with bacteria and have potent immunostimulatory properties. Endotoxins have profound inflammatory properties and high exposure is specifically associated with some occupational respiratory diseases, such as in swineries. However, there is also data that exposure to high levels of endotoxin in infancy may protect against the later development of allergic disease, albeit while increasing nonallergic wheeze. Endotoxins are usually measured using a LAL assay [numerous assays are available, with Bio-Whittaker QCL-1000 (Walkersville, Maryland, U.S.A.) being widely used] or more recently by a chromogenic assay using recombinant Factor C (130) also from Bio–Whittaker. Large variations in exposure assessment between laboratories have been reported (131), and numerous technical issues remain to be standardized or overcome.

2. *1–3 beta glucans*: These are mainly derived from fungal walls, although other microbial sources occur. They are recognized to be inflammatory, although the role in allergies and asthma is uncertain, partly due to confounding by co-exposures.

3. *Environmental causes of idiopathic rhinitis*: In a large subgroup of patients with negative allergy tests, nasal challenge with allergen can result in significant symptoms (132) suggesting either unrecognized allergic disease or non-allergic mechanisms are involved. Non-allergen components of mite extracts also trigger NO responses (9). The environmental, but non-allergic, triggers of both asthma and rhinitis have not been widely explored.

Measuring Exposure to Allergens

There are numerous and complex issues to be considered prior to embarking on a plan to sample and measure allergens. Table 1 identifies issues previously raised for developing a strategy for occupational sampling (133), which are considered here for allergens, in order to assist in rationalizing decisions.

Methods of Collecting Reservoir Allergen Sources

Reservoir Samples (Settled Dust)

The quantity of allergen in dust recovered from reservoir items, such as bedding, carpets, soft furniture, is commonly used as a surrogate for exposure. Dust reservoirs are usually chosen on the basis of their proximity to the person, their capacity to function as relevant sources of aeroallergens, and that they

Table 1 Items to Consider Prior to Embarking on a Program to Sample Allergens. There is no Single Standard Way to Perform Such Sampling Nor the Associated Assays and Numerous Precedents Occur. In Addition to the Practical Considerations, There Are Limitations On The Clinical Application of the Information Obtained

Issues	Aspects to consider in study design
Why sample?	Assessment of risk, identify causes of symptoms, relate exposures to outcomes (allergy, symptoms), assess an intervention, clarification of disease model, epidemiological study
What level of approach?	The type of information is required; the level of allergen specificity, whether allergens are to be quantified or identified, what is feasible within practical constraints (budget, time, access, etc.), what assays to use and their detection limits
What to measure?	Airborne (volumetric, inhaled, static, personal, or settling), total mass or size fractionated or reservoir samples, settling (Petri) dust. Single allergens, multiple allergens, total allergens, nonallergen contributors/modulators
Whose exposure should be measured?	Decide to what extent an individual's exposure is a proxy for other people, whether a group of individuals is a proxy for community
Where to collect the sample?	Multiple or single sites in room, different rooms, indoor and outdoor, plus as above—static or personal sampling
When to measure?	Dependence of symptoms on timing of exposure (early and late responses), likely temporal changes in exposure over timeframes of minutes, hours, season
How long to sample for?	Chronic or acute exposure; whether to collect separate samples for each exposure event or integrate these within a sample; what is known about the time-course of exposure
How many measurements?	How accurate an assessment is any single measurement of "relevant" exposure? What is the variance, how many samples are required, and is it practical to collect?
How often to sample?	What frequency along some time-course, what is the effect of season, interventions, changes in the subject's environment
What to do with the data?	Options for units for expression of data
What to record?	Establish data recording of additional information; why, when, and where and any other circumstances involved, as these get lost as a study progresses

<u>Factors affecting loss and generation of aeroallergen from reservoirs</u>
Presence of sources in the room
Different reservoirs in the room
    quantity of allergen
    concentration of allergen
    3D distribution of allergen
Intensity of disturbance of sources
Interaction of dust and surface
    texture, electrostatics
Air movement
    thermal, mechanical
Mechanical removal of dust from room
Rate of biological breakdown of allergen
Aeroallergen sources outside the room
    ventilation between rooms
    penetration of outside air

Figure 1 Some factors that affect the loss and generation of particles from reservoir sources within a room and from outside a room.

will contain sufficient allergenic dust to assay. Some of the factors involved in the generation of aeroallergens from reservoirs are shown in Fig. 1.

The nature and quantity of the dust recovered from these sites varies, in part, depending on details of the sampling procedure. The First Mite Workshop outlined a standardized protocol, and expanded on this in the Second Workshop (134). These guidelines were not exhaustive and many studies use variations that have an unknown influence on the outcome. The area used for collection is usually $2\,m^2$ for mattress and bedding, and $1\,m^2$ for carpet and other soft items, and these are usually sampled for a fixed time (2 min). The power of the vacuum cleaner can make a difference (135), and this has not been standardized. Dust is usually sieved (400 μm) to obtain a fine fraction, although this practice is not followed in some studies. Extraction buffers, times, and temperatures vary, and each of these influences the recovery of mite allergen (136). The assay standard used also differs (137). The influence of the immunoassay is discussed elsewhere.

It has been shown repeatedly that the concentration of allergen in dust collected from different locations of a surface may have wide variations over short distances and over time (138–140) and collection of multiple samples is recommended. Marks et al. provided estimates of numbers of samples required to show differences in allergen between population groups.

There is also variation in the ways that data for reservoirs are expressed. For indoor allergens, data are usually expressed in units of μg of allergen/g of original or of sieved dust, following the earlier practice of reporting mite populations in mites/g of dust. For some purposes, such as assessing an intervention, or with some research groups, μg of allergen per unit area is used (141). Expression as μg/g is important in studies where the "biological richness" of the dust is of interest, such as relating allergen levels to microclimate or the number of cats in a house. In other cases, for example, when a powdered acaricide is added to carpets and which dilutes any existing dust and automatically results in a reduction in concentration, μg/area is more appropriate. Decisions as to the appropriate unit become more difficult where an intervention is involved, such as addition of an encasing. Here, the quantity of dust that can be recovered declines dramatically, while the concentration in μg/g declines by much less. Expression of this outcome in μg of allergen/area, which is the product of these, indicates dramatic reductions. Thus, the extent that reservoirs (however expressed) can act as proxies for actual exposure becomes increasingly unreliable and in these circumstances, in our view, only collection of airborne antigen can indicate the true benefit of the intervention. Incidentally, when aeroallergen is measured, the benefit of encasings is small, compared to changes in reservoirs (142). In our experience, μg/g correlates better with aeroallergen than μg/area (143). All these factors need to be taken into account when comparing data between different laboratories.

In our group, for epidemiological field studies, we use a battery-powered vacuum cleaner for convenience, whereas for intervention studies, where the quantity of recovered dust may be small, we use a mains-powered model. To help account for spatial variation in allergen on floors, we sample several smaller sites to make up the total area (144). Dust is collected near the nozzle of the cleaning head, in two tapered nylon bags each of surface area $\sim$50 cm^2 held in series: the first has pores of 0.5 mm and this coarse fraction is discarded; the second bag has pores of 20 μm and this constitutes the "fine" dust fraction used for analysis. Extracts are usually stored frozen before analysis, and this results in a small loss of allergen.

Swabs and Cloth Samplers

An alternative to collection of reservoir samples by vacuuming is to collect dust using wipe cloths, swabs, or adhesive tape. This method is commonly used for domestic pesticides and lead, but has only seldom been used for allergen. These are illustrated in the upper panels of Fig. 2. We have used a small paint roller to collect surface dust by covering the roller with adhesive tape and then rolling it on the surfaces. Some types of electrostatic dust-cleaning cloths can also be integrated into a simple, portable, and convenient device for patients to self-collect samples (Sercombe, in preparation).

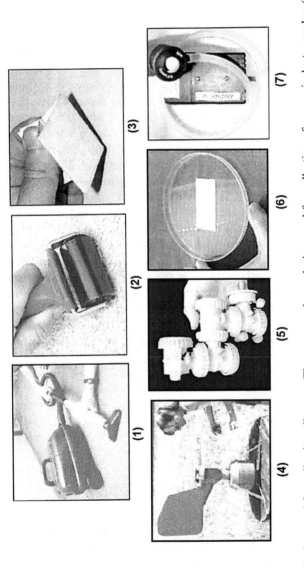

Figure 2 Devices used for collecting allergens. The top row shows devices used for collection of reservoir dust samples: (1) a vacuum cleaner, in this case fitted with a collection device attached directly to the nozzle, (2) a roller sampler coated with adhesive tape, and (3) an electrostatic cloth sampler, which can be rubbed by hand on surfaces to collect dust samples. The bottom row shows devices used for the collection of aeroallergen samples: (4) a Burkard spore trap in use in the field to sample spores and pollens, (5) a Cascade impactor which fractionates particles according to their aerodynamic size, (6) a Petri dish, which is used to passively sample settling airborne dust, and (7) a battery operated pump unit connected to a sampling head containing an air filter.

Methods of Collecting Aeroallergens

A Primer on Aeroallergen Collection

The quantity of allergen that is airborne in a domestic room is measured in units of nanograms, while the total amount of reservoir allergen is measured in the million-fold greater units of milligrams. Numerous authors have questioned the relevance of reservoir measurements as a guide to personal exposure (37,145,150) as many studies have failed to find an association. In 32 such studies listed in a recent review (5), few showed any correlation. Both aeroallergen itself and measures of reservoir involve numerous and different variables. As mentioned, Fig. 1 lists some of the variables that determine the movement of allergens-between reservoir and aeroallergen pools, while Fig. 3 describes factors influencing the amount of aeroallergen either inhaled or collected at any time. Given these, this lack of correlation is perhaps not surprising. No systematic attempt has been made to integrate these factors into predictive models of exposure. The influence of subtle factors on aeroallergen exposure is demonstrated by one study, which showed that the type of fiber in a carpet (wool vs. synthetic) was more important than the concentration of allergen in the dust (147).

Many methods have evolved to collect particles from the air and some of these are shown in Figs. 2 and 4. These range from large, mechanically powered devices to small samplers worn in the nostrils and operated by respiration. Each has advantages and characteristics that need to be matched to the nature of the analysis proposed and the timeframes of interest.

Collection of aeroallergen requires an initial decision to collect either static samples or personal samples. Static sampling is where the sampler is located in a fixed position in a room, whereas personal sampling refers to those samples collected continuously from within the "breathing zone" of the subject. Static sampling can range from short duration/low volume sampling approximately equivalent to human respiration (100), to the collection of very high volumes of air over periods of days or weeks (100). Samplers like a Hirst-type spore trap collect particles onto a tape so that hourly fluctuations over the period of a week can be observed. In some circumstances, high volume samplers may be the only way to get enough aeroallergen to detect.

Personal samplers are considered to best reflect the dose of exposure that an individual receives (148). These generally use a lapel-mounted sampler head attached to a battery-powered pump worn in the belt or in a backpack. During active indoor sampling situations, such samplers may collect up to 2–10 times more allergen per unit volume of air, than static samplers in the same general location (100,149,150). This reflects that personal exposure is closely associated with activity and dust disturbance. The nature of such personal measurements also is that they can demonstrate wide

Factors affecting quantity of aeroallergen collected or inhaled at a location at any point of time

Airborne concentration of particles carrying allergens in the immediate vicinity of the sampling device or subject
Physical properties of these particles
aerodynamic properties: size, shape, density
distribution of electrostatic charge on particles
allergen content / particle

Sampler characteristics
relative movement of sampler in the air
orientation of sampler (vertical / horizontal)
shape of sampler inlet
air velocity at the inlet

Human factors
respiration rate and activity of the person
distribution of mouth / nose breathing
distribution of inhalation between left / right nostrils

Figure 3   Some factors that affect the quantity of aeroallergen either collected or inhaled at a location. Some of these factors change with time and location within an environment.

variation over short distances. In two studies, measurements of aeroallergens made with pairs of personally worn pumps showed variations of up to two fold between the pairs of samples (151,152). In another study, the quantities of inhaled indoor fungi, measured with nasal samplers, showed greater variation between four members of each family than between the families in different houses (153). Here, the main determinant of exposure was the type and level of activity of the people.

Although data from air sampling are expressed as quantity of allergen per unit volume of air, numerous factors operate during sampling to select only a subset of particles originally contained in that volume. These include the combination of inlet orifice shape and flow rate, and movement of the sampler head relative to the air, and the different shapes and sizes of the particles. Collection efficiency of suspended particles per volume of air, decreases with both increasing airflows and with increasing size of particles. Particles of $>10\,\mu m$ diameter are more influenced by gravity and inertia and thus escape being sampled, while those smaller than <2.5 are more influenced by drag forces and follow air streamlines into a sampling head. Under these circumstances, the orientation and movement of the filter head all make a difference. True measurement of the concentration requires isokinetic sampling, where the movement of air onto the face of the sampler is equal to the movement of the sampler orifice into the air; an ideal that is

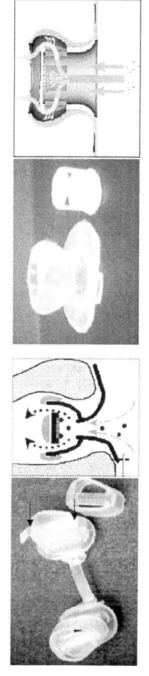
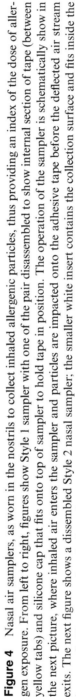

Figure 4 Nasal air samplers, as worn in the nostrils to collect inhaled allergenic particles, thus providing an index of the dose of allergen exposure. From left to right, figures show Style 1 sampler with one of the pair disassembled to show internal section of tape (between yellow tabs) and silicone cap that fits onto top of sampler to hold tape in position. The operation of the sampler is schematically show in the next picture, where inhaled air enters the sampler and particles are impacted onto the adhesive tape before the deflected air stream exits. The next figure shows a dissembled Style 2 nasal sampler; the smaller white insert contains the collection surface and fits inside the larger soft silicone cap that fits into the nose with the flat flange outside. The principle of operation of the Style 2 sampler is shown schematically in the final picture.

seldom practiced. There is considerable literature comparing the performances of differently shaped sampling heads when used in simulated occupational situations and at different airflows (148,154).

To further complicate matters, the human nose also behaves as a particular type of sampling system to select particles from air. On normal inhalation, the flow of air into the human nose occurs with sharply fluctuating and reversing flow (inhaled breaths) through small downward-facing orifices (nostrils). Our data from using nasal air samplers, shows that at the normal resting respiration rate of $\sim$10 L/min, people inhale (within a factor of $\sim$2) the same quantity of allergen as collected by a vertically oriented IOM sampling head worn on the lapel and operating with constant flow of 2 L/min (70,80).

The pattern of inhalation also varies over time and with physical activity. The volume of air inhaled when inactive is usually around 8–10 L/min, and shifts from nose breathing to include some mouth breathing at around 35 L/min, which occurs with moderate physical activity. The respiration rate may rise to peak at 200–300 L/min in extremes. Airflow is not evenly distributed between the nostrils at any time and in most adults, but few children, the dominant nostril alternates every 2–6 hr. Despite appearances, while some people have their mouths slightly open at rest, they are usually nose breathing; reinforcing the role of the nose in conditioning inhaled air.

Types of Air Samplers

Impaction/Impingers

These samplers operate on the principle of arranging a collision between aspirated particles and an adhesive-coated collection surface. Usually a column of air carrying the particles of interest is drawn through a jet and directed onto an adhesive-coated collection surface such that the air diverts around the surface and the inertia of the particles carries them forward, so the particles are impacted onto the surface. The flow of air is regulated and so such sampling is volumetric. In a well-designed sampler, the air velocity of the orifice jet and the aerodynamic diameter of the particle mainly determine the size cutoff for these samplers. Hirst-type spore traps (Burkard, Lanzoni) operate with a single jet and collection surface, and are suitable to collect particles down to $\sim$4μm.

Cascade samplers are a type of impactor that have a series of jets of decreasing size that collect the largest particles on the first stage and successively smaller particles are collected on the following stages. These can be either static samplers (Anderson spore trap, Casella cascade) or personally worn samplers (Marple Personal Sampler).

Impingement samplers utilize a similar principle by directing a jet of air carrying the particles into an impaction surface within an enclosed container where the surface is submerged in liquid. In some cases, the airflow is directed around the inner wall of a circular vessel. These are mainly used to collect micro-organisms that can be cultured. They can be used for allergens, but the samples may need concentration for assay and the sampling efficiency is questionable.

In RotorRod samplers, the adhesive collecting surface is attached to two swinging arms that are rotated at high speed by a small motor and particles in the surrounding air are impacted onto the adhesive. Such samplers are popular and widely used, but are non-quantitative and under-sample smaller spores.

Mechanical Mesh Filters

These operate on the principle that the gaps between the fibers are smaller than the diameter of the particle, and particles are sieved from the air stream as it is drawn through the sampler. In practice, with filters of some depth, such as bonded glass fiber filters, much smaller particles are also collected because they impact or impinge onto the fibers themselves. Non-fibrous filters, such as polycarbonate track-etched filters, comprise a thin film with precise and perpendicular pores through the membrane. These also collect particles below their pore size due to the behavior of air entering the pores. Two advantages with polycarbonate membranes are their low protein binding capacity and the ability to view particles collected on them; however, their capacity is low. On the other hand, glass fiber filters have a high capacity, but some will avidly bind proteins and the particles are difficult to view. The binding of soluble allergens to nitrocellulose and PVDF membranes is exceptionally high and this property is utilized in the Halogen assay, whereas protein binding to Teflon (PTFE) membranes is very low and the latter are commonly used for air sampling where good recovery is required for subsequent immunoassay.

Ionic Air Samplers

Airborne particles, particularly when freshly disturbed, may carry either residual positive or negative charges, or can have such a charge induced on them, and can be attracted to electrostatic samplers comprising two or more metal plates carrying high voltages of the opposite charge. The principle, which is widely applied in air cleaners; can also be adopted for air sampling. Some samplers use passive charge (155) or generate an "ionic breeze" and such samples in one study showed a good correlation with those collected with a filter and pump (39). The advantage is that relatively large (although imprecise) volumes of air are sampled with low use of energy and minimal noise, providing samples large enough to easily detect allergen in. This is adequate for many comparative studies.

Settling Dust (Petri Dish)

This uses large Petri dishes left open in a room for 1–2 weeks to collect settling airborne dust (156–158). The method is a simple and inexpensive way to collect accumulating allergen that has been airborne over this period. However, experience with spores shows that such sampling over-represents large particles and is sensitive to wind currents. Both these issues are less of a problem with indoor aeroallergens, as most allergen is carried by relatively large particles and air currents are uncommon. The plate data correlate with air pump samples and between paired samples in a room (143) and the sum of separate daily samples was closely related to a single weekly sample (157).

Nasal Air Samplers

These are small devices worn inside each nostril to collect the particles that are inhaled. These are collected by impaction onto an adhesive layer. Two of the types of nasal air samplers developed by our group are shown in Fig. 4. Such samples have been analyzed by Halogen assay, amplified ELISA, and for endotoxin. The currently available samplers collect virtually all particles over 10 μm and about 50% of those ~5 μm. In a number of reported studies (30,33,70,80,159–163), they have been worn for periods of 10–120 min. Two styles of nasal sampler are shown: Style 1 is used for both Halogen and ELISA assay, whereas Style 2 is used for amplified Enzyme–linked immuno sorbent assay (ELISA) assays; however other applications are under development. The samplers have been used for a range of domestic (mite, cat, dog, cockroach) and outdoor (pollens and fungi) allergens, although the area where nasal samplers may find ready application is in the monitoring of inhaled occupational exposure. Here, they have been used for rat (160), latex (80,164) and flour proteins (Renstrom, personal communication) as well as endotoxin (Palmberg, personal communication). The practical advantages of nasal samples are that they are intuitive to use, silent, discreet, simple, and inexpensive and the samplers can be easily stored and distributed. Because they are located within the nasal orifice, by definition they sample from what is actually inhaled. They also provide some concurrent prophylactic protection from exposure. The main problem is that the currently available models do not efficiently collect small airborne particles such as the smaller fungi, but they do collect the majority of most allergens, which are carried by particles >5 μm in diameter.

Measurement of Allergens and Visual Identification of Their Sources

Immunoassays

Immunoglobulins provide highly specific instruments for the precise quantification of allergens. The primary immunoglobulins used can be human

Table 2 Simplified View of Some Issues Involved in Choosing Assay Systems. There are Usually Practical Considerations, such as what is available and at what Cost, as well as the Precision of the Type of Information Obtained

Assay	Commercial availability	Sensitivity	Quantitative	Labor cost	Reagent cost
ELISA	Yes	High	High	Low–moderate	Low–moderate
RAST inhibition	No	Medium–high	Moderate–high	Moderate	Moderate–high
CRIE	No	Low	Low	High	Moderate–high
Rapid	Yes	High	Moderate–(threshold)	Low	Low–moderate
Halogen	No	Very high	Moderate	Low–moderate	Moderate

IgE, hyperimmune polyclonal antibodies raised against the antigen (less common now), or highly specific monoclonal antibodies directed against a single epitope on a specific allergen. A simplified overview comparing some practical issues of using different immunoassay methods is shown in Table 2.

ELISA

ELISA is the most widely used form of immunoassay for allergens. Such assays are available for many common allergens in kitset form from Indoor Biotechnology (www.inbio.com). Numerous other ELISA assays for individual allergens have been established by individual research groups and can be found via literature searches. Conventional sandwich ELISA assays generally have a lower level of sensitivity of about 1–2 ng allergen/mL, and this sensitivity can be boosted to about 10 pg/mL by using additional amplification steps. Different assay formats (inhibition, direct, competitive, double-antibody sandwich assays) can be employed, determined by availability of antibodies and antigens.

RAST Inhibition Immunoassays

Radioallergosorbent (RAST) inhibition assays have been widely used to measure a range of allergens in dust reservoirs and airborne samples, and such use still occurs, particularly where no alternative monoclonal-based assays are available (165–170). These can be run in an ELISA plate format or using solid-phase bound antigens. At times the correlation between inhibition and monoclonal-based assays has been low (167,171). Such assays compare the competition between a population of solid-phase bound allergens to another population of soluble allergens (either standards and unknown), using a pool of allergen-specific antibodies, often from human allergic serum. The advantage is that the effect of all the allergens in a mixture may be accommodated simultaneously, while the disadvantages are that any comparison is relative to the reference allergens and the serum used. The assays can be difficult to interpret precisely and may be expensive in terms of technical resources.

Halogen™

Halogen is one of the techniques that enables allergens associated with particles to be visualized; analogous assays include the press-blotting of the allergens to a solid phase (172,173), immunoprecipitation (90), and the fixation of allergens to membranes in the periphery of carrier particles (174).

In its original form, Halogen assays collected airborne particles onto a nitrocellulose membrane coated with a very thin film of agar and then held the particles in place by recoating on top of the particles (175). The more common embodiment, as shown in Fig. 5, either collects particles onto an adhesive (by impaction, or tape lift), which is then laminated with a protein-binding membrane, or alternatively the particles are collected by suction onto the protein-binding membrane which is then laminated with the adhesive–film (61,176). This formation of a permanent sandwich is followed by wetting to facilitate elution of the allergens, which bind to the membrane in the periphery of the particle. Subsequent immunostaining of these allergens using either IgE or an allergen-specific monoclonal as the primary antibody is similar to protein blotting. On microscopic examination through the clear adhesive, the particles that were carriers of allergens can be identified by the "halo" of immunostain around them. The method is exquisitely sensitive and shows the size, shape, and appearance of particles carrying allergens, as well as a visual estimate of their allergen content. However, attempts to make the assay quantitative for allergen by image analysis have proved technically frustrating. The assay can also be modified to show germination of fungi (66). Halogen assays have been used to measure mite (28,161,177) cat, cockroach, latex (178), and rat aeroallergens (179), as well as pollens and fungi (61,185). While most samples have been collected by nasal air sampling or on membrane filters attached to pumps, samples can also be collected by rolling adhesive tape over a surface or by using the adhesive tape in a Burkard spore trap.

Rapid/Dipstick

The format of rapid assays is familiar to most people as an over-the-counter method to determine pregnancy, where such assays provide yes/no result in about 5 min. They function by initially complexing soluble allergen in a sample with gold-labeled antibody, which then passes laterally through

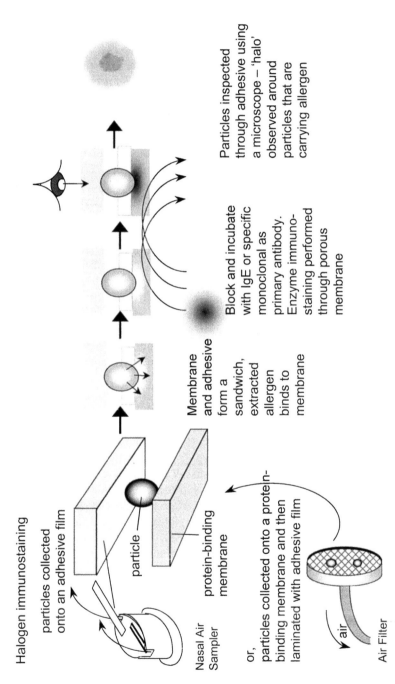

Figure 5 A schematic representation of the Halogen assay. As the text on the figure describes, particles may be collected by either impaction onto the adhesive film or by suction onto the protein-binding membrane, which after collection is laminated with the membrane/film, respectively. Solubilized allergens bind to the membrane and are probed with a primary antibody (monoclonal or IgE), which is then detected using a labeled second antibody. The color generated by the label forms a "halo," which is visible around the particle when viewed through the tape.

the membrane where the complex is captured by a region of a membrane-bound second antibody resulting in the appearance of a visible line of bound gold on the assay strip. Two commercial kitsets are available, either to measure mite allergen in a sample of dust collected with a vacuum cleaner (181) or as a direct test that incorporates the sampling device into the assay cassette (182). The intensity of the colored line that is produced is approximately proportional to allergen concentration sampled. The assays are designed to operate around a threshold of approximately 0.5–2 µg/g at which they provide a "positive" response. Several other "dipstick" assays that use sequential incubation, rather than chromatography, are available, although these take a couple of hours to complete.

Biological Assays

Biological assays using allergen extracts are commonly used as a diagnostic test to quantify allergy, and this format can be used in the converse manner to measure allergens. Such assays include skin prick test, histamine release from sensitized basophils, or direct challenge of an end-organ (nose, lung, eye). Such assays are also a valuable addition to understanding the relevance of exposure to symptoms or to characterize the biological potency of the allergens. One such study using pure recombinant grass allergens demonstrated that individual allergens differed markedly in their clinical potency as assessed by nasal challenge and skin test compared to IgE binding in in vitro assays (183). Where skin testing with extracts has been used to measure allergens after interventions (such as tannic acid denaturation), the results differ from those obtained with in vitro tests (184,185), and it could be argued that the in vivo assay are more relevant, even if less precise than the monoclonal antibody-based in vitro tests.

Biochemical and Chemical Assays

A few allergens or materials present with allergens can be quantified using biochemical markers, providing an indirect measure. Guanine is an excretory product of mites, and its chemical measurement using a dipstick-based assay forms the basis of the Acarex test (186). The enzymic components of mite extracts also provide the basis for assays to estimate allergens (187), and recently such a test has been marketed in the U.K. (www.acaris.com). The measurement of ergosterol, a common component of fungal cell walls, by HPLC, has been used as a measure of total fungi in dust samples (188). The latter is relevant as it is difficult to quantify the diversity of fungi present.

PCR for Allergen Sources

While the quantification of some fungal species that produce large and distinctive spores can be performed by microscopy, such methods cannot be used with the smaller spores, and these require time-consuming culture to identify. An alternative, which is both specific and enables batch processing, is to perform PCR. This uses primers based on conserved regions of the fungal mitochondrial DNA and then sequences into the non–conserved intron regions that form novel identifiers for a species or genera (189–192). Such techniques are becoming increasingly common with the application of RT-PCR to provide some semiquantitative information. Such a method does not differentiate between nonviable and viable spores, nor is it a direct method of measuring allergens.

Microscopy and Culture

Both fungi spores and pollen grains have traditionally been enumerated from collection slides by microscopic techniques, at times in combination with culture-based methods for fungi. There are numerous specialist texts that are well worth studying (193,194). For air samples, chemical stains are used to differentiate spores and pollens from other components in the samples, and from each other. It is outside the objectives of a chapter on allergens to provide details. The most common stain for pollens is Calberla's solution (194). Numerous stains are used for fungi, to some extent depending on the species sought. Recently, fluorescent-labeled recombinant chitinase has been used to specifically stain the wall components of fungal spores and hyphae (195). Image analysis, including with confocal microscopy and spectral analysis, has been used to explore the automated and real-time identification of spores and pollen grains. Such efforts have been accelerated by renewed interest in the rapid and specific identification of the agents of biological warfare.

The ability of airborne fungal propagules to germinate and develop into colony forming units (CFUs) on synthetic culture media is dependant on a number of variables particularly the type of nutrient source and culture temperature. Traditionally, fungal spores have been collected onto a variety of culture mediums, in particular Sabourand's dextrose (SAB) and malt extract (MALT) agars (196). Comparative studies conducted by Burge et al. (197) and Pei-Chih (198) have also shown that V8 juice (V8), potato dextrose (PDA) and dichloran glycerol–18 (DG 18) agars are just as effective at recovering fungal CFUs. Nutrient media, in particular SAB, can also be used to selectively recover specific fungal genera as in the case for *Aspergillus* spp (196,199,200) as well as yield more allergenically potent extracts (201,202). Furthermore, some fungal genera including *Aspergillus fumigatus* and *Candida albicans* are thermotolerant and are adapted to growth at higher temperatures (37°C); however, temperatures between 24°C and

25°C are considered optimal for culturing most species of the Deuteromycetes (203,204).

Extraction of Allergens into Solution

Allergens are usually readily extracted from their source material, however, the quantity recovered is partly determined by the methods used. This has been explored for several allergens. For mite allergens, although most allergen is rapidly extracted (27), both the extraction temperature and buffer used can each make a difference of up to twofold (136). With both pollen and fungi, the effect of buffer and time on the profile of extracted (or induced) allergens has long been recognized (203–206). For rodent allergens, the addition of Tween and BSA to the buffer can increase the recovery of allergen by 10–fold (207), for additional protocols for rat see Ref. (208) and for peanut allergens see Ref. (209).

For most, if not all, allergens the extraction process is not standardized, and differences in the following can all make a difference to the final amount recovered: the content of different anions and cations in buffers, pH, times, temperatures, the type and concentration of detergents, the presence of carrier proteins such as BSA, enzyme inhibitors and anti-bacterial agents. In addition, agents such as glycerol can increase recovery during extraction and stabilize extracts, but may also interfere with ELISA assays and need to be diluted out. Storage conditions such as the freezing temperature, and cycles of freeze-thawing, can lead to some loss of activity.

Sampling Protocols

The protocols adopted for aeroallergen sampling are partly determined by the practical considerations of performing the study, weighed against the type of information needed (Table 3). Important considerations are the need to collect samples that can be accommodated within the limits of detection and the time that is available to collect the samples within. Where samples are going to be immunoassayed (lower level of detection usually ~1 ng allergen), it may be necessary to use very long sampling times, active dust disturbance and/or static samplers operating with high flow rates. Here, the relevance to personal exposure may be reduced. Conversely, in the case of measuring fungal exposure assayed by culture, where the airborne density of spores is high ($\sim10^4/m^3$), then very short times may be required to avoid overloading culture plates. However, such brief "grab-samples" also cannot be expected to accurately reflect exposure occurring over a longer period. It has been suggested that 27–36 samples per home would be required for the reliable estimation of average exposure with less than 10% bias (210).

The nature of some aeroallergen exposures is that they can be highly variable over time if any significant dust disturbance is involved. Sakaguchi

Table 3 Simplified View of Different Types of Allergen Measurements that Have Commonly Been Applied in Different Types of Studies

Study-type	Allergen measurement
Cross-sectional study of exposure or sensitization within a community	Reservoir allergen levels
Effectiveness of an allergen avoidance intervention on symptoms	Serial measurement of inhaled or airborne allergen measured at the site of the intervention, with controls
Patient education	Rapid assay for mite performed by the patient or by commercial laboratory assay with patient–collected dust.
Longitudinal cohort study of effectiveness of allergen avoidance on sensitization	Repeated reservoir in bedroom and lounge room, plus aeroallergen by Petri dish (7 days) or static air sampling (24 hr), several times a year
Panel study of relationship between allergen exposure and symptoms	Serial measurement of inhaled or airborne allergens—for both specific allergens and with the subject's IgE for total allergen

et al. (211) found more than a thousand-fold differences between aeroallergen concentrations in an unoccupied room compared with the same room when a bed was actively being made in it. This represents an extreme, and we have observed only about threefold increase in inhaled aeroallergen when a person is normally active within a room compared with when they are sedentary within the same room (70,212). Further, where repeated samples under similar circumstances are involved, the differences between these may be quite small. For example, in another study (5), a series of eight consecutive air samples, each of 10 min collected once a week for 6 weeks. Here, the mean quantity collected was 13 units of allergen with a standard deviation of 3.38 and a coefficient of variation of 26%.

Numerous other practical considerations occur: the costs of the sampling and analytical equipment, particularly if simultaneous collections are required, noise, and interruption generated by sampling pumps; the provision of a power source; the need for expert technical assistance; the need for repeated visits to a sampling site; etc. These practical requirements limit the collection and interpretation of the data in terms of understanding differences in actual personal exposure occurring during an activity or event.

Comments in Conclusion

The prevalence of reported asthma and rhinitis continue to increase in children. The goals of research include the understanding of disease etiology with the intention of preventing its incidence and reversing its progression. An important component of this includes unraveling the interactions of environmental allergic and non-allergic stimuli and genetic susceptibilities, better understanding of the role that allergens and allergies play in the exacerbation of symptoms, and a more rational approach to methods to avoid exposure. In order to achieve this, comprehensive, valid, and reliable methods of measuring human exposure are required.

In the last 5–10 years, new methods to assist this have been developed. These include methods to collect air samples that reflect acute human exposure to inhaled particles, assays that will identify and quantify many of the allergens involved, and methods to measure the physical characteristics of the particles. This provides a basis to develop and test more relevant models of the important characteristics of allergen exposure and to apply these to observations of their clinical effects in allergic diseases. Such relationships are complex as the clinical outcomes are additionally determined by issues of timing, susceptibility, variations between individuals, interactions with multiple genes, and numerous other modulating effects and non-allergen exposures. If the changes in our thinking about asthma in the last 10 years are indicative, then many other new elements and directions can be anticipated in the future.

These developments in sampling aeroallergens will also have broader health applications. These will include application in a range of respiratory and occupational diseases, exposures to microbes in various formats, and to other airborne products of our 21st century lifestyle.

Acknowledgments

Many thanks to our colleagues Jason Sercombe and Brett Green, John Cherrie in the U.K., and Anne Renstrom in Sweden for discussion and suggestions of material in this chapter.

References

1. Blackley C. Experimental researchers on the causes and nature of Catarrhus Aestivus (hay– fever or hay–asthma). Bailliere Tindall and Cox, 1873 (Republished 1988 by Oxford Historical Books).
2. Strachan D, Sibbald B, Weiland S, et al. Worldwide variations in prevalence of symptoms of allergic rhinoconjunctivitis in children: the International Study of Asthma and Allergies in Childhood (ISAAC). Pediatr Allergy Immunol 1997; 8:161–176.
3. Renstrom A. Exposure to airborne allergens: a review of sampling methods. J Environ Monit 2002; 4(5):619–622.

4. Solomon WR. How ill the wind? Issues in aeroallergen sampling. J Allergy Clin Immunol 2003; 112:3–8.
5. O'Meara T, Tovey E. Monitoring personal allergen exposure. Clin Rev Allergy Immunol 2000; 18:341–395.
6. Platts–Mills TA. Local production of IgG, IgA and IgE antibodies in grass pollen hay fever. J Immunol 1979; 122:2218–2225.
7. Wang JE, Warris A, Ellingsen EA, et al. Involvement of CD14 and toll-like receptors in activation of human monocytes by *Aspergillus fumigatus* hyphae. Infect Immun 2001; 69:2402–2406.
8. Epton MJ, Smith W, Hales BJ, Hazell L, Thompson PJ, Thomas WR. Non-allergenic antigen in allergic sensitization: responses to the mite ferritin heavy chain antigen by allergic and non-allergic subjects. Clin Exp Allergy 2002; 32:1341–1347.
9. Peake H, Currie A, Stewart G, McWilliam A. Nitric oxide production by alveolar macrophages in response to house dust mite fecal pellets and the mite allergens, Der p 1 and Der p 2. J Allergy Clin Immunol 2003; 112:531–537.
10. Nelson HS. The importance of allergens in the development of asthma and the persistence of symptoms. J Allergy Clin Immunol 2000; 105:S628–S632.
11. Sluyter R, Tovey ER, Duffy DL, Britton WJ. Limited genetic control of specific IgE responses to rye grass pollen allergens in Australian twins. Clin Exp Allergy 1998; 28:322–331.
12. Tovey E, Sluyter R, Duffy D, Britton W, Woolcock A. Genetic control of specificity of mite- IgE shown by immunoblotting twin sera. Aust N Z J Med 1994; 24:474.
13. King T, Hoffman D, Lowenstein H, Marsh D, Platts–Mills T, Thomas W. Allergen nomenclature. Allergy 1995; 50:765–774.
14. Chapman MD, Platts–Mills TAE. Purification and characterization of the major allergen from Dermatophagoides pteronyssinus-antigen P1. J Immunol 1980; 125:587–592.
15. Colloff M, Stewart G. House dust mites. In: Barnes PJ, Grunstein MM, Leff AR, Woolcock AJ, eds. Asthma. Vol. 2. Philadelphia: Lippincott–Raven, 1997:1089–1104.
16. Arlian L, Platts–Mills TAE. The biology of dust mites and the remediation of mite allergens in allergic disease. J Allergy Clin Immunol 2001; 107(3 Suppl):S406–S413.
17. Platts–Mills TAE, Chapman MD. Dust mites: immunology, allergic disease, and environmental control. J Allergy Clin Immunol 1987; 80:755–775.
18. Platts–Mills TAE, de Weck AL, et al. Dust mite allergens and asthma—a worldwide problem. Report of an International Workshop, Bad Kreuznach, Federal Republic of Germany, Sep 1987. J Allergy Clin Immunol 1989; 83:416–427.
19. Platts–Mills TAE, Vervloet D, Thomas WR, Aalberse RC, Chapman MD. Indoor allergens and asthma: Report of the Third International Workshop. J Allergy Clin Immunol 1997; 100:S1–S24.
20. Zhang L, Chew FT, Soh SY, et al. Prevalence and distribution of indoor allergens in Singapore. Clin Exp Allergy 1997; 27:876–885.

21. Arruda LK, Rizzo MC, Chapman MD, et al. Exposure and sensitization to dust mite allergens among asthmatic children in Sao Paulo, Brazil. Clin Exp Allergy 1991; 21:433–439.

22. Thomas WR, Smith WA, Hales BJ, Mills KL, O'Brien RM. Characterization and immunobiology of house dust mite allergens. Int Arch Allergy Immunol 2002; 129:1–18.

23. Smith WA, Hales BJ, Jarnicki AG, Thomas WR. Allergens of wild house dust mites: environmental Der p 1 and Der p 2 sequence polymorphisms. J Allergy Clin Immunol 2001; 107:985–992.

24. Nandy A, Graefe L, Bormann I, et al. European variants of house dust mite allergen Der f 2. J Allergy Clin Immunol 2003; 111:S204 (Abs 544).

25. Tovey ER, Baldo BA. Localisation of antigens and allergens in thin section of the house dust mite *Dermatophagoides pternoyssinus* (Acari: Pyroglyphidae). J Med Entomol 1990; 27:368–376.

26. Stewart G, McWilliam A. Endogenous function and biological significance of aeroallergens: an update. Curr Opin Allergy Clin Immunol 2001; 1(1):47–50.

27. Tovey ER, Chapman MD, Platts–Mills TAE. Mite faeces are a major source of house dust allergens. Nature 1981; 289:592–593.

28. De Lucca S, Sporik R, O'Meara T, Tovey E. Mite Allergen (Der p 1) is not only carried on mite feces. J Allergy Clin Immunol 1999; 103:174–175.

29. Custovic A, Woodcock H, Craven M, et al. Dust mite allergens are carried on not only large particles. Pediatr Allergy Immunol 1999; 10:258–260.

30. O'Rourke SD, Tovey ER, O'Meara TJ. Personal exposure to mite and cat allergens. J Allergy Clin Immunol 2002; 109:S47.

31. Eggleston PA, Arruda LK. Ecology and elimination of cockroaches and allergens in the home. J Allergy Clin Immunol 2001; 107:S422–S429.

32. de Blay F, Sanchez J, Hedelin G, et al. Dust and airborne exposure to allergens derived from cockroach (*Blatella germanica*) in low-cost public housing in Strasbourg (France). J Allergy Clin Immunol 1997; 99:107–112.

33. De Lucca S, Taylor D, O'Meara T, Jones A, Tovey E. Measurement and characterisation of cockroach allergens detected during normal domestic activity. J Allergy Clin Immunol 1999; 104:672–680.

34. Arbes SJ, Sever M, Archer J, et al. Abatement of cockroach allergen (Bla g 1) in low–income, urban housing: a randomized controlled trial. J Allergy Clin Immunol 2003; 112:339–345.

35. Roost HP, Kunzli N, Schindler C, et al. Role of current and childhood exposure to cat and atopic sensitization. J Allergy Clin Immunol 1999; 104: 941–947.

36. Luczynska CM, Li Y, Chapman MD, Platts–Mills TAE. Airborne concentrations and particle size distribution of allergen derived from domestic cat (*Felis domesticus*). Am Rev Respir Dis 1990; 141:361–367.

37. Custovic A, Simpson B, Simpson A, Hallam C, Craven M, Woodcock A. Relationship between mite, cat, and dog allergens in reservoir dust and ambient air. Allergy 1999; 54:612–616.

38. Custovic A, Simpson A, Pahdi H, Green RM, Chapman MD, Woodcock A. Distribution, aerodynamic characteristics, and removal of the major cat allergen Fel d 1 in British homes. Thorax 1998; 53:33–38.

39. Custis NJ, Woodfolk JA, Vaughan JW, Platts–Mills TAE. Quantitative measurement of airborne allergens from dust mites, dogs, and cats using an ion–charging device. Clin Exp Allergy 2003; 33:986–991.

40. Custovic A, Fletcher A, Pickering CA, et al. Domestic allergens in public places III: house dust mite, cat, dog and cockroach allergens in British hospitals. Clin Exp Allergy 1998; 28:53–59.

41. Chew GL, Perzanowski MS, Miller RL, et al. Distribution and determinants of mouse allergen exposure in low-income New York City apartments. Environ Health Perspect 2003; 111:1348–1351.

42. Custovic A, Hallam C, Simpson B, Craven M, Simpson A, Woodcock A. Decreased prevalence of sensitization to cats with high exposure to cat allergen. J Allergy Clin Immunol 2001; 108(4):537–539.

43. Platts–Mills T, Vaughan JW, Squillace SP, Woodfolk J, Sporik R. Sensitisation, asthma, and a modified Th2 response in children exposed to cat allergen: a population-based cross-sectional study. Lancet 2001; 357:752–756.

44. Svanes C, Heinrich J, Jarvis D, et al. Pet-keeping in childhood and adult asthma and hay fever: European Community Respiratory Health Survey. J Allergy Clin Immunol 2003; 112:289–300.

45. Langley SJ, Goldthorpe S, Craven M, Morris J, Woodcock A, Custovic A. Exposure and sensitization to indoor allergens: association with lung function, bronchial reactivity, and exhaled nitric oxide measures in asthma. J Allergy Clin Immunol 2003; 112:362–368.

46. Almqvist C, Egmar AC, van Hage-Hamsten M, et al. Heredity, pet ownership, and confounding control in a population–based birth·cohort. J Allergy Clin Immunol 2003; 111:800–806.

47. Perzanowski MS, Ronmark E, Platts-Mills TAE, Lundback B. Effect of cat and dog ownership on sensitization and development of asthma among preteenage children. Am J Respir Crit Care Med 2002; 166:696–702.

48. Ownby DR, Johnson CC, Peterson EL. Exposure to dogs and cats in the first year of life and risk of allergic sensitization at 6 to 7 years of age. JAMA 2002; 288:963–972.

49. Ford SA, Tovey ER, Baldo BA. Identification of orchard grass (*Dactylis glomerata*) pollen allergens following electrophoretic transfer to nitrocellulose. Int Arch Allergy Appl Immunol 1985; 78:15–21.

50. Marks GB, Colquhoun JR, Girgis ST, et al. Thunderstorm outflows preceding epidemics of asthma during spring and summer. Thorax 2001; 56:468–471.

51. Knox RB. Grass pollen, thunderstorms and asthma. Clin Exp Allergy 1993; 23:354–359.

52. Taylor PE, Flagan RC, Valenta R, Glovsky MM. Release of allergens as respirable aerosols: a link between grass pollen and asthma. J Allergy Clin Immunol 2002; 109:51–56.

53. Girgis ST, Marks GB, Downs SH, Kolbe A, Car GN, Paton R. Thunderstorm–associated asthma in an inland town in south-eastern Australia. Who is at risk? Eur Respir J 2000; 16:3–8.

54. Dechamp C, Penel V. Results of pollen counts for 2001 from the Rhone–Alpes ragweed pollen-monitoring network (SARA). Rev Fr Allergol Immunol Clin 2002; 42:539–542.

55. Hirano M, Katoh T. Pollen information providing system. NTT Rev 2001; 13:49–55.

56. Davies HJ. Exposure of hay fever subjects to an indoor environmental grass pollen challenge system. Clin Allergy 1985; 15:419–427.

57. Sicherer S, Wood R, Eggleston P. Determinants of airway responses to cat allergen: comparison of environmental challenge to quantitative nasal and bronchial allergen challenge. J Allergy Clin Immunol 1997; 99:798–805.

58. Platts-Mills TA, Hayden ML, Chapman MD, Wilkins SR. Seasonal variation in dust mite and grass-pollen allergens in dust from the houses of patients with asthma. J Allergy Clin Immunol 1987; 79:781–791.

59. Reed CE, Swanson MC, Yunginger JW. Measurement of allergen concentration in the air as an aid in controlling exposure to aeroallergens. J Allergy Clin Immunol 1986; 78:1028–1030.

60. Stewart GA, Holt PG. Submicronic airborne allergens (Letter). Med J Aust 1985; 143:426–427.

61. Razmovski V, O'Meara TJ, Taylor DJ, Tovey ER. A new method for simultaneous immunodetection and morphologic identification of individual sources of pollen allergens. J Allergy Clin Immunol 2000; 105:725–731.

62. Bush RK, Portnoy JM. The role and abatement of fungal allergens in allergic diseases. J Allergy Clin Immunol 2001; 107:S430–S440.

63. Burge HA. An update on pollen and fungal spore aerobiology. J Allergy Clin Immunol 2002; 110:544–552.

64. Kauffman HF, van der Heide S. Exposure, sensitization, and mechanisms of fungus-induced asthma. Curr Allergy Asthma Rep 2003; 3(5):430–437.

65. Braun H, Buzina W, Freudenschuss K, Beham A, Stammberger H. 'Eosinophilic fungal rhinosinusitis': a common disorder in Europe? Laryngoscope 2003; 113:264–269.

66. Green BJ, Mitakakis TZ, Tovey ER. Allergen detection from 11 fungal species before and after germination. J Allergy Clin Immunol 2003; 111:285–289.

67. Doring G, Bellon G, Knight R. Immunology of cystic fibrosis. In: Geddes Ha, ed. Cystic Fibrosis. London: Arnold, 2000:109–140.

68. Barnes C, Schreiber K, Pacheco F, Landuyt J, Hu F, Portnoy J. Comparison of outdoor allergenic particles and allergen levels. Ann Allergy Asthma Immunol 2000; 84:47–54.

69. Sporik RB, Arruda LK, Woodfolk J, Chapman MD, Platts-Mills TAE. Environmental exposure to *Aspergillus fumigatus* allergen (Asp fI). Clin Exp Allergy 1993; 23:326–331.

70. Mitakakis T, Tovey E, Xuan W, Marks G. Personal exposure to allergenic pollen and mould spores in inland New South Wales, Australia. Clin Exp Allergy 2000; 30:1733–1739.

71. Verhoeff AP, Burge HA. Health risk assessment of fungi in home environments. Ann Allergy Asthma Immunol 1997; 78:544–554.

72. Garrett MH, Rayment PR, Hooper MA, Abramson MJ, Hooper BM. Indoor airborne fungal spores, house dampness and associations with environmental factors and respiratory health in children. Clin Exp Allergy 1998; 28:459–467.

73. Zock JP, Jarvis D, Luczynska C, Sunyer J, Burney P. European Community Respiratory Health Survey. Housing characteristics, reported mold exposure,

and asthma in the European Community Respiratory Health Survey. J Allergy Clin Immunol 2002; 110:285–292.

74. Zureik M, Neukirch C, Leynaert B, et al. Sensitisation to airborne moulds and severity of asthma: cross sectional study from European Community respiratory health survey. BMJ 2002; 325:411–414.

75. Chew GL, Rogers C, Burge HA, Muilenberg ML, Gold DR. Dustborne and airborne fungal propagules represent a different spectrum of fungi with differing relations to home characteristics. Allergy 2003; 58:13–20.

76. Verhoeff AP, Vanreenenhoekstra ES, Samson RA, Brunekreef B, Vanwijnen JH. Fungal propagules in house dust. 1. Comparison of analytic methods and their value as estimators of potential exposure. Allergy 1994; 49: 533–539.

77. Lieutier–Colas F, Meyer P, Pons F, et al. Prevalence of symptoms, sensitization to rats, and airborne exposure to major rat allergen (Rat n 1) and to endotoxin in rat-exposed workers: a cross-sectional study. Clin Exp Allergy 2002; 32:1424–1429.

78. Lieutier-Colas F, Meyer P, Larsson P, et al. Difference in exposure to airborne major rat allergen (Rat n 1) and to endotoxin in rat quarters according to tasks. Clin Exp Allergy 2001; 31:1449–1456.

79. Laoprasert N, Swanson MC, Jones RT, Schroeder DR, Yunginger JW. Inhalation challenge testing of latex-sensitive health care workers and the effectiveness of laminar flow HEPA-filtered helmets in reducing rhinoconjunctival and asthmatic reactions. J Allergy Clin Immunol 1998; 102:998–1004.

80. Poulos LM, O'Meara TJ, Hamilton RG, Yeang HY, Tovey ER. Inhaled latex allergen. J Allergy Clin Immunol 2001; 107:sl30.

81. Goodno LE, Stave GM. Primary and secondary allergies to laboratory animals. J Occup Environ Med 2002; 44:1143–1152.

82. Krakowiak A, Palczynski C, Walusiak J, et al. Allergy to animal fur and feathers among zoo workers. Int Arch Occup Environ Health 2002; 75:S113–S116.

83. Brisman J, Lillienberg L, Belin L, Ahman M, Jarvholm B. Sensitisation to occupational allergens in bakers' asthma and rhinitis: a case-referent study. Int Arch Occup Environ Health 2003; 76:167–170.

84. Vissers M, Doekes G, Heederik D. Exposure to wheat allergen and fungal alpha-amylase in the homes of bakers. Clin Exp Allergy 2001; 31:1577–1582.

85. Sarlo K. Control of occupational asthma and allergy in the detergent industry. Ann Allergy Asthma Immunol 2003; 90:32–34.

86. Platts-Mills TAE. Allergen avoidance in the treatment of asthma and rhinitis. N Engl J Med 2003; 349:207–208.

87. Terreehorst I, Hak E, Oosting AJ, et al. Evaluation of impermeable covers for bedding in patients with allergic rhinitis. N Engl J Med 2003; 349:237–246.

88. Thatcher T, Layton D. Deposition, resuspension and penetration of particles within a residence. Atmos Environ 1995; 29:1487–1497.

89. Appendix A: Theoretical considerations relevant to the influence of ventilation and air–cleaning on exposures to indoor-generated pollutants. Clearing the air. Washington DC: National Academic Press, 2000; 10: 409–414.

90. Tovey ER, Chapman MD, Platts-Mills TAE. The distribution of house dust mite allergen in the houses of patients with asthma. Am Rev Respir Dis 1981; 124:630–635.

91. Swanson MC, Agarwal MK, Reed CE. An immunochemical approach to indoor aeroallergen quantitation with a new volumetric air sampler: studies with mite, roach, cat, and guinea pig antigens. J Allergy Clin Immunol 1985; 76:724–729.

92. Platts-Mills TAE, Heymann PW, Longbottom JL, Wilkins SR. Airborne allergens associated with asthma: particle sizes carrying dust mite and rat allergens measured with a cascade impactor. J Allergy Clin Immunol 1986; 77:850–857.

93. de Blay F, Heymann P, Chapman M, Platts-Mills T. Airborne mite allergens: comparison of group II allergens with group 1 mite allergen and cat Fel d I. J Allergy Clinical Immunol 1991; 88:919–926.

94. Woodfolk JA, Luczynska CM, de Blay F, Chapman MD, Platts-Mills TAE. The effect of vacuum cleaners on the concentration and particle size distribution of airborne cat allergen. J Allergy Clin Immunol 1993; 91:829–837.

95. Wood RA, Laheri AN, Eggleston PA. The aerodynamic characteristics of cat allergen. Clin Exp Allergy 1993; 23:733–739.

96. Tovey E, De Lucca S, Pavlicek P, Sercombe J, Taylor D, O'Meara T. The morphology of particles carrying mite, dog, cockroach and cat aeroallergens affects their efficiency of collection by nasal samplers and cascade impactors. J Allergy Clin Immunol 2000; 105:S228.

97. Custovic A, Green R, Pickering CAC, et al. Major dog allergen Can f 1: distribution in homes, airborne levels and particle sizing. J Allergy Clin Immunol 1996; 97:478.

98. Custovic A, Green R, Fletcher A, et al. Aerodynamic properties of the major dog allergen Can f 1: distribution in homes, concentration, and particle size of allergen in the air. Am J Respir Crit Care Med 1997; 155:94–98.

99. Sarpong SB, Wood RA, Eggleston PA. Aerodynamic properties of cockroach allergens (Abstract). J Allergy Clin Immunol 1995; 95:262.

100. Price JA, Longbottom JL. ELISA method for measurement of airborne levels of major laboratory animal allergens. Clin Allergy 1988; 18:95–107.

101. Van Metre TE, Marsh DG, Adkinson NF, et al. Dose of cat (*Felis domesticus*) allergen 1 (Fel d 1) that induces asthma. J Allergy Clin Immunol 1986; 78:62–75.

102. Wood RA, Phipatanakul W, Hamilton RG, Eggleston PA. A comparison of skin prick tests, intradermal skin tests, and RASTs in the diagnosis of cat allergy. J Allergy Clin Immunol. 1999; 103:773–779.

103. Lieutier–Colas F, Purohit A, Meyer P, et al. Bronchial challenge tests in patients with asthma sensitized to cats—the importance of large particles in the immediate response. Am J Respir Crit Care Med 2003; 167:1077–1082.

104. Arshad SH, Hamilton RG, Adkinson NF Jr. Repeated aerosol exposure to small doses of allergen. A model for chronic allergic asthma. Am J Respir Crit Care Med 1998; 157:1900–1906.

105. Altounyan REC. Changes in histamine and atropine responsiveness as a guide to diagnosis and evaluation of therapy in obstructive airways disease. In:

Pepys J, Frankland AW, eds. Disodium Chromoglycate in Allergic Airways Disease. London: Butterworth, 1970:43–47.

106. Platts-Mills TAE, Mitchell EB, Nock P, Tovey ER, Moszoro H, Wilkins SR. Reduction of bronchial hyperreactivity during prolonged allergen avoidance. Lancet 1982; 2:675–677.

107. Korsgaard J. Mite asthma and residency. A case–control study on the impact of exposure to house-dust mites in dwellings. Am Rev Respir Dis 1983; 128:231–235.

108. Warner AM, Bjorksten B, Munir AKM, Moller C, Schou C, Kjellman NIM. Childhood asthma and exposure to indoor allergens: low mite levels are associated with sensitivity. Pediatr Allergy Immunol 1996; 7:61–67.

109. Matsui EC, Wood RA, Rand C, et al. Cockroach allergen exposure and sensitization in suburban middle-class children with asthma. J Allergy Clin Immunol 2003; 112:87–92.

110. Assessing exposure and risk. In: Pope A, Patterson, R and Burge H, eds. Indoor Allergens: Assessing and Controlling Adverse Health Effects. Washington DC: National Academy Press, 1993:185–205.

111. Wahn U, Lau S, Bergmann R, et al. Indoor allergen exposure is a risk factor for sensitization during the first three years of life. J Allergy Clin Immunol 1997; 99:763–769.

112. Platts-Mills TAE. Is there a dose–response relationship between exposure to indoor allergens and symptoms of asthma? (Editorial). J Allergy Clin Immunol 1995; 96:435–440.

113. Gelber LE, Seltzer LH, Bouzoukis JK, Pollart SM, Chapman MD, Platts-Mills TAE. Sensitization and exposure to indoor allergens as risk factors for asthma among patients presenting to hospital. Am Rev Respir Dis 1993; 147:573–578.

114. Ingham JM, Sporik R, Rose G, Honsinger R, Chapman MD, Platts–Mills TAE. Quantitative assessment of exposure to dog (Can f I) and cat (Fel d I) allergens: relationship to sensitization and asthma among children living in Los Alamos, New Mexico. J Allergy Clin Immunol 1995; 96:449–456.

115. Baur X. Are we closer to developing threshold limit values for allergens in the workplace? Ann Allergy Asthma-Immunol 2003; 90:11–18.

116. Green RM, Custovic A, Sanderson G, Hunter J, Johnston SL, Woodcock A. Synergism between allergens and viruses and risk of hospital admission with asthma: case–control study. BMJ 2002; 324:763.

117. Tunnicliffe WS, Fletcher TJ, Hammond K, et al. Sensitivity and exposure to indoor allergens in adults with differing asthma severity. Eur Respir J 1999; 13:654–659.

118. Pearce N, Pekkanen J, Beasley R. How much asthma is really attributable to atopy? Thorax 1999; 54:268–272.

119. Douwes J, Gibson P, Pekkanen J, Pearce N. Non-eosinophilic asthma: importance and possible mechanisms. Thorax 2002; 57:643–648.

120. Martin JG, Duguet A, Eidelman DH. The contribution of airway smooth muscle to airway narrowing and airway hyperresponsiveness in disease. Eur Respir J 2000; 16:349–354.

121. Nagao K, Tanaka H, Komai M, Masuda M, Narumiya S, Nagai H. Role of prostaglandin 12 in airway remodeling induced by repeated allergen challenge in mice. Am J Respir Cell Mol Biol 2003; 29:314–320.

122. Sun G, Stacey MA, Schmidt M, Mori L, Mattoli S. Interaction of mite allergens Der P3 and Der P9 with protease–activated receptor-2 expressed by lung epithelial cells. J Immunol 2001; 167:1014–1021.

123. Wahlstrom J, Gigliotti D, Roquet A, Wigzell H, Eklund A, Grunewald J. T cell receptor V beta expression in patients with allergic asthma before and after repeated low-dose allergen inhalation. Clin Immunol 2001; 100:31–39.

124. Duffy DL, Battistutta D, Martin NG, Hopper JL, Mathews JD. Genetics of asthma and hayfever in Australian twins. Am Rev Respir Dis 1990; 142:1351–1358.

125. Savilahti R, Uitti J, Roto P, Laippala P, Husman T. Increased prevalence of atopy among children exposed to mold in a school building. Allergy 2001; 56:175–179.

126. Baur X, Chen Z, Liebers V. Exposure–response relationships of occupational inhalative allergens. Clin Exp Allergy 1998; 28:537–544.

127. Heederik D, Doekes G. Exposure–response relationships for airborne allergens. Clin Exp Allergy 1999; 29:423–424.

128. Douwes J, Thome P, Pearce N, Heederik D. Bioaerosol health effects and exposure assessment: progress and prospects. Ann Occup Hyg 2003; 47:187–200.

129. Roy SR, Schiltz AM, Marotta A, Shen YQ, Liu AH. Bacterial DNA in house and farm–barn dust. J Allergy Clin Immunol 2003; 112:571–578.

130. Ding J, Ho B. A new era in pyrogen testing. Trends Biotechnol 2001; 19: 277–281.

131. Reynolds S, Thome P, Donham K, et al. Interlaboratory comparison of endotoxin assays using agricultural dusts. Am Ind Hyg Assoc J 2002; 63:430–438.

132. Carney AS, Powe DG, Huskisson RS, Jones NS. Atypical nasal challenges in patients with idiopathic rhinitis: more evidence for the existence of allergy in the absence of atopy? Clin Exp Allergy 2002; 32:1436–1440.

133. Gardiner K. Sampling strategies. In: Harrington JG, ed. Occupational Hygiene. Oxford: Blackwell Scientific, 1995:287–307.

134. Platts-Mills TA, Thomas WR, Aalberse RC, Vervloet D, Chapman MD. Dust mite allergens and asthma: report of a second international workshop. J Allergy Clin Immunol 1992; 89:1046–1060.

135. Lewis RD, Breysse PN. A comparison of the sampling characteristics of two vacuum surface samplers for the collection of dust mite allergen. Appl Occup Environ Hyg 1998; 13(7):536–541.

136. Siebers R, Luey B, Crane J, Fitzharris P. The effects of temperature and buffer on the extraction of Der p 1–from dust (let). J Allergy Clin Immunol 1997; 100:580.

137. Yasueda H, Saito A, Akiyama K, et al. Estimation of Der p and Der f I quantities in the reference preparations of *Dermatophagoides* mite extracts. Clin Exp Allergy 1994; 24:1030–1035.

138. Hirsch T, Kuhlisch E, Soldan W, Leupold W. Variability of house dust mite allergen exposure in dwellings. Environ Health Perspect 1998; 106:659–664.

139. Simpson A, Hassall R, Custovic A, Woodcock A. Variability of house dust mite allergen levels within carpets. Allergy 1998; 53:602–607.
140. Marks GB, Tovey ER, Peat JK, Salome C, Woolcock AJ. Variability and repeatability of house dust mite allergen measurement: implications for study design and interpretation. Clin Exp Allergy 1995; 25:1190–1197.
141. Carswell F, Chavarria JF, Oliver J, Clifford F. A sampling standard for mite allergens: surface area ir dust ratio? J Allergy Clin Immunol 1991; 87:322.
142. O'Meara TJ, Vasram R, Moses C, Tovey ER. Bed washing and mattress encasing result in only a small reduction in personal allergen exposure. ACI Int 2000; Suppl 2:57.
143. Tovey ER, Mitakakis TZ, Sercombe JK, Vanlaar CH, Marks GB. Four methods of sampling for dust mite allergen: differences in 'dust'. Allergy 2003; 58:790–794.
144. Mitakakis TZ, Mahmic A, Tovey ER. Comparison of vacuuming procedures for reservoir dust mite allergen on carpeted floors. J Allergy Clin Immunol 2002; 109:122–124.
145. Bollinger ME, Eggleston PA, Flanagan E, Wood RA. Cat antigen in homes with and without cats may induce allergic symptoms. J Allergy Clin Immunol 1996; 97:907–914.
146. Swanson MC, Campbell AR, Klauck MJ, Reed CE. Correlations between levels of mite and cat allergens in settled and airborne dust. J Allergy Clin Immunol 1989; 83:776–783.
147. Price JA, Pollock I, Little SA, Longbottom JL, Warner JO. Measurement of airborne mite antigen in homes of asthmatic children. Lancet 1990; 336:895–897.
148. Kenny LC, Aitken R, Chalmers C, et al. A collaborative European study of personal inhalable aerosol sampler performance. Ann Occup Hyg 1997; 41:135–153.
149. Gordon S, Tee R, Nieuwenhuijsen M, Lowson D, Harris J, Newman TA. Measurement of airborne rat urinary allergen in an epidemiological study. Clin Exp Allergy 1994; 24:1070–1077.
150. Swanson M, Bubak M, LW H, Yunginger J, Warner M, Reed C. Quantification of occupational latex aeroallergens in a medical centre. J Allergy Clin Immunol 1994; 94:445–51.
151. Renstrom A, Larsson P, Malmberg P, Bayard C. A new amplified monoclonal rat allergen assay used for evaluation of ventilation improvements in animal rooms. J Allergy Clin Immunol 1997; 100:649–655.
152. Vaughan N, Chalmers C, Botham R. Field comparison of personal samplers for inhalable dust. Ann Occup Hyg 1990; 34:553–573.
153. Mitakakis T, Graham JAH, Marks GB, Tovey ER. Comparison of indoor and outdoor Altemaira exposure using IRM intra-nasal samplers and IOM filter samplers. J Allergy Clin Immunol 1999; 103:S188.
154. Bartley D. Inhalable aerosol samplers. Appl Occup Environ Hyg 1998; 13:274–278.
155. Parvaneh S, Ahlf E, Elfman LHM, van Hage-Hamsten M, Elfman L, Nybom R. A new method for collecting airborne allergens (correction: 56:1229). Allergy 2000; 55:1148–1154.

156. Tovey ER, Marks GB, Matthews M, Green WF, Woolcock A. Changes in mite allergen Der p I in house dust following spraying with a tannic acid/acaricide solution. Clin Exp Allergy 1992; 22:67–74.

157. Karlsson AS, Hedren M, Almqvist C, Larsson K, Renstrom A. Evaluation of Petri dish sampling for assessment of cat allergen in airborne dust. Allergy 2002; 57:164–168.

158. Carswell F, Birmingham K, Oliver J, Crewes A, Weeks J. The respiratory effects of reduction of mite allergen in the bedrooms of asthmatic children– a double-blind controlled trial. Clin Exp Allergy 1996; 26:386–396.

159. De Lucca SD, Tovey ER. Quantitative modelling of domestic allergen (Der p1) using amplified ELISA assays and nasal sampling. J Allergy Clin Immunol 2001; 107:721.

160. Renstrom A, Karlsson AS, Manninen A, Tovey E. Measuring inhaled occupational allergens: a comparison between nasal sampling and conventional air sampling on filters using pumps. Eur Respir J 1999; 14(30):538s.

161. Gore RB, Hadi EA, Craven M, et al. Personal exposure to house dust mite allergen in bed: nasal air sampling and reservoir allergen levels. Clin Exp Allergy 2002; 32:856–859.

162. Gore RB, Bishop S, Durrell B, Curbishley L, Woodcock A, Custovic A. Air filtration units in homes with cats: can tey reduce personal exposure to cat allergen? Clin Exp Allergy 2003; 33:765–769.

163. Gore RB, Durrell B, Bishop S, Curbishley L, Woodcock A, Custovic A. High-efficiency particulate arrest–filter vacuum cleaners increase personal cat allergen exposure in homes with cats. J Allergy Clin Immunol 2003; 111:784–787.

164. Mitakakis TZ, Tovey ER, Yates DH, et al. Particulate masks and non-powdered gloves reduce latex allergen inhaled by healthcare workers. Respirology 2002; 7:A23.

165. Fernandez-Caldas E, Codina R, Ledford DK, Trudeau WL, Lockey RF. House dust mite, cat, and cockroach allergen concentrations in daycare centers in Tampa, Florida. Ann Allergy Asthma Immunol 2001; 87:196–200.

166. Cruz MJ, Rodrigo MJ, Anto JM, Morell F. An amplified ELISA inhibition method for the measurement of airborne soybean allergens. Int Arch Allergy Immunol 2000; 122:42–48.

167. Renstrom A, Gordon S, Larsson PH, Tee RD, Taylor AJN, Malmberg P. Comparison of a radioallergosorbent (RAST) inhibition method and a monoclonal enzyme linked immunosorbent assay (ELISA) for aeroallergen measurement. Clin Exp Allergy 1997; 27:1314–1321.

168. Gordon S, Wallace J, Cook A, Tee RD, Taylor AJN. Reduction of exposure to laboratory animal allergens in the workplace. Clin Exp Allergy 1997; 27: 744–751.

169. Wahl R, Heutelbeck A, Musken H. Comparison between EAST, CRIE, skin prick test and intracutaneous test at cat-allergic patients. Allergologie 1996; 19:356–360.

170. Wasserfallen JB, Aubert V, Mosimann B, Leuenberger P. Bronchial provocation with cat allergen—long-term outcome of the late allergic reaction and the individual IgE CRIE pattern. J Invest Allergol Clin Immunol 1995; 5: 134–141.

171. Swanson M, Campbell A, Klauck M, Reed C. Correlations between levels of mite and cat allergens in settled and airborne dust. J Allergy Clin Immunol. 1989; 83:776–783.
172. Takahashi Y, Nillson S, Berggren B. Aeroallergen immunoblotting with human IgE antibody. Grana 1995; 34:357–360.
173. Schumacher M, Griffith R, O'Rourke M. Recognition of pollen and other particulate aeroantigens by immunoblot microscopy. J Allergy Clin Immunol 1988; 82:608–616.
174. Acevedo F, Vesterberg O, Bayard C. Visualization and quantification of birch-pollen allergens directly on air-sampling filters. Allergy 1998; 53(6):594–601.
175. O'Meara T, DeLucca S, Sporik R, Graham A, Tovey E. Detection of inhaled cat allergen. Lancet 1998; 351:1488–1489.
176. Razmovski V, O'Meara T, Hjelmroos M, Marks G, Tovey E. Adhesive tapes as capturing surfaces in Burkard sampling. Grana 1998; 37:305–310.
177. De Lucca SD, O'Meara T J, Tovey ER. Exposure to mite and cat allergens on a range of clothing items at home and the transfer of cat allergen in the work-place. J Allergy Clin Immunol 2000; 106:874–879.
178. Poulos LM, O'Meara TJ, Hamilton RG, Tovey ER. Inhaled latex allergen (Hev b 1). J Allergy Clin Immunol 2002; 109:701–706.
179. Renstrom A, Karlsson AS, Tovey E. Nasal air sampling used for the assessment of occupational allergen exposure and the efficacy of respiratory protection. Clin Exp Allergy 2002; 32:1769–1775.
180. Mitakakis TZ, Barnes C, Tovey ER. Spore germination increases allergen release from Alternaria. J Allergy Clin Immunol 2001; 107:388–390.
181. Chapman MC, Tsay A, Vailes LD. Home allergen monitoring and control–improving clinical practice and patient benefits. Allergy 2001; 56:604–610.
182. Polzius R, Wuske T, Mahn J. Wipe test for the detection of indoor allergens. Allergy 2002; 57:143–145.
183. Niederberger V, Stubner P, Spitzauer S, et al. Skin test results but not serology reflect immediate type respiratory sensitivity: a study performed with recombinant allergen molecules. J Invest Dermatol 2001; 117:848–851.
184. Price JA, Marchant JL, Warner JO. Allersearch DMS in the control of domestic allergens. Clin Exp Allergy 1990; 20:65.
185. Green WF, Nicholas NR, Salome CM, Woolcock AJ. Reduction of house dust mites and mite allergens: effects of spraying carpets and blankets with Aller-search DMS, an acaricide combined with an allergen reducing agent. Clin Exp Allergy 1989; 19:203–207.
186. Haouichat H, Pauli G, Ott M, et al. Controlling indoor mite exposure: The relevance of the Acarex test. Indoor Built Environ 2001; 10:109–115.
187. Stewart GA, Bird CH, Krska KD, Colloff MJ, Thompson PJ. A comparative study of allergenic and potentially allergenic enzymes from *Dermatophagoides pteronyssinus*, *Dermatophagoides farinae* and *Euroglyphus maynei*. Exp Appl Acarol 1992; 16:165–180.
188. Dharmage S, Bailey M, Raven J, et al. Current indoor allergen levels of fungi and cats, but not house dust mites, influence allergy and asthma in adults with high dust mite exposure. Am J Respir Crit Care Med 2001; 164:65–71.

189. Shin EJ, Guertler N, Kim E, Lalwani AK. Screening of middle ear effusion for the common sinus pathogen Bipolaris. Eur Arch Otorhino laryngol 2003; 260:78–80.
190. Arlorio M, Coisson JD, Martelli A. Identification of *Saccharomyces cerevisiae* in bakery products by PCR amplification of the ITS region of ribosomal DNA. Eur Food Res Technol 1999; 209:185–191.
191. Urata T, Kobayashi M, Imamura J, et al. Polymerase chain reaction amplification of Asp f I and alkaline protease genes from fungus balls: clinical application in pulmonary aspergillosis. Intern Med 1997; 36:19–27.
192. Gaskell GJ, Carter DA, Britton WJ, Tovey ER, Benyon FHL, Lovborg U. Analysis of the internal transcribed spacer regions of ribosomal DNA in common airborne allergenic fungi. Electrophoresis 1997; 18:1567–1569.
193. Gregory P. The microbiology of the atmosphere. In: Polunin PN, ed. Plant Science Monographs. Bucks: Leonard Hill, 1973.
194. Smith G. Sampling and Identifying Allergenic Pollens and Molds. San Antonio, Texas: Bluestone Press, 1990:196.
195. Taylor MJ, Ponikau JU, Sherris DA, et al. Detection of fungal organisms in eosinophilic mucin using a fluorescein-labeled chitin-specific binding protein. Otolaryngol Head Neck Surg 2002; 127:377–383.
196. Einarsson R, Aukrust L. Allergens of the fungi imperfecti. Clin Rev Allergy 1992; 10:165–190.
197. Burge HP, Solomon WR, Boise JR. Comparative merits of eight popular media in aerometric studies of fungi. J Allergy Clin Immunol 1977; 60: 199–203.
198. Pei-Chih W, Huey-Jen S, Hsiao-Man H. A comparison of sampling media for environmental viable fungi collected in a hospital environment. Environ Res Sect A 2000; 82:253–257.
199. Noble WC, Clayton YM. Fungus in the air of hospital wards. J Gen Microbiol 1963; 32:397.
200. Noble WC. Sampling airborne microbes–handling the catch. In: Noble WC, ed. Airborne Microbes. Cambridge: University Press, 1967:81–101.
201. Bisht V, Singh BP, Arora N, Sridhara S, Gaur SN. Allergens of *Epicoccum nigrum* grown in different media for quality source material. Allergy 2000; 55:274–280.
202. Gupta R, Singh BP, Sridhara S, Gaur SN, Chaudhary VK, Arora N. Allergens of *Curvularia lunata* during cultivation in different media. J Allergy Clin Immunol 1999; 104:857–862.
203. Cadot P, Lejoly M, Stevens EAM. The effect of sucrose on the quality of ryegrass (*Lolium perenne*) pollen extracts. Allergy 1995; 50:941–951.
204. Carnes J, Femandez-Caldas E, Boluda L, et al. Rapid release of Ole e 1 from olive pollen using different solvents. Allergy 2002; 57:798–804.
205. Gupta N, Sriramarao P, Kori R, Rao PVS. Immunochemical characterization of rapid and slowly released allergens from the pollen of *Parthenium hysterophorus* (Reprinted). Int Arch Allergy Immunol 1995; 107:557–565.
206. Portnoy J, Pacheco F, Ballam Y, Barnes C. The effect of time and extraction buffers on residual protein and allergen content of extracts derived from 4 strains of Alternaria. J Allergy Clin Immunol 1993; 91:930–938.

207. Renström A, Gordon S, Hollander A, et al. Comparison of methods to assess airborne rat and mouse allergen levels. II. Factors influencing antigen detection. Allergy 1999; 54:150–157.
208. Hollander A, Gordon S, Renstrom A, et al. Comparison of methods to assess airborne rat and mouse allergen levels. I. Analysis of air samples. Allergy 1999; 54:142–149.
209. Pomes A, Helm RM, Bannon GA, Burks AW, Tsay A, Chapman MD. Monitoring peanut allergen in food products by measuring Ara h 1. J Allergy Clin Immunol 2003; 111:640–645.
210. Heederik D, Attfield M. Characterisation of dust exposure for the study of chronic occupational lung disease: a comparison of different exposure assessment strategies. Am J Epidemiol 2000; 151:982–990.
211. Sakaguchi M, Inouye S, Yasueda H, Irie T, Yoshizawa S, Shida T. Measurement of allergens associated with dust mite allergy. Int Arch Allergy Appl Immunol 1989; 90:190–193.
212. Tovey E, de Dreu A, Verspaandonk M, et al. Personal exposure to mite and cat allergens. J Allergy Clin Immunol 1999; 103:S32.

9

Monitoring Asthma in the Workplace

JEAN-LUC MALO, CATHERINE LEMIERE, ANDRÉ CARTIER, MANON LABRECQUE, and DENYSE GAUTRIN

Department of Chest Medicine, Hôpital du Sacré-Cœur de Montréal, Montréal, Québec, Canada

Introduction and Background

Asthma in the Workplace

Asthma can be caused or worsened by exposure to agents present in the workplace, Several interesting population-based studies have ascertained the frequency of symptomatic worsening of asthma and/or of asthma caused by the workplace, without distinguishing between the two entities. A community survey conducted in 12 industrialized countries and including more than 15,000 people aged 20–44 years showed that 5–10% of adult-onset asthma could be attributed to the workplace (1). A meta-analysis quotes similar figures (2). This does notprove that the workplace causes or exacerbates asthma. Confirmation should be obtained by objective testing and monitoring.

The general topic of asthma in the Workplace can be subdivided into different entities as illustrated in Fig. 1. Occupational asthma (OA) is defined as follows: "*Occupational asthma is a disease characterized by variable airflow limitation and/or airway hyper-responsiveness due to causes and conditions attributable to a particular occupational environment and not*

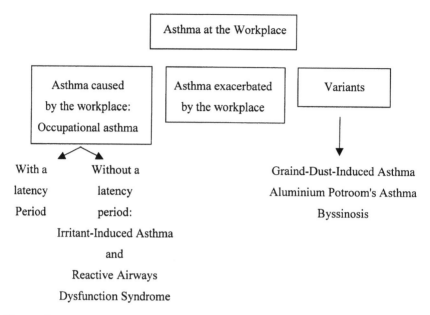

Figure 1 Types of asthmatic situations that can occur at the workplace.

to stimuli encountered outside the workplace." **(3)**. OA can occur after a latency period necessary for acquiring immunological sensitization or without a latency period, such as after an inhalational accident. There are also cases of workers with non-occupational asthma who may experience exacerbations of their asthma while at work due to exposures to non-specific stimuli such as dust, cold air, and fumes. In the latter instance, such exposures may cause a transient increase in asthma symptoms that are relieved by the use of inhaled bronchodilator. It is unlikely that such exposures, contrary to OA, result in permanent airway inflammation and remodelling. They act as triggers or inciters as opposed to inducers (4). There is no evidence that they lead to long-lasting changes in bronchial responsiveness (5) or airway inflammation (6). Clear distinction between OA and exacerbations of asthma at work should be made for medico–legal purposes and proper management (7,8). It is clear that exacerbation of asthma at work caused by nonspecific stimuli can be managed by reducing exposure to these irritants to recommended levels (9), and by more adequate asthma treatment by adjusting the medication. Typically, exacerbations of asthma at work signal an uncontrolled asthmatic situation, in which symptoms are exacerbated not only at work but in daily life when the subject is exposed to non-specific stimuli (unconditioned air, fumes, smoke, etc.). Better control of asthma by adjusting medication usually resolves the problem. The asthmatic worker can then tolerate workplace exposure even if the concentrations of a product exceed threshold limit values. By contrast, OA should be managed by advising the worker to avoid exposure to the causal agent; otherwise the asthma will worsen (10,11). Finally, there are variants of asthma in the workplace, like byssinosis (12), potroom or grain-dust-induced asthma (13), that share some similarities with asthma but are more likely to lead to fixed chronic obstructive lung disease.

From Airway Physiology to Airway Physiopathology

The definition of asthma proposed in the 1960s and frequently used is based on clinical and physiological items: episodic respiratory symptoms of shortness of breath, cough, and wheeze with airway obstruction that shows partial or complete recovery spontaneously or as a result of treatment, together with non-specific airway hyper-responsiveness (14).

Ascertainment of airway caliber is most often based on the volume of air maximally blown in the first second (the FEV_1) and the total volume of air blown (the vital capacity); their ratio is known as Tiffeneau's index after the French physiologist who suggested its use (15,16). This index is still the gold standard for assessing airway calibre. Other indices that also reflect airway obstruction, such as flows at different portions of the vital capacity, especially the non-effort-dependent part, and indices derived from the nitrogen washout curve (slope of Phase III, closing volume and capacity), were proposed by highly knowledgeable physiologists in the 1960s and 1970s, but have been almost entirely forgotten by today's practitioners. Airway resistance (or it's related value, specific conductance) is used by some physicians to assess airway caliber although it is less reliable than FEV_1. Because fluctuations in airway caliber are a critical element in asthma, it has been proposed that airway caliber be assessed with an effort-dependent index (an index almost totally disregarded in the 1960s and 1970s because of its effort-dependent nature), peak expiratory flow (PEF), which could be readily assessed using inexpensive, portable instruments (17,18). Such monitoring, carried out by the patient, is suggested in difficult cases of asthma. Treatments "action plans" using such values are recommended now and then, but they cannot be suggested in all asthma cases due to poor compliance (19). Serial monitoring of PEF (Sec. Rationale for selection of monitoring techniques: Tools to be applied for different purposes) was proposed by Burge et al. in 1979 (20,21) in the investigation of asthma in the workplace and has since been developed by this group. It is often used in the investigation of asthma in the workplace.

Assessment of airway hyper-responsiveness in humans with pharmacological agents was proposed in the 1940s (22,23), although standardized methods did not become available until the 1970s (24,25). Pharmacological agents such as methacholine and histamine are still the preferred means to evaluate non-specific bronchial responsiveness (Sec. Assessment of impairment/disability), although other physical and chemical agents such as exercise, cold air, and adenosine 5'-monophosphate can be used. This testing is particularly useful and meaningful when conducted at a time when airway caliber is normal. Its use was proposed in the investigation of work-related asthma in the 1980s (26,27).

With the advance in our knowledge of the physiopathology of asthma, it was suggested that we include a physiopathological item—"eosinophilic bronchitis"—in the definition of asthma. Flexible fibreoptic instruments made it possible to perform bronchoscopy and lavage with relative ease, making the assessment of inflammatory status more tolerable for patients. Methodologies for reliably obtaining and examining induced sputum were proposed in the 1980s (Sec. Non-invasive Monitoring of Airway Inflammation and Remodeling). Recent information suggests that asthma is more accurately managed through the use of the information obtained from induced sputum than from clinical and lung physiology (28). It is therefore possible that pneumologists and physicians who started their careers in the 1970s by asking their asthmatic patients to "blow hard" will ask them in the future to "expectorate hard." This evolving management is even more relevant with rapid advances in molecular biology that make it possible to examine the mediators of airway inflammation and the activity status of the key cells such as eosinophils, lymphocytes, and neutrophils. The only limitations, for the time being, are that induced sputum cannot be obtained from all individuals and that examination is time consuming and costly, and does not yield results rapidly enough to advise outpatients at the time of their visit. The same comments in terms of relevance and applicability can be made for another methodology aimed at assessing airway inflammation, the analysis of exhaled NO and other gases (Sect. Non-invasive Monitoring of Airway Information and Remodeling).

Natural History of Occupational Asthma with a Latency Period: Tools to be Applied at Different Steps

The natural history of the development of OA with a latency period is illustrated in Fig. 2 modified from Ref. (29). The first steps are characterized by initiation of immunological sensitization, at which time it is important to use reliable immunological tools that address IgE-dependent reactions, especially for high-molecular-weight (HMW) agents. The target organs are affected afterwards, often beginning with the nose and the eyes (30,31). At this step, tools that reflect physiopathological changes (cell types, quantity and activation; chemokines and mediators of airway inflammation, etc.) are a sensitive way to detect these changes. Thereafter, bronchial hyper-responsiveness appears, followed by airway obstruction. Lung-function tests are then required to measure these effects. At this step,

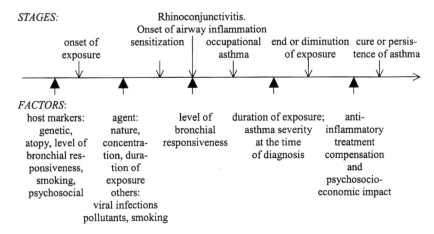

Figure 2 Steps and factors (at each step) of the natural history of occupational asthma. *Source*: Modified from Ref. 29.

it is important to make the most reliable diagnosis so as to advise the worker to leave his/her job or carry on working. Proper assessment of permanent disability after leaving exposure to the causal agent is often required for medico–legal purposes and is based on a combination of tools (questionnaire and physiological tests).

Rationale for Selection of Monitoring Techniques: Tools to be Applied for Different Purposes

Tools should be selected in relation to the use for which they are intended. For surveillance programs, tools need to be sensitive, simple, safe, and not costly. Questionnaires such as the one validated by the European Respiratory Society in the case of asthma (32) are a good example of such tools. Skin-prick testing with HMW proteinaceous agents is also a simple tool devoid of side effects in the detection of IgE sensitization (33). Assessment of bronchial responsiveness to methacholine is a longer procedure that is more costly, though safe in clinical and epidemiological settings (34). PEF monitoring is useful on an individual basis for the clinical investigation of work-related asthma (35), but it is more difficult for field studies in which contamination of data can occur (subjects may tell each other what values should be reported) and supervision is less stringent than for clinical investigation. Specific inhalation challenges with occupational agents are reserved for strictly clinical purposes (36,37). Assessing disability requires a proper assessment of asthma severity, for which information on asthma control, need for medication, baseline spirometry, and airway responsiveness need to be considered (38).

Monitoring

General Considerations

Monitoring of asthma that may be related to the workplace is based on a decision tree in which various steps are followed and specific tools are proposed. This decision tree suggests using simple and sensitive tests for the initial procedures and adding more complex and specific tests in a progressive way.

Figure 3 presents a proposed decision tree for surveillance programs in high-risk workplaces. The combination of a questionnaire and assessment of specifc-IgE status is first proposed in the case of high-molecular- and some low-molecular-weight (LMW) agents for which skin-prick testing is feasible (male rat urine, which is a strong antigen in the case of laboratory animal handlers (39,40); cereals and flour; enzymes; platinum salts). Assessment of bronchial responsiveness can be reserved for those with positive skin tests. It is even doubtful whether responses to the questionnaire should be kept in the decision tree. In a surveillance program among hospital nurses, Vandenplas et al. (41) identified seven nurses with OA to latex. Whereas all of them had positive skin tests, two did not report symptoms suggestive of asthma or OA. It is known that subjects with positive skin tests

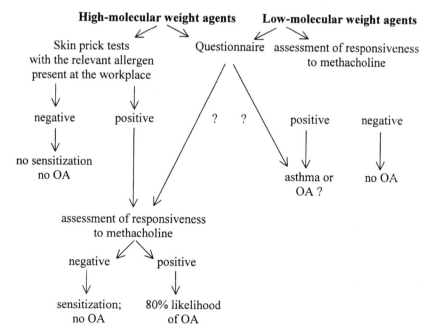

Figure 3 Algorithm for the investigation of OA in a surveillance program. Question marks indicate questionable steps.

and bronchial hyper-responsiveness have an 80% chance of developing an asthmatic reaction on exposure to the relevant antigen in the laboratory (42,43). In the case of LMW agents, for which, in the majority of cases, skin-prick tests cannot be performed, a combination of questionnaire and assessment of bronchial responsiveness is suggested, although the validity of such an approach has not been tested. Also untested is the validity of a medical interview at this step. The medical questionnaire administered to subjects referred to a clinic for suspected OA is indeed a sensitive tool (44). At least, if there is no airway hyper-responsiveness, this reasonably excludes asthma and OA.

In the case of clinical investigation of work-related asthma, an algorithm has been proposed (45) (Fig. 4). Since this publication, new tools that assess airway inflammation have been proposed. Exhaled NO was found to

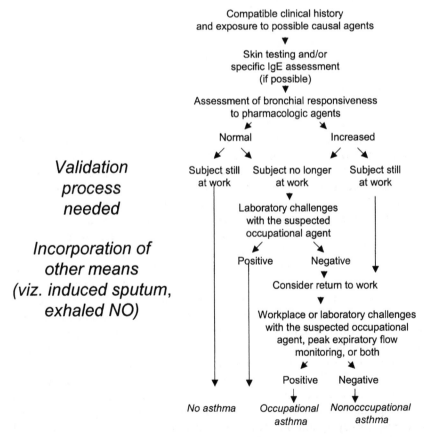

Figure 4 Algorithm for the investigation of OA in a clinical setting. *Source*: From Ref. 45.

be significantly increased 24 hrs after challenges with plicatic acid (46). Increase in sputum eosinophils has also been documented in subjects with OA after bronchial inhalation challenges (46,47,6). While an increase in sputum eosinophils is typical after an asthmatic reaction following challenge with an occupational agent, recent work suggests that there might be an increase in neutrophils in asthmatic subjects without OA exposed for several days in their workplace (48). It is therefore our opinion that inflammatory monitoring of induced sputum cells represents a useful adjunct to the functional monitoring provided by serial PEF and assessment of bronchial responsiveness in the investigation of OA. Moreover, induced sputum should be performed together with the assessment of bronchial responsiveness after performing inhalation challenges with occupational agents.

Questionnaires

For Epidemiological Surveys and Surveillance Programs

In epidemiological field studies of populations of workers or apprentices at risk of developing OA, a respiratory symptom questionnaire (32) and a work history questionnaire are of great value for the detection of possible early markers of OA. These questionnaires can be administered by a nurse or another health-care worker during face-to-face interviews. Shorter versions of these questionnaires have been developed for self-administration (49). The bronchial symptoms questionnaire developed for epidemiological studies on asthma (50) has been tested for its validity and reproducibility, translated into several languages, and assessed internationally (32). Questions on respiratory symptoms under normal and specific conditions, such as cold, exercise, exposure to heavy dust and fumes, and to such environmental allergens as pollens, pets, or dust mites, are useful for identifying subjects who may be at increased risk of developing OA, as are questions on rhinitis, whether perennial, seasonal, or on contact with pets (31). Two questions from the bronchial symptoms questionnaire (*Have you ever had asthma? Was this confirmed by a doctor?*) are commonly used in epidemiological studies to assess the presence of asthma. A number of questionnaires have been developed to obtain information on work history, including type of industry, job title, duration of work for each employment, work sensitizers used, use of personal protective equipment, and subjective assessment of level and duration (usually on a weekly basis) of exposure; these questionnaires are adapted to each particular working environment but have not been standardized. A series of questions makes it possible to document the presence of work-related skin symptoms, nasal symptoms (runny nose, sneezing, stuffy nose), ocular symptoms (itchy eyes, watery eyes, red eyes), and respiratory symptoms (wheezing, cough, and chest tightness); to be considered as work-related, the symptoms have to be present at work and improve on weekends and/or on holidays.

Although no questionnaire has been validated specifically in the case of OA, similar questionnaires have been used in different epidemiological study designs and in surveillance programs. In prevalence, or cross-sectional studies in workforces at risk, the questionnaires enable us to determine the prevalence of work-related nasal and/or respiratory symptoms and to identify those subjects who are more susceptible to have, or develop other features of OA and are therefore candidates for further investigation. In longitudinal prospective studies of large workforces (i.e., prospective cohort studies), the information collected makes it possible to determine the incidence of work-related symptoms (51,52) and, eventually, of probable OA, if information is also available on skin-prick-test reactivity to occupational sensitizers (when applicable) and/or on the status of non-specific airway responsiveness (31,53). Although such a "questionnaire-based" approach is sensitive, some cases can still be missed in asymptomatic subjects; therefore, coupling questionnaires with other tools has been suggested (54).

The methods used for the purpose of medical surveillance do not differ significantly from those used in cross-sectional and longitudinal epidemiological surveys. Short self-administered questionnaires containing key questions on common respiratory symptoms and work-related symptoms can be used. Further investigation, more specific for OA, is indicated for subjects selected on the basis of their responses to this questionnaire. The problems with these questionnaires are that workers may be illiterate or may answer certain questions dishonestly for fear that they will lose their jobs.

For Clinical Purposes

The questionnaire still represents a key element in a diagnostic and therapeutic endeavor. An open, physician-driven questionnaire, complemented by systematic adherence to key questions, is a powerful tool that will not be replaced. It represents a very sensitive, though not very specific tool (44). Indeed, we previously found that 65/75 subjects (sensitivity of 87%) with OA had a very likely or likely diagnosis based on an open, physician-driven questionnaire. Only 9/33 subjects (specificity of 27%) without asthma and OA had what was considered to be a negative questionnaire. The sensitivity of the questionnaire in the clinical assessment of OA has also been estimated to be 87% by Vandenplas et al. (55), as assessed in a group of symptomatic workers exposed to natural rubber latex. However, in the quoted study, skin-prick test to latex was 100% sensitive and coupling skin-prick test and history proved to have greater sensitivity (94%) than history alone.

All adult subjects with asthma should be questioned about past and current occupations. In the vast majority of cases, subjects with OA start having symptoms as adults, but an asthma history as a child is not impossible. Past exposure to a potential workplace causal agent should be explored. Stopping exposure to an agent causing OA results in improvement of symptoms, but generally, the asthma persists. Current occupational history is crucial. A combination of self-reported occupational exposure and information about present occupation makes it possible to build a job-exposure matrix that can be useful (56). Information on job title is useful: knowing that a worker is a nurse should alert the physician to the possibility of exposure to latex, glutaraldehyde, psyllium, and various pharmaceutical powders, all known sensitizing agents. Working in a plastic company exposes workers to many potential sensitizing agents. It is as important to get material safety data (MSD) sheets on all products handled at the workplace and not only by the worker. Reference to a published list of agents causing OA with a latency period can greatly ease searches (asmanet; asthme.csst.qc.ca). MSD sheets have recently been criticized on the grounds that they do not distinguish between the irritant and sensitizing properties of the ingredient, nor do they provide an exhaustive list of the contents of all of the product's ingredients (57), particularly when the proportion of an agent represents less than 1%. In some cases, then, it is worthwhile to call the product's manufacturer for further information. Key elements of the occupational history have been proposed by Bernstein (58). Besides recording employment history, symptoms should be documented in terms of their nature, temporality, and possible improvement or worsening in relation to work (58). The question regarding improvement on weekends and holidays is sensitive but not specific. Modification of asthma treatment throughout the course of symptomatology should be taken into account in the interpretation. Nasoconjunctival symptoms should be questioned as they may precede or coincide with the development of OA, more so in the case of HMW than LMW agents, and are most often present in irritant-induced asthma. Moreover, it has recently been found that occupational rhinitis may increase the risk of developing asthma (59).

In the cases of asthma exacerbated by the workplace and of irritant-induced asthma, it is relevant to determine whether exposure to irritant levels has occurred and whether other workers have also complained of symptoms. Documentation of exposure to irritant levels that exceed acceptable levels (9) can sometimes be obtained from surveys carried out by industrial hygienists. Diagnosis of irritant-induced asthma most often depends on a reliable clinical history in which a worker, most often with no previous respiratory disease, states that he or she was exposed to abnormally high levels of an irritant material and developed upper and lower airway symptoms within minutes or hours (60), or, at the latest, during the following days (61). The abrupt onset of an intense burning sensation in the nose after the inhalation of a substance (often referred to as a "puff) is a common symptom in respiratory upper airways dysfunction syndrome

(RUDS) and reactive airways dysfunction syndrome (RADS). Often, other workers present in the vicinity are affected as well. Symptoms are more frequent and intense in those workers who are closer to the source (62,63). Accidental inhalations lead to visits to the first-aid unit of the workplace or to emergency rooms. Workers are too often discharged without a control visit at which the status of airway responsiveness can be assessed. Administering parenteral (64) followed by inhaled steroids is a valuable treatment in case of RADS. Vapors, such as chlorine and ammonia, the two most common agents causing RUDS and RADS, and aerosols, cause irritant-induced asthma more often than dry particles (63). There are also instances of workers repeatedly exposed to irritant material who experience mini-RADS "puffs" symptoms. These workers do not necessarily go to the first-aid unit but may experience functional changes (65). The transience or permanence of these changes merits further exploration.

Monitoring of Antibodies

Skin-prick testing is easy to carry out both in field studies and during clinical assessment. Interpretation of positive skin-prick tests to common inhalants is blurred by the fact that, currently, 50% of young adults are "atopic" (66). There are no standardized extracts for agents causing OA (67). LMW agents, chemicals, cannot be tested on the skin. Generally, practitioners and researchers have to rely on antigenic preparations made in laboratories of experts in the field, and these preparations may not have been approved by regulatory agencies. The presence of an immediate reaction means that the worker has immunological sensitization, but not necessarily the disease. Of approximately 100 apprentices who acquired sensitization to an animal-derived allergen, only one-third developed bronchial hyper-responsiveness and were labelled subjects with probable OA in the study by Gautrin et al. (68). Sensitization can exist on its own or accompanied by nasoconjunctival, cutaneous, or respiratory symptoms. Assessment of specific IgE to occupational allergens by in vitro tests bears no benefit over simple skin-prick testing in the case of HMW agents. For some LMW agents, specific IgE and IgG can be assessed. This is the case for isocyanates for which increased specific IgE levels at the time of exposure is specific though not very sensitive not only for the presence of OA (69,70) but also for the persistence of symptoms and bronchial responsiveness after removal from exposure. An increase in specific IgG may reflect sensitization (71) and/ or exposure. Recently, increase in antigen-stimulated monocyte chemo attract ant protein-1 synthesis has been shown to have greater test efficiency than specific IgE and IgG antibodies for OA due to isocyanates (70).

Lung Function Tests

If FEV_1, the Tiffeneau index (FEV_1/forced vital capacity) and the concentration of methacholine or histamine causing a 20% fall in FEV_1 (PC20) are normal when the worker is at work, whether he/she has respiratory symptoms or not, OA is virtually excluded. If FEVl is reduced and significantly improved after the use of a bronchodilator, it is a strong support for a diagnosis of asthma, although it does not tell if the asthma is caused or exacerbated by the workplace. Airway hyper-responsiveness is present in active asthma, but can also exist in subjects with rhinitis and chronic bronchitis associated with tobacco smoking, although, in the latter instances the level of bronchial hyper-responsiveness is generally mild. Most studies have found that variations in airway hyper-responsiveness, as determined by comparing periods at work and away from work, are not satisfactorily associated with OA. However, having a so-called positive PC20 value while at work and a negative PC20 while away from work is suggestive of OA. It is unlikely that exacerbations of asthma at work by exposure to irritant stimuli would be accompanied by changes in bronchial hyper-responsiveness.

For Surveillance Programs

Assessment of FEV_1 can be done at the workplace. However, the ideal timing in relation to work should be towards the end of a work shift. This is not always feasible. Moreover, theoretically, pre and postshift FEV_1 would pick up significant fluctuations suggestive of OA. However, this does not seem to be the case (72). Assessment of airway responsiveness to methacholine can be performed at the workplace. Serial monitoring of PEF has been used in surveillance programs, but we do not know if it is as useful as in a clinical setting. Close^ supervision of the worker is needed to ensure that he/she does the monitoring accurately.This is not always feasible and workers have a tendency to "contaminate" their results (73) by telling each other what values to write in their diaries.

For Clinical Purposes

Before claiming that someone has workplace-exacerbated asthma, it must be demonstrated that the worker does in fact suffer from asthma. As with non-occupational asthma, this can easily be done by having the subject perform a spirometry. If the spirometry is significantly reduced a bronchodilator is given; if it is normal, methacholine responsiveness is assessed.

In order to show that someone suffers from OA, Burge initially proposed using PEF monitoring in the investigation of OA in the same way it had been used previously for assessing asthma (20). Burge and his colleagues have subsequently carried out many studies using PEF in the assessment of OA. This team developed a computer-assisted program (OASYS) that provides automated readings of PEF and states a likelihood score for the presence of OA (74). The sensitivity and specificity of this method of assessment by comparison with specific inhalation challenges are 75% each. While this method is simple and cheap, it does present pitfalls in terms of compliance and falsification, and these can affect the interpretation of data. Moreover, in many instances, it cannot differentiate between asthma exacerbated by, and asthma caused by the workplace.

Exposing the worker to an agent suspected of causing asthma and present in the workplace can be done either at work or in a hospital laboratory under close supervision by a technician. The methodology of these tests, first proposed by Pepys (75), has been extensively covered (36,76). These tests are time-consuming but are still considered to be the gold standard. They are safe when preformed in specialized centres and under the close supervision of an expert physician. When performed in the laboratory, they also allow identification of the offending agent (making recommendations for rehabilitation easier). Exposing subjects to low concentrations of a product makes it possible to disclose any irritant reactions and to avoid too-serious asthmatic reactions (77). These tests can be done with closed-circuit equipment that can generate low and stable concentrations; this is possible with several but not all agents (36). Specific inhalation tests can be falsely negative if the subject is not exposed to the right agent in the laboratory or if the causal agent is no longer used at work. If the tests are negative and OA is suspected, there should be a provision to return the worker to his/her usual workplace and monitor PEF to make sure that no worsening of asthma appears. The tests generally remain positive even years after cessation of exposure, although the dose of occupational sensitizer required to elicit a positive reaction is generally larger (78).

Non-invasive Monitoring of Airway Inflammation and Remodeling

Induced Sputum

The first papers reporting the use of induced sputum in the investigation of OA were published in the 1990s. They showed that the subjects with OA had higher eosinophil counts when they were at work compared with periods away from work (47). Recent data suggest that the analysis of induced sputum yields additional information beyond PEF monitoring during periods at work and away from work, thus facilitating the diagnosis of OA (48).

Changes in sputum cell counts after exposure to various occupational agents during specific inhalation challenges in the laboratory have also been studied and described in a number of case reports (79–81). As in asthma, eosinophils are the cells that are most often increased in the sputum of subjects with occupational asthma. Sputum eosinophils can be induced by exposure to both HMW (6,81) and LMW agents (82,83). However, both sputum eosinophilia and neutrophilia have been reported after exposure to LMW agents. Some agents, such as isocyanates, seem to induce a neutrophilic, rather than an eosinophilic inflammation following specific challenges (84,85,89).

Exposure to occupational agents per se does not seem to induce non-specific changes in airway inflammation in subjects not sensitized to these agents (6). Indeed, asthmatic subjects without OA showed no change in their sputum cell counts after exposure to occupational agents such as flour or acrylates. One potentially interesting role of induced sputum in OA is the early diagnosis of the condition—that is, before the occurrence of respiratory symptoms and pulmonary function changes. As in asthma (86,87), changes in induced sputum can precede functional changes in FEV_1 and PC20 after exposure to occupational agents (88). However, the use of induced sputum in the early diagnosis of OA in workers exposed to sensitizers remains to be assessed.

Induced sputum may also be beneficial for following workers after removal from exposure. Indeed, Chan-Yeung et al. (89) showed that the percentage of sputum eosinophils was correlated inversely with FEV_1 and positively with the class of respiratory impairment. Therefore, induced sputum provides more information than FEV_1 and PC20 and may be an asset for the diagnosis and follow-up of subjects with OA.

Exhaled NO

Relatively few studies have investigated the changes in exhaled NO in OA. The results are not consistent throughout the different studies published. Some authors found higher exhaled NO levels in subjects with OA to laboratory animals compared with asymptomatic exposed subjects (90). Others failed to show any difference in exhaled NO after work exposure to latex in latex-sensitive subjects (91). A non-specific increase in exhaled NO was shown in subjects without OA exposed to plicatic acid, whereas subjects with OA did not show any change in exhaled NO after exposure to plicatic acid (46). A significant positive correlation between sputum eosinophils and exhaled NO has been shown (89); however, exhaled NO was not correlated with functional parameters (FEV_1, PC20) or respiratory impairment.

More recently, exhaled NO was measured before and after specific challenges to methylene diphenyldiisocyanate (MDI) and latex, as well as before and after challenge to methacholine (92). The changes in exhaled NO were not consistent throughout the different inhalation challenges.

Since it is relatively simple to measure exhaled NO, this procedure has been proposed as a potentially valuable epidemiological tool for the early detection of occupational asthma. Lund et al. (93) have investigated whether exhaled NO could be an early marker of potroom asthma. They investigated 186 subjects employed in potrooms and 40 controls. The 99 non-smokers exposed to potrooms had higher levels of exhaled NO than the 30 non-smoking controls. Although statistically significant, the difference between exposed and non-exposed subjects was minimal and its clinical significance unclear. Moreover, there was no difference between groups when the smokers were included. Therefore, exhaled NO may have some value for the early detection of OA in the workplace, but the factors affecting its measurement, such as smoking, inhaled-steroid treatment, or suboptimal bronchodilation are likely to limit its usefulness in clinical practice.

An example of investigation of an individual case of workplace asthma is proposed in Table 1 (Box A), whereas discussion on a surveillance program in a high-risk workplace is presented in Table 2 (Box B).

Assessment of Impairment/disability

It is often necessary to assess impairment and disability for insurance or medico–legal purposes. Some subjects are affected with severe asthma, and asthma may lead to severe obstruction of the airways. These subjects may not be able to work, justifying insurance assessment.

Impairment is functional decrement by comparison with normal values, whereas disability (work disability in this instance) is a compromised capacity for work (94). When the diagnosis of OA with a latency period is made, the worker is considered 100% impaired, as he/she cannot return to his/her normal work. Rehabilitation programs should help workers to find another job, either with the same company or another, with or without training, and with a satisfactory quality of life (95).

In approximately 75% of cases of OA with a latency period, and probably an equivalent proportion of subjects with irritant-induced asthma, there is persistent airway hyper-responsiveness that causes permanent asthmatic symptoms (94). Most often, the impairment is mild to moderate. The causes and mechanism of this permanent impairment are unknown. Recent findings show that there is often persistent inflammatory influx of eosinophils and neutrophils with elevated levels of IL-8 and myeloperoxidase (MPO) (Maghni K et al., in preparation), in parallel with the degree of the asthmatic condition at the time the diagnosis of OA is made. Information on the nature and magnitude of the persisting inflammatory status is lacking in the case of irritant-induced asthma. Although exposing subjects with asthma to occupational agents to which they are sensitized in a realistic way does not cause influx of inflammatory cells in induced sputum, more detailed exploration of the inflammatory status including chemokines is warranted to ensure that exposing asthmatic subjects to non-specific stimuli in the workplace does not increase airway inflammation.

The best time to assess permanent impairment/disability in relation to cessation of exposure is questionable. It was first assumed that the

Table 1 Example of Investigation of an Individual Case of Workplace Asthma

A worker is exposed accidentally to a "spill" of isocyanate that is normally used at work in acceptable concentrations. In the following hours, he develops symptoms of coughing, wheezing and shortness of breath. He pays a visit to an emergency room where he is given oxygen and a wet aerosol of bronchodilator. He is discharged a few hours later. He is away from work for two weeks and becomes asymptomatic. On returning to work, he experiences wheezing and a burning sensation in the eyes and nose every time he is exposed to isocyanates, which are present at apparently acceptable concentrations (no evidence of recurrence of spill).

What tools will you propose to diagnose one of the following: OA due to isocyanate with a latency period or irritant-induced asthma or exacerbation of asthma in the workplace?

Comments and Answer

Confirmation of asthma as defined by reversible airflow obstruction and/or bronchial hyper-responsiveness (as assessed by a methacholine or histamine bronchial challenge) should first be considered. This worker had no assessment of airway caliber when evaluated in the emergency room, as this could have probably confirmed airflow obstruction. The diagnosis of OA without a latency period is based on history of exposure to a toxic chemical and documentation of persistent asthma. On his discharge from the emergency room, this worker might have warranted treatment with oral or inhaled steroids and a follow-up visit to make sure that he was not left with airway hyper-responsiveness.

Recurrence of symptoms upon return to a working environment where exposure to irritants is usually at low concentrations, makes the diagnosis of OA with a latency period also possible. Documentation of asthma should be made by asking the subject to record his PEF ideally every two hours at work, and asking for a methacholine test at the end of a two-week period at work. If PEF shows fluctuations suggestive of asthma and the methacholine test reveals significant bronchial responsiveness, provision should be made to have the worker off work for two weeks and compare PEF values with the period at work. If PEF values away from work show less fluctuation, specific inhalation challenges with isocyanates in a laboratory (if this service is available) or monitoring of spirometry at work under supervision by a technician should be considered. If this testing is positive, the diagnosis is OA with a latency period. There is indeed a suggestion that isocyanate spills might increase the risk of acquiring "sensitization" to isocyanate and OA with a latency period. If this testing is negative, it suggests that the worker has suffered sequelae from irritant-induced asthma. He should be treated for his asthma and returned to work, in which case exposure to non-specific irritants will probably no longer cause symptoms or changes in PEF.

improvement in OA and irritant-induced asthma reaches a plateau two years after leaving work. In the case of OA with a latency period, the data were based on a follow-up study that included 31 workers previously

Table 2   Discussion of a Surveillance Program in a High-Risk Workplace

A 29-year-old man has been working in a poultry slaughterhouse for 13 years. For the past five years, he has had a runny nose and, for the last seven months, asthma symptoms, principally at work. The diagnosis of OA due to hens' feathers is subsequently proven by specific inhalation challenges. The company's physician mentions that two other workers in this company of 100 employees have reported nasal and respiratory symptoms. The local Health and Safety Committee asks you to conduct a survey at the plant. What decision tree and tools will you propose to conduct that survey?

Comments and Answer

OA has been reported in poultry slaughterhouses and hens' feathers are the causal agent. The aim of the survey should be to assess the prevalence of respiratory symptoms suggestive of OA, immunologic sensitization and OA, and to identify possible cases. Hens' feathers are considered a HMW agent. Therefore, besides a surveillance questionnaire, it would be appropriate to include a skin-prick test with hens' feathers as a first investigation tool. To improve the success rate of such a survey, it is essential that both the employer and the employees are aware of it's aims and that a proper readaptation–relocation program is agreed upon for those workers in whom OA will be confirmed.

The enclosed decision tree illustrates one possibility.

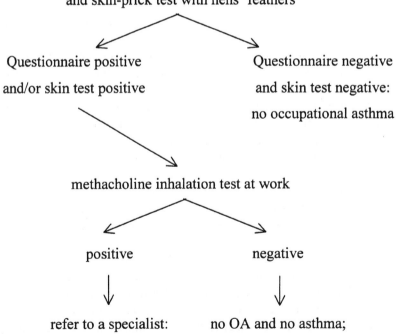

Surveillance questionnaire
and skin-prick test with hens' feathers

Questionnaire positive and/or skin test positive

Questionnaire negative and skin test negative: no occupational asthma

methacholine inhalation test at work

positive

negative

refer to a specialist: asthma or OA

no OA and no asthma; follow-up to be done in those with positive skin test

(*Continued*)

Table 2 Discussion of a Surveillance Program in a High-Risk Workplace (*Continued*)

Subjects with a positive questionnaire and/or skin test reactivity to hens' feathers will be invited to participate in a further investigation. The next step would be to assess bronchial responsiveness to methacholine during a regular working day or in the following 3–4 hr. Then, subjects with positive methacholine test will be referred to a specialist who will consider specific inhalation challenges. In this case, they can be performed at the workplace by monitoring FEV_1 hourly during a work shift and, by comparison, after a day away from work. Alternatively, monitoring of PEF at work, coupled with assessment of PC20 methacholine may be sufficient to document OA. The latter approach is, however, more time consuming than performing monitoring of spirometry at work. Those with a negative methacholine test, but positive skin test to hens' feathers, should be followed to see whether OA at a later stage.

---

exposed, though only seasonally, to snow-crab (96). These results were extrapolated to all cases of OA with a latency period. However, more recent works show that, although the improvement is probably steeper in the first two years after cessation of exposure, there is still improvement afterwards and even many years after cessation of exposure (97,98),. In the case of irritant-induced asthma, improvement was noticed from approximately six months to two-and-a-half years after stopping exposure (99), though the outcome at a later stage is unknown.

The tools to assess impairment/disability need to be appropriate for the type of condition. Until 1993, the tools proposed for respiratory diseases were specifically inadequate for asthma (100). Exercise testing was required, but exercise performance is meaningless in this situation. Moreover, no consideration was made for the level of airway hyperresponsiveness, which is a key aspect of asthma. New tools specifically addressing impairment/disability for asthma were proposed by the American Thoracic Society in 1993 (38). The asthmatic situation should be clinically stable as judged by the absence of nocturnal awakenings and minimal need for extra-bronchodilator. Scales are presented and take into account three main factors: the type of medication required to maintain satisfactory asthma control, the level of bronchial obstruction and acute reversibility after bronchodilator and the level of airway responsiveness. Although this guide represents a major improvement, some items warrant revision. For example, the level of airway obstruction considered is the one obtained after administering a bronchodilator. Should the pre- or post- or average value be used? The dose of inhaled steroids to control asthma and the use of new anti-inflammatory preparations and long-acting bronchodilators should be further considered in the assessment.

Table 3 Assessment of Impairment/Disability

A worker with OA with a latency period is reassessed two years after leaving work. She is told that she warrants class II impairment/disability according to suggested scales (Ref. 100). What tools were used to assess her impairment/disability? How does the worker's case fit in these scales?

Comments and answer

Tools to be used to assess impairment/disability include need for medication to control asthma, baseline spirometry, and non-specific airway responsiveness. By referring to Ref. 100, this worker still has airway obstruction and hyper-responsiveness and needs regular anti-inflammatory medication.

An example of a subject with OA in whom impairment/disability needs to be assessed is proposed in Table 3 (Box C).

Conclusion

Although clinical and physiological tools have been the preferred means to assess asthma in the workplace, there is now a tendency to add assessment of airway inflammation through non-invasive means. To date, information has been obtained primarily in cases of OA with a latency period. More work needs to be done in cases of OA without a latency period (irritant-induced asthma) and the consequences of non-specific worsening of asthma in the workplace. Improvement is also needed in the specific case of the assessment of impairment/disability after stopping exposure to an agent present in the workplace.

Acknowledgment

The authors express their gratitude to Lori Schubert for reviewing this article.

References

1. Kogevinas M, Anto JM, Sunyer J, Tobias A, Kromhout H, Burney P, Group and the European Community Respiratory Health Survey Study. Occupational asthma in Europe and other industrialised areas: a population-based study. Lancet 1999; 353:1750–1754.
2. Blanc PD, Toren K. How much asthma can be attributed to occupational factors? Am J Med 1999; 107:580–587.
3. Bernstein IL, Chan-Yeung M, Malo JL, Berstein D. Asthma in the Workplace. 2nd ed. New York, NY: Marcel Dekker Inc., 1999.
4. Dolovich J, Hargreave FE. The asthma syndrome: inciters, inducers, and host characteristics. Thorax 1981; 36:641–644.

5. De Luca S, Caire N, Cloutier Y, Cartier A, Ghezzo H, Malo JL. Acute exposure to sawdust does not alter airway calibre and responsiveness to histamine in asthmatic subjects. Eur Respir J 1988; 1:540–546.

6. Lemière C, Chaboillez S, Malo JL, Cartier A. Changes in sputum cell counts after exposure to occupational agents: What do they mean? J Allergy Clin Immunol 2001; 107:1063–1068.

7. Wagner GR, Wegman DH. Occupational Asthma: Prevention by Definition. Am J Ind Med 1998; 33:427–429.

8. Malo JL, Chan-Yeung M. Comment on the editorial: Occupational asthma: Prevention by definition. Am J Ind Med 1999; 35:207.

9. American Conference of Governmental Industrial Hygienists. 2001 TLVs and BEIs. Threshold Limit Values for Chemical Substances and Physical Agents. Cincinnati, OH 2001.

10. Côté J, Kennedy S, Chan-Yeung M. Outcome of patients with cedar asthma with continuous exposure. Am Rev Respir Dis 1990; 141:373–376.

11. Moscato G, Dellabianca A, Perfetti L, Brame B, Galdi E, Niniano R, Paggiaro P. Occupational asthma. A longitudinal study on the clinical and socioeconomic outcome after diagnosis. Chest 1999; 115:249–256.

12. Merchant JA, Bernstein II, Pickering A. Cotton and other textile dusts. In: Bernstein IL, Chan-Yeung M, Malo JL, Bernstein DI, eds. Asthma in the Workplace. New York: Marcel Dekker Inc., 1999:595–616.

13. Chan-Yeung M, Kennedy S, Schwartz DA. Grain dust-induced lung diseases. In: Bernstein IL, Chan-Yeung M, Malo JL, Bernstein DI, eds. Asthma in the Workplace. New York: Marcel Dekker Inc., 1999:617–634.

14. American Thoracic Society. Chronic bronchitis, asthma, and pulmonary emphysema. Statement by the committee on diagnostic standards for nontuberculous respiratory diseases. Am Rev Respir Dis 1962; 85:762–768.

15. Tiffeneau R, Bousser J, Drutel P. Capacité vitale et capacité pulmonaire utilisable à l'effort. Critères statique et dynamique de la ventilation pulmonaire. Paris Méd 1949:543–547.

16. Yernault JC. The birth and development of the forced expiratory manoeuvre: a tribute to Robert Tiffeneau (1910–1961). Eur Respir J 1997; 10:2704–2710.

17. Flint FJ, Khan MO. Clinical use of peak flow meter. Br Med J 1962: 1231–1233.

18. Turner-Warwick M. On observing patterns of airflow obstruction in chronic asthma. Br J Dis Chest 1977; 71:73–86.

19. Verschelden P, Cartier A, L'Archevêque J, Trudeau C, Malo JL. Compliance with and accuracy of daily self-assessment of peak expiratory flows (PEF) in asthmatic subjects over a three month period. Eur Respir J 1996; 9:880–885.

20. Burge PS, O'Brien IM, Harries MG. Peak flow rate records in the diagnosis of occupational asthma due to isocyanates. Thorax 1979; 34:317–323.

21. Burge PS, O'Brien IM, Harries MG. Peak flow rate records in the diagnosis of occupational asthma due to colophony. Thorax 1979; 34:308–316.

22. Dautrebande L, Philippot E. Crise d'asthme experimental par aérosols de carbaminoylcholine chez l'homme traitée par dispersat de phénylaminopropane. Presse Médicale 1941; 49:942–946.

23. Tiffeneau R, Beauvallet M. Épreuve de bronchoconstriction et de bronchodi-latation par aérosols. Emploi pour le dépistage, la mesure et le contrôle des insuffisances respiratoires chroniques. Bull Acad Natl Méd (Paris) 1945; 129:165–168.

24. Chai H, Fair RS, Froehlich LA, Mathison DA, McLean JA, Rosenthal RR, Sheffer AL, Spector SL, Townley RG. Standardization of bronchial inhalation challenge procedures. J Allergy Clin Immunol 1975; 56:323–327.

25. Cockcroft DW, Killian DN, Mellon JJA, Hargreave FE. Bronchial reactivity to inhaled histamine: a method and clinical survey. Clinical Allergy 1977; 7:235–243.

26. Hargreave FE, Ramsdale EH, Pugsley SO. Occupational asthma without bronchial hyperresponsiveness. Am Rev Respir Dis 1984; 130:513–515.

27. Cartier A, L'Archevêque J, Malo JL. Exposure to a sensitizing occupational agent can cause a long-lasting increase in bronchial responsiveness to hista-mine in the absence of significant changes in airway caliber. J Allergy Clin Immunol 1986; 78:1185–1189.

28. Green RH, Brighting CE, McKenna S, Hargadon B, Parker D, Bradding P, Wardlaw AJ, Pavord ID. Asthma exacerbations and sputum eosinophil counts: a randomised controlled trial. Lancet 2002; 360:1715–1721.

29. Malo JL, Ghezzo H, D'Aquino C, L'Archevêque J, Cartier A, Chan-Yeung M. Natural history of occupational asthma: relevance of type of agent and other factors in the rate of development of symptoms in affected subjects. J Allergy Clin Immunol 1992; 90:937–944.

30. Malo JL, Lemière C, Desjardins A, Cartier A. Prevalence and intensity of rhinoconjunctivitis in subjects with occupational asthma. Eur Respir J 1997; 10:1513–1515.

31. Gautrin D, Ghezzo H, Infante-Rivard C, Malo JL. Natural history of sensiti-zation, symptoms and diseases in apprentices exposed to laboratory animals. Eur Respir J 2001; 17:904–908.

32. Burney PGJ, Laitinen LA, Perdrizet S, Huckauf H, Tattersfield AE, Chinn S, Poisson N, Heeren A, Britton JR, Jones T. Validity and repeatability of the IUATLD (1984) bronchial symptoms questionnaire: an international compar-ison. Eur Respir J 1989; 2:940–945.

33. Barbee RA, Lebowitz MD, Thompson HC, Burrows B. Immediate skin-test reactivity in a general population sample. Ann Intern Med 1976; 84:129–133.

34. Troyanov S, Malo JL, Cartier A, Gautrin D. Frequency and determinants of exaggerated bronchoconstriction during shortened methacholine challenge tests in epidemiological and clinical set-ups. Eur Respir J 2000; 16:9–14.

35. Burge PS, Moscato G. Physiologic assessment: Serial measurements of lung function. In: Bernstein IL, Chan-Yeung M, Malo JL, Bernstein DL, eds. Asthma in the Workplace. 2nd ed. New York: Marcel Dekker Inc., 1999:193–210.

36. Vandenplas O, Malo JL. Inhalation challenges with agents causing occupa-tional asthma. Eur Respir J 1997; 10:2612–2629.

37. Cartier A, Malo JL. Occupational challenge tests. In: Bernstein IL, Chan-Yeung M, Malo JL, Bernstein DL, eds. Asthma in the Workplace. 2nd ed. New York: Marcel Dekker Inc., 1999:211–233.

38. American Thoracic Society. Guidelines for the evaluation of impairment/disability in patients with asthma. Am Rev Respir Dis 1993; 147:1056–1061.
39. Gordon S, Taylor AJ Newman. Animal, insect, and shellfish allergy. In: Bernstein IL, Chan-Yeung M, Malo JL, Bernstein DL, eds. Asthma in the Workplace. New York: Marcel Dekker Inc., 1999:399–424.
40. Gautrin D, Ghezzo H, Infante-Rivard C, Malo JL. Incidence and determinants of IgE- mediated sensitization in apprentices: a prospective study. Am J Respir Crit Care Med 2000; 162:1222–1228.
41. Vandenplas O, Delwiche JP, Evrard G, Aimont P, Brempt X Van der, Jamart J, Delaunois L. Prevalence of occupational asthma due to latex among hospital personnel. Am J Respir Crit Care Med 1995; 151:54–60.
42. Cockcroft DW, Ruffin RE, Frith PA, Cartier A, Juniper EF, Dolovich J, Hargreave FE. Determinants of allergen-induced asthma: dose of allergen, circulating IgE antibody concentration, and bronchial responsiveness to inhaled histamine. Am Rev Respir Dis 1979; 120:l053–1058.
43. Malo JL, Cartier A, L'Archevêque J, Ghezzo H, Lagier F, Trudeau C, Dolovich J. Prevalence of occupational asthma and immunologic sensitization to psyllium among health personnel in chronic care hospitals. Am Rev Respir Dis 1990; 142:1359–1366.
44. Malo JL, Ghezzo H, L'Archevêque J, Lagier F, Perrin B, Cartier A. Is the clinical history a satisfactory means of diagnosing occupational asthma? Am Rev Respir Dis 1991; 143:528–532.
45. Chan-Yeung M, Malo JL. Occupational asthma. N Engl J Med 1995; 333:107–112.
46. Obata H, Cittrick M, Chan H, Chan-Yeung M. Sputum eosinophils and exhaled nitric oxide during late asthmatic reaction in patients with western red cedar asthma. Eur Respir J 1999; 13:489–495.
47. Lemière C, Pizzichini MMM, Balkissoon R, Clelland L, Efthimiadis A, O'Shaughnessy D, Dolovich J, Hargreave FE. Diagnosing occupational asthma: use of induced sputum. Eur Respir J 1999; 13:482–488.
48. Girard F, Côté J, Boulet LP, Tarlo S, Hargreave FE, Lemière C. Role of induced sputum in the investigation of occupational asthma. Am J Respir Crit Care Med 2003; 167:A685.
49. Venables KM, Farrer N, Sharp L, Graneek BJ, Taylor AJ Newman. Respiratory symptoms questionnaire for asthma epidemiology: validity and reproducibility. Thorax 1993; 48:214–219.
50. Burney PGJ, Luczynska C, Chinn S, Jarvis D. The European Community Respiratory Health Survey. Eur Respir J 1994; 7:954–960.
51. Cullinan P, Cook A, Gordon S, Nieuwenhuijsen MJ, Tee RD, Venables KM, McDonald JC, Taylor AJ Newman. Allergen exposure, atopy and smoking as determinants of allergy to rats in a cohort of laboratory employees. Eur Respir J 1999; 13:1139–1143.
52. Rodier F, Gautrin D, Ghezzo H, Malo JL. Incidence of occupational rhinoconjunctivitis and risk factors in animal-health apprentices. J Allergy Clin Immunol 2003; 112:1105–1111.

53. El-Zein M, Malo JL, Infante-Rivard C, Gautrin D. Incidence of probable occupational asthma and of changes in airway calibre and responsiveness in apprentice welders. Eur Respir J 2003; 22:513–518.

54. Gordon SB, Curran AD, Murphy J, Sillitoe C, Lee G, Wiley K, Morice AH. Screening questionnaires for bakers' asthma-are they worth the effort? Occup Med 1997; 47:361–366.

55. Vandenplas O, Cangh F Binard-Van, Brumagne A, Caroyer JM, Thimpont J, Sohy C, Larbanois A, Jamart J. Occupational asthma in symptomatic workers exposed to natural rubber latex: Evaluation of diagnostic procedures. J Allergy Clin Immunol 2001; 107:542–547.

56. Le Moual N, Bakke P, Orlowski E, Heederik D, Kromhout H, Kennedy SM, Rijcken B, Kauffmann F. Performance of population specific job exposure matrices (JEMs): European collaborative analyses on occupational risk factors for chronic obstructive pulmonary disease with job exposure matrices (ECOJEM). Occup Environ Med 2000; 57:126–132.

57. Bernstein JA. Material safety data sheets: are they reliable in identifying human hazards? J Allergy Clin Immunol 2002; 110:35–38.

58. Bernstein DI. Clinical assessment and management of occupational asthma. In: Bernstein IL, Chan-Yeung M, Malo JL, Bernstein DI, eds. Asthma in the Workplace. 2nd ed. New York: Marcel Dekker Inc., 1999:145–157.

59. Karjalainen A, Martikainen R, Klaukka T, Saarinen K, Uitti J. Risk of asthma among Finnish patients with occupational rhinitis. Chest 2003; 123:283–288.

60. Brooks SM, Weiss MA, Bernstein IL. Reactive airways dysfunction syndrome (RADS). Persistent asthma syndrome after high level irritant exposures. Chest 1985; 88:376–84.

61. Brooks SM, Hammad Y, Richards I, Giovinco-Barbas J, Jenkins K. The spectrum of irritant-induced asthma. Chest 1998; 113:42–49.

62. Kern DG. Outbreak of the reactive airways dysfunction syndrome after a spill of glacial acetic acid. Am Rev Respir Dis 1991; 144:1058–1064.

63. Gautrin D, Bernstein IL, Brooks S. Reactive airways dysfunction syndrome, or irritant-induced asthma. In: Bernstein IL, Chan-Yeung M, Malo JL, Bernstein DI, eds. Asthma in the Workplace. New York: Marcel Dekker Inc., 1999:565–593.

64. Demnati R, Fraser R, Martin JG, Plaa G, Malo JL. Effects of dexamethasone on functional and pathological changes in rat bronchi caused by high acute exposure to chlorine. Toxicol Sci 1998; 45:242–246.

65. Gautrin D, Leroyer C, Infante-Rivard C, Ghezzo H, Dufour JG, Girard D, Malo JL. Longitudinal assessment of airway caliber and responsiveness in workers exposed to chlorine. Am J Respir Crit Care Med 1999; 160: 1232–1237.

66. Gautrin D, Infante-Rivard C, Dao TV, Magnan-Larose M, Desjardins D, Malo JL. Specific IgE-dependent sensitization, atopy and bronchial hyperresponsiveness in apprentices starting exposure to protein-derived agents. Am J Respir Crit Care Med 1997; 155:1841–1847.

67. Moscato G, Malo JL, Bernstein D. Diagnosing occupational asthma: how, how much, how far? Eur Repir J 2003; 21:879–885.

68. Gautrin D, Infante-Rivard C, Ghezzo H, Malo JL. Incidence and host determinants of probable occupational asthma in apprentices exposed to laboratory animals. Am J Respir Crit Care Med 2001; 163:899–904.

69. Tee RD, Cullinan P, Welch J, Burge PS, Newman-Taylor AJ. Specific IgE to isocyanates: A useful diagnostic role in occupational asthma. J Allergy Clin Immunol 1998; 101:709–715.

70. Bernstein DI, Cartier A, Cote J, Malo JL, Boulet LP, Warmer M, Milot J, L'Archeveque J, Trudeau C, Lummus Z. Diisocyanate antigen-stimulated monocyte chemoattractant protein-1 synthesis has greater test efficiency than specific antibodies for identification of diisocyanate asthma. Am J Respir Crit Care Med 2002; 166:445–450.

71. Cartier A, Grammer L, Malo JL, Lagier F, Ghezzo H, Harris K, Patterson R. Specific serum antibodies against isocyanates: association with occupational asthma. J Allergy Clin Immunol 1989; 84:507–514.

72. Burge PS. Single and serial measurements of lung function in the diagnosis of occupational asthma. Eur J Respir Dis 1982; 63(suppl 123):47–59.

73. Cartier A, Malo JL, Forest F, Lafrance M, Pineau L, St-Aubin JJ, Dubois JY. Occupational asthma in snow crab-processing workers. J Allergy Clin Immunol 1984; 74:261–269.

74. Gannon PFG, Newton DT, Belcher J, Pantin CFA, Burge PS. Development of OASYS-2: a system for the analysis of serial measurement of peak expiratory flow in workers with suspected occupational asthma. Thorax 1996; 51: 484–489.

75. Pepys J, Bernstein IL. Historical aspects of occupational asthma. In: Bernstein IL, Chan-Yeung M, Malo JL, Bernstein DI, eds. Asthma in the Workplace. 2nd ed. New York: Marcel Dekker Inc., 1999:5–26.

76. Sterk PJ, Fabbri LM, Quanjer PH, Cockcroft DW, O'Byrne PM, Anderson SD, Juniper EF, Malo JL. Airway responsiveness. Standardized challenge testing with pharmacological, physical and sensitizing stimuli in adults. Report working party standardization of lung function tests European Community for Steel and Coal. Official statement of the European Respiratory Society. Eur Respir J 1993; 6(suppl 16):53–83.

77. Malo JL, Cartier A, Lemière C, Desjardins A, Labrecque M, L'Archevèque J, Perrault G, Lesage J, Cloutier Y. Exaggerated bronchoconstriction due to inhalation challenges with occupational agents. Eur Respir J 2004; 23:300–303..

78. Lemière C, Cartier A, Malo JL, Lehrer SB. Persistent specific bronchial reactivity to occupational agents in workers with normal nonspecific bronchial reactivity. Am J Respir Crit Care Med 2000; 162:976–980.

79. Lemière C, Weytjens K, Cartier A, Malo JL. Late asthmatic reaction with airway inflammation but without airway hyperresponsiveness. Clin Exp Allergy 2000; 30:415–417.

80. Leigh R, Hargreave FE. Occupational neutrophilic asthma. Can Respir J 1999; 6:194–196.

81. Alvarez MJ, Castillo R, Rey A, Ortega N, Blanco C, Carrillo T. Occupational asthma in a grain worker due to Lepidoglyphus destructor, assessed by bronchial provocation test and induced sputum. Allergy 1999; 54:884–889.

82. Quirce S, Baeza ML, Tornero P, Blasco A, Barranco R, Sastre J. Occupational asthma caused by exposure to cyanoacrylate. Allergy 2001; 56:446–449.

83. Maestrelli P, Calcagni PG, Saetta M, Stefano A Di, Hosselet JJ, Santonastaso A, Fabbri LM, Mapp CE. Sputum eosinophilia after asthmatic responses induced by isocyanates in sensitized subjects. Clin Exp Allergy 1994; 24:29–34.

84. Park HS, Jung KS, Kim HY, Nahm DH, Kang KR. Neutrophil activation following TDI bronchial challenges to the airway secretion from subjects with TDI-induced asthma. Clin Exp Allergy 1999; 29:1395–1401.

85. Lemiére C, Romeo P, Chaboillez S, Tremblay C, Malo JL. Airway inflammation and functional changes after exposure to different concentrations of isocyanates. J Allergy Clin Immunol 2002; 110:641–646.

86. Pizzichini MMM, Pizzichini E, Clelland L, Efthimiadis A, Pavord I, Dolovich J, Hargreave FE. Prednisone-dependent asthma: inflammatory indices in induced sputum. Eur Respir J 1999; 13:15–21.

87. Jatakanon A, Lim S, Barnes PJ. Changes in sputum eosinophils predict loss of asthma control. Am J Respir Crit Care Med 2000; 161:64–72.

88. Lemiére C, Chaboilliez S, Trudeau C, Taha R, Maghni K, Martin JG, Hamid Q. Characterization of airway inflammation after repeated exposures to occupational agents. J Allergy Clin Immunol 2000; 106:1163–1170.

89. Chan-Yeung M, Obata H, Dittrick M, Chan H, Abboud R. Airway inflammation, exhaled nitric oxide, and severity of asthma in patients with western red cedar asthma. Am J Respir Crit Care Med 1999; 159:1434–1438.

90. Adisesh LA, Kharitonov SA, Yates DH, Snashell DC, Newman-Taylor AJ, Barnes PJ. Exhaled and nasal nitric oxide is increased in laboratory animal allergy. Clin Exp Allergy 1998; 28:876–880.

91. Tan K, Bruce C, Birkhead A, Thomas PS. Nasal and exhaled nitric oxide in response to occupational latex exposure. Allergy 2001; 56:627–632.

92. Allmers H, Chen Z, Barbinova L, Marcynski B, Kirschman V, Baur X. Challenge from methacholine, natural rubber latex, or 4,4'-diphenylmethane diisocyanate in workers with suspected sensitization affects exhaled nitric oxide (change in exhaled NO levels after allergen challenges). Int Arch Occup Environ Health 2000; 73:181–186.

93. Lund MB, Oksne PI, Hamre R, Kongerud J. Increased nitric oxide in exhaled air: an early marker of asthma in non-smoking aluminium potroom workers? Occup Environ Med 2000; 57:274–278.

94. Malo JL, Blanc P, Chan-Yeung M. Evaluation of impairment/disability in subjects with occupational asthma. In: Bernstein IL, Chan-Yeung M, Malo JL, Bernstein DI, eds. Asthma in the workplace. New York: Marcel Dekker Inc., 1999:299–313.

95. Malo JL, Dewitte JD; Cartier A, Ghezzo H, L'Archeveque J, Boulet LP, Côté J, Bédard G, Boucher S, Champagne F, Tessier G, Contandriopoulos AP. Quality of life of subjects with occupational asthma. J Allergy Clin Immunol 1993; 91:1121–1127.

96. Malo JL, Cartier A, Ghezzo H, Lafrance M, Mccants M, Lehrer SB. Patterns of improvement of spirometry, bronchial hyperresponsiveness, and specific IgE antibody levels after cessation of exposure in occupational asthma caused by snow-crab processing. Am Rev Respir Dis 1988; 138:807–812.

97. Perfetti L, Cartier A, Ghezzo H, Gautrin D, Malo JL. Follow-up of occupational asthma after removal from or diminution of exposure to the responsible agent. Chest 1998; 114:398–403.

98. Padoan M, Pozzato V, Simon M, Zedda L, Milan G, Bononi J, Piola C, Maestrelli P, Boschetto P, Mapp CE. Long-term follow-up of toluene diisocyanate-induced asthma. Eur Respir J 2003; 21:637–640.

99. Malo JL, Cartier A, Boulet LP, L'Archeveque J, Saint-Denis F, Bherer L, Courteau JP. Bronchial hyperresponsiveness can improve while spirometry plateaus two to three years after repeated exposure to chlorine causing respiratory symptoms. Am J Respir Crit Care Med 1994; 150:1142–1145.

100. American Thoracic Society. Evaluation of impairment/disability secondary to respiratory disorders. Am Rev Respir Dis 1986; 133:1205–1209.

10

Monitoring Airway Hyperresponsiveness: Pharmacological Stimuli

ALAN JAMES

West Australian Sleep Disorders Research Institute,
  Sir Charles Gairdner Hospital, and School of Medicine and
  Pharmacology, University of Western Australia,
Nedlands, Western Australia, Australia

Introduction

The role of airway challenge tests using pharmacologic stimuli in asthma has fluctuated in importance over the last 40 years. Initially proposed as diagnostic tests for asthma, they have not found widespread use in this regard. These tests remain useful in the detection of asthma in epidemiological surveys and have been included in the definition of asthma. As our knowledge of the pathology and "natural" history of asthma has increased and the focus of asthma treatment has gradually extended beyond days, weeks, and months to years, the use of direct challenge with pharmacologic stimuli is likely to increase. There are two reasons for this. Firstly, direct airway challenges may be useful to ensure the adequacy of current therapy and secondly, to determine the long-term efficacy of treatment, analogous to the use of the glycosylated hemoglobin in managing diabetes.

Pharmacologic stimuli are classified as direct if they cause airflow limitation by acting on airway smooth muscle without involving intermediate pathways. This chapter focusses on the two stimuli that have been studied most extensively, methacholine and histamine. Other pharmacologic stimuli

Table 1 Frequency of Use of Challenge Agents in U.S. Laboratories (28)

Type of challenge	Number	Percentage of total
Methacholine	10,858	62
Histamine	3,012	17
Exercise	1,442	8
Specific antigen	800	5
Acetylcholine	360	2
Occupational agents	314	2
Distilled water	258	2
Hyperventilation	148	1
Hyperosmolar saline	97	1
Other	238	1

such as pilocarpine, carbachol, acetylcholine, prostaglandin D2, and leuko-trienes C4/D4/E4 have all been shown to have direct effects on airway smooth muscle in vitro or in vivo, however, they are used rarely in the clinical or epidemiologic setting. They are predominantly used for mechanistic studies and will be dealt with only very briefly. Pharmacologic stimuli with indirect effects include adenosine, tachykinins, bradykinins, metabisulfite, sulfur dioxide, and propranolol, and will be discussed only to compare with the direct pharmacologic stimuli. Methacholine is used most often for direct challenges in clinical laboratories in the United States (Table 1). Exercise testing is used most frequently as an indirect challenge. These findings are reflected in the focus of recent ATS guidelines (1).

Properties of Methacholine and Histamine

Methacholine

Methacholine is a beta-methyl synthetic analog of acetylcholine, which acts throughout the body via cholinergic receptors. It is metabolized by the cholinesterases, although more slowly than acetylcholine. Since there is very little metabolism by the plasma butyryl-cholinesterase, the actions of methacholine are of longer duration than acetylcholine. Exogenous methacholine induces airway smooth muscle contraction by direct stimulation of muscarinic (M3) receptors on the cell surface. Receptor stimulation leads to the release of calcium from intracellular stores via a G-protein coupled activation of phospholipase C and inositol-1,4,5-triphosphate. The bronchoconstrictive response to inhaled methacholine is reduced in sensitivity by prior inhalation of anticholinergic agents (2,3) and by beta-agonists (2,4,5), and variably by sodium cromoglycate (6,7). Bronchoconstriction following inhaled methacholine is reversible with inhaled beta-agonists including isoproterenol and salbutamol, and with anti-cholinergic agents such as ipratropium bromide (8,9).

Bronchoconstriction induced by inhalation of methacholine is prevented, attenuated, or rapidly reversed by atropine (2,3) and beta-agonists (2,8). Using standard protocols, the onset and peak of effect are rapid and the spontaneous recovery occurs at approximately 45 min (Table 2) (10). The time course may be longer in non-asthmatic subjects and may be dose dependent. The use of higher doses is associated with a greater duration of effect in some individuals. After premedication with inhaled ipratropium bromide and inhalation of concentrations of methacholine between 128 and 362 mg/mL, 4 of 12 asthmatic subjects complained of wheeze, chest tightness, or breathlessness 5–12 hr later (2). Tolerance has been observed where repeat methacholine challenges have been administered within 24 hr or less (11–13), The mechanisms remain unclear but appear to be related to the administration of high doses to non-asthmatic subjects (12).

Histamine

Histamine is a naturally occurring biogenic amine, which is formed by the decarboxylation of L-histidine in numerous tissues. The highest organ levels are observed in the lung at $33 \pm 10 \, \mu g/gm$ of tissue (14), It is released from mast cells after IgE cross-linking by antigen, with direct effects on end organs such as airway smooth muscle and mucous glands. The effects of

Table 2 Properties of Methacholine and Histamine (References)

Property	Methacholine chloride	Histamine diphosphate
Molecular weight	197.5	325.2
Stability	4 months at or below room temperature (224)	8 months in opaque container at or below 12°C (225)
Action on airways	Direct on smooth muscle	Direct on smooth muscle indirect via nerves and mediators
Time course of action mean [range] (226)		
onset	2 [1–4] min	2 [1–4] min
duration	75 [12–150]	17 [4–37]
recovery	57 [14–97]	26 [5–35]
Tachyphylaxis[a]	Yes (11,13)	Yes (227,228)

[a]The degree of tachyphylaxis is generally less complete than observed with indirect stimuli (229).

histamine are mediated via three receptor subtypes. Contraction of non-vascular smooth muscle occurs through interaction of histamine with H_1 receptors coupled to intracellular G-protein and phospholipase C. Stimulation of the H_1 receptor results in the formation of IP_3 (inositol-1,4,5-triphosphate) and the release of stored intracellular calcium. H_2 receptors are important in gastric secretion and H_3 receptors have inhibitory feedback effects. The effects of histamine are opposed by H_1 receptor blockers and the first- and second-generation anti-histamines. The simultaneous administration of histamine and methacholine by inhalation has little additive effect on airway function (15). Refer to Table 2 and time course of effect.

Adverse Effects

Direct agents (methacholine and histamine) have a very good history of safety with an extensive experience of use in man published in the medical literature. There are no reported fatalities associated with their use and very few serious side effects.

Systemic administration of methacholine causes diffuse muscarinic effects: (a) cardiovascular—vasodilatation, bradycardia, reduced systemic blood pressure (usually accompanied by a compensatory tachycardia that masks any bradycardia); (b) gastrointestinal—salivation, increased peristalsis and secretion; (c) respiratory—bronchoconstriction, increased tracheobronchial secretions; (d) ocular—miosis and increased tear production. The systemic administration of histamine is poorly tolerated due to headache, flushing, sweats, tachycardia, and hypotension (16). These side effects may also be observed after inhalation of histamine at high doses. The bronchoconstrictive action of inhaled methacholine and histamine produces symptoms of airway narrowing in 30—70% of subjects (17,18). The symptoms include breathlessness, chest tightness, wheeze, and cough, and they correlate only poorly with the degree of bronchoconstriction that is induced (17,18). They are almost universally described as mild to moderate and alleviated rapidly by inhaled beta-agonists. Non-airway reactions include excess salivation, headache, facial flushing, and sweating and are seen in less than 2% of subjects using standard protocols for methacholine (17). These symptoms are seen more often when higher doses are used (9,19), are short-lived, and are described as mild to moderate (9,19). Dizziness, fatigue, and nausea (9,19,20) may also be reported and are probably due to the repetitive respiratory maneuvers needed during the standard tests since they occur more commonly in older subjects and are less common when less strenuous maneuvers are used (9,19,20).

One study (18) was undertaken to specifically examine the adverse effects of methacholine inhalation challenge and has been published in abstract form. Patients with asthma (n = 68, aged 11–78 yr) with normal lung function were given a standard challenge and 32 had $\geq 20\%$ fall in FEV_1 (responders) while 36 patients had only a fall in FEV_1 of 0–16% (non-responders). Responders reported symptoms of cough, chest tightness, throat irritation, dyspnea, and dizziness (28–72%) more often than non-responders (19–44%). Flushing, headache, salivation, and sweating were "less common." There were statistically significant but small changes in heart rate, blood pressure, and oxygen saturation in responders. Immediate symptoms lasted for a mean of 16 min and FEV_1 was reversible to 92% of the baseline value by two inhalations of isoetharine. After 12–24 hr, five subjects reported a mild increase in cough or chest tightness that did not require additional medication. The authors concluded that methacholine challenge was a safe procedure in subjects with normal lung function, and is associated with mild and reversible symptoms.

In the Lung Health Study (17), methacholine challenge was performed on 5877 current cigarette smokers, aged 35–59 years with borderline to moderate airflow obstruction and side effects were assessed. In the open-ended enquiry, 246 (5%) subjects reported side effects from inhalation of methacholine. When direct questioning was used, 37% reported one or more symptoms, which included cough (25%), shortness of breath (21%), wheeze (10%), dizziness (6%), headache (2%), nausea ($<1\%$), and "other" (4%). Only a "few" subjects had their test terminated by the technician due to symptoms, or required evaluation by a physician. After leaving the study center, "several" subjects complained of headache, one subject had a recurrence of chest tightness, and one subject was found to have a pneumothorax several days after the study was completed. The use of methacholine challenge in 78 sedated infants has recently been reported to show good tolerability and safety (21).

Townley et al. (10) reported their experience using a modification of the dosimeter technique in over 1500 methacholine challenges in children and adults and noted: (a) no reaction severe enough to require hospitalization; (b) reversal to normal pulmonary function within 5 min in most subjects after a bronchodilator, or within 30–45 min without a bronchodilator (c) and; no incidences of delayed reactions.

Using standard protocols, histamine was reported to cause laryngeal irritation with cough or a hoarse voice although these effects were uncommon and mild (22).

Comparisons of Responses to Methacholine and Histamine

In general, the reproducibility of airway responses to histamine is comparable with the responses to methacholine (2,10,23,24) although one study has suggested that methacholine more reliably distinguishes subjects with asthma (25). Considerable variation in sensitivity to histamine and methacholine may exist within individual subjects (10,26). In children, one study showed that airway responses to histamine were reduced compared with methacholine on a molar basis (10,26). In another community study, the reproducibility of methacholine was similar to that of histamine although more subjects responded to methacholine than histamine (27). Some studies have suggested that histamine responses may be less reproducible than those for methacholine (23,25,27).

The site of action of methacholine appears to be confined to the large airways, whereas histamine is said to stimulate both small and large airways (28), and cause changes in the mechanical properties of the lung parenchyma (29). A study in adults showed no differences in changes in ventilation–perfusion distribution and respiratory system resistance induced by either histamine or methacholine (30). The ventilatory responses (tidal volume, inspiratory time, and frequency) to methacholine and histamine are reportedly similar (31). Both agents cause comparable falls in arterial oxygen saturation in relation to bronchoconstriction (32), although in the same study, histamine caused increases in inspiratory and expiratory times whereas methacholine did not.

Methods of Testing

The Development of Formal Tests of Airway Responsiveness

Dautrebaude and Philpott (33) and Tiffeneau and Beauvallet (34) showed in the early 1940s that patients with asthma had increased airway responses to histamine and cholinergic agents. The studies of Curry (35) in 1946 and Parker et al. (36) in 1965 showed that, like acetylcholine and histamine, inhaled methacholinc produced exaggerated airway responses in asthmatic patients compared with non-asthmatic individuals.

The study of Parker et al. (36) included a total of 80 individuals with a variety of illnesses including asthma, hay fever, bronchiectasis, hyperventilation syndrome, emphysema, and chronic bronchitis. Adults and children were studied, including siblings of subjects with asthma. The reproducibility of the test was examined by performance of a second test in 17 individuals within a short period and repeating the test 15 times over a 2-year period in the same subject. They concluded that the test was highly reproducible, that it identified patients with asthma who had greater responses than normal subjects, and that patients with other respiratory diseases had increased responses to inhaled methacholine but not as marked as seen in patients with asthma.

Administration of bronchoconstrictors was initially by intramuscular or intravenous injection (35). Most early inhalation tests were undertaken using fixed concentrations or doses nebulized into a reservoir in a tidal breathing circuit (37). This fixed dosage schedule occasionally resulted in the sudden onset of symptoms that were sometimes severe and associated with large reductions in lung function (37). Parker et al. (36) administered nebulized methacholine (25 mg/mL) during a single inspiratory capacity breath. If there was less than a 20% fall in FEV_1, then four more inhalations of the same solution were taken and the response was measured. They found this stepped approach to be safe and free of systemic side effects in 400 different subjects although three asthmatic subjects had sudden moderately severe responses to the initial dose, which could be reversed immediately with subcutaneous epinephrine. Since then a number of protocols, using lower starting doses, have been developed for inhalation challenge with methacholine and other agents, although no single method has been universally adopted.

Standard Methodologies

Guidelines for methacholine (and exercise) challenge testing have recently been published (1) and guidelines for a range of challenge tests were published in 1993 by the European Respiratory Society (8).

Tidal Breathing Method

This method (23,38) has been thoroughly standardized with attention to the technical and non-technical factors that might affect the test variability (39). During the test, subjects are asked to breath quietly (tidal breaths) for a fixed period (usually 2 min) while inhaling aerosols through a mask or mouthpiece from a reservoir, nebulizer, or circuit. After inhalation of a neutral, control solution (normal saline or diluent), increasing concentrations or doses of methacholine are delivered at 5-min intervals. The airway response (usually FEV_1) is measured at 30 and 90 sec after each period of tidal breathing. The usual range of concentrations that is given is from 0.03 to 32 mg/mL. The test continues until there is a 20% fall in FEV_1 or until all doses have been given. To shorten the procedure, doses can be omitted if there is less than 10% fall in FEV_1 and the starting dose can be adjusted as below.

Most testing of this method has been carried out by Hargreave et al. (39). They have conducted bronchial provocation tests using histamine and methacholine in a large number of subjects and shown it to be a safe method (40). To avoid sudden, large responses in very sensitive subjects, the starting concentration of methacholine is adjusted according to a number of criteria (8):

1. FEV_1/FVC >80% *and* FEV_1 >70% predicted *and* FEV_1 falls <10% after control *and* symptoms are well controlled, starting concentration is between 0.125 and 2.0 mg/mL depending on current medication:

Corticosteroids   0.125 mg/mL
Daily bronchodilators   0.25 mg/mL
Occasional bronchodilators   1.0 mg/mL
No medication   2.0 mg/mL

2. FEV_1/FVC <80% *or* FEV_1 <70% predicted *and* FEV_1 falls <10% after control *and* symptoms are well controlled, starting concentrations are between 0.03 and 0.125 mg/mL depending on current medication:

Corticosteroids   0.03 mg/mL
Other or no medication   0.125 mg/mL

3. If the FEV_1 falls > 10% after control, or if asthma symptoms are not well controlled, starting concentration is 0.03 mg/mL *and* no concentration steps are skipped.

Dosimeter Method

This test has also been well standardized (8,41). Subjects inhale nebulized control solution and increasing concentrations of methacholine or histamine (0.03–32 mg/mL) using five consecutive inspiratory capacity breaths—from functional residual capacity to total lung capacity. The dosimeter delivers aerosol for a set time (usually 0.6 sec) whilst the subject takes an inspiratory breath. It is activated by the subject's inspiratory flow. Doses are administered at 5-min intervals and the response (FEV_1) is measured at 30 and 90 sec after inhalation. Starting doses and end points are the same as for the tidal breathing method.

Yan (Or Rapid) Method

This method (42) was developed to give a safe and portable procedure with a short time required for its completion. Hand-held nebulizers are used to deliver a variable number of puffs of control and methacholine or histamine solutions (3.15, 6.25, 25, and 50 mg/mL) during inspiratory breaths. The breath is held for 3 sec at Total Lung Capacity after each inhalation. The number of breaths delivered for each concentration of methacholine varies to give a range of delivered doses from 0.03 to 7.8 µmol. FEV_1 is measured 60 sec after each dose and the next dose is then administered. The test is stopped if there is a 20% fall in FEV_1. The protocol is dependent upon initial lung function, severity of symptoms, medication use, and the response at each dose, as for the tidal breathing and dosimeter methods.

"Squeeze" Method for Infants

Aerosolized methacholine (or histamine) is delivered to a sleeping or sedated infant (usually less than 12 months old) in doubling concentrations from 0.125 mg/mL to 16 mg/mL (43,44). The response is measured as changes in the maximum expiratory flow at a given lung volume such as functional residual capacity (V_{max}FRC). The test is continued until all doses are given or until a predetermined change in lung function occurs—usually a 40% change in V_{max}FRC.

Variations

The tidal breathing, dosimeter, and Yan methods have been best characterized and are recommended for routine clinical testing (8). A survey of current practice has shown that the tidal breathing method and dosimeter methods are used in roughly equal numbers in the clinical laboratory setting (45). However, numerous variations in methodology have been used and continue to be developed, depending on the requirements of research aims and protocols or for measurements of airway responsiveness in particular settings such as large epidemiological studies, specific occupational exposures, or varying age groups of subjects. These variations include: use of increasing numbers of inhalations of a fixed concentration of methacholine (46,47); delivery of aerosol from a dosimeter during tidal breathing (48); use of inspiratory capacity breaths but continuous nebulization of methacholine (49); longer time for actuation of dosimeter (10); activation of the dosimeter by the operator (13,17); use of higher doses of methacholine (13,17,50,51); use of higher end point for change in lung function (13,17,50,51); omissionof control and low doses based on carefully defined asthma severity (19); and inclusion of subjects with severe airflow obstruction (52).

Despite these variations there are several features that remain common to all protocols:

1. Low starting doses for subjects with symptoms, abnormal lung function, or current medication use;
2. Increments of dose adjusted according to the response;
3. Defined end points;
4. Specific exclusion criteria (see below); and
5. Parameters of responsiveness should not be extrapolated beyond the data (53).

Precautions

The precautions, derived from the known systemic cholinergic effects of methacholine, are listed above. In general, these include uncontrolled acute asthma, recent or unstable cardiac or coronary artery disease, and current, untreated peptic ulceration. In addition, it is usually recommended that methacholine or histamine are not routinely administered in the following circumstances: (a) severe airflow obstruction; (b) recent myocardial infarction (<3 months); (c) recent cerebral ischemia (<3 months); (d) known arterial aneurysm; (e) pregnancy; and (f) epilepsy.

Challenge agents should be administered incrementally commencing with an appropriate starting dose, adjusted according to the severity of respiratory disease of the subject. Oxygen and a bronchodilator should be available. It is advisable to give an inhaled bronchodilator to all subjects who have a measurable airway response. Administration of inhaled doses higher than those used in standardized protocols should be under the supervision of a doctor experienced in respiratory diseases and with resuscitation equipment available. Subjects should be warned of the possibility of persistent symptoms (cough or shortness of breath) for up to 12 hr following the use of doses of methacholine greater than those used in standardized protocols.

Factors Affecting Airway Responsiveness

The technical and non-technical factors (23,38,39,54–57) that may affect airway responsiveness are summarized in Table 3. Standardization of the methods of measuring airway responsiveness involves control of these factors to maximize the reproducibility of the test. The technical aspects of the commonly used methods are now well standardized (8) and will not be discussed further here.

Sex, Age, and Body Size

In most, but not all, studies of adults, women have increased airway responsiveness compared with men (17,58,59). In children, males have increased

Table 3 Factors Affecting Airway Responsiveness

Technical	Non-technical
Preparation of solutions	Sex
Nebuliser output	Age
Droplet size	Body size
Breathing pattern	Allergen exposure
Measurement of response	Baseline lung function
	Smoking
	Drug treatment
	Diurnal variation
	Viral infection

responsiveness compared with females (49). Responsiveness decreases from infancy (60) through childhood to adulthood and increases after middle age (61). The effect of age and sex may be related to body size, and therefore to dose reaching the airways, to properties or amount of smooth muscle, or to differences in starting airway caliber (62). Correction for body size has been suggested (63) but at present, there are no standardized methods in use.

Smoking and Airway Caliber

Airway responsiveness is generally increased in smokers compared with non-smokers (59,64,65), probably due to differences in baseline lung function (66). Other explanations may include a common association of smoking and sputum eosinophilia with airway hyperresponsiveness (67). There is a demonstrable relationship between baseline lung function and airway responsiveness (17,52,64,65,68). However, airway responsiveness may vary greatly between subjects with similar levels of starting airway caliber (69,70), or may be increased in subjects with normal baseline lung function (36,38) so that it is not possible to "correct" for the starting airway caliber, except in selected subjects (71a). Changes in airway responsiveness over time correlate with changes in lung function (71b). Finally, a large population study has shown that in addition to sex, age, smoking, and atopic status, airway responsiveness has a non-linear relationship to airway size (71c). These observations confound the interpretation and limits the usefulness of tests of airway responsiveness in subjects with airflow obstruction.

Allergen Exposure

Increased airway responses to methacholine or histamine are seen in subjects with positive skin prick tests to common allergens in cross-sectional studies of non-selected populations (72–74) and in selected populations such as college students (75,76) and occupational groups (77). Seasonal increases in airway responsiveness have been observed in atopic subjects who are sensitive to plant pollens (78,79), and allergen avoidance (80,81) results in reduced airway responsiveness to inhaled histamine or methacholine.

Respiratory Infection

Patients with acute respiratory infections (36), non-asthmatic subjects with "colds" (82), and asthmatic subjects exposed experimentally to viruses (83) have increased airway responses to inhaled methacholine or histamine. In non-asthmatic subjects, exposure to virus resulted in increased airway responsiveness in some studies (84,85) but not others (86,87). Current recommendations suggest avoiding measurement of airway responses within 6 weeks of a clinical viral respiratory illness, although in occupational (66) and community-based (65,88) studies, the presence of subjects with current or recent "colds" has not been shown to be an independent determinant of airway responsiveness.

Expression of Results and Reproducibility

Changes in lung function to inhaled doses of bronchoconstrictor are best illustrated by the dose–response curve (DRC), which may be described in a number of ways. The most commonly used derivative is the provocative dose (PD) or concentration (PC) that causes a fall in lung function (most often measured by FEV_1) of a predetermined percentage (usually 20%) from the control value; the $PD_{20}FEV_1$ (38). However, many subjects may not achieve a fall in FEV_1 of 20%, or even 6% (58) in response to the usual doses of inhaled methacholine or histamine. Therefore, continuous parameters have been derived from the DRC by calculating the area under the dose–response curve (AUC) (46), by fitting mathematical models to obtain slope or position of the DRC (89–91), or by calculating the slope between the origin and the final data point, the dose–response slope (DRS) (92). All of these except the DRS require more time-consuming or difficult calculations than the PD_{20} or PC_{20}.

When technical and non-technical factors are controlled for, the reproducibility (internal validity) of airway responses to histamine and methacholine for PD_{20} or PC_{20} has been reported as ± 1 doubling dose under ideal conditions (23,56,93) and ± 2 or 3 doubling doses in the field (94–96) in inexperienced subjects (97) or when standardization is less than optimal (98). The DRS has been shown to be more reproducible than the PD_{20} in large populations (26,92,99) although its reproducibility is less in non-responsive subjects with a low slope (100). The DRS is related to asthma symptoms even in subjects who do not have a measurable $PC_{20}FEV_1$, and has been shown to differentiate subjects with different asthma severity better than the $PC_{20}FEV_1$ (101). To improve sensitivity, other measures of airway caliber have been used. Measurement of changes in specific airway conductance (SGaw) avoids the bronchodilatory effect of taking a big breath for maximum expiratory maneuvers, however, compared with the $PC_{20}FEV_1$, is less reproducible. Similarly, if responsiveness is expressed as slope of the DRC using all data points, as PD_{10} (94) or as the plateau response (13), sensitivity is increased but reproducibility is reduced. In general, the reproducibility of responses to histamine and methacholine is comparable (10,23,24). However, considerable variation in sensitivity to histamine and methacholine may exist within individual subjects (10,26).

The Use of Direct Stimuli to Diagnose Asthma

The lack of a "gold standard" for the diagnosis of asthma limits the assessment of any test for asthma. Some clinical validity has been established by Hargreave et al. (39), who showed that airway responsiveness was related to medication requirements, diurnal variation of peak flow measurements, and ease of provocation of asthma symptoms by other stimuli such as cold air or exercise. Early studies suggested that airway responsiveness was a sensitive and specific test for asthma (38) but (like most tests) when applied to a wider spectrum of people (i.e., epidemioiogical surveys) many subjects without any history of asthma or respiratory symptoms were hyperresponsive and some supposedly asthmatic subjects were not (49,102).

A search of "Pubmed" from 1983 to 2003 was undertaken using the search phrase "[methacholine (mh) OR histamine (mh)] AND [sensitivity (mh) AND specificity (mh)]." From the studies obtained and from their reference lists, 22 studies were reviewed (Table 4). The studies included a wide spectrum of patients, ranging from random samples of general populations to highly selected groups of patients. Some studies included conditions that might be confused with asthma such as chronic airflow limitation, bronchitis, breathlessness on exertion, and non-specific cough (38,103).

Airway responsiveness was compared with the results of questionnaire responses with "asthma" being variably diagnosed as wheeze (ever or within the last 12 months), asthma diagnosed by a doctor, attacks of asthma or combinations of symptoms (ever or within the last 12 months, or currently). In two studies of occupational asthma (104,105), disease was defined as a positive response to a specific occupational agent. This resulted in tests of the point prevalence of airway responsiveness being compared to the cumulative prevalence of a history of diagnosed asthma or the period prevalence of symptoms such as wheeze (106).

The diagnostic test varied between studies with regard to the agent used, the definition of a response and the cut-off dose used to define a response although there were no apparent differences between methacholine and histamine. The DRS was similar in sensitivity and specificity to the PD_{20} (107,108). The cut-offs used to define normal and abnormal in these studies are to some extent arbitrary. Changes in the cut-off level result in changes in sensitivity and specificity (109). A lower PC_{20} was less sensitive and more specific (76,110). No consistent value that best separated asthmatic from non-asthmatic subjects was evident across the studies. Godfrey et al. (111) performed an analysis of large random populations in the literature. They found that a PD_{20} of 6.6 μmol gave the best sensitivity (92%) and specificity (89%) for the diagnosis of asthma.

Using a cut-off value of 8 mg/mL or 8 μmol of histamine or methacholine and disease diagnosed by symptoms, the average sensitivity was 56%

Table 4 Studies to Assess Validity of Testing Airway Responsiveness

Reference	No.	Population group	Disease	Parameter	Sensitivity (%)	Specificity (%)	Prevalence (%)
109	165	Children	Asthma	PD_{20} M	89	89	33
230	32	Children	Asthma	PD_{20} M	95	83	64
231	70	4–16 yrs	Reactive[a]	PD_{20} M	77	82	30
24	2,363	8–11 yrs	Wheeze	PD_{20} H	40	89	24
110	633	Adults	Wheeze	PD_{20} H 8 μmol	68	81	20
			Wheeze	PD_{20} H 1 μmol	35	95	20
			Attack	PD_{20} H 8 μmol	86	76	10
			Attack	PD_{20} H 1 μmol	57	93	10
232	654	15–64 yrs	Asthma	PD_{15} M	79	89	4
			Asthma	DRS M	46	97	4
103	339	General	Wheeze	PC_{20} H	35	77	12
				DRS H	51	80	12
102	2,053	7–10 yrs	Asthma	PC_{20} H	52	90	14
104	23	Red Cedar workers	Plicatic acid challenge	PC_{20}M	62	78	50
233	495	7–16 yrs	Wheeze	PC_{20} H	57	98	11
108	1,777	7–11 yrs	Asthma	PC_{20} M	43	87	6
				DRS M	46	82	6
				AUC M	59	72	6
76	500	Students		PC_{20} H 8 mg/mL	100	93	10
		Current		PC_{20} H 1 mg/mL	41	100	10
			Wheeze	FEV_{50} M	28	87	10
9	201	Adults	Asthma	PD_{20} M	20	94	10

(Continued)

Table 4 Studies to Assess Validity of Testing Airway Responsiveness (*Continued*)

Reference	No.	Population group	Disease	Parameter	Sensitivity (%)	Specificity (%)	Prevalence (%)
114	40	Adults	EIA	PD$_{15}$ M	55	100	50
				PD$_{20}$ M	35	100	50
71	82	Adults	Asthma and COPD	PD$_{20}$ M	92	93	30
48	791	Adults	Asthma	PD$_{20}$ M	89	76	40
234	211	Adults	1 Symptom	PD$_{20}$ H	90	70	41
			3 Symptoms	PD$_{20}$ H	69	94	16
105	75	Workers	TDI challenge	PD$_{15}$ M	76	51	40
115	1,777	Children	Asthma	PD$_{20}$ M	72	52	6
				Any			
235	247	Children	Asthma	PD$_{20}$ M	47	97	14
236	645	Children	7 yrs	PC$_{20}$ H	46	93	9
		Current	Wheeze	Reservoir			
237	102	Childern	Asthma	PD$_{20}$ M	56–73	87–94	19
	84	Adults					

[a]Reactive refers to a variety of non-specific symptoms suggesting airway disease.

Abbreviations: H, histamine; M, methacholine; EIA, exercise induced asthma; FEV$_{50}$, 50% change in FEV$_1$; TDI, toluene di-isocyanate.

(range 22–100%) and specificity was 86% (range 70–100%). The use of an occupational challenge to define disease gave sensitivities of 76% (105) and 62% (104) and specificities of 51% (105) and 78% (104). A recent review of studies that compared symptoms of asthma to tests of airway responsiveness (112) gave summary values for sensitivity of 36% and for specificity of 94%, similar to the values estimated above.

Detection of Asthma in Different Populations

Sensitivity and specificity are inherent properties of a test, independent of the prevalence of disease, but do not predict the odds of asthma being present. Knowledge of the prevalence of asthma, however, defined in the population under study allows the positive (PPV) and negative (NPV) predictive values to be calculated. This may be illustrated in two examples: (i) a general population where the prevalence of asthma will be around 10%; and (ii) a group of patients who present for investigation of possible asthma where the actual prevalence of asthma may be around 50%. If values of 60% and 90% for sensitivity and specificity (from the studies reviewed above) are used and a population of 100 subjects is studied, it can be seen from Table 5 that the PPV and NPV vary with disease prevalence.

In populations where the prevalence is relatively low (as in epidemiological studies), a negative result is likely to be more useful in excluding the disease and other tests may be necessary to confirm the presence of asthma. In populations where the prevalence is higher (as in clinical laboratories or selected groups), a positive result is more useful in diagnosing asthma but a

Table 5 Predictive Values of Airway Hyperresponsiveness in Different Populations

	Low prevalence (general population)			High prevalence (laboratory subjects)		
	Asthma			Asthma		
	Yes	No	Total	Yes	No	Total
Test Positive	6	9	15	30	5	35
Test Negative	4	81	85	20	45	65
Total	10	90	100	50	50	100
	Prevalence = 10% PPV = 40%, NPV = 95%			Prevalence = 50% PPV = 86%, NPV = 69%		

Abbreviations: PPV, true positive tests / all positive tests; NPV, true negative tests / all negative tests.

negative result will occur in approximately 30% of subjects where the disease is present.

Another method of using the results of a diagnostic test is to calculate the likelihood ratio (LR) (113). This is the ratio of the likelihood that a given result will occur when the disease is present over the likelihood that the same result will occur when the disease is absent. Its advantages are that it is relatively independent of disease prevalence, it can be used for multiple cut-off points (76,109,110) for a positive response and it can be used to calculate the probability that disease is present (the post-test probability) based on the result of the test and the pre-test probability that the disease is present. The prevalence of disease can be taken as the pre-test probability but clinicians will usually estimate a pre-test probability dependent on clinical features that make better use of the result. When there are only two outcomes (positive or negative) for a test, as above, the post-test probabilities for one or other result are the same as the positive and negative predictive values.

The contribution of other tests to the diagnosis of asthma as well as airway responsiveness has not been established. In children, assessment of airway responsiveness was less useful as a screening test for asthma in the community than a history of doctor-diagnosed asthma from the parents (102). However, compared with histamine or methacholine, "specific" challenges with cold air or exercise were less useful in the detection of exercise-induced asthma (114). Peak flow measurements may be more useful than airway responsiveness in following trends in asthma severity (115).

The aims of the investigator will ultimately determine how testing of airway responsiveness will be performed and interpreted. In epidemiological studies, the definition of disease and the cut-off values for a required airway response will be varied. The test may also be used to define "normality" for a variety of purposes. For example, if it is considered desirable to absolutely exclude all those with asthma from taking on certain work or from going diving, the cut-off could be set so that the sensitivity is high, despite specificity being low. This would result in all asthmatic subjects being detected at the expense of needlessly excluding some normal subjects from activity. Alternatively, to avoid giving a potentially harmful treatment to non-asthmatic subjects, one might set the cut-off value for the test so that only asthmatics subjects are detected, low sensitivity and high specificity. This, of course, would result in the test failing to detect many cases of asthma. It has been suggested that the use of indirect stimuli to assess airway responsiveness may improve specificity, in relation to airway inflammation and exercise-induced asthma, in populations of athletes or those seeking employment in diving or service industries (116).

Increased airway responsiveness may also be included in the definition of asthma (117). A potential advantage of this is that it adds an objective component to the definition of asthma, which is usually based predominantly on symptoms that may themselves vary in frequency for a variety of reasons not related to the actual prevalence of disease (118). It may be preferable to assess the prevalence of airway responsiveness separately from symptoms since, like allergy, airway hyperresponsiveness may have separate genetic determinants (119) and be associated with the expression of asthma symptoms through as yet unknown mechanisms.

Occupational Asthma

Methacholine and histamine inhalation challenges are useful to test "non-specific" airway responsiveness in the occupational setting (120) for the following reasons: (a) to help confirm the diagnosis of asthma; (b) to document that the airways have become sensitized to agents at work; (c) to estimate the initial dose of allergen that an individual can safely be exposed to during specific challenge testing; and (d) to estimate the prevalence of airway disease, including asthma, in an occupational setting for comparison to the general population. Two studies have shown that measurements of methacholine responsiveness did not improve the sensitivity or specificity of peak flow measurements in the diagnosis of occupational asthma, defined using a specific challenge (104,121). In these studies, a history of symptoms in the workplace was more sensitive than a methacholine inhalation challenge.

A long list of low and high molecular weight substances have been associated with occupational asthma (122). Those most carefully documented exposures and those that involve the most numbers of subjects include Western Red Cedar (123), toluene di-isocyanate (19), grain dust (124), and potroom asthma (125) in the aluminum smelting industry. In a review of the topic (122), 14,246 subjects were reported, with an estimated 50% undergoing bronchial challenge with histamine or methacholine. In a review of 1392 subjects from sawmills, grain elevators, and foundries (126), it was found that responsiveness to methacholine was more closely associated with doctor-diagnosed asthma than asthma-like symptoms. Increased responsiveness to methacholine was present in 16 workers previously exposed to toluene di-isocyanate, suggesting permanent airway injury (127). Repeated bronchial challenge with methacholine has been used to investigate the effects of occupational exposures over time (122,128). Although responses to methacholine may not necessarily reflect airway responses to specific occupational agents (129), a negative response to methacholine may be used to exclude occupational asthma and avoid the need for laborious challenges with specific agents (130).

Comparisons with Indirect Challenge Agents

Exercise, Cold Air, Non-Isotonic Solutions and Adenosine

In general, there is a correlation between responsiveness to methacholine and to exercise testing or tests that involve hyperventilation, cold air, non-isotonic solutions, and adenosine (116,127,131,132). When tested in patients with symptoms that suggest asthma, direct challenges are more sensitive and less specific than indirect challenges such as exercise testing, hypertonic saline, and adenosine (25,111,133–138). Since indirect challenges act through the release of mediators, predominantly from mast cells (116), they are thought to be more specific as markers of airway inflammation, a characteristic of asthma (139–147). This is supported by comparisons of the correlations of direct and indirect challenges with inflammatory markers in sputum (148–151). Indirect markers may also be more useful for discriminating other airway diseases from asthma (152–154). Airway responses to inhaled methacholine and histamine correlate with those to a variety of inhaled agents such as leukotriene D4 (155), prostaglandin F2α (156), and occupational agents (127). Recently, a protocol for the use of inhaled lysine aspirin (116) for the purpose of confirming aspirin-sensitive asthma was published.

Tests of responsiveness to agents other than methacholine or histamine have not been as extensively standardized with regard to technical aspects, methodology, reproducibility, and correlation with asthma severity. They tend to be less discriminatory in populations of asthmatic and non-asthmatic subjects and the methodology is usually more cumbersome and time-consuming. The airway response is less predictable in some subjects. The tests may be more useful however, in the determination of the contribution of specific factors to a patient's symptoms, for the detection of specific sensitising or triggering factors and for the discrimination of asthmatic subjects from those with chronic obstructive pulmonary disease (COPD) (153). The use of adenosine monophosphate has been shown to be more sensitive to the anti-inflammatory effects of inhaled corticosteroids, compared with methacholine or bradykinin (157) and responsiveness to exercise showed greater change after treatment with a leukotriene antagonist than responsiveness to methacholine (158). It has been suggested that, following treatment with corticosteroids, changes in airway responsiveness to direct and indirect challenges may provide complementary information regarding airway pathology (116).

Allergen

As discussed above, exposure to allergen increases the airway responsiveness to methacholine or histamine. This has been shown in studies of allergic subjects in and out of pollen season or in subjects studied in allergen-free environments. Boonsawat et al. (51) also showed that allergen challenge increased the maximal airway narrowing that was induced by high-dose methacholine challenge. Cockcroft et al. (159) showed many years ago that the airway response to inhaled allergen was largely explained by two variables, the airway responsiveness to inhaled histamine and the size of the skin weal induced by skin prick testing with the same allergen.

Relation of Direct Challenge Responses to Asthma Severity and Treatment

There is in general, a relationship between the magnitude of the airway response to direct challenge agents and the clinical severity of asthma seen in selected laboratory populations and in general population studies (38,39,57,90,101,102,160,161a,161b). The relation to severity and increased sensitivity of the direct challenge agents may make them a better screening tool in population studies (162). A study of children in New Zealand (49) which used an abbreviated protocol showed that the proportion of subjects with a positive response to methacholine increased in relation to asthma severity, defined mainly by symptoms (Fig. 1), and early validation studies showed that the level of airway responsiveness was also related to treatment requirements and peak flow variability (38,57). Interestingly, airway responsiveness may correlate not with markers of severity in the recent

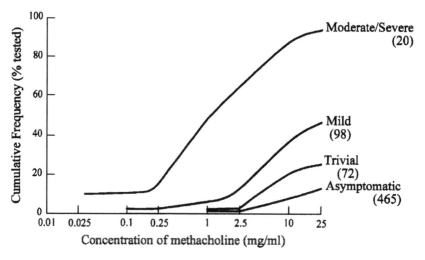

Figure 1 Cumulative frequency of airway responsiveness to increasing concentrations of methacholine in children with and without symptoms who did not have resting airflow obstruction. Numbers in brackets indicate numbers of children tested in each group. *Source*: Adapted from Ref. 49.

past but with those over periods of weeks or months (163a). Responsiveness to inhaled methacholine correlates with markers of airway inflammation such as exhaled nitric oxide and induced sputum eosinophils (163b).

Numerous studies have shown that treatments with anti-inflammatory agents, predominantly inhaled or oral corticosteroids, result in improvement in airway hyperresponsiveness to direct challenge agents (161a,164–166). There is accumulating evidence that the magnitude of the effect of inhaled corticosteroids on airway responsiveness is both time- and dose dependent (167–174) with periods of treatment of 6–18 months required to achieve maximum improvement (174). The changes in airway responsiveness following therapy lag considerably behind the changes observed in symptoms, FEV_1, morning peak flows, and requirements for reliever medications (Fig. 2) (174).

The effects of treatment on airway responsiveness to direct agents do not always correlate strongly with the effects on responses to indirect agents (157,175), and it has been suggested that the early changes in airway responses to indirect agents after treatment with inhaled corticosteroids best reflects the improvements in airway inflammation (176). The level of the maximal response is decreased by the use of inhaled corticosteroids (177).

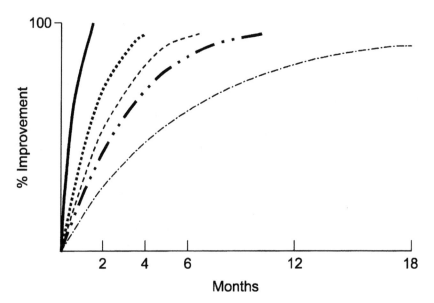

Figure 2 Time course of changes (percentage of improvement) in different measures of asthma control over 18 months of treatment with inhaled corticosteroids. Symptoms at night (*solid line*), FEV_1 (*dotted line*), morning peak flow (*dashed line*), use of short acting bronchodilators (dashed and double dotted line), and airway responsiveness (*dashed and dotted line*). *Source*: From Ref. 174.

Relation and Relevance to Airway Pathology

Factors Affecting the Measured Response to an Inhaled Agonist

Moreno et al. (178) elucidated the chain of events that will influence the magnitude of the airway response to an inhaled bronchoconstrictor agonist. In summary, inhaled particles must deposit on the airway surface, transit the airway mucus and inner airway wall, and interact with the appropriate receptor on the airway smooth muscle. This interaction will stimulate the smooth muscle, with the development of tension which results in shortening around the circumference of the airway wall. The shortening leads to narrowing of the airway lumen which, acting in concert with other airways in parallel or in series, increases total airway resistance. The additional effects of changes in tissue resistance, airway wall compliance, and dynamic effects of a forced expiration from total lung capacity will all contribute to the measured FEV_1.

All of these elements are subject to a number of modifying influences (178). The amount of stimulation/activation of the airway smooth muscle that arises from an inhaled dose will depend on factors that affect deposition, clearance of agonist from the airway wall, opposing anti-agonist neural or humoral influences, agonist–receptor interactions, receptor numbers, and intrinsic airway smooth muscle properties. The amount of shortening that occurs in the stimulated smooth muscle will be determined by the balance between the tension that the muscle can develop and the forces that oppose the tendency to shorten. The latter include internal resistive loads within the tissues in the airway wall, including the smooth muscle, extracellular matrix elements, and cartilage, the elastic recoil of the lung parenchyma that surrounds the airway and the degree to which this is transmitted to the airway smooth muscle via the outer airway wall. The amount that a given degree of shortening causes the airway lumen to narrow will depend on the proportion of the airway circumference that is surrounded by smooth muscle (usually 100% in all but the first two or three generations of airways in man) and the thickness of structures between the outer border of the smooth muscle and the airway lumen. These structures include the airway smooth muscle itself, the loose connective tissue below the basement membrane, the reticular basement membrane, the epithelium, and the mucus and surface lining fluid on the epithelial surface.

The Pathology of Asthma

Asthma is characterized pathologically by an inflammatory infiltrate consisting of T-lymphocytes with a low CD8+/CD4+ ratio, macrophages, eosinophils, and neutrophils (139–147) (Fig. 3). Mast cell numbers may or may not be increased (144,179) but they are most prominent on the airway smooth muscle and submucosal mucous glands and show increased

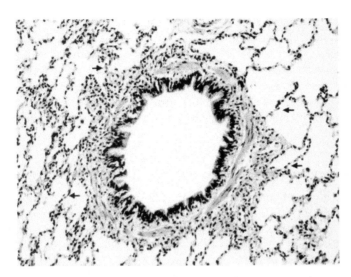

Figure 3 Membranous bronchiole from a case of asthma showing prominent smooth muscle and an inflammatory infiltration composed predominantly of mononuclear cells and occasional eosinophils. The direct connection of the smooth muscle to the lung parenchyma via the outer airway wall and alveolar attachments (*arrows*) can readily be seen.

degranulation in relation to asthma severity (180). Vascular enlargement is seen in large and small airways (181). Hyperplasia of goblet cells and increased production of mucus (182) are documented although there is debate regarding the degree of epithelial desquamation that occurs in asthma (183). The airway wall is increased in thickness in asthma due to increased areas of epithelium, inner airway wall, airway smooth muscle, outer airway wall, and submucosal mucous glands (183–192). These structural changes are referred to collectively as "remodeling." Lastly, there are changes in the constituents and therefore the physical properties (such as compliance) of components of the airway wall. These include alterations of the extracellular proteins in the airway wall with deposition of collagens I, III, V, fibronectin, and tenascin below the basement membrane (193) and changes in the mucin, glycoprotein and lipid composition of mucus (194,195), which result in a more tenacious mucus. A number of studies have not shown consistent changes in the responsiveness of airway smooth muscle from cases of asthma in vitro (196) or a relationship between airway responsiveness in vivo and airway smooth muscle responsiveness in vitro (197–199). However, recent studies have shown, compared with non-asthmatic cases, increased numbers of mast cells on airway smooth muscle from patients with atopic sensitization (200), increased degranulation of mast cells on the smooth muscle from patients with mild and fatal asthma

(144), and increased in vitro proliferation of airway smooth muscle from asthmatic subjects in response to mitogenic stimuli (201). Lastly, changes in the forces, which act on smooth muscle within the airway wall, may alter the mechanical behavior of the smooth muscle. Reduced cyclical stretch of the smooth muscle has been suggested as a mechanism for the development of a latch state of the smooth muscle, resulting in excessive narrowing of the airway, increased responsiveness, and abnormal airway narrowing following a big breath (202–204).

Characteristics of the Dose–Response Curve in Asthma

The dose at which the first discernible response occurs is known as the threshold dose (90). Following this, the response continues to increase as the dose increases. The slope of the line that describes the relationship between dose and response is the reactivity or rate of response. The position, or sensitivity, of the curve at any particular dose is determined both by the threshold dose and the reactivity. Eventually there will be no further response despite the administration of higher doses, the plateau or maximal response. Increased airway responsiveness in patients with asthma is characterized not only by a steep DRC that is shifted to the left but also by a greater or absent maximal response (9,90). Whereas a plateau of response occurs in subjects without asthma, the response shows no plateau in patients with moderate or severe asthma (9,90). In other words, airway narrowing is normally limited in non-asthmatic subjects and it has been suggested that asthma occurs when the factors that normally limit narrowing are altered or lost (205). The mechanisms for the increased maximal response do not seem to be neurological or pharmacological (206) but are likely to be mechanical (191,205,207). The level of the plateau response correlates inversely with the PD_{20} (9). It should be stressed that, in patients with asthma of mild and moderate clinical severity, all of these abnormal airway responses may occur at a time when the patients resting lung function is normal and even in the virtual absence of symptoms. In normal subjects airway narrowing induced by inhalation of a bronchoconstrictor is partly or completely reversed by taking a deep breath (208). Avoidance of deep breaths can result in asthmatic-type responses in normal individuals (209). In patients with asthma, a deep breath results in very little reversal of the induced narrowing or may even exaggerate it (29,208,210–212).

The various properties of airway responses to inhaled direct agents may change with time within individuals and vary between patients with asthma in relation to clinical severity and treatment—as described in more detail above. In general, airway responsiveness increases with asthma severity although the temporal relationship may not be only with recent symptoms (163a). Treatment with beta-agonists may alter the position of the DRS but tends not to affect reactivity or the maximal response (177).

Treatment with inhaled corticosteroids results in reduced sensitivity and reactivity (reflected in reduced PC_{20} or PD_{20} or DRS) and a reduction in the maximal response, or its emergence where it was not previously measurable (174). These improvements in airway responsiveness following treatment with inhaled corticosteroids take several months to reach their maximum (171,174). This parallels the prolonged treatment with higher doses required to achieve changes in the thickness of the reticular basement membrane (169,170). In contrast, treatment with lower doses of inhaled corticosteroid can achieve marked improvements in lung function (peak flows and FEV_1) over short periods which are paralleled by decreased numbers of eosinophils within the airway wall (169,171,176,213–215).

Airway Pathology and The Dose–Response Curve

The pathology of asthma is reflected in the altered characteristics of the DRC as follows:

Dose–Response curve	Pathology
Increased sensitivity	
Greater access/deposition of agonist	Higher gas velocities (216)
	Increased permeability (217)
Reduced removal of agonist from the airway wall	Altered airway blood flow (218)
Increased release of mast cell products	Greater mast cell degranulation (144)
Increased reactivity	
Amplified narrowing response	Increased airway wall thickness (219)
Increased force development	Increased thickness of muscle (124)
Increased maximal response	
Excessive narrowing response	Increased airway wall thickness (219)
Increased force development	Increased thickness of muscle (124)
Reduced loads opposing shortening of smooth muscle	Altered airway wall mechanics
	Increased outer airway wall area (183)
Relationship with severity	
	Increased remodeling with severity (183)
	Increased inflammation with severity (144,145)
Temporal relationship to severity (163)	Cumulative effects of remodeling
Temporal relationship to treatment	
Response to bronchodilators and non-specific response to range of bronchoconstrictors	Dependence on smooth muscle shortening for effects of remodeling to be evident (191)
Rapid (days and weeks) changes in symptoms, lung function and	Rapid changes in airway inflammatory cells with corticosteroids (173)

(Continued)

Dose–Response curve	Pathology
responses to indirect challenges	
Longer-term (months) changes in airway responses to direct challenges	Longer-term changes in remodeling (220)
Deep breath effect	Dissociation of airway smooth muscle from recoil of lung parenchyma by increased area of outer airway wall

Non-specific responses
  Qualitatively and quantitatively similar changes in airway response to smooth muscle shortening due to effects of airway dimensions rather than agonist–receptor interactions or intrinsic smooth muscle properties. Therefore, response is dependent on strength of stimulus, not type of stimulus.

Airway hyperresponsiveness in the presence of normal lung function
  Increased airway wall thickness has minimal effects on airway lumen dimensions per se, but is only apparent when smooth muscle shortens (178,191). This theoretical analysis is supported by CT scan studies (221,222) of proximal airways showing that, compared with non-asthmatic subjects, the area of the airway wall was increased in both cases of asthma and cases with COPD due to smoking. The airway lumen was normal however, only in the cases of COPD, whereas in the asthma cases the airway lumen was not different from control cases.

Summary

The use of direct stimuli in the investigation of airway disease has been well standardized and has proven to be safe when correctly administered. They are sensitive tests for asthma for doctor-diagnosed asthma. However, direct stimuli are only specific tests for asthma when low cut-off levels for a positive response are used, in which case sensitivity will be sacrificed. They are not reliable in the presence of reduced baseline airway caliber, where their use should be avoided. Responses to direct stimuli reflect the pathology of asthma. Although it is impossible to separate inflammatory from remodeling effects based on a test that induces airway narrowing, the evidence suggests that indirect stimuli may predominantly reflect airway inflammation and direct stimuli may predominantly reflect airway remodeling. The relationships of responses to direct challenge stimuli and long-term (rather than recent) severity of asthma on the one hand, and effects of treatment on the other, support this contention. In this respect, it seems likely that symptoms, lung function, use of short-acting bronchodilators, measures of airway inflammation, challenges with indirect stimuli, and challenges with direct stimuli will have complementary roles in monitoring asthma (79,223). However, as the management of asthma, a disease of persistent and possibly life-long airway pathology, moves to long-term goals such as avoidance of exacerbations and excessive decline in lung function, the intermittent use of direct stimuli to monitor long-term treatment regimens may increase in importance.

Acknowledgment

The invaluable assistance of Peta Maxwell in the preparation of the manuscript for this chapter is gratefully acknowledged. A/Prof James is a National Health and Medical Research Council (NHMRC) Research Practitioner.

References

1. Crapo RO, Casaburi R, Coates AL, et al. Guidelines for methacholine and exercise challenge testing-1999. This official statement of the American Thoracic Society was adopted by the ATS Board of Directors, July 1999. Am J Respir Crit Care Med 2000; 161(l):309–329.
2. Bandouvakis J, Carrier A, Roberts R, Ryan G, Hargreave FE. The effect of ipratropium and fenoterol on methacholine–histamine-induced bronchoconstriction. Br J Dis Chest 1981; 75(3):295–305.
3. Thomson NC, O'Byrne P, Hargreave FE. Prolonged asthmatic responses to inhaled methacholine. J Allergy Clin Immunol 1983; 71(4):357–362.
4. Nair N, Bewtra A, Townley RG. Protection by SCH-1000 and metaproterenol against bronchoconstriction. 1977; 38:9.
5. Chung KF, Dent G, Barnes PJ. Effects of salbutamol on bronchoconstriction, bronchial hyperresponsiveness, and leucocyte responses induced by platelet activating factor in man. Thorax 1989; 44(2):102–107.
6. Griffin MP, MacDonald N, McFadden ER Jr. Short- and long-term effects of cromolyn sodium on the airway reactivity of asthmatics. J Allergy Clin Immunol 1983; 71(3):331–338.
7. Weiner P, Saaid M, Reshef A. Isotonic nebulized disodium cromoglycate provides better protection against methacholine- and exercise-induced bronchoconstriction. Am Rev Respir Dis 1988; 137(6):1309–1311.
8. Sterk PJ, Fabbri LM, Quanjer PH, et al. Airway responsiveness. Standardized challenge testing with pharmacological, physical and sensitizing stimuli in adults. Report Working Party Standardization of Lung Function Tests, European Community for Steel and Coal. Official Statement of the European Respiratory Society. Eur Respir J suppl l993; 6(16):53–83.
9. James A, Lougheed D, Pearce-Pinto G, Ryan G, Musk B. Maximal airway narrowing in a general population. Am Rev Respir Dis 1992; 146(4):895–899.
10. Townley RG, Bewtra AK, Nair NM, Brodkey FD, Watt GD, Burke KM. Methacholine inhalation challenge studies. J Allergy Clin Immunol 1979; 64(6 pt 2):569–574.

11. Beckett WS, McDonnell WF III, Wong ND. Tolerance to methacholine inhalation challenge in nonasthmatic subjects. Am Rev Respir Dis 1988; 137(6):1499–1501.

12. Stevens WH, Manning PJ, Watson RM, O'Byrne PM. Tachyphylaxis to inhaled methacholine in normal but not asthmatic subjects. J Appl Physiol 1990; 69(3):875–879.

13. Lougheed MD, Pearce-Pinto G, de Klerk NH, Ryan G, Musk AW, James A. Variability of the plateau response to methacholine in subjects without respiratory symptoms. Thorax 1993; 48(5):512–517.

14. van Aradel PP, Beall BN. The metabolism and functions of histamine. Arch Int Med 1960; 106:714–733.

15. Nogrady SG, Bevan C. Inhaled antihistamines—bronchodilatation and effects on histamine- and methacholine-induced broncho constriction. Thorax 1978; 33(6):700–704.

16. Weiss ST, Robb GP, Ellis LB. The systemic effects of histamine in man. Arch Int Med 1932; 49:360–396.

17. Tashkin DP, Altose MD, Bleecker ER, et al. The lung health study: airway responsiveness to inhaled methacholine in smokers with mild to moderate airflow limitation. The Lung Health Study Research Group. Am Rev Respir Dis 1992; 145(2 Pt 1):301–310.

18. Braman SS, Corrao WM, Fregault R, Hasan FM. Methacholine bronchoprovocation: adverse effects and clinical safety. Am Rev Respir Dis 1984; 129:A28.

19. Hendrick DJ, Fabbri LM, Hughes JM, et al. Modification of the methacholine inhalation test and its epidemiologic use in polyurethane workers. Am Rev Respir Dis 1986; 133(4):600–604.

20. Connolly MJ, Kelly C, Walters EH, Hendrick DJ. An assessment of methacholine inhalation tests in elderly asthmatics. Age Ageing 1988; 17(2):123–128.

21. Bez C, Sach G, Jarisch A, Rosewich M, Reichenbach J, Zielen S. Safety and tolerability of methacholine challenge in infants with recurrent wheeze. J Asthma 2003; 40(7):795–802.

22. Toelle BG, Li J, Dalton M, Devadason SG. Subject discomfort associated with the histamine challenge in a population study. Respir Med 2002; 96(12):990–992.

23. Juniper EF, Frith PA, Dunnett C, Cockcroft DW, Hargreave FE. Reproducibility and comparison of responses to inhaled histamine and methacholine. Thorax 1978; 33(6):705–710.

24. Salome CM, Peat JK, Britton WJ, Woolcock AJ. Bronchial hyperresponsiveness in two populations of Australian school children. I. Relation to respiratoy symptoms and diagnosed asthma. Clin Allergy 1987; 17(4):271–281.

25. Chatham M, Bleecker ER, Smith PL, Rosenthal RR, Mason P, Norman PS. A comparison of histamine, methacholine, and exercise airway reactivity in normal and asthmatic subjects. Am Rev Respir Dis 1982; 126(2):235–240.

26. Peat JK, Salome CM, Bauman A, Toelle BG, Wachinger SL, Woolcock AJ. Repeatability of histamine bronchial challenge and comparability with

methacholine bronchial challenge in a population of Australian school children. Am Rev Respir Dis 1991; 144(2):338–343.

27. Higgins BG, Britton JR, Chinn S, et al. Comparison of histamine and methacholine for use in bronchial challenge tests in community studies. Thorax 1988; 43(8):605–610.

28. Sekizawa K, Yanai M, Shimizu Y, Sasaki H, Takishima T. Serial distribution of bronchoconstriction in normal subjects. Methacholine versus histamine. Am Rev Respir Dis 1988; 137(6):1312–1316.

29. Pellegrino R, Violante B, Crimi E, Brusasco V. Effects of deep inhalation during early and late asthmatic reactions to allergen. Am Rev Respir Dis 1990; 142(4):822–825.

30. Echazarreta AL, Gomez FP, Ribas J, et al. Pulmonary gas exchange responses to histamine and methacholine challenges in mild asthma. Eur Respir J 2001; 17(4):609–614.

31. Savoy J, Louis M, Kryger MH, Forster A. Respiratory response to histamine- and methylcholine-induced bronchospasm in nonsmokers and asymptomatic smokers. Eur Respir J 1988; l(3):209–216.

32. Stewart IC, Parker A, Catterall JR, Douglas NJ, Flenley DC. Effect of bronchial challenge on breathing patterns and arterial oxygenation in stable asthma. Chest 1989; 95(l):65–70.

33. Dautrebaude L, Philpott E. Asthmatic crisis produced by aerosols of carbaminoylcholine in man treated by aerosols of amphetamine: study of action of these substances on respiration by determination of useful respiratory volume. Presse Med 1941; 49:942–946.

34. Tiffeneau R, Beauvallet M. Test of bronchial constriction and dilatation produced by aerosols (acetylcholine and epinephrine): use for detection, evaluation and control of chronic respiratory insufficiency. Bull Acad Med 1945; 26:430–438.

35. Curry JJ. The action of histamine on the respiratory tract in normal and asthmatic subjects. J Clin Invest 1946; 25:785–791.

36. Parker CD, Bilbo RE, Reed CE. Methacholine aerosol as test for bronchial asthma. Arch Intern Med 1965; 115:452–458.

37. Herxheimer H. Bronchial obstruction induced by allergens, histamine and acetyl-beta-methylcholinechloride. Int Arch Allergy 1957; 2:27–39.

38. Cockcroft DW, Killian DN, Mellon JJ, Hargreave FE. Bronchial reactivity to inhaled histamine: a method and clinical survey. Clin Allergy 1977; 7(3):235–243.

39. Hargreave FE, Ryan G, Thomson NC, et al. Bronchial responsiveness to histamine or methacholine in asthma: measurement and clinical significance. J Allergy Clin Immunol 1981; 68(5):347–355.

40. Cockcroft DW, Berscheid BA. Measurement of responsiveness to inhaled histamine: comparison of FEV_1 and SGaw. Ann Allergy 1983; 51(3):374–377.

41. Chai H, Farr RS, Froehlich LA, et al. Standardization of bronchial inhalation challenge procedures. J Allergy Clin Immunol 1975; 56(4):323–327.

42. Yan K, Salome C, Woolcock AJ. Rapid method for measurement of bronchial responsiveness. Thorax 1983; 38(10):760–765.

43. Montgomery GL, Tepper RS. Changes in airway reactivity with age in normal infants and young children. Am Rev Respir Dis 1990; 142(6 Pt l):1372–1376.

44. Stick SM, Turner DJ, LeSouef PN. Lung function and bronchial challenges in infants: repeatability of histamine and comparison with methacholine challenges. Pediatr Pulmonol 1993; 16(3):177–183.

45. Scott GC, Braun SR. A survey of the current use and methods of analysis of bronchoprovocational challenges. Chest 1991; 100(2):322–328.

46. Townley RG, Ryo UY, Kolotkin BM, Kang B. Bronchial sensitivity to methacholine in current and former asthmatic and allergic rhinitis patients and control subjects. J Allergy Clin Immunol 1975; 56(6):429–442.

47. Chatham M, Bleecker ER, Norman P, Smith PL, Mason P. A screening test for airways reactivity. An abbreviated methacholine inhalation challenge. Chest 1982; 82(l):15–18.

48. Nieminen MM, Lahdensuo A, Kellomaeki L, Karvonen J, Muittari A. Methacholine bronchial challenge using a dosimeter with controlled tidal breathing. Thorax 1988; 43(11):896–900.

49. Sears MR, Jones DT, Holdaway MD, et al. Prevalence of bronchial reactivity to inhaled methacholine in New Zealand children. Thorax 1986; 41(4): 283–289.

50. Sterk PJ, Daniel EE, Zamel N, Hargreave FE. Limited bronchoconstriction to methacholine using partial flow–volume curves in nonasthmatic subjects. Am Rev Respir Dis 1985; 132(2):272–277.

51. Boonsawat W, Salome CM, Woolcock AJ. Effect of allergen inhalation on the maximal response plateau of the dose–response curve to methacholine. Am Rev Respir Dis l992; 146(3):565–569.

52. Ramsdell JW, Nachtwey FJ, Moser KM. Bronchial hyperreactivity in chronic obstructive bronchitis. Am Rev Respir Dis 1982; 126(5):829–832.

53. Agalliu I, Eisen EA, Hauser R, et al. Truncating the dose range for methacholine challenge tests: three occupational studies. J Occup Environ Med 2003; 45(8):841–847.

54. Cockcroft DW. Measurement of airway responsiveness to inhaled histamine or methacholine: method of continuous aerosol generation and tidal breathing inhalation. In: Hargreave FE, Woolcock AJ, eds. Airway Responsiveness: Measurement and Interpretation. Ontario: Astra Pharmaceuticals, 1985:22–28.

55. Ryan G, Dolovich MB, Obminski G, et al. Standardization of inhalation provocation tests: influence of nebulizer output, particle size, and method of inhalation. J Allergy Clin Immunol 1981; 67(2):156–161.

56. Ryan G, Dolovich MB, Roberts RS, et al. Standardization of inhalation provocation tests: two techniques of aerosol generation and inhalation compared. Am Rev Respir Dis l981; 123(2):195–199.

57. Ryan G, Latimer KM, Dolovich J, Hargreave FE. Bronchial responsiveness to histamine: relationship to diurnal variation of peak flow rate, improvement after bronchodilator, and airway calibre. Thorax 1982; 37(6):423–429.

58. Malo JL, Pineau L, Cartier A, Martin RR. Reference values of the provocative concentrations of methacholine that cause 6% and 20% changes in

forced expiratory volume in one second in a normal population. Am Rev Respir Dis 1983; 128(1):8–11.

59. Rijcken B, Schouten JP, Weiss ST, Speizer FE, van der Lende R. The relationship of nonspecific bronchial responsiveness to respiratory symptoms in a random population sample. Am Rev Respir Dis 1987; 136(1):62–68.

60. Le Souef PN, Geelhoed GC, Turner DJ, Morgan SE, Landau LI. Response of normal infants to inhaled histamine. Am Rev Respir Dis 1989; 139(1):62–66.

61. Hopp RJ, Bewtra A, Nair NM, Townley RG. The effect of age on methacholine response. J Allergy Clin Immunol 1985; 76(4):609–613.

62. Le Souef PN. Validity of methods used to test airway responsiveness in children. Lancet 1992; 339(8804):1282–1284.

63. Peat JK, Xuan W, Woolcock AJ. Importance of adjusting measurements of airway responsiveness for lung size and airway caliber. Am J Respir Crit Care Med 1995; 151:A132.

64. Sparrow D, O'Connor G, Colton T, Barry CL, Weiss ST. The relationship of nonspecific bronchial responsiveness to the occurrence of respiratory symptoms and decreased levels of pulmonary function. The Normative Aging Study. Am Rev Respir Dis 1987; 135(6):1255–1260.

65. Woolcock AJ, Peat JK, Salome CM, et al. Prevalence of bronchial hyperresponsiveness and asthma in a rural adult population. Thorax 1987; 42(5): 361–368.

66. Kennedy SM, Burrows B, Vedal S, Enarson DA, Chan-Yeung M. Methacholine responsiveness among working populations. Relationship to smoking and airway caliber. Am Rev Respir Dis 1990; 142(6 Pt 1):1377–1383.

67. Petays T, von Hertzen L, Metso T, et al. Smoking and atopy as determinants of sputum eosinophilia and bronchial hyper-responsiveness in adults with normal lung function. Respir Med 2003; 97:947–954.

68. de Vries K, Booy-Nord H, Lende Rv, van Lookeren Campagne JG, Orie NG. Reactivity of the bronchial tree to different stimuli. Bronches 1968; 18(6):439–452.

69. Chung KF, Snashall PD. Effect of prior bronchoconstriction on the airway response to histamine in normal subjects. Thorax 1984; 39(1):40–45.

70. Rubinfeld AR, Pain MC. Relationship between bronchial reactivity, airway caliber, and severity of asthma. Am Rev Respir Dis 1977; 115(3):381–387.

71a. Greenspon LW, Gracely E. A discriminant analysis applied to methacholine bronchoprovocation testing improves classification of patients as normal, asthma, or COPD. Chest 1992; 102(5):1419–1425.

71b. Wise RA, Kanner RE, Lindgren P, Connett JE, Altose MD, Enright PL, Tashkin DP for Lung Health Study Research Group. The effect of smoking intervention and an inhaled bronchodilator on airways reactivity in COPD. Chest 2003; 124:449–458.

71c. Schwartz J, Schindler C, Zemp E, Perruchoud AP, Zellweger J-P, Wuthrich B, Leuenberger P, Ackermann-Liebrich U, SAPALDIA Team. Predictors of methacholine responsiveness in a general population. Chest 2002; 122: 812–820.

72. Burrows B, Lebowitz MD, Barbee RA. Respiratory disorders and allergy skin-test reactions. Ann Intern Med 1976; 84(2):134–139.

73. O'Connor GT, Sparrow D, Segal MR, Weiss ST. Smoking, atopy, and metha-choline airway responsiveness among middle-aged and elderly men. The Nor-mative Aging Study. Am Rev Respir Dis 1989; 140(6):1520–1526.

74. Witt C, Stuckey MS, Woolcock AJ, Dawkins RL. Positive allergy prick tests associated with bronchial histamine responsiveness in an unselected popula-tion. J Allergy Clin Immunol 1986; 77(5):698–702.

75. Cookson WO, Musk AW, Ryan G. Associations between asthma history, atopy, and non-specific bronchial responsiveness in young adults. Clin Allergy 1986; 16(5):425–432.

76. Cockcroft DW, Murdock KY, Berscheid BA, Gore BP. Sensitivity and speci-ficity of histamine PC20 determination in a random selection of young college students. J Allergy Clin Immunol 1992; 89(1 Pt 1):23–30.

77. Enarson DA, Chan-Yeung M, Tabona M, Kus J, Vedal S, Lam S. Predictors of bronchial hyperexcitability in grainhandlers. Chest 1985; 87(4):452–455.

78. Hensley MJ, Scicchitano R, Saunders NA, et al. Seasonal variation in non-specific bronchial reactivity: a study of wheat workers with a history of wheat associated asthma. Thorax 1988; 43(2):103–107.

79. Beier J, Beeh KM, Kornman O, Morankic E, Ritter N, Buhl R. Dissimilarity between seasonal changes in airway responsiveness to adenosine-5-monopho-sphate and methacholine in grass pollen allergic rhinitis: relation to induced sputum. Int Arch Allergy Immunol 2003; 132(l):76–81.

80. Platts-Mills TA, Tovey ER, Mitchell EB, Moszoro H, Nock P, Wilkins SR. Reduction of bronchial hyperreactivity during prolonged allergen avoidance. Lancet 1982; 675–678.

81. Marks GB, Tovey ER, Green W, Shearer M, Salome CM, Woolcock AJ. The effect of changes in house dust mite allergen exposure on the severity of asthma. Clin Exp Allergy 1995; 25(2):114–118.

82. Empey DW, Laitinen LA, Jacobs L, Gold WM, Nadel JA. Mechanisms of bronchial hyperreactivity in normal subjects after upper respiratory tract infection. Am Rev Respir Dis 1976; 113(2):131–139.

83. Cheung D, Dick EC, Timmers MC, de Klerk EPA, Spaan WJM, Sterk PJ. Rhinovirus inhalation causes prolonged excessive airway narrowing to metha-choline in asthmatic subjects in vivo. Am J Respir Crit Care Med 1994; 149:A47.

84. Halperin SA, Eggleston PA, Beasley P, et al. Exacerbations of asthma in adults during experimental rhinovirus infection. Am Rev Respir Dis 1985; 132(5):976–980.

85. Lemanske RF Jr. Dick EC, Swenson CA, Vrtis RF, Busse WW. Rhinovirus upper respiratory infection increases airway hyperreactivity and late asth-matic reactions. J Clin Invest 1989; 83(1):1–10.

86. Bush RK, Busse W, Flaherty D, Warshauer D, Dick EC, Reed CE. Effects of experimental rhinovirus 16 infection on airways and leukocyte function in normal subjects. J Allergy Clin Immunol 1978; 61(2):80–87.

87. Summers QA, Higgins PG, Barrow IG, Tyrrell DA, Holgate ST. Bronchial reactivity to histamine and bradykinin is unchanged after rhinovirus infection in normal subjects. Eur Respir J 1992; 5(3):313–317.

88. Burney PG, Britton JR, Chinn S, et al. Descriptive epidemiology of bronchial reactivity in an adult population: results from a community study. Thorax 1987; 42(l):38–44.

89. Bellia V, Rizzo A, Amoroso S, Mirabella A, Bonsignore G. Analysis of dose–response curves in the detection of bronchial hyperreactivity. Respiration 1983; 44(1):10–18.

90. Woolcock AJ, Salome CM, Yan K. The shape of the dose–response curve to histamine in asthmatic and normal subjects. Am Rev Respir Dis 1984; 130(l):71–75.

91. Orehek J, Gayrard P, Smith AP, Grimaud C, Charpin J. Airway response to carbachol in normal and asthmatic subjects: distinction between bronchial sensitivity and reactivity. Am Rev Respir Dis 1977; 115(6):937–943.

92. O'Connor G, Sparrow D, Taylor D, Segal M, Weiss S. Analysis of dose–response curves to methacholine. An approach suitable for population studies. Am Rev Respir Dis 1987; 136(6):1412–1417.

93. Juniper EF, Syty-Golda M, Hargreave FE. Histamine inhalation tests: inhalation of aerosol via a facemask versus a valve box with mouthpiece. Thorax 1984; 39(7):556–557.

94. Dehaut P, Rachiele A, Martin RR, Malo JL. Histamine dose–response curves in asthma: reproducibility and sensitivity of different indices to assess response. Thorax 1983; 38(7):516–522.

95. Chinn S, Britton JR, Burney PG, Tattersfield AE, Papacosta AO. Estimation and repeatability of the response to inhaled histamine in a community survey. Thorax 1987; 42(1):45–52.

96. Britton J, Mortagy A, Tattersfield A. Histamine challenge testing: comparison of three methods. Thorax 1986; 41(2):128–132.

97. Knox AJ, Wisniewski A, Cooper S, Tattersfield AE. A comparison of the Yan and a dosimeter method for methacholine challenge in experienced and inexperienced subjects. Eur Respir J 1991; 4(4):497–502.

98. Balzano G, Delli Carri I, Gallo C, Cocco G, Melillo G. Intrasubject between-day variability of PD20 methacholine assessed by the dosimeter inhalation test. Chest 1989; 95(6):1239–1243.

99. Abramson MJ, Saunders NA, Hensley MJ. Analysis of bronchial reactivity in epidemiological studies. Thorax 1990; 45:924–929.

100. Chinn S, Burney PGJ, Britton JR, Tattersfield AE, Higgins BG. Measures of response to bronchial challenge for us in epidemiological studies: a comparison. Eur Respir J 1992; 5(suppl):493s.

101. Peat JK, Salome CM, Berry G, Woolcock AJ. Relation of dose–response slope to respiratory symptoms in a population of Australian school children. Am Rev Respir Dis 1991; 144(3 Pt l):663–667.

102. Pattemore PK, Asher MI, Harrison AC, Mitchell EA, Rea HH, Stewart AW. The interrelationship among bronchial hyperresponsiveness, the diagnosis of asthma, and asthma symptoms. Am Rev Respir Dis 1990; 142(3):549–554.

103. Rijcken B, Schouten JP, Weiss ST, Meinesz AF, de Vries K, van der Lende R. The distribution of bronchial responsiveness to histamine in symptomatic and in asymptomatic subjects. A population-based analysis of various indices of responsiveness. Am Rev Respir Dis 1989; 140(3):615–623.

104. Cote J, Kennedy S, Chan-Yeung M. Sensitivity and specificity of PC20 and peak expiratory flow rate in cedar asthma. J Allergy Clin Immunol 1990; 85(3):592–598.

105. Moscato G, Dellabianca A, Corsico A, Biscaldi G, Gherson G, Vinci G. Bronchial responsiveness to ultrasonic fog in occupational asthma due to toluene diisocyanate. Chest 1993; 104(4):1127–1132.

106. CockGroft DW, Hargreave FE. Airway hyperresponsiveness. Relevance of random population data to clinical usefulness. Am Rev Respir Dis 1990; 142(3):497–500.

107. Beckett WS, Pace PA, Sferlazza SJ, Carey VJ, Weiss ST. Annual variability in methacholine responsiveness in nonasthmatic working adults. Eur Respir J 1997; 10(11):2515–2521.

108. Forastiere F, Pistelli R, Michelozzi P, et al. Indices of nonspecific bronchial responsiveness in a pediatric population. Chest 1991; 100(4):927–934.

109. Hopp RJ, Bewtra AK, Nair NM, Townley RG. Specificity and sensitivity of methacholine inhalation challenge in normal and asthmatic children. J Allergy Clin Immunol 1984; 74(2):154–158.

110. Burney PG, Chinn S, Britton JR, Tattersfield AE, Papacosta AO. What symptoms predict the bronchial response to histamine? Evaluation in a community survey of the bronchial symptoms questionnaire (1984) of the International Union Against Tuberculosis and Lung Disease. Int J Epidemiol 1989; 18(1):165–173.

111. Godfrey S, Springer C, Bar-Yishay E, Avital A. Cut-off points defining normal and asthmatic bronchial reactivity to exercise and inhalation challenges in children and young adults. Eur Respir J 1999; 14(3):659–668.

112. Toren K, Brisman J, Jarvholm B. Asthma and asthma-like symptoms in adults assessed by questionnaires. A literature review. Chest 1993; 104(2):600–608.

113. Jaeschke R, Guyatt G, Sackett DL. Users' guides to the medical literature. III. How to use an article about a diagnostic test. A. Are the results of the study valid? Evidence-Based Medicine Working Group. J Am Med Assoc 1994; 271(5):389–391.

114. Eliasson AH, Phillips YY, Rajagopal KR, Howard RS. Sensitivity and specificity of bronchial provocation testing. An evaluation of four techniques in exercise-induced bronchospasm. Chest 1992; 102(2):347–355.

115. Josephs LK, Gregg I, Mullee MA, Holgate ST. Nonspecific bronchial reactivity and its relationship to the clinical expression of asthma. A longitudinal study. Am Rev Respir Dis 1989; 140(2):350–357.

116. Joos GF, O'Connor B, Anderson SD, et al. Indirect airway challenges. Eur Respir J 2003; 21(6):1050–1068.

117. Toelle BG, Peat JK, Salome CM, Mellis CM, Woolcock AJ. Toward a definition of asthma for epidemiology. Am Rev Respir Dis 1992; 146(3):633–637.

118. Peat JK, Haby M, Spijker J, Berry G, Woolcock AJ. Prevalence of asthma in adults in Busselton, Western Australia. Br Med J 1992; 305:1326–1329.

119. Postma DS, Bleecker ER, Amelung PJ, et al. Genetic susceptibility to asthma—bronchial hyperresponsiveness coinherited with a major gene for atopy. N Engl J Med 1995; 333(14):894–900.

120. Robertson CF, Bishop J, Dalton M, et al. Prevalence of asthma in regional Victorian school children. Med J Aust 1992; 156(12):831–833.
121. Perrin B, Lagier F, L'Archeveque J, et al. Occupational asthma: validity of monitoring of peak expiratory flow rates and non-allergic bronchial responsiveness as compared to specific inhalation challenge. Eur Respir J 1992; 5(1):40–48.
122. Chan-Yeung M, Lam S. Occupational asthma. Am Rev Respir Dis 1986; 133(4):686–703.
123. Vedal S, Enarson DA, Chan H, Ochnio J, Tse KS, Chan-Yeung M. A longitudinal study of the occurrence of bronchial hyperresponsiveness in western red cedar workers. Am Rev Respir Dis 1988; 137(3):651–655.
124. James A, Carroll N. Airway smooth muscle in health and disease; methods of measurement and relation to function. Eur Respir J 2000; 15(4):782–789.
125. Abramson MJ, Wlodarczyk JH, Saunders NA, Hensley MJ. Does aluminum smelting cause lung disease? Am Rev Respir Dis 1989; 139(4):1042–1057.
126. Enarson DA, Vedal S, Schulzer M, Dybuncio A, Chan-Yeung M. Asthma, asthmalike symptoms, chronic bronchitis, and the degree of bronchial hyperresponsiveness in epidemiologic surveys. Am Rev Respir Dis 1987; 136(3):613–617.
127. Paggiaro PL, Vagaggini B, Dente FL, et al. Bronchial hyperresponsiveness and toluene diisocyanate. Long-term change in sensitized asthmatic subjects. Chest 1993; 103(4):1123–1128.
128. Chan-Yeung M, Desjardins A. Bronchial hyperresponsiveness and level of exposure in occupational asthma due to western red cedar (*Thuja plicata*). Serial observations 53 before and after development of symptoms. Am Rev Respir Dis 1992; 146(6):1606–1609.
129. Banks DE, Sastre J, Butcher BT, et al. Role of inhalation challenge testing in the diagnosis of isocyanate-induced asthma. Chest 1989; 95(2):414–423.
130. Baur X, Huber H, Degens PO, Allmers H, Ammon J. Relation between occupational asthma case history, bronchial methacholine challenge, and specific challenge test in patients with suspected occupational asthma. Am J Ind Med 1998; 33(2):114–122.
131. Aquilina AT. Comparison of airway reactivity induced by histamine, methacheline, and isocapnic hyperventilation in normal and asthmatic subjects. Thorax 1983; 38(10):766–770.
132. Roach JM, Hurwitz KM, Argyros GJ, Eliasson AH, Phillips YY. Eucapnic voluntary hyperventilation as a bronchoprovocation technique. Comparison with methacholine inhalation in asthmatics. Chest 1994; 105(3):667–672.
133. Smith CM, Anderson SD. Inhalational challenge using hypertonic saline in asthmatic subjects: a comparison with responses to hyperpnoea, methacholine and water. Eur Respir J 1990; 3(2):144–151.
134. Filuk RB, Serrette C, Anthonisen NR. Comparison of responses to methacholine and cold air in patients suspected of having asthma. Chest 1989; 95(5):948–952.
135. Eggleston PA. A comparison of the asthmatic response to methacholine and exercise. J Allergy Clin Immunol 1979; 63(2):104–110.

136. Fourie PR, Joubert JR. Determination of airway hyper-reactivity in asthmatic children: a comparison among exercise, nebulized water, and histamine challenge. Pediatr Pulmonol 1988; 4(l):2–7.

137. Lin CC, Wu JL, Huang WC, Lin CY. A bronchial response comparison of exercise and methacholine in asthmatic subjects. J Asthma 1991; 28(l):31–40.

138. Vasar M, Braback L, Julge K, Knutsson A, Riikjarv MA, Bjorksten B. Prevalence of 54 bronchial hyperreactivity as determined by several methods among Estonian school children. Pediatr Allergy Immunol 1996; 7(3): 141–146.

139. Poulter LW, Norris A, Power C, Condez A, Schmekel B, Burke C. T-cell dominated inflammatory reactions in the bronchi of asthmatics are not reflected in matched bronchoalveolar lavage specimens. Eur Respir J 1992; 5(2):182–189.

140. Poston RN, Chanez P, Lacoste JY, Litchfield T, Lee TH, Bousquet J. Immunohistochemical characterization of the cellular infiltration in asthmatic bronchi. Am Rev Respir Dis 1992; 145(4 Pt 1):918–921.

141. Azzawi M, Bradley B, Jeffery PK, et al. Identification of activated T lymphocytes and eosinophils in bronchial biopsies in stable atopic asthma. Am Rev Respir Dis 1990; 142(6Pt l):1407–1413.

142. Bradley BL, Azzawi M, Jacobson M, et al. Eosinophils, T-lymphocytes, mast cells, neutrophils, and macrophages in bronchial biopsy specimens from atopic subjects with asthma: comparison with biopsy specimens from atopic subjects without asthma and normal control subjects and relationship to bronchial hyperresponsiveness. J Allergy Clin Immunol 1991; 88(4):661–674.

143. Beasley R, Roche WR, Roberts JA, Holgate ST. Cellular events in the bronchi in mild asthma and after bronchial provocation. Am Rev Respir Dis 1989; 139(3):806–817.

144. Carroll NG, Mutavdzic S, James AL. Distribution and degranulation of airway mast cells in normal and asthmatic subjects. Eur Respir J 2002; 19(5):879–885.

145. Carroll N, Cooke C, James A. The distribution of eosinophils and lymphocytes in the large and small airways of asthmatics. Eur Respir J 1997; 10(2):292–300.

146. Djukanovic R, Roche WR, Wilson JW, et al. Mucosal inflammation in asthma. Am Rev Respir Dis 1990; 142(2):434–457.

147. Vignola AM, Chanez P, Chiappara G, et al. Evaluation of apoptosis of eosinophils, macrophages, and T lymphocytes in mucosal biopsy specimens of patients with asthma and chronic bronchitis. J Allergy Clin Immunol 1999; 103(4):563–573.

148. Van Den Berge M, Meijer RJ, Kerstjens HA, et al. PC(20) adenosine 5'-monophosphate is more closely associated with airway inflammation in asthma than PC(20) methacholme. Am J Respir Crit Care Med 2001; 163(7):1546–1550.

149. Yoshikawa T, Shoji S, Fujii T, et al. Severity of exercise-induced bronchoconstriction is related to airway eosinophilic inflammation in patients with asthma. Eur Respir J 1998; 12(4):879–884.

150. in't Veen JC, Smits HH, Hiemstra PS, Zwinderman AE, Sterk PJ, Bel EH. Lung function and sputum characteristics of patients with severe asthma during an induced exacerbation by double-blind steroid withdrawal. Am J Respir Crit Care Med 1999; 160(l):93–99.

151. van den Berge M, Kerstjens HA, Meijer RJ, et al. Corticosteroid-induced improvement in the PC20 of adenosine monophosphate is more closely associated with reduction in airway inflammation than improvement in the PC20 of methacholine. Am J Respir Crit Care Med 2001; 164(7):1127–1132.

152. Carlsen KH, Engh G, Mork M, Schroder E. Cold air inhalation and exercise–induced bronchoconstriction in relationship to methacholine bronchial responsiveness: different patterns in asthmatic children and children with other chronic lung diseases. Respir Med 1998; 92(2):308–315.

153. Woolcock AJ, Anderson SD, Peat JK, et al. Characteristics of bronchial hyperresponsiveness in chronic obstructive pulmonary disease and in asthma. Am Rev Respir Dis 1991; 143(6):1438–1443.

154. Sanchez-Toril F, Prieto L, Peris R, Perez JA, Millan M, Marin J. Differences in airway responsiveness to acetaldehyde and methacholine in asthma and chronic bronchitis. Eur Respir J 2000; 15(2):260–265.

155. Bel EH, van der Veen H, Kramps JA, Dijkman JH, Sterk PJ. Maximal airway narrowing to inhaled leukotriene D4 in normal subjects. Comparison and interaction with methacholine. Am Rev Respir Dis 1987; 136(4):979–984.

156. Thomson NC, Roberts R, Bandouvakis J, Newball H, Hargreave FE. Comparison of bronchial responses to prostaglandin F2 alpha and methacholine. J Allergy Clin Immunol 1981; 68(5):392–398.

157. Doull J, Sandall D, Smith S, Schreiber J, Freezer NJ, Holgate ST. Differential inhibitory effect of regular inhaled corticosteroid on airway responsiveness to adenosine 5' monophosphate, methacholine, and bradykinin in symptomatic children with recurrent wheeze. Pediatr Pulmonol 1997; 23(6):404–411.

158. Leff JA, Busse WW, Pearlman D, et al. Montelukast, a leukotriene–receptor antagonist, for the treatment of mild asthma and exercise-induced bronchoconstriction. N Engl J Med 1998; 339(3):147–152.

159. Cockcroft DW, Murdock KY, Kirby J, Hargreave F. Prediction of airway responsiveness to allergen from skin sensitivity to allergen and airway responsiveness to histamine. Am Rev Respir Dis 1987; 135(l):264–267.

160. Gibson PG, Saltos N, Borgas T. Airway mast cells and eosinophils correlate with clinical severity and airway hyperresponsiveness in corticosteroid-treated asthma. J Allergy Clin Immunol 2000; 105(4):752–759.

161a. Juniper EF, Kline PA, Vanzieleghem MA, Ramsdale EH, O'Byme PM, Hargreave FE. Long-term effects of budesonide on airway responsiveness and clinical asthma severity in inhaled steroid-dependent asthmatics. Eur Respir J 1990; 3(10):1122–1127.

161b. Weiss ST, Van Natta ML, Zeiger RS, for the Childhood Asthma Management Research Group. Relationship between increased airway responsiveness and asthma severity in the childhood asthma management program. Am J Respir Crit Care Med 2000; 162:50–56.

162. Fowler SJ, Dempsey OJ, Sims EJ, Lipworth BJ. Screening for bronchial hyperresponsiveness using methacholine and adenosine monophosphate.

Relationship to asthma severity and beta(2)-receptor genotype. Am J Respir Crit Care Med 2000; 162(4 Pt 1):1318–1322.

163a. Makino S. Clinical significance of bronchial sensitivity to acetylcholine and histamine in bronchial asthma. J Allergy 1966; 38(3):127–142.

163b. Jatakanon A, Lim S, Kharitonov SA, Chung KF, Barnes PJ. Correlation between exhaled nitric oxide, sputum eosinophils, and methacholine responsiveness in patients with mild asthma. Thorax 1998; 53:91–95.

164. Juniper EF, Frith PA, Hargreave FE. Airway responsiveness to histamine and methacholine: relationship to minimum treatment to control symptoms of asthma. Thorax 1981; 36(8):575–579.

165. van Essen-Zandvliet EE, Hughes MD, Waalkens HJ, Duiverman EJ, Pocock SJ, Kerrebijn KF. Effects of 22 months of treatment with inhaled corticosteroids and/or beta-2–agonists on lung function, airway responsiveness, and symptoms in children with asthma. The Dutch Chronic Non-specific Lung Disease Study Group. Am Rev Respir Dis 1992; 146(3):547–554.

166. Jenkins CR, Woolcock AJ. Effect of prednisone and beclomethasone dipropionate on airway responsiveness in asthma: a comparative study. Thorax 1988; 43(5):378–384.

167. Juniper EF, Kline PA, Vanzieleghem MA, Ramsdale EH, O'Byrne PM, Hargreave FE. Effect of long-term treatment with an inhaled corticosteroid (budesonide) on airway hyperresponsiveness and clinical asthma in nonsteroid-dependent asthmatics. Am Rev Respir Dis 1990; 142(4):832–836.

168. Kraan J, Koeter GH, van der Mark TW, et al. Dosage and time effects of inhaled budesonide on bronchial hyperreactivity. Am Rev Respir Dis 1988; 137(1):44–48.

169. Ward C, Pais M, Bish R, et al. Airway inflammation, basement membrane thickening and bronchial hyperresponsiveness in asthma. Thorax 2002; 57(4):309–316.

170. Sont JK, Willems LN, Bel EH, van Krieken JH, Vandenbroucke JP, Sterk PJ. Clinical control and histopathologic outcome of asthma when using airway hyperresponsiveness as an additional guide to long-term treatment. The AMPUL Study Group. Am J Respir Crit Care Med 1999; 159(4 Pt l):1043–1051.

171. Haahtela T, Jarvinen M, Kava T, et al. Comparison of a beta 2-agonist, terbutaline, with an inhaled corticosteroid, budesonide, in newly detected asthma. N Engl J Med 1991; 325(6):388–392.

172. Currie GP, Fowler SJ, Lipworth BJ. Dose response of inhaled corticosteroids on bronchial hyperresponsiveness: a meta-analysis. Ann Allergy Asthma Immunol 2003; 90(2):194–198.

173. Currie GP, Stenback S, Lipworth BJ. Effects of fluticasone vs. fluticasone/salmeterol on airway caliber and airway hyperresponsiveness in mild persistent asthma. Br J Clin Pharmacol 2003; 56(1):11–17.

174. Reddel HK, Jenkins CR, Marks GB, et al. Optimal asthma control, starting with high doses of inhaled budesonide. Eur Respir J 2000; 16(2):226–235.

175. Leuppi JD, Salome CM, Jenkins CR, et al. Markers of airway inflammation and airway hyperresponsiveness in patients with well-controlled asthma. Eur Respir J 2001; 18(3):444–450.

176. Prosperini G, Rajakulasingam K, Cacciola RR, et al. Changes in sputum counts and airway hyperresponsiveness after budesonide: monitoring anti–inflammatory response on the basis of surrogate markers of airway inflammation. J Allergy Clin Immunol 2002; 110(6):855–861.

177. Bel EH, Timmers MC, Zwinderman AH, Dijkman JH, Sterk PJ. The effect of inhaled corticosteroids on the maximal degree of airway narrowing to methacholine in asthmatic subjects. Am Rev Respir Dis 1991; 143(1):109–113.

178. Moreno RH, Hogg JC, Pare PD. Mechanics of airway narrowing. Am Rev Respir Dis 1986; 133(6):1171–1180.

179. Brightling CE, Bradding P, Symon FA, Holgate ST, Wardlaw AJ, Pavord ID. Mast-cell infiltration of airway smooth muscle in asthma. N Engl J Med 2002; 346(22):1699–1705.

180. Carroll NG, Mutavdzic S, James AL. Increased mast cells and neutrophils in submucosal mucous glands and mucus plugging in patients with asthma. Thorax 2002; 57(8):677–682.

181. Carroll NG, Cooke C, James AL. Bronchial blood vessel dimensions in asthma. Am J Respir Crit Care Med 1997; 155(2):689–695.

182. Aikawa T, Shimura S, Sasaki H, Ebina M, Takishima T. Marked goblet cell hyperplasia with mucus accumulation in the airways of patients who died of severe acute asthma attack. Chest 1992; 101(4):916–921.

183. Carroll N, Elliot J, Morton A, James A. The structure of large and small airways in nonfatal and fatal asthma. Am Rev Respir Dis 1993; 147(2):405–410.

184. Dunnill MS, Massarella GR, Anderson JA. A comparison of the quantitative anatomy of the bronchi in normal subjects, in status asthmaticus, in chronic bronchitis, and in emphysema. Thorax 1969; 24(2):176–179.

185. Huber HL, Koessler KK. The pathology of fatal asthma. Arch Intern Med 1922; 30:689–760.

186. Kuwano K, Bosken CH, Pare PD, Bai TR, Wiggs BR, Hogg JC. Small airways dimensions in asthma and in chronic obstructive pulmonary disease. Am Rev Respir Dis 1993; 148(5):1220–1225.

187. Sobonya RE. Quantitative structural alterations in long-standing allergic asthma. Am Rev Respir Dis 1984; 130(2):289–292.

188. Takizawa T, Thurlbeck WM. Muscle and mucous gland size in the major bronchi of patients with chronic bronchitis, asthma, and asthmatic bronchitis. Am Rev Respir Dis 1971; 104(3):331–336.

189. Heard BE, Hossain S. Hyperplasia of bronchial muscle in asthma. J Pathol 1973; 110:319–331.

190. Ebina M, Takahashi T, Chiba T, Motomiya M. Cellular hypertrophy and hyperplasia of airway smooth muscles underlying bronchial asthma. A 3-D morphometric study. Am Rev Respir Dis 1993; 148(3):720–726.

191. James AL, Pare PD, Hogg JC. The mechanics of airway narrowing in asthma. Am Rev Respir Dis 1989; 139(1):242–246.

192. Saetta M, Di Stefano A, Rosina C, Thiene G, Fabbri LM. Quantitative structural analysis of peripheral airways and arteries in sudden fatal asthma. Am Rev Respir Dis 1991; 143(1):138–143.

193. Laitinen A, Altraja A, Kampe M, Linden M, Virtanen I, Laitinen LA. Tenascin is increased in airway basement membrane of asthmatics and decreased by an inhaled steroid. Am J Respir Crit Care Med 1997; 156(3 Pt l):951–958.

194. Bhaskar KR, O'Sullivan DD, Coles SJ, Kozakewich H, Vawter GP, Reid LM. Characterization of airway mucus from a fatal case of status asthmaticus. Pediatr Pulmonol 1988; 5(3):176–182.

195. Sheehan JK, Richardson PS, Fung DC, Howard M, Thornton DJ. Analysis of respiratory mucus glycoproteins in asthma: a detailed study from a patient who died in status asthmaticus. Am J Respir Cell Mol Biol 1995; 13(6):748–756.

196. Goldie RG, Spina D, Henry PJ, Lulich KM, Paterson JW. In vitro responsiveness of human asthmatic bronchus to carbachol, histamine, beta-adrenoceptor agonists and theophylline. Br J Clin Pharmacol 1986; 22(6): 669–676.

197. Armour CL, Lazar NM, Schellenberg RR, et al. A comparison of in vivo and in vitro human airway reactivity to histamine. Am Rev Respir Dis 1984; 129(6):907–910.

198. Cerrina J, Le Roy Ladurie M, Labat C, Raffestin B, Bayol A, Brink C. Comparison of human bronchial muscle responses to histamine in vivo with histamine and isoproterenol agonists in vitro. Am Rev Respir Dis 1986; 134(1): 57–61.

199. Vincenc KS, Black JL, Yan K, Armour CL, Donnelly PD, Woolcock AJ. Comparison of in vivo and in vitro responses to histamine in human airways. Am Rev Respir Dis 1983; 128(5):875–879.

200. Ammit AJ, Bekir SS, Johnson PR, Hughes JM, Armour CL, Black JL. Mast cell numbers are increased in the smooth muscle of human sensitized isolated bronchi. Am J Respir Crit Care Med 1997; 155(3):1123–1129.

201. Johnson PR, Roth M, Tamm M, et al. Airway smooth muscle cell proliferation is increased in asthma. Am J Respir Crit Care Med 2001; 164(3): 474–477.

202. Solway J, Fredberg JJ. Perhaps airway smooth muscle dysfunction contributes to asthmatic bronchial hyperresponsiveness after all. Am J Respir Cell Mol Biol 1997; 17(2):144–146.

203. Fredberg JJ. Airway smooth muscle in asthma: flirting with disaster. Eur Respir J 1998; 12(6):1252–1256.

204. Fredberg JJ, Inouye D, Miller B, et al. Airway smooth muscle, tidal stretches, and dynamically determined contractile states. Am J Respir Crit Care Med 1997; 156(6):1752–1759.

205. Macklem PT. Bronchial hyporesponsiveness. Chest 1987; 91(6 suppl):189S–191S.

206. Sterk PJ, Daniel EE, Zamel N, Hargreave FE. Limited maximal airway narrowing in nonasthmatic subjects. Role of neural control and prostaglandin release. Am Rev Respir Dis 1985; 132(4):865–870.

207. Ding DJ, Martin JG, Macklem PT. Effects of lung volume on maximal methacholine-induced bronchoconstriction in normal humans. J Appl Physiol 1987; 62(3):1324–1330.

208. Fish JE, Ankin MG, Kelly JF, Peterman VI. Regulation of bronchomotor tone by lung inflation in asthmatic and nonasthmatic subjects. J Appl Physiol 1981; 50(5):1079–1086.

209. Skloot G, Permutt S, Togias A. Airway hyperresponsiveness in asthma: a problem of limited smooth muscle relaxation with inspiration. J Clin Invest 1995; 96(5):2393–2403.

210. Ingram RH. Relationships among airway–parenchymal interactions, lung responsiveness, and inflammation in asthma. Chest 1995; 107(3):148S–152S.

211. King GG, Moore BJ, Seow CY, Pare PD. Time course of increased airway narrowing caused by inhibition of deep inspiration during methacholine challenge. Am J Respir Crit Care Med 1999; 160(2):454–457.

212. Scichilone N, Permutt S, Togias A. The lack of the bronchoprotective and not the bronchodilatory ability of deep inspiration is associated with airway hyperresponsiveness. Am J Respir Crit Care Med 2001; 163(2):413–419.

213. Laitinen LA, Laitinen A, Haahtela T. A comparative study of the effects of an inhaled corticosteroid, budesonide, and a beta 2-agonist, terbutaline, on airway inflammation in newly diagnosed asthma: a randomized, double-blind, parallel–group controlled trial. J Allergy Clin Immunol 1992; 90(l):32–42.

214. Jeffery PK, Godfrey RW, Adelroth E, Nelson F, Rogers A, Johansson SA. Effects of treatment on airway inflammation and thickening of basement membrane reticular collagen in asthma. A quantitative light and electron microscopic study. Am Rev Respir Dis 1992; 145(4 Pt l):890–899.

215. Djukanovic R, Wilson JW, Britten KM, et al. Effect of an inhaled corticosteroid on airway inflammation and symptoms in asthma. Am Rev Respir Dis 1992; 145(3):669–674.

216. Guillemi S, James AL, Pare PD. Effect of breathing pattern during inhalation challenge on the shape and position of the dose–response curve. Lung 1989; 167(2):95–106.

217. Ilowite JS, Bennett WD, Sheetz MS, Groth ML, Nierman DM. Permeability of the bronchial mucosa to 99mTc–DTPA in asthma. Am Rev Respir Dis 1989; 139(5):1139–1143.

218. Kelly L, Kolbe J, Mitzner W, Spannhake EW, Bromberger-Barnea B, Menkes H. Bronchial blood flow affects recovery from constriction in dog lung periphery. J Appl Physiol 1986; 60(6):1954–1959.

219. James AL. Relationship between airway wall thickness and airway hyperresponsiveness. In: Stewart AG, ed. Airway wall remodeling in asthma. New York, U.S.A.: CRC Press Inc;, 1997:1–28.

220. Sont JK, Han J, van Krieken JM, et al. Relationship between the inflammatory infiltrate in bronchial biopsy specimens and clinical severity of asthma in patients treated with inhaled steroids. Thorax 1996; 51(5):496–502.

221. Niimi A, Matsumoto H, Amitani R, et al. Airway wall thickness in asthma assessed by computed tomography. Relation to clinical indices. Am J Respir Crit Care Med 2000; 162(4 Pt 1):1518–1523.

222. Nakano Y, Muller NL, King GG, et al. Quantitative assessment of airway remodeling using high-resolution CT. Chest 2002; 122(6 suppl):271S–275S.

223. Strunk RC, Szefler SJ, Phillips BR, et al. Relationship of exhaled nitric oxide to clinical and inflammatory markers of persistent asthma in children. J Allergy Clin Immunol 2003; 112(5):883–892.

224. Pratter MR, Woodman TF, Irwin RS, Johnson B. Stability of stored methacholine chloride solutions: clinically useful information. Am Rev Respir Dis 1982; 126(4):717–719.

225. Marwaha RK, Johnson BF. Long-term stability study of histamine in sterile bronchoprovocarion solutions. Am J Hosp Pharm 1986; 43(2):380–383.

226. Cartier A, Malo JL, Begin P, Sestier M, Martin RR. Time course of the bronchoconstriction induced by inhaled histamine and methacholine. J Appl Physiol 1983; 54(3):821–826.

227. Manning PJ, Jones GL, O'Byrne PM. Tachyphylaxis to inhaled histamine in asthmatic subjects. J Appl Physiol 1987; 63(4):1572–1577.

228. Strban M, Manning PJ, Watson RM, O'Byme PM. Effect of magnitude of airway responsiveness and therapy with inhaled corticosteroid on histamine tachyphylaxis in asthma. Chest 1994; 105(5):1434–1438.

229. Van Schoor J, Joos GF, Pauwels RA. Indirect bronchial hyperresponsiveness in asthma: mechanisms, pharmacology and implications for clinical research. Eur Respir J 2000; 16(3):514–533.

230. Galdes-Sebaldt M, McLaughlin FJ, Levison H. Comparison of cold air, ultrasonic mist, and methacholine inhalations as tests of bronchial reactivity in normal and asthmatic children. J Pediatr 1985; 107(4):526–530.

231. Spiropoulos K, Stevens J, Eigen H, Spiropoulos A. Specificity and sensitivity of methacholine challenge test in children with normal and hyperreactive airways. Acta Paediatr Scand 1986; 75(5):737–743.

232. Bruschi C, Cerveri I, Zoia MC, Maccarini L, Grassi M, Rampulla C. Bronchial responsiveness to inhaled methacholine in epidemiological studies: comparison of different indices. Eur Respir J 1989; 2(7):630–636.

233. Backer V, Groth S, Dirksen A, et al. Sensitivity and specificity of the histamine challenge test for the diagnosis of asthma in an unselected sample of children and adolescents. Eur Respir J 1991; 4(9):1093–1100.

234. Venables KM, Fairer N, Sharp L, Graneek BJ, Newman Taylor AJ. Respiratory symptoms questionnaire for asthma epidemiology: validity and reproducibility. Thorax 1993; 48(3):214–219.

235. Remes ST, Pekkanen J, Remes K, Salonen RO, Korppi M. In search of childhood asthma: questionnaire, tests of bronchial hyperresponsiveness, and clinical evaluation. Thorax 2002; 57(2):120–126.

236. Niggemann B, Illi S, Madloch C, et al. Histamine challenges discriminate between symptomatic and asymptomatic children. MASS-tudy Group. Multicentre Allergy Study. Eur Respir J 2001; 17(2):246–253.

237. Xu X, Niu T, Chen C, et al. Association of airway responsiveness with asthma and persistent wheeze in a Chinese population. Chest 2001; 119(3):691–700.

11

Monitoring Airway Hyperresponsiveness: Indirect Stimuli—Exercise, Hypertonic Saline, Mannitol, and Adenosine Monophosphate

SANDRA D. ANDERSON and JOHN D. BRANNAN

Department of Respiratory Medicine, Royal
    Prince Alfred Hospital,
Camperdown, Australia

JÖRG D. LEUPPI

Respiratory Medicine, University Hospital
    Basel,
Basel, Switzerland

HEIKKI KOSKELA

Department of Respiratory Medicine, Kuopio
    University Hospital,
Kuopio, Finland

Overview

Tests of airway hyperresponsiveness (AHR) using stimuli that act indirectly to cause airway narrowing are becoming increasingly popular to identify and monitor asthma (1–3). AHR to an indirect stimulus may identify a person with active airway inflammation who would likely benefit from treatment with inhaled corticosteroids (ICS). Identification of AHR is of significant clinical value particularly if the person has normal spirometry and/or few symptoms, is well controlled, or has a past history of asthma. The documentation of a response to an indirect stimulus, within the normal healthy range, indicates quiescence of asthma and provides an end-point for treatment and a starting point for back titration of inhaled steroids.

The indirect stimuli include exercise, eucapnic voluntary hyperpnea (EVH), hypertonic (4.5%) saline, mannitol, and adenosine monophosphate. All these stimuli have been used to identify AHR and to assess its severity and to monitor response to treatment with inhaled steroids (4–11). Some have been used to monitor AHR in response to a change in environmental allergen exposure (12) or change due to seasonal exposure (13–15), and some have been used in epidemiological studies to document prevalence of active asthma (16–22).

Indirect stimuli provide a non-immunological stimulus resulting in the release of mediators from inflammatory cells and possible sensory nerves (23–26). The indirect stimuli have many characteristics in common. A positive airway response to one indirect stimulus predicts a positive response to another indirect stimulus. The airway responses to the indirect stimuli are all similarly modified by the same therapeutic interventions. The indirect stimuli differ in the complexity of the equipment required to administer them. For example, exercise requires an ergometer and controlled environment if responses are to be compared over time. A special gas mixture or a gas analyzer is required for testing with eucapnic voluntary hyperpnea. A large volume ultrasonic nebulizer with a high output of aerosol is required for administering hypertonic saline. For adenosine, solutions need to be made up and nebulizers are used for generation and delivery of the aerosol. For mannitol, a dry powder inhaler is required to administer the capsules. An advantage of an indirect challenge using a dose–response protocol is that the investigator has more control over the challenge.

The procedures for administering these stimuli have now been standardized (27), improving their utility for monitoring changes over time or for comparing data between different laboratories or between different populations. The ready availability of inexpensive equipment to measure changes in FEV_1 and the use of simple hand-held spirometers allow some of these procedures to be carried out at the point of need.

Definition of Indirect Stimuli

These "indirect" stimuli are so named because they do not act directly on bronchial smooth muscle to cause contraction and airway narrowing, but rather they act indirectly by releasing mediators (histamine, prostaglandins, leukotrienes) from inflammatory or neuronal cells (neuropeptides) (2). The stimuli known to act indirectly to cause the airways of asthmatics to narrow include hyperpnea with dry air (exercise, or eucapnic voluntary hyperpnea), hypertonic aerosols (saline and mannitol), and the pharmacologic agent adenosine monophosphate. A proposed pathway for dry air and hyperosmolar challenge is given in Figure 1. The severity of AHR to an indirect stimulus is not closely associated with baseline lung function, and many asthmatics with normal lung function are very responsive to these stimuli (Fig. 2) (28). In an asthmatic whose disease is active, it is thought that the number of inflammatory cells and the concentration of mediators is sufficient to cause the bronchial smooth muscle to contract and the airways to narrow in response to these indirect stimuli.

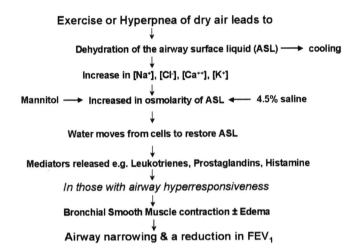

Exercise or Hyperpnea of dry air leads to
↓
Dehydration of the airway surface liquid (ASL) ⟶ **cooling**
↓
Increase in [Na⁺], [Cl⁻], [Ca⁺⁺], [K⁺]
↓
Mannitol ⟶ **Increased in osmolarity of ASL** ⟵ **4.5% saline**
↓
Water moves from cells to restore ASL
↓
Mediators released e.g. Leukotrienes, Prostaglandins, Histamine
↓
In those with airway hyperresponsiveness
↓
Bronchial Smooth Muscle contraction ± Edema
↓
Airway narrowing & a reduction in FEV₁

Figure 1   Flow chart relating indirect stimuli involving hyperpnea with dry air, as occurs with exercise or eucapnic voluntary hyperpnea, and osmotic stimuli (mannitol and 4.5% saline) to the events that occur in the airways of an asthmatic with airway inflammation and AHR, both hallmarks of asthma.

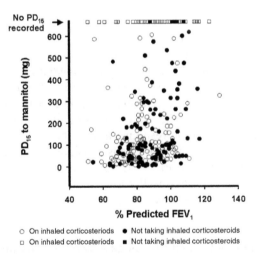

| ○ On inhaled corticosteriods | ● Not taking inhaled corticosteroids |
| □ On inhaled corticosteriods | ■ Not taking inhaled corticosteroids |

Figure 2   Individual values for the provoking dose of mannitol to cause a 15% reduction (PD₁₅) in forced expiratory volume in one second (FEV₁) in relation to the pre-challenge FEV₁ expressed as a percentage of predicted normal. There was no relationship between baseline lung function and sensitivity to the inhalation of mannitol and the majority of subjects who recorded a positive response, i.e., a PD₁₅ had values for FEV₁ within the normal range. *Source:* From Ref. 28. Closed circles are those responsive who were not taking inhaled corticosteroids (ICS) and open circles are those taking ICS. Open squares are those were not responsive to mannitol (i.e., No PD₁₅) and taking ICS and closed squares are those not responsive and not taking ICS.

The Coming of Age for Indirect Stimuli

In 1983, the recommendations of the European Society for Clinical Physiology Working Group on Bronchial Hyperreactivity stated that "Bronchial hyperresponsiveness denotes an increased bronchial response to inhaled substances which produce airways obstruction in normal subjects if given in adequate doses... it may be used for research into the pathogenesis and therapeutic manipulation of asthma" (29). Histamine and methacholine were considered the best validated substances at the time. The difference between the tests recommended in 1983 and the indirect stimuli discussed here in 2004 is that normal subjects seldom respond to an indirect stimulus and research on indirect stimuli has provided more useful information than direct stimuli in reference to "the pathogenesis and the therapeutic manipulation of asthma" (29).

It is now known that asthma is a disease that involves inflammation of the airways and that inhaled corticosteroids are the most suitable therapeutic agents to modify the disease itself (30,31). Treatment with inhaled steroids has given investigators the opportunity to study AHR in people with good lung function and values for FEV_1 within the normal predicted range. The reason that indirect stimuli are becoming more widely used is that in most studies they have been reported to be more sensitive for monitoring a change in AHR in response to treatment with ICS compared with direct stimuli such as histamine and methacholine (8,11,32–34). This is probably a result of the airway response to these indirect stimuli being dependent on the presence of inflammatory cells and their mediators in addition to the bronchial smooth muscle (BSM) being sensitive. A positive response to an indirect stimulus indicates that inflammation is active in that there are sufficient numbers of cells and concentrations of mediators to cause the BSM to contract. A negative response means that either there are not an adequate number of inflammatory cells (eosinophils, mast cells) or that the concentration of mediators is insufficient, or that the BSM does not respond to the mediators. It is well known that the BSM in asthmatics will respond to the mediators when they are administered directly to the airways, even if the asthmatic is well controlled on ICS alone (8,35–38).

Reasons to Use Indirect Stimuli as a Monitor of Asthma

There are a number of reasons that indirect stimuli are useful to monitor response to ICS. First, the reduction in AHR to indirect stimuli is rapid and 50% of asthmatics are likely to require the standard daily dose for 8 weeks or less. Second, the dose and duration of treatment with ICS can be better selected on the initial severity of the airway response. Third, the end-point for treatment is clearly defined as a response within the healthy range (e.g., fall in FEV_1 <10% after exercise or EVH). A higher dose or longer period of treatment is required for those with more severe AHR on initial assessment. Fourth, for those well controlled on ICS, who have a response within the healthy range, the response–dose ratio can be used to predict successful reduction of steroid dose.

The indirect stimuli play a valuable role in the evaluation of people with a past history of asthma who wish to pursue a sport (diving with scuba) (39) or occupation (police, fire fighting, defense force) that could bring on an attack (40). Many people free of EIA but with a past history of asthma, would still be expected to be responsive to a pharmacological agent, perhaps as a result of airway remodelling. Thus, responsiveness to an indirect challenge would also seem to be a fairer test for a risk assessment for asthma that is active. The same argument may apply for entry into occupation (41).

Background to the Use of These Indirect Stimuli for Monitoring Airway Hyperresponsiveness

Exercise

Exercise was the first indirect stimulus used for demonstrating AHR and monitoring treatment for asthma and has been widely used in both children and adults (42). Exercise has the advantage of inducing the symptoms of asthma as well as the classical physiological signs of an asthma attack, i.e., airway narrowing, hypoxemia, and hyper-inflation (43,44). Exercise became an excellent model to study the effect of drugs used in the treatment of asthma (45–47). The original exercise protocol (48,49) was developed to identify those with exercise-induced attacks of asthma (EIA) and to evaluate the prophylactic effect of beta$_2$-agonists and sodium cromoglycate (46,50).

In the early 1980s, exercise was used not only to demonstrate the efficacy of ICS in reducing AHR (51), but also for demonstrating that only very small doses of beta$_2$-agonists were required to prevent EIA in the presence of ICS (52). The findings in this and other studies have alerted investigators to the clinical significance of EIA in identifying airway inflammation. Reducing inflammation by treatment with ICS also reduced severity of EIA (4,38,53). Direct evidence for airway inflammation in EIA has been provided by the finding of significantly more eosinophils in the sputum of asthmatics with EIA compared with asthmatics without EIA (54,55). This is important because the presence of eosinophils is accepted as a sign of active asthma.

Exercise was also used to demonstrate the superiority of aerosol formulations of beta$_2$-adrenoceptor agonists compared with oral formulations of the same class of drug in preventing attacks of asthma (56). Later exercise was used to demonstrate the prolonged protective effect of the long-acting beta$_2$-agonists (LABA) (57,58). More recently exercise has been used

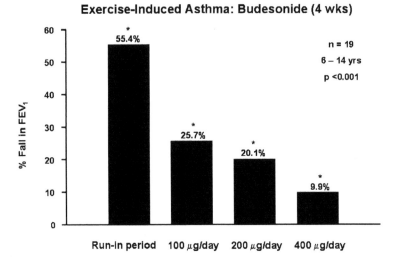

Figure 3 Mean values for the fall in FEV_1, expressed as a percentage of the baseline value for FEV_1 after exercise, in 19 asthmatic children who received different doses of budesonide in random order for 4 weeks. The data demonstrate a dose–response relationship between severity of exercise-induced asthma and the dose of inhaled steroid. *Source:* From Ref. 53.

to demonstrate the tolerance to the protective effect of SABAs (59) and LABAs that is now recognized as a consequence of daily use (60–62). Exercise has also been used to demonstrate the acute modifying effects of drugs such as nedocromil sodium (63) and montelukast (64,65).

The findings in epidemiological studies suggest that EIA is one of the first signs of asthma to develop (16). EIA also appears to be the last sign of asthma to resolve in response to treatment with ICS (53). Exercise was the first stimulus to be used successfully to demonstrate a dose–response curve to inhaled steroids (Fig. 3) (53).

Exercise has been a difficult test to standardize for use between laboratories and experienced personnel are required (66,67). Subjects need to be encouraged to reach the appropriate intensity of exercise and the environmental conditions need to be controlled or a source of dry air provided if the test is to be repeated to monitor the effects of treatment (68).

Eucapnic Voluntary Hyperpnea

As increasing numbers of athletes, defense force recruits, and otherwise "healthy individuals" started to report EIA, there was a need to develop a protocol that permitted the generation of high ventilation (V_E) in a laboratory setting. For this reason, a test of eucapnic voluntary hyperpnea with dry air was developed as a surrogate for exercise (69–72).

The profound advantage of using EVH over exercise is the ability to achieve and sustain a high rate of V_E (70–72). The V_E reached and sustained with EVH is considerably higher ($> 75\%$ maximum voluntary V_E) than that achieved with exercise ($< 65\%$ maximum voluntary V_E) in normal healthy subjects. This makes EVH a sensitive test for identifying EIA in the laboratory and reducing the chance of false-negative tests for EIA (73). The EVH test can be performed easily in those who are difficult to evaluate using the ergometers available in a laboratory. Further, with EVH the conditions under which a person exercises (temperature, duration, ventilation) can be simulated easily. EVH requires less expensive equipment than exercise but does require a special gas mixture or the monitoring of inspired and expired carbon dioxide (72).

Like exercise, EVH has been used to evaluate drugs used to prevent EIA, and to evaluate their duration of action (74–76). Given the potency of the challenge, EVH is probably one of the most sensitive of the indirect stimuli to evaluate the effect of ICS on AHR. The effect of both short- (5) and long-term treatment (77) with ICS has been demonstrated. For the long-term study, the EVH was performed inhaling cold dry air (77). EVH has also been used to evaluate benefit from ICS in very young children (78).

Hypertonic Saline

Hypertonic aerosols were introduced for routine use in the laboratory when it was realized that they probably mimicked the effects of evaporative water loss during exercise and EVH (79,80). Asthmatics with positive responses to exercise and EVH also responded to hypertonic saline (81,82) and the test with hypertonic saline was simpler to perform. The airway responses to different concentrations of hypertonic saline (1.8%, 2.7%, 3.6%, 4.5%) were similar to those provoked by different intensities of exercise (83). The concentration of hypertonic saline now used most commonly is 4.5% (27,84). The response to 4.5% saline relates to the presence of inflammatory cells in the airways (85).

Rodwell et al. (6) were the first to demonstrate that hypertonic saline could be used to monitor AHR in response to treatment with ICS for the first time or to monitor a change in dose of ICS. Du Toit et al. (8) were the first to compare systematically the modifying effects of ICS on both an indirect and direct stimulus to evaluate changes in AHR. The time course of the improvement in AHR to 4.5% saline was compared with improvement in AHR to histamine in the same subjects. The airway response to 4.5% saline was reduced to within the normal healthy ranges in half the subjects after only 8–12 weeks of treatment and at a time when all the subjects remained hyper-responsive to histamine (Fig. 4). The

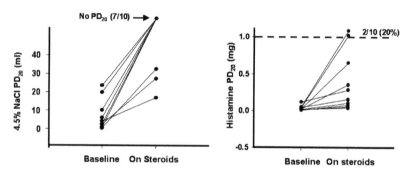

Figure 4   Individual values for the provoking dose to cause a 20% fall in FEV_1 (PD_{20}) to 4.5% saline (NaCl) and to histamine at baseline and after treatment with budesonide (1000 µg/day) for 4–12 weeks. Most of the subjects became unresponsive to saline but remained within the hyper-responsive range (1 mg is equivalent to 5 µmol or 100 breath units) for histamine. *Source:* From Ref. 8.

subjects who became non-responsive to hypertonic saline were usually those who were less responsive at baseline (PD_{20} >3 mL). This finding suggested that severity of the airway response at baseline could be used to predict dose of steroid required to normalize AHR.

Hypertonic saline was also used to demonstrate that the airway response to an indirect stimulus could plateau in the presence of drugs like nedocromil sodium. The plateau was most likely to occur in those subjects who were taking ICS and who had a PD_{20} >3 mL (86). A similar observation has been reported for mannitol with those with a PD_{15} >200 mg taking ICS becoming unresponsive in the presence of nedocromil (87). Of interest is the finding that the acute inhibitory effect of sodium cromoglycate on response to 4.5% saline, expressed as fold-change in PD_{20}, was significantly related to the fold-change in PD_{20} after 24–56 days treatment with budesonide 1000 µg/day ($r = 0.88$, $p < 0.01$), suggesting that the same cells were involved in the action of these two drugs (7). For example, mast cell release of mediators may be inhibited by the acute administration of SCG and the mast cell number or concentration of the mast cell mediators may be markedly reduced with long-term treatment with ICS. Hypertonic saline has also been used to evaluate treatment with ICS with and without combination with a beta$_2$-agonist (88). AHR to hypertonic saline can be reduced with an acute dose of steroids (89).

Hypertonic saline has been used to monitor AHR in many population studies (17–19) and in the work place (90). It has been successfully used to study those with a past history of asthma but no current symptoms. Of 180 potential divers with scuba, who had been medically cleared fit to dive pending investigation of their asthma due to a past history, 29 had a positive response hypertonic saline and a further 11 a borderline response (39). Hypertonic saline has also been used as a challenge to evaluate potential recruits to the Police Force (91). With few exceptions, this highly motivated group has demonstrated that compliance to treatment with ICS for 8–12 weeks also results in AHR to an indirect stimulus within the healthy range.

Mannitol

As it became obvious that hypertonic saline was a useful test to monitor the benefits of ICS, attention was focused on developing an easier test to deliver a hypertonic stimulus. Initially, a dry powder preparation of sodium chloride was prepared for inhalation. This was successfully used for performing a challenge test (92), but concerns were raised about the stability of the powder under conditions of high humidity. Mannitol was chosen as an alternative, as it resists absorption of water and is stable at a relative humidity of less than 86%. The mannitol powder is prepared by spray drying and more than 40% of the particles are less than 7 μm when measured by dispersion through the inhaler device. The powder is encapsulated and administered from a dry powder inhaler (93). The mannitol test is portable and easy to administer (28,94). Mannitol is faster and easier to deliver than hypertonic saline, as it requires only a single inhalation per capsule to deliver the dose.

The mannitol challenge takes a median time of 12 min to perform in those who are positive and less than 20 min in those who are negative (93). The response is repeatable within one doubling dose over 2 weeks (10). The results of a Phase III trial of a preparation of mannitol for inhalation, known as Aridol^{TM} (Pharmaxis Ltd, Sydney, Australia), are currently being reviewed by regulatory authorities. The advantage provided by mannitol over the other indirect stimuli is that it would come as a test kit—providing a common operating standard for use worldwide.

Mannitol has been used in a number of studies to study the effects of drugs used in the treatment of asthma for the first time, and inhaled steroids in particular (Figs. 5 and 6) (10,77,87,95–98). Details of these studies are given below.

Relationship Between One Indirect Stimulus and Another

The people who respond positively to one indirect stimulus also respond positively to another. Thus, those found positive to hypertonic saline are positive to mannitol (Fig. 7) (93). Those positive to exercise are likewise positive to mannitol (Fig. 8) (94), and those positive to EVH are positive to exercise (73), and saline (82). Those positive to EVH are positive to

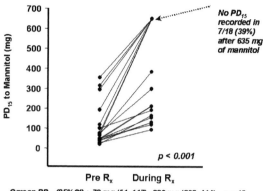

Figure 5   Individual values for the provoking dose to cause a 15% fall in FEV_1 (PD_{15}) to mannitol at baseline and after treatment with budesonide (800–2400 µg/ day) for 6–9 weeks. The subjects who remained responsive had values for PD_{15} at baseline usually less than 100 mg, suggesting those who were more responsive may require a longer duration of treatment or a higher dose on inhaled steroid to become unresponsive. *Source:* From Ref. 10.

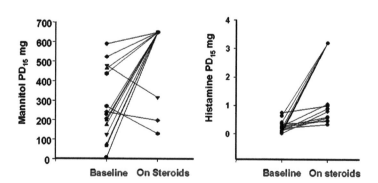

Figure 6   Individual values for the provoking dose to cause a 15% fall in FEV_1 (PD_{15}) to mannitol and to histamine at baseline and after treatment with budesonide (1000 µg/day) for 3–6 months. More subjects became unresponsive to mannitol than histamine and half the group remained in the hyper-responsive range (1 mg is equivalent to 5 µmol or 100 breath units) for histamine. *Source:* From Ref. 9.

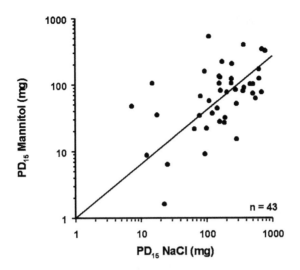

Figure 7 Individual values for the provoking dose of dry powder mannitol to cause a 15% fall in FEV_1 (PD_{15}) in relation to the values obtained for PD_{15} to saline (NaCl) delivered as a wet aerosol at a dose of 45 mg/mL. The data demonstrate that those individuals who are sensitive to salt are also sensitive to mannitol inhalation. *Source:* From Ref. 93.

mannitol (Fig. 9) (99). Those positive to adenosine are also positive to mannitol (Fig. 10) (100). In only a few cases of mild responsiveness have the responses been discordant in the same subjects between two indirect stimuli (17,94).

Role of Mediators in the Differences Between Indirect Stimuli and Direct Stimuli

Indirect stimuli are more specific for identifying asthma and are probably more sensitive for assessing AHR than previously thought (77,98). There are now a number of studies reporting that some people have a positive response to an indirect challenge yet a negative response to a direct challenge such as methacholine or histamine (16,101–103). In a study on athletes, it was reported that methacholine had a sensitivity of only 36% to identify people with AHR to EVH (103). In a study in children, AHR to histamine was only found in 50% of a group of children with EIA (16).

This unexpected finding may be explained by the custom of only a single agonist being inhaled when using a direct stimulus (usually histamine or methacholine), whereas a number of different and more potent mediators (leukotrienes and prostaglandins) are involved in the response to an indirect stimulus. Further, whilst mast cells contain all the mediators implicated in

**Relationship between PD₁₅ to mannitol and
maximum % fall in FEV₁ following exercise**

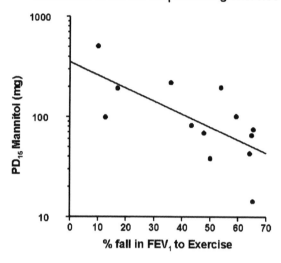

Figure 8 Individual values for the provoking dose of dry powder mannitol to cause a 15% fall in FEV_1 (PD_{15}) in relation to the fall in FEV_1 after exercise values expressed as a percentage of the pre-exercise value (% fall). Those who were the most responsive to exercise were also the most sensitive to mannitol. *Source:* From Ref. 94.

indirect stimuli, the eosinophils contain only leukotrienes (104). It is known that a hyper-osmolar stimulus can cause release of leukotrienes from eosinophils (105) and this may explain why some investigators have found discordant AHR responses between direct and indirect stimuli.

Significant changes in levels of leukotrienes and prostaglandins have been measured in both lavage fluid and in urine following these indirect challenges (23–25,106). However, the release of histamine has been difficult to document in all subjects in response to the indirect stimuli such as exercise and EVH (106–108). Evidence for sensory nerve and epithelial cell stimulation comes from findings of hyper-osmolar challenge in the nose (26,109).

The recognition that leukotrienes are important in sustaining the response to an indirect stimulus has been a "break through" in our understanding of AHR. Previously, it has been thought that all the provocative stimuli were measuring the same thing and the type of stimulus was unimportant for measuring AHR (29). The fact that a leukotriene antagonist can reduce the duration of the airway response to exercise (110) and the hypertonic stimuli (95) (Fig. 11), while having no effect on response to methacholine (65), has changed our thinking in this regard.

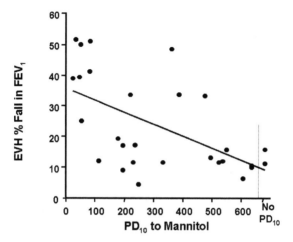

Figure 9 Individual values for the provoking dose of dry powder mannitol to cause a 15% fall in FEV_1 (PD_{15}) in relation to the fall in FEV_1 after eucapnic voluntary hyperpnea (EVH) expressed as a percentage of the pre-challenge value (% fall in FEV_1). Those who were most responsive to EVH were also the most sensitive to mannitol. *Source:* From Ref. 99.

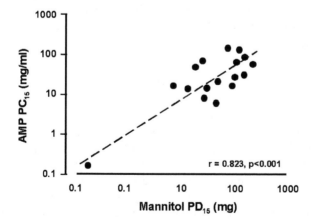

Figure 10 Individual values for the provoking dose of dry powder mannitol to cause a 15% fall in FEV_1 (PD_{15}) in relation to the values obtained for the concentration of adenosine monophosphate (AMP) required to induce a 15% fall in FEV_1 (PC_{15}) fall in asthmatic subjects. There was a good relationship between the sensitivity to the two indirect stimuli. *Source:* From Ref. 100.

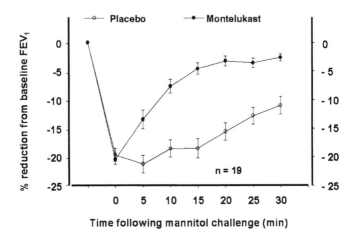

Figure 11   The reduction in FEV_1 expressed as a percentage of the baseline value in relation to time following a challenge with mannitol in the presence of montelukast, given in a dose of 10 mg 5, 11, and 24 hr before challenge and its corresponding placebo. The area above the $FEV_1/\%$ reduction time curve is significantly reduced indicating a rapid recovery from bronchoconstriction in the presence of the leukotriene antagonist montelukast. This demonstrates that leukotrienes are important in sustaining the airway response to mannitol. *Source:* From Ref. 95.

Today, AHR to a direct stimulus in the absence of AHR to an indirect one may be a sign of airway remodelling. AHR to an indirect stimulus in the absence of AHR to a direct one may be interpreted as a difference in potency of the agonists delivered or released—and the affinity and number of receptors available.

Indications for Use of Indirect Stimuli

There are many indications for using indirect stimuli. The major indications are to identify AHR that (1) is consistent with a diagnosis of active asthma, (2) will respond to treatment with steroids, and (3) is consistent with exercise-induced bronchoconstriction. These indirect stimuli are also useful (4) to follow response to treatment with inhaled steroids and for back titration of steroid dose, (5) to identify the efficacy of drugs (e.g., nedocromil sodium, sodium cromoglycate, and leukotriene antagonists) in the prevention of exercise-induced bronchoconstriction and other forms of provoked asthma, (6) for collecting sputum, (7) to evaluate cough-variant asthma, (8) to identify those who may have airway narrowing while diving with scuba, (9) to identify those subjects who would benefit from the therapeutic use of hypertonic aerosols for clearance of unwanted secretions without airway narrowing as a side effect, and (10) to document airway responsiveness in pregnancy (27).

Administering the Stimulus and Measuring the Response

The details for administering the indirect stimuli are published elsewhere and are described below only briefly (2,27,66–68,72). Some protocols, like exercise, require complex equipment such as ergometers and electrocardiographs as well as personnel experienced in exercise testing. Eucapnic voluntary hyperpnea requires a special gas mixture and a means of delivery. Hypertonic saline requires a large volume (400 mL) ultrasonic nebulizer to generate the aerosol. Adenosine monophosphate (AMP) is administered via inexpensive hand-held nebulizers, but the different solutions need to be made up regularly and the substance is not readily available for use by inhalation. Mannitol is delivered as a dry powder from a hand-held inhaler device.

Technical Aspects of Interpretation of Indirect Stimuli in General

When using indirect stimuli to challenge, one must be aware of cross refractoriness and the time since the last drugs were taken. Thus, the response to indirect stimuli can be affected by recent exposure to either the same stimulus or another indirect stimulus. About 50% of asthmatics will have significant (> 50%) protection against repeated challenge with stimuli such as exercise, EVH, AMP, and hypertonic saline (111–114). Further, challenge with hypertonic saline can reduce response to exercise, and vice versa (115).

Drugs used in the treatment of asthma and allergies also affect the responses and the investigator may choose to study the subject either on the medication or after the medication has been withdrawn for a suitable time, which is always less than 48 hr.

Osmotic challenges are self-limiting because the volume of airway surface liquid beyond the 12th generation is so great that the evaporation of water or deposition of a small amount of hypertonic aerosol is likely to be negligible (79). Another advantage of using osmotic stimuli is that when the stimulus ceases water will move rapidly to restore normal tonicity of the airway surface fluid.

Measurement and Expression of the Airway Response to Indirect Stimuli

The forced expiratory volume in 1 sec (FEV_1) has become the most commonly used measure of AHR over the last 20 years because it has good repeatability (coefficient of variation is $< 6\%$) (116), it can be measured repeatedly and the equipment is readily available (117,118). Spirometry is usually measured in triplicate at baseline and the FEV_1 only is measured in duplicate after the delivery of the stimulus. Because it is required to measure the FEV_1 so frequently, subjects are discouraged from prolonging the forced expiration beyond 2 sec because multiple maneuvers can be tiring.

The response to challenge with exercise and eucapnic voluntary hyperpnea is expressed as the % fall in FEV_1. The classification of severity of the response is given in Table 1 and calculated, e.g.,

$$\% \text{ fall index} = 100 \times \frac{(\text{pre-exercise } FEV_1 - \text{lowest } FEV_1 \text{ post-exercise})}{\text{pre-exercise } FEV1}$$

A value of 10% or more is outside the range for healthy non-asthmatics (119), although a value of 13% has been suggested in children (120).

The area above the FEV_1 time-recovery curve (AAC 0–30 or 0–60 min) can also be measured in response to hyperpnea. It is particularly useful for evaluating drugs that limit the duration of the response, leukotriene antagonists for example (Fig. 11).

A fall in FEV_1 of 15% to saline and mannitol is consistent with a diagnosis of active asthma and exercise-induced asthma. The provoking dose of saline or mannitol to cause a 15% fall in FEV_1, known as the PD_{15}, is calculated. The value for PD_{15} defines severity (see Table 1) and is obtained by linear interpolation from a graph relating the % fall in FEV_1 to the cumulative dose of aerosol inhaled. A PD_{10} to mannitol is consistent with 10% reduction in response to hyperpnea (99) and identifies those with exercise-induced bronchoconstriction.

The response–dose ratio (RDR) (also known as the dose–response slope) is also used as an index because all the population can be included (19,22). This index has also proven to be valuable for monitoring treatment with inhaled steroids (10,77,97,98). The RDR is particularly useful for describing responses to agents such as hypertonic saline and mannitol where the dose delivered is easily measured.

The provoking concentration of AMP required to cause a 20% fall in FEV_1 is the index most commonly used to measure response to AMP, but PC_{15} has also been used for comparison of response to mannitol (100).

Spontaneous recovery of lung function after indirect stimuli has been documented. Most subjects recover to within 5% of baseline FEV_1 within 30 min. When the % fall in FEV_1 in response to challenge exceeds 25%, the recovery usually takes 60 min. It is usual for airway narrowing in response to all the indirect stimuli to reverse rapidly in response to the administration of a standard dose of beta$_2$-agonist given by inhalation.

Table 1 Grading of the Severity of the Airway Response to Indirect Stimuli

	Index	Normal	Mild	Moderate	Severe
Exercise	% Fall				
on ICS		< 10	10–20	20–30	> 30
not on ICS		< 10	10–25	25–50	> 50
Eucapnic voluntary hyperpnea	% Fall				
6 min at V_E > 50% MVV[a]	> 60% MVV	< 10	< 20	20–30	30+
	< 60% MVV	< 10	—	10–30	30+
4.5% Saline	PD_{15} mL	> 23.3	> 6.0	2.0–6.0	< 2.0
Mannitol	PD_{15} mg	> 635	> 155	35–155	< 35

[a]MVV is maximum voluntary ventilation and taken as $35 \times FEV_1$ (L).

Exercise

In order to provoke EIB and for the response to be repeatable, a standard protocol is required (66–68,121). The air inspired during exercise should be dry—preferably from a cylinder or source of medical air, the V_E should reach 17–21 times the FEV_1 and be sustained for at least 4 min and preferably 6. To fulfill this criterion, a duration of exercise in a young child of 6 min, and in older children and adults a duration of 8 min, is required. In the absence of a measure of ventilation, the heart rate can be used to check intensity of exercise. In children, the heart rate in the last 4 min of exercise should be 95% (121) of calculated maximum (220—age in years) and in adults 80–90% predicted [210—(0.65 × age in years)].

To achieve the V_E or heart rate recommended for testing, an estimate of the workload is required from graphs relating oxygen consumption to ventilation and workload. In the laboratory, exercise is most commonly performed by cycling or by running. For treadmill exercise, this usually requires running at 6 km/hr (3.3 mph) at a > 10% gradient for the average adult and 9 km/hr at a gradient of 5.5% for children. Sustaining these workloads will depend on the fitness and the weight of the subject.

Exercise by cycling is a safer option in most laboratories. A target workload for an untrained subject expressed in watts is (53.76 × predicted FEV_1) − 11.07. The load is set to 60% of target for the first minute, increasing to 70, 90, then 100% in the second, third, fourth minutes. This progressive increase is used because it is easier for the subject to achieve and the protocol is easily repeated. The maximum workload should ideally be sustained for 4–5 min, but some subjects find this difficult and it is often reduced by 10% in the last few minutes. The workload increments remain the same, if possible, for any subsequent assessment—particularly when a drug effect is being evaluated. Other ergometers can be used to assess EIB if available in the laboratory. The same intensity and duration of exercise and inspired air content are recommended as for cycling and running. The intensity and duration of exercise and inspired temperature, however, might be altered to simulate the conditions that provoke the symptoms in the person being evaluated. The conditions should be carefully noted if the exercise is to be repeated after treatment. FEV_1 is measured in triplicate before and in duplicate at 1, 3, 5, 7, 10, 15, and 30 or even 60 min after exercise at each time point. The highest value for FEV_1 is recorded at each time point.

Eucapnic Voluntary Hyperpnea

The protocol that is best standardized is that which the subject is required to breathe dry air containing 5% carbon dioxide at a V_E equivalent to 30 × measured FEV_1 for 6 min (71,72,122). This protocol provides a more potent stimulus than exercise, probably as a result of V_E increasing rapidly to the target rate and being sustained for a longer period (73).

In brief, the spirometry is measured in triplicate at baseline. The target V_E is calculated and the reservoir bag filled with dry gas mixture containing 21% O_2, 5% CO_2, and balance N_2. The subject inhales the mixture via a two-way non-rebreathing valve and is encouraged to keep the reservoir balloon at a constant volume, which is maintained by being refilled at target V_E, usually from a gas tank. If CO_2 is being added, it is mandatory to have a measure of end-tidal CO_2. The FEV_1 is measured in duplicate immediately after challenge and then again 5, 10, 15, and 20 min later. If a comparison is to be made of recovery of lung function, the follow-up is to 30 min.

Indications for Specific Use for Exercise and EVH

The same indications apply for use of EVH and for exercise in that both tests are primarily used to identify those with exercise-induced bronchoconstriction. EVH is more potent than exercise for provoking airway narrowing and is useful to assess military recruits, elite athletes, and well-controlled asthmatics. This protocol is most appropriately used for those without known asthma with normal lung function or for those with well-controlled asymptomatic asthma. For less well-controlled asthmatics, either the time of the test (4 rather than 6 min) or the target V_E ($21 \times FEV_1$ rather than 30) can be reduced or a multistage protocol can be used with greater safety (94,123).

Technical Aspects Exercise and EVH with Respect to Monitoring Asthma

Protocols using hyperpnea have an advantage over aerosols in that particle deposition is unimportant. However, these tests may be less suitable than the hypertonic aerosols for assessing the benefits of treatment because the protocols using hyperpnea do not produce a dose–response curve. Further, the airway response to dry air hyperpnea is necessarily limited by the ability to ventilate enough to cause significant dehydration of the airways. This may be the reason that older people are insensitive to this stimulus relative to younger people (124,125). It should also be noted that the EVH protocol using a fixed concentration of CO_2 (4.9–5.1%) can only be used in a person with an $FEV_1 > 1.5$ L.

Measurement of V_E is recommended in order to assess severity of the response and in order for the test to be repeated. For EVH, the ventilation of $30 \times FEV_1$ is a target ventilation and the test is valid for a non-athlete if the rate is greater than $22 \times FEV_1$, which is the ventilation usually achieved on exercise. For elite athletes, values for $V_E > 85\%$ of their maximum voluntary ventilation predicted would be expected to be achieved (73,99).

It is not necessary for the air to be cooled unless the room temperature air test is negative in a person who complains of symptoms specifically in the cold. When cold air is used, usually only 4 min is required (126–128). However, the 4 min cold air protocol is not sensitive for identifying adults (9,124) suspected of having asthma. By contrast, the 6 min room temperature protocol for EVH identified all but a few athletes who responded to exercise in the field in cold air conditions (73).

When using exercise or EVH to monitor treatment, it needs to be understood that the person may be so improved by therapy that challenging them at the same work load or ventilation may result in a negative test. The treated person may have no problem repeating the workload performed at the same workload or target ventilation, but still have severe EIA at a higher workload or ventilation. To assess the complete success of therapy, the target workload or ventilation needs to be recalculated, based on the post-treatment FEV_1.

Hypertonic Saline

Spirometry is performed in triplicate at baseline. The 4.5% solution is placed in the canister and the canister and tubing, but not the valve, are weighed. The subject breathes normally and inhales the aerosol by mouth (with a nose clip in place) through a non-rebreathing valve (Hans Rudolph 2700, or 1400 for children). Measurements of FEV_1 are made in duplicate 60 sec after progressively increasing times of exposure (0.5, 1.0, 2.0, 4.0, 8.0 min). If the fall in FEV_1 is more than 10% for a single exposure, the exposure time is repeated rather than doubled. The test is terminated when the FEV_1 falls 15% or the minimum dose of 23 g (for a child) and 18.6 g for an adult has been delivered in 15.5 min (1.5 and 1.2 mL/min, respectively). To ensure that the aerosol is being delivered to the inspired port of the valve at the correct rate, the canister and tubing but not the valve are weighed before and again at the end of the challenge. The rate of delivery of the aerosol is the change in weight divided by the time the aerosol was delivered expressed in mL/min. This protocol has been performed safely on thousands of children and adults (17,18,27,90).

Technical Aspects with Respect to Monitoring Asthma

The inhalation of hypertonic saline is associated with increased production of secretions and the big advantage of hypertonic saline is the ability to collect sputum at the same time as testing for AHR (129).

However, these secretions also have the potential to alter airway caliber as measured by changes in FEV_1 and this has been demonstrated in people with cystic fibrosis (130). This would not appear to be a problem in healthy subjects, as the mean % fall in FEV_1 for this group is low (2–3%).

It is important to ensure that the nebulizer output is adequate when the person is inspiring through the valve. The dose delivered can be quite variable in children and the output needs to be higher as impaction occurs on the smaller valve (Hans Rudolph 1400). In adults, air is entrained during tidal breathing and the dose of aerosol delivered is less variable than in children. Less impaction of the aerosol occurs on the larger Hans Rudolph valve (2700), so the rate of delivery to the inspired port of the valve can be a minimum of 1.2 mL/min.

The concentration of 4.5% saline is used for challenge because it provides an adequate osmotic stimulus for the test to be carried out in a reasonable time. It is rate of change of osmolarity that is the determining factor for an osmotic stimulus to cause the airways to narrow, so it is important that the time taken to perform the FEV_1 after each exposure is short and no more than 1 min. If sputum is being collected, it should occur after the completion of the challenge to determine airway responsiveness (131).

As with delivery of other wet aerosols, the precise dose of 4.5% saline that reaches the lower airways is not known. It is likely to be 15–35% of the dose reaching the mouth (132). The rate and depth of tidal breathing could potentially affect deposition of the aerosol in the lower respiratory tract. The normal range of values for RDR needs to be established for the laboratory equipment used.

Mannitol

Spirometry is performed in triplicate at baseline. Initially, the subject is given an empty capsule to inhale through a dry powder inhaler (Cyclohaler RSO1, Plastiape, Italy) while wearing a nose clip. Patients are encouraged to hold their breath for 5 sec after inhalation while still wearing the nose clip for all inhalations. The first capsule acts as a "placebo" and the inhalation serves to familiarize the subject to the inspiratory resistance provided by the device. Measurements of FEV_1 are made in duplicate 60 sec after progressively increasing doses of mannitol are inhaled (5, 10, 20, 40, 80, 160, 160, 160 mg). The doses of 80 and 160 are given as 2×40 and 4×40 mg capsules. The capsules are given one immediately after the other. If the % fall in FEV_1 is more than 10% for a single dose then the dose is repeated rather than doubled. The test is terminated when the FEV_1 falls 15% from the highest value measured after the empty capsule, or when a cumulative dose of 635 mg has been inhaled (10,27,87,93). The test has been carried in children as well as adults (133,134).

Technical Aspects Mannitol

Some cough is experienced during the mannitol challenge. The cough is often confined to the 60-sec period after inhalation, either on inhalation but more often after inhalation in association with the deposition of the mannitol in the airways. In some cases, at the 40 mg dose a second inhalation may be required to empty the capsule. Static electricity can sometimes present a problem with capsule adhering to the device. To minimize this, following decontamination the device should be washed in detergent and dried.

Adenosine 5'-Monophosphate (AMP)

Bronchial provocation testing using AMP (135) has been used in for research studies over the last 10 years and it is not a stimulus commonly offered by routine lung function laboratories (2,136). Spirometry is performed in triplicate at baseline. The test begins with the subject inhaling 0.9% saline aerosol generated by a hand-held nebulizer. The aerosol is inhaled with either a 5-breath technique from functional residual capacity to total lung capacity using a dosimeter or 2 min of tidal breathing. The FEV_1 is measured in duplicate 60 and 180 sec after progressively increasing concentrations (3.125, 6.26, 12.5, 25, 50, 100, 200, and 400 mg/mL). The test is terminated when a 20% fall in FEV_1 is documented or the highest concentration has been inhaled.

Adenosine Monophosphate

AMP is different from the other indirect stimuli discussed here as its mode of action is via a specific adenosine$_{2B}$ receptor (137). These receptors are on mast cells and this test is regarded as specific to identify presence of mast cells (138). This is in contrast to the other stimuli, where there is potential for all cells in the airways to be affected by the dehydrating and osmotic effects of hyperpnea and hypertonic aerosols. However, the airway response and the profile of drug effects for AMP are similar to the other indirect stimuli (96,139).

Technical Aspects

The atopic status of a person would appear to be important in determining a positive response to AMP. Atopic healthy people can respond with a 20% fall in FEV_1 as can smokers with chronic obstructive pulmonary disease (COPD). This makes AMP responses in non-asthmatic healthy subjects different to the other indirect stimuli (135,140,141).

The AMP normally comes as a dry powder and needs to be stored in a desiccator. The solubility of the adenosine at the higher concentrations can be a problem. The jet nebulizers need to generate particles sized between 1 and 3.6 μm and deliver approximately 9 μL per 0.6 sec of inhalation. Differences in particle occur size with different flow rates. The rate and depth of tidal breathing or each single breath could potentially affect deposition of the aerosol.

Clinical Evaluation Using Indirect Stimuli

Comparing Responses to Indirect with Other Outcome Measures After Treatment with Inhaled Steroids

It has long been recognized that ICS provide beneficial effects on symptoms, lung function, and various parameters of airway inflammation (142–144). It has also been recognized for some time that measurement of AHR is a useful technique for monitoring the response to asthma treatment with ICS (6–8,52,145). A special feature of airway responsiveness to most indirect stimuli is that it can be reduced to within the normal healthy range in a substantial proportion of asthmatic subjects during long-term treatment with ICS (Figs. 3–6) (4,8,10,32,38,53,77,78). To understand the significance of the change in airway responsiveness to indirect stimuli by ICS treatment, its relationship to changes in various other parameters describing the asthma severity needs to be understood.

Changes in Airway Responsiveness

The decrease in AHR to various indirect stimuli after a long-term (several weeks or more) treatment with ICS is usually 2–3 doubling doses or concentration of mannitol (Figs. 5 and 6), hypertonic saline (Fig. 4), adenosine, bradykinin, and distilled water (6,8,10,11,33,77,146–150). In addition, treatment with ICS can increase the provocative ventilation required to cause a 20% fall in FEV_1 by 76% (5) and decrease the exercise-induced fall in FEV_1 or PEF by 50–70% (5,51,52,151,152). However, in two studies treatment with ICS did not change the bronchoconstriction provoked by cold air hyperpnea significantly when the airway response was measured by a whole-body plethysmograph or spirometry (77,153). The effect of ICS on responsiveness to cold air could be detected using impulse oscillation or interrupter technique to measure the airway response (153,154). There are only a few studies comparing the sensitivity of indirect stimuli to detect changes in AHR in response to ICS. Challenge with mannitol is more sensitive than cold air to detect changes in AHR (77) and adenosine appears to be more sensitive than bradykinin and sodium metabisulfite challenges (32,148). Hypertonic saline appears to be more sensitive than histamine (8).

Symptoms

There are a number of studies describing a decrease in symptom severity and a change in responsiveness to various indirect stimuli during treatment with ICS (10,11,53,77,78,152). Most indicate, that after introduction of ICS into the treatment of asthma, symptoms improve rapidly and the response usually reaches its maximum within a few weeks (143,144). The concomitant change in responsiveness to indirect stimuli may not occur simultaneously with resolution of symptoms.

It should be kept in mind, however, that just a single high dose of steroids can diminish responsiveness to adenosine (155). The dose required to increase the threshold for a response to AMP 2.7 doubling doses was 1000 μg dose of fluticasone propionate (155), the same drug and dose were used less successfully for exercise (156), although a single dose of 2400 μg budesonide increased PD_{20} to saline 2.2-fold in 6 hr (89). Importantly, with adenosine there was no additional benefit of three or seven inhalations, taken every 12 hr, over one inhalation, suggesting a plateau after just one dose. By contrast, a decrease in responsiveness to hypertonic aerosols continues up to 2–6 months (8,77). A plateau in symptom improvement was observed after 3 months of treatment with budesonide in one study, whereas the decrease in mannitol responsiveness continued up to 6 months (Fig. 6) (77). Symptom control can be achieved with much lower doses of ICS than those required to protect against exercise-induced asthma (Fig. 12) (53). This suggests that responses to indirect stimuli are more sensitive and reliable than symptoms to demonstrate the effects of ICS in preventing against provoked attacks of asthma. This concept is supported by the findings of significant reduction in airway responsiveness to an indirect stimulus even in the absence of changes in symptom scores (146,153). As a whole, these studies suggest that measurement of AHR using indirect stimuli provides additional information about the "healing" of asthma during ICS treatment, compared with relying on symptoms only.

Recently, a significant correlation was found between change in symptom frequency and change in responsiveness to mannitol and cold air over

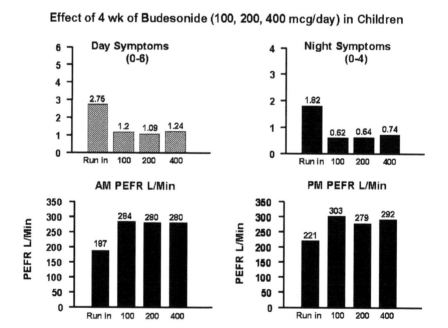

Figure 12   The change in symptoms, peak expiratory flow in relation to dose of inhaled budesonide in asthmatic children who also performed an exercise challenge as shown in Figure 3. The data illustrate that symptoms and Peak flow rapidly resolved at low doses of budesonide, whereas exercise-induced asthma was usually only resolved at the higher doses. *Source:* From Ref. 53.

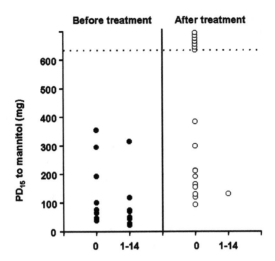

Figure 13   The values for PD_{15} to mannitol in 18 asthmatic subjects who took 800–1600 µg budesonide for 6–9 weeks in relation to the frequency of a positive or negative response to the question "How many days over the past 2 weeks have you had morning wheeze or chest tightness?" prior to testing with mannitol before and after treatment. These data illustrate that this important symptom, consistent with a classification of moderate to severe asthma (157) is absent in some subjects with moderate responsiveness to mannitol either before or after treatment. The values above the dashed line represent the subjects who no longer recorded a positive response to mannitol, i.e., a PD_{15} after treatment.

the same time interval in patients treated with budesonide (77). The individual analysis showed that the responsiveness to these indirect stimuli decreased most in the asthmatic subjects with the greatest improvement in symptoms. This finding suggests that these tests were valid in demonstrating the "healing" of asthma by ICS. Such a significant association could not be found between the change in symptoms and the change in responsiveness to histamine, a direct stimulus (77). Similarly, Brannan et al. (10) demonstrated an improvement in symptoms including severity, frequency, and use of beta$_2$-agonists. As the PD_{15} to mannitol improved some of the symptoms, e.g., nighttime wakening, completely disappeared (Fig. 13).

Spirometry

In general, substantial improvements in AHR to various indirect stimuli can be observed without significant changes in spirometry (33,77,146,148,149). This means that a measurement of AHR using indirect stimuli is likely to provide additional information about the "healing" of asthma during ICS treatment. The improvement in lung function reaches its plateau usually 6 weeks–few months after introducing treatment with ICS in asthma (77,143,144,158,159). Further, many asthmatic patients have normal spirometry at the start of treatment with ICS, in which case FEV_1 is not a sensitive index to show the effects of the therapy on AHR. Morning peak expiratory flow (PEF) and diurnal PEF variation may be more sensitive indices to demonstrate the effect of ICS than spirometry (77,146). However, in one study, responsiveness to mannitol continued to improve up to 6 months after the start of treatment, while the daily PEF variation reached its plateau at 3 months of therapy (77). In the same study, the decrease in daily PEF variation correlated closely with the decrease in cold air hyperpnea responsiveness. A highly significant association has been found between daily PEF variation and response to exercise challenge in ICS-treated children (151). These findings emphasize the validity of the cold air and exercise challenges in demonstrating the "healing" of asthma by ICS. However, it must be kept in mind that improvement in morning PEF values can be achieved with considerably lower ICS doses than protection against exercise-induced bronchoconstriction (53). Improvement in spirometry can also be achieved with lower ICS doses than protection against adenosine-induced bronchoconstriction (160) or saline-induced bronchoconstriction (8).

Relationship of Airway Responsiveness to Indices of Airway Inflammation

Since asthma is a disease characterized by airway inflammation (161), it is of interest to know if AHR to an indirect stimulus could act as a surrogate marker of airway inflammation during treatment with ICS. In a study by Prosperini et al. (149), a significant decrease in adenosine responsiveness could be observed after just 1 week's therapy with budesonide, while a decrease in the induced sputum eosinophils could not be detected before 4 weeks. A decrease in the sputum epithelial cells did not occur before 6 weeks from the start of therapy. This study corroborates the very rapid change in adenosine responsiveness after an introduction of ICS therapy (155). This finding raises the question as to whether a decrease in adenosine responsiveness is a valid index of the improvement in airway inflammation by ICS or if it is just an indicator of the presence of ICS therapy. However, in the study of Prosperini et al. (149), the association between sputum eosinophils and adenosine PC_{20} value was maintained during the budesonide treatment, suggesting the validity of adenosine challenge to demonstrate the "healing" of asthma by ICS in their study.

Dose of Steroids

Two studies have reported a dose-dependent reduction in responsiveness to adenosine by ICS. Treatment with a novel ICS, ciclesonide, given in a daily dose range of 100–1600 μg, was associated with a dose-dependent reduction in the responsiveness to adenosine. Though ciclesonide also reduced the percentage of eosinophils and eosinophilic cationic protein in the induced sputum, these changes were not dose-dependent (33). Similarly, budesonide induced a dose-dependent reduction in the responsiveness to adenosine in a daily dose range of 400–1600 μg (160). In one study, the decrease in exhaled nitric oxide showed a plateau after the lowest dose of steroid (400 μg dose). These studies suggest usefulness of adenosine challenge in the evaluation of ICS responses in a wide range of daily doses. By contrast, hypertonic saline challenge is modified by higher doses of ICS ($\geq$800 μg) (7,8,88), and it may not be as useful in the evaluation of ICS responses in the low range of daily ICS doses. For example, Jones et al. (162) treated uncontrolled asthmatic patients for 8 weeks with inhaled beclomethasone of 50, 100, 200, and 500 μg/day (162). They did not find a significant change in saline responsiveness at any dose of beclomethasone and a change was only suggestive after the largest daily dose. Linear dose–response relationships could be found, however, between the dose of beclomethasone and changes in exhaled nitric oxide and sputum eosinophils. The findings of Jones et al. (162) may reflect the greater severity of asthma that is often recorded in this part of the world and lower doses of steroids may be effective on hypertonic stimuli in patients with milder asthma.

Hypertonic saline is however useful in assessing the effects of budesonide in doses of $\geq$800 μg or its equivalent (7,8,88). Gibson et al. (85) have found that following 8 weeks of therapy with a large dose of 2000 μg/day beclomethasone mast cells still persist in the airways (85). At that stage, airway responsiveness to hypertonic saline correlated with the number of mast cells in bronchial brush biopsy. This finding is important since persistent elevations in airway mast cells during ICS treatment seems to predict treatment failure in patients who discontinue the treatment (163). In addition, responsiveness to hypertonic saline correlated with sputum eosinophilia following 8 weeks of 2000 μg/day beclomethasone therapy (85). The special feature of hypertonic aerosols is the possibility to assess airway responsiveness and induce sputum simultaneously.

A treatment period with inhaled budesonide 800–2400 μg for 6–9 weeks results in a significant decrease in AHR to mannitol, which was associated with a significant reduction in symptoms and bronchodilator use in all asthmatic patients (10). Further, responsiveness to mannitol appears to be useful for determining adequacy in dosing with inhaled steroids. While 60% of subjects remained responsive to mannitol, 40% did not (Fig. 5), suggesting that for those who became unresponsive, the dose of steroid was sufficient to reduce the inflammatory cell number and concentration of mediators to less than that required to cause airway narrowing under provoked conditions.

Thus, different indirect challenges reflect the response to long-term treatment with ICS in different ways. Adenosine responsiveness decreases rapidly, probably faster than the improvements in symptoms and lung function. Adenosine is sensitive even to small daily doses of ICS and large changes in AHR to adenosine can occur within hours after a single dose suggesting that its mode of action is different in preventing adenosine-induced constriction compared with the osmotic challenges. By contrast, exercise and hypertonic aerosol responsiveness decrease more slowly, in response to chronic dosing with ICS, and require relatively high daily doses of ICS ($\geq 800\,\mu g$ of budesonide or its equivalent). This may be due to the osmotic challenge reflecting the presence of a wider variety of inflammatory cells compared with adenosine, which acts on specific receptors on mast cells. More studies are needed to investigate if a decrease in responsiveness to indirect stimuli reflects airway remodelling in asthma in addition to the presence of inflammation. If they did, their measurement would be useful in monitoring the disease in the long term.

There is good evidence that treatment with inhaled corticosteroids improves asthma and their use is recommended in current guidelines (30). ICS are most effective in preventing asthma attacks, improving symptoms, increasing lung function and reducing death from asthma (164). The correct dose necessary and the best way to monitor response to ICS is still a matter of debate. A recent meta-analysis suggested that, for the majority of patients, the optimum ICS effect is achieved at equivalent dose of 200 μg fluticasone daily (165). This may be so for control of symptoms, but the data presented above suggest that a measurement of AHR using indirect stimuli is warranted even when symptoms are under control. Higher doses of ICS at the start of treatment may lead to a faster reduction in AHR (37); however, introducing doses higher than equivalent doses of 800 μg budesonide does not seem to be useful (98). These studies may need to be repeated using responses to indirect stimuli before drawing conclusions about optimal dose effect.

Before commencement of ICS treatment, significant correlation is described between sputum eosinophils and FEV_1 percentage of predicted, between sputum eosinophils and AHR methacholine, or between exhaled nitric oxide (eNO) and AHR methacholine (36). During ICS treatment, all these parameters (sputum eosinophils, lung function, AHR methacholine, and eNO) improve, but these improvements do not correlate with each other (36). Even in clinically well-controlled asthmatics using ICS for many years, the correlations can no longer be found (98). Therefore, which non-invasive parameter of airway inflammation is best to monitor asthma is still not clear. It is however clear that if a patient remains responsive to a stimulus, such as exercise, their asthma cannot claim to be under control. For this reason, indirect stimuli provide an opportunity to improve monitoring of asthma.

Back Titration of Steroids and Monitoring Exacerbations

Asthma as a chronic inflammatory airway disease characterized by recurrent episodes of symptoms of wheezing, and chest tightness is associated with variable airways obstruction. According to the present guidelines (30), the level and adjustment of ICS is solely guided by symptoms and lung function. However, it has been shown that in clinically controlled patients, AHR and airway inflammation persist (167,168). Under a stepwise ICS reduction, neither symptoms nor lung function including peak flow (lowest percentage of recent best) had any predictive value for later asthma exacerbation (98). Therefore, there is a clear need for other non-invasive parameters to monitor asthma treatment other than relying on symptoms and lung function.

Higher levels of eNO have been found in adults and children with allergies and asthma than in the rest of the population (169,170). Exhaled NO can distinguish between atopic children in those with AHR and those without AHR (171), and eNO can successfully be decreased with ICS (172). However, looking on bronchoscope studies, eNO levels do not seem to be suitable for the assessment of asthma control or airway inflammation (173), and the measurement of eNO has no predictive value for later asthma exacerbation once patients are treated with ICS (97).

Sputum eosinophils play an important role in the pathogenesis of asthma. Eosinophils and their mediators are very frequently found in asthmatic but not in healthy airways and can be suppressed by steroids (174,175). Asthma attacks due to thunderstorms are characterized by an elevation in sputum eosinophils; however, the patients used less ICS, which might have been an important confounder affecting inflammatory indices in this study (176). However, the measurement of sputum eosinophils has potential for monitoring asthma. Green et al. (177) used normalization of sputum eosinophils as an additional treatment guide and reached a significant lower level of sputum eosinophils and—importantly—fewer severe asthma exacerbations and hospital admissions than the control group using only the British Thoracic Society asthma guidelines (178). In an ICS step-down regimen, we were able to show that increased sputum eosinophils were, next to AHR to mannitol, a clear predictor for asthma exacerbations (Table 2) (97). Although there is good evidence that sputum eosinophils are helpful in monitoring asthmatic patients, it has to be taken into account that the sputum induction and even more so the sputum analysis is a labor- and time-consuming investigation.

AHR is a characteristic feature of asthma and is thought to be related to airway inflammation (21,179), and its severity changes with ICS treatment. However, it appears that in clinically well-controlled patients, AHR to direct agents and airway inflammation persist (168,180). Sont et al. (35) compared AHR to methacholine as an additional treatment guide to current recommendations (30) and found a significantly improvement in

Table 2 Visit Before the Last Successful Reduction in Dose of Inhaled Corticosteroids Compared with the Visit Before the Failed Reduction in Dose in 26 Subjects

	Successful reduction	Failed reduction	p-Value
RDR mannitol	0.05 (0.03–0.08)	0.09 (0.06–0.15)	0.003
Exhaled NO (ppb)	18.4 (14.9–22.8)	18.5 (12.9–26.4)	0.95
FEV$_1$ predicted (%)	87.4 (81.1–93.8)	86.9 (79.7–92.5)	0.84
FVC predicted (%)	88.7 (82.7–92.7)	87.5 (81.2–94.2)	0.73
PEF predicted (%)	84.3 (80.5–92.1)	82.6 (79.4–83.7)	0.65
PEF (lowest % best)	85.5 (81.9–87.8)	82.9 (78.3–86.5)	0.57
Sputum neutrophils (%)	26 (13.5–38.5)	18.6 (8.5–28.7)	0.23
Sputum eosinophils (%)	7.9 (3.9–11.8)	22.5 (11.4–33.6)	0.03
Sputum macrophages (%)	56.8 (45.5–68)	58.6 (47.5–69.7)	0.62
Sputum lymphocytes (%)	3.2 (0.4–6.1)	0.53 (0.1–0.9)	0.13
Sputum mast cells (%)	0.09 (−0.03 to 0.2)	0.4 (−0.4 to −1.2)	0.42

Mean values (95% confidence interval).
RDR: % fall FEV$_1$ at the last dose/cumulative dose mg.

FEV$_1$ and 1.8-fold lower rate of mild exacerbations in the AHR strategy group. The changes of AHR in both their strategy groups correlated well with eosinophils in the biopsies. Interestingly, this finding was accompanied by a greater reduction in thickness of the sub-epithelial reticular layer in the AHR strategy group after 2 years of ICS treatment. This might even indicate a possible reversal of airway remodelling. It should be noted that in the AHR strategy group of Sont et al. (35) the PC$_{20}$ to methacholine only improved by 1.1 doubling doses from a baseline of 0.47 mg/mL (SD 2.0) so that most subjects remained hyper-responsive at a time other changes noted above were documented. Even so, the study demonstrated that measuring AHR was a useful guide to treatment. The potential for AHR to an indirect stimulus to change more significantly or move into a healthy range makes it likely that the indirect tests will prove an even more valuable guide to monitor therapy. This finding of Sont et al. has been supported by those of Ward et al. (159), who showed an improvements of the basement membrane thickening under ICS treatment. In that study, reticular basal membrane thickening was also the strongest single predictor for AHR to methacholine.

As one of the primary outcomes of treatment with ICS is a decrease in the inflammatory cell number, it has been suggested that "indirect" BPTs may better reflect the inflammatory status of the airway following treatment (34,181). Although asthma treatment with ICS is highly effective (30,182), there is also a clear concern about side effects. Inhaled corticosteroids can cause or at least be an additional risk factor for cataract, glaucoma, osteoporosis, or adrenal insufficiency (183). The aim should be to achieve the lowest dose of ICS necessary to control the disease. However, there is still not clear at which time or treatment point, it might be safe to reduce the ICS. Clinical studies have shown that once the ICS treatment has been stopped, an asthma exacerbation can occur (97,184,185). However, if patients have been using a high dose of ICS, their dose can usually be halved safely without an exacerbation. In the study by Hawkins et al. (186), the mean dose of 1430 µg beclomethasone dipropionate/day was either halved or continued for a 1-year follow-up. The proportion of patients with asthma exacerbations and the numbers of visits to the general practice or hospitals was not significantly different between the two groups. This finding is supported by our recent study (97), in which patients using a median dose of 1000 µg beclomethasone dipropionate/day could halve their ICS dose without experiencing an asthma exacerbation. Some subjects remained unresponsive to mannitol, as measured by a PD$_{15}$, for the duration of the study, whilst others who were unresponsive at baseline became responsive over the period that ICS dose was reduced (Fig. 14). However, further halving of the ICS dose could cause an asthma exacerbation. Being hyper-responsive to both direct (histamine) and indirect (mannitol) challenge test at baseline and hyper-responsive to mannitol during dose-reduction phase (Fig. 15) were clear predictors for failure of inhaled

Return of the PD₁₅ in previously well controlled subjects after stepwise dose reduction of ICS

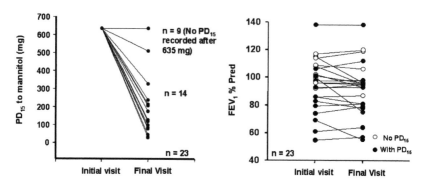

Figure 14   Individual values for the provoking dose of dry powder mannitol to cause a 15% fall in FEV₁ (PD₁₅) and the FEV₁ % predicted after stepwise reduction of dose of inhaled steroid. Fourteen of the 23 subjects became hyper-responsive and the median time taken to achieve a PD₁₅ was 126 days. There were no significant changes in FEV₁ % predicted for most subjects over this time. The data demonstrate that measuring response to mannitol was more useful than measuring FEV₁ for documenting an important outcome of back-titration of steroids (i.e., return of AHR and active asthma). *Source:* From Ref. 97.

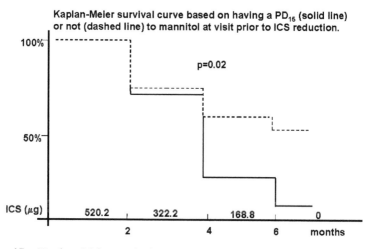

Figure 15   Kaplan–Meier survival curve based on having a PD₁₅ to mannitol (*solid line*) or not (*dashed line*) at the visit prior to reduction of inhaled steroid dose. *Source:* From Ref. 97.

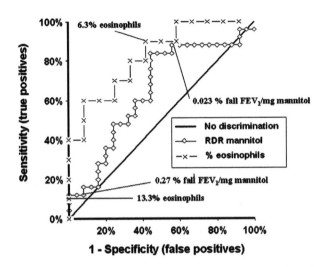

Figure 16 Receiver operator characteristic (ROC) curves showing the sensitivity and 1-specificity over a range of cut-points for response–dose ratio for mannitol (*open triangles*) and % eosinophils (*crosses*) for predicting failure of inhaled corticosteroids reduction in 26 subjects. The solid line indicates no discrimination. *Source:* Ref. 97.

corticosteroid reduction. The responsiveness to inhaled mannitol as measured by the response–dose ratio during the ICS-reduction phase had 70% sensitivity for predicting failure to reduce inhaled steroids successfully (Fig. 16). Further, an increase in sputum eosinophilia during back-titration of ICS was also a predictor for later asthma exacerbation (Fig. 16). In the same study, sputum eosinophilia was also shown to be a predictor of failed reduction in dose of steroids. The subjects studied were clinically well controlled and symptom-free before the failed reduction of inhaled corticosteroids, suggesting that mannitol responsiveness and sputum eosinophils provide information additional to that provided by symptoms alone. The conclusion from these studies is that measurement of AHR and sputum eosinophils are the best surrogate markers to monitor asthma. Whereas the sputum analysis is a labor- and time-consuming investigation, measurement of AHR—especially if a common operating standard such as the dry powder mannitol could be used—might be the best tool to monitor asthmatic patients.

Monitoring Changes to Allergen Avoidance and Exposure

While many studies have investigated airway responsiveness to direct stimuli after inhalation of allergen and found increased responsiveness, surprisingly few studies have assessed the effects of allergen exposure on responses to indirect stimuli. Responsiveness to exercise has been shown to increase after allergen challenge (187). Thus, the percentage fall in FEV_1 after exercise in the asthmatic children was more severe after allergen challenge in contrast to responses seen with a direct challenge (187). This enhanced response to exercise was not dependent on the presence of a late response to the allergen challenge (187). Increases in sensitivity to AMP also occur after allergen challenge (188). The reason that the responses to indirect stimuli are influenced by exposure to allergen is likely to be a result of an increase in inflammatory cell number. It is known that acute responses to allergen are responsible for increases in the number of airway mast cells (189), eosinophils, and basophils (190).

Further, indirect stimuli such as exercise have been also used to study exposure to or avoidance of allergen (13). Controlled trials in patient's homes using allergen avoidance measures (191), and studies where patients have spent time living in high-altitude environments (15,192,193) or in allergen-free hospital rooms (194) have demonstrated improvements in AHR and all support allergen avoidance as a treatment for asthma. It is suggested that the efficacy of the high-altitude environments in improving asthma are due to lower allergen levels, particularly dust mite, compared to levels at sea level. There is also evidence that dust mites do not survive at high altitudes due to the low levels of humidity (195–197), although other factors such as other allergens or pollutants may also be reduced at altitude providing a cleaner environment for persons with asthma.

Studies at high altitude are difficult to perform, requiring relocation, and they are also difficult to perform in a blinded manner. It is clear, however, from many studies, that, together with improvements in AHR, improvements occur in symptoms and quality of life, spirometry, allergic status, and a variety of markers of airway inflammation in the blood, sputum, and urine (15,192,193). Similar improvements in AHR have been documented using both indirect and direct stimuli following a reduction in allergen exposure. Responsiveness to an indirect challenge appears to improve more rapidly when compared to a direct challenge upon avoidance of allergen. A 1-month stay at altitude demonstrated significant decreases in airway sensitivity to AMP but not to methacholine (Fig. 17) (12,15). These findings suggest that, like the response to inhaled steroids, the indirect stimulus adenosine was more sensitive to detect early changes in AHR in response to allergen avoidance when compared to a direct stimulus. The difference in changes in responses to allergen avoidance as measured by direct and indirect stimuli were less evident for longer-term studies (192,193). Improvements in AHR to both AMP and histamine were seen after 1-month in asthmatic children taking high doses of inhaled steroids (193). It is also evident that continued benefits of allergen avoidance at altitude are associated with longer duration at altitude. Children with moderate-to-severe asthma, after weaning off ICS, demonstrate continued improvement in AHR to exercise over 9 months, which was associated with

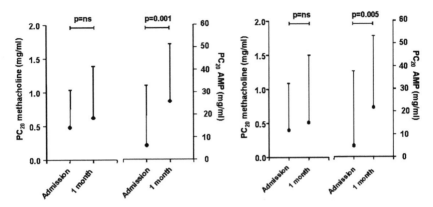

Figure 17 Mean values for the provoking concentration of methacholine required to cause a 20% fall in FEV_1 (PC_{20}) and mean values for the concentration of adenosine monophosphate (AMP) required to induce a 20% fall in FEV_1 (PC_{20}) fall in asthmatic subjects at admission and 1 month after residence at high altitude. The data demonstrate that there is a significant change in responsiveness to AMP but not to methacholine over this time period during which allergen levels would be predicted to be low. *Source:* From Refs. 12, 15.

similar reductions in serum IgE (192). On reintroduction to life at sea level and recommencement of inhaled steroids, the airway response to exercise after 3 months were at the pre-altitude levels, in association with increased levels of serum IgE. The results of these studies not only reinforce the importance of allergen avoidance in combination with inhaled steroids improving treatment of asthma but also demonstrate that allergen exposure can have a direct effect on response to indirect challenge in the presence of treatment.

Conclusions

The significance of challenge with indirect stimuli is that a positive response, usually defined as a 15% fall in FEV_1, to any of the indirect stimuli, is consistent with a diagnosis of active inflammation consistent with a diagnosis of asthma. Thus, all people with a positive response to the indirect stimuli would be expected to benefit from daily treatment with inhaled corticosteroids for 8–12 weeks. All people positive to these stimuli would also expect to suffer EIA. People with a positive response could expect their responses to exercise or other indirect stimuli would be markedly inhibited or even abolished by the acute administration of aerosols of sodium cromoglycate, nedocromil sodium, or a beta$_2$-adrenoceptor agonist and/or tablets of a leukotriene antagonist. Some people might benefit from pre-medication with a histamine antagonist. Indirect stimuli provide a non-immunological event resulting in the release of mediators from cells and possibly sensory nerves. For the osmotic challenges, a wide variety of cells are involved and the mediators released include leukotrienes, prostaglandins, histamine, and possibly sensory neuropeptides. The documentation of a response to an osmotic stimulus within the normal healthy range indicates that asthma is not active and it provides a goal for chronic treatment with inhaled corticosteroids and a starting point for back titration of inhaled steroids.

References

1. Van Schoor J, Joos GF, Pauwels RA. Indirect bronchial hyperresponsiveness in asthma: mechanisms, pharmacology and implications for clinical research. Eur Respir J 2000; 16:514–533.
2. Joos GF, O'Connor B, Anderson SD, Chung F, Cockcroft DW, Dahlén B, DiMaria G, Foresi A, Hargreave FE, Holgate ST, Inman M, Lötvall J, Magnussen H, Polosa R, Postma DS, Riedler J. ERS task force. Indirect airway challenges. Eur Respir J 2003; 21:1050–1068.
3. Riedler J. Nonpharmacological challenges in the assessment of bronchial responsiveness. Eur Respir Monogr 1997; 5:115–135.
4. Jonasson G, Carlsen KH, Hultquist C. Low-dose budesonide improves exercise-induced bronchospasm in schoolchildren. Pediatr Allergy Immunol 2000; 11:120–125.
5. Vathenen AS, Knox AJ, Wisniewski A, Tattersfield AE. Effect of inhaled budesonide on bronchial reactivity to histamine, exercise, and eucapnic dry air hyperventilation in patients with asthma. Thorax 1991; 46:811–816.
6. Rodwell LT, Anderson SD, Seale JP. Inhaled steroids modify bronchial responses to hyperosmolar saline. Eur Respir J 1992; 5:953–962.
7. Anderson SD, du Toit JI, Rodwell LT, Jenkins CR. Acute effect of sodium cromoglycate on airway narrowing induced by 4.5 percent saline aerosol. Outcome before and during treatment with aerosol corticosteroids in patients with asthma. Chest 1994; 105:673–680.
8. du Toit JI, Anderson SD, Jenkins CR, Woolcock AJ, Rodwell LT. Airway responsiveness in asthma: bronchial challenge with histamine and 4.5% sodium chloride before and after budesonide. Allergy Asthma Proc 1997; 18:7–14.
9. Koskela H, Hyvärinen L, Brannan JD, Chan HK, Anderson SD. Responsiveness to three bronchial provocation tests in patients with difficult to diagnose asthma. Chest 2003; 124:2171–2177.
10. Brannan JD, Koskela H, Anderson SD, Chan HK. Budesonide reduces sensitivity and reactivity to inhaled mannitol in asthmatic subjects. Respirology 2002; 7:37–44.
11. Holgate S, Arshad H, Stryszak P, Harrison JE. Mometasone furoate antagonizes AMP-induced bronchoconstriction in patients with mild asthma. J Allergy Clin Immunol 2000; 105:906–911.
12. Benckhuijsen J, van den Bos JW, van Velzen E, de Bruijn R, Aalbers R. Differences in the effect of allergen avoidance on bronchial hyperresponsive-

ness as measured by methacholine, adenosine 5'-monophosphate, and exercise in asthmatic children. Pediatr Pulmonol 1996; 22:147–153.

13. Henriksen JM. Exercise-induced bronchoconstriction. Seasonal variation in children with asthma and in those with rhinitis. Allergy 1986; 41:468–470.

14. Karjalainen J, Lindqvist A, Laitenen LA. Seasonal variability of exercise-induced asthma especially out-doors. Effect of birch pollen allergy. Clin Exp Allergy 1989; 19:273–279.

15. van Velzen E, van den Bos JW, Benckhuijsen JAW, van Essel T, de Bruijn R, Aalbers R. Effect of allergen avoidance at high altitude on direct and indirect bronchial hyperresponsiveness and markers of inflammation in children with allergic asthma. Thorax 1996; 51:582–584.

16. Haby MM, Anderson SD, Peat JK, Mellis CM, Toelle BG, Woolcock AJ. An exercise challenge protocol for epidemiological studies of asthma in children: comparison with histamine challenge. Eur Respir J 1994; 7:43–49.

17. Riedler J, Reade T, Dalton M, Holst DI, Robertson CF. Hypertonic saline challenge in an epidemiological survey of asthma in children. Am J Respir Crit Care Med 1994; 150:1632–1639.

18. Riedler J, Gamper A, Eder W, Oberfeld G. Prevalence of bronchial hyperresponsiveness to 4.5% saline and its relation to asthma and allergy symptoms in Austrian children. Eur Respir J 1998; 11:355–360.

19. Lis G, Pietrzyk JJ. Response–dose ratio as an index of bronchial responsiveness to hypertonic saline in an epidemiological survey of asthma in Polish children. Pediatr Pulmonol 1998; 25:375–382.

20. Nicolai T, Mutius EV, Reitmeir P, Wjst M. Reactivity to cold-air hyperventilation in normal and in asthmatic children in a survey of 5,697 schoolchildren in southern Bavaria. Am Rev Respir Dis 1993; 147:565–572.

21. Gibson PG, Wlodarczyk J, Hensley MJ, Gleeson M, Henry PL, Cripps AW, Clancy R. Epidemiological association of airway inflammation with asthma symptoms and airway hyperresponsiveness in childhood. Am J Respir Crit Care Med 1998; 158:36–41.

22. de Meer G, Hoes AW, Brunekreef B. Measures of Airway Responsiveness to Hypertonic Saline in Children: PD$_{15}$FEV$_1$ or Dose–Response Slope? Airway Responsiveness to Direct and Indirect Stimuli. A Population Based Approach. Thesis, Institute for Risk Assessment Sciences (RAS) Division Environmental & Occupational Health, Utrecht University, Utrecht, 2002:35–48.

23. Reiss TF, Hill JB, Harman E, Zhang J, Tanaka WK, Bronsky E, Guerreiro D, Hendeles L. Increased urinary excretion of LTE$_4$ after exercise and attenuation of exercise-induced bronchospasm by montelukast, a cysteinyl leukotriene receptor antagonist. Thorax 1997; 52:1030–1035.

24. O'Sullivan S, Roquet A, Dahlén B, Larsen F, Eklund A, Kumlin M, O'Byrne PM, Dahlén SE. Evidence for mast cell activation during exercise-induced bronchoconstriction. Eur Respir J 1998; 12:345–350.

25. Brannan JD, Gulliksson M, Anderson SD, Chew N, Kumlin M. Evidence of mast cell activation and leukotriene release after mannitol inhalation. Eur Respir J 2003; 22:491–496.

26. Baraniuk JN, Ali M, Yuta A, Fang SY, Naranch K. Hypertonic saline nasal provocation stimulates nociceptive nerves, substance P release, and glandular

mucous exocytosis in normal humans. Am J Respir Crit Care Med 1999; 160:655–662.

27. Anderson SD, Brannan JD. Methods for 'indirect' challenge tests including exercise, eucapnic voluntary hyperpnea and hypertonic aerosols. Clin Rev Allergy Immunol 2003; 24:63–90.

28. Leuppi JD, Brannan JD, Anderson SD. Bronchial provocations tests: The rationale for using inhaled mannitol as a test for airway hyperresponsiveness. Swiss Med Wkly 2002; 132:151–158.

29. Eiser NM, Kerrebijn KF, Quanjer PH. Guidelines for standardization of bronchial challenge with (nonspecific) bronchoconstricting agents. Working Group on Bronchial Hyperreactivity SEPCR. Bull Eur Physiolopathol Respir 1983; 19:495.

30. Global Initiative for Asthma. Global strategy for asthma management and prevention. In: US. Department of Health and Human Services. Public Health Service NIoH, National Heart, Lung, and Blood Institute, ed. NHLBI/WHO Workshop Report. Bethesda, MD: Medical Communications Resources, Inc., 1995:1–8.

31. van Asperen PP, Mellis CM, Sly PD. The role of corticosteroids in the management of childhood asthma. Med J Aust 2002; 176:168–173.

32. Doull L, Sandall D, Smith S, Schrieber J, Freezer NJ, Holgate ST. Differential inhibitory effect of regular inhaled corticosteroid on airway responsiveness to adenosine $5'$ monophosphate, methacholine, and bradykinin in symptomatic children with recurrent wheeze. Pediatr Pulmonol 1997; 23:404–411.

33. Taylor DA, Jensen MW, Kanabar V, Engelstätter R, Steinijans VW, Barnes PJ, O'Connor BJ. A dose-dependent effect of the novel inhaled corticosteroid ciclesonide on airway responsiveness to adenosine-$5'$-monophosphate in asthmatic patients. Am J Respir Crit Care Med 1999; 160:237–243.

34. van den Berge M, Kerstjens HA, Meijer RJ, de Reus DM, Koëter GH, Kauffman HF, Postma DS. Corticosteroid-induced improvement in the PC_{20} of adenosine monophosphate is more closely associated with reduction in airway inflammation than improvement in the PC_{20} of methacholine. Am J Respir Crit Care Med 2001; 164:1127–1132.

35. Sont JK, Willems LN, Bel EH, van Krieken JH, Vandenbroucke JP, Sterk PJ. Clinical control and histopathologic outcome of asthma when using airway hyperresponsiveness as an additional guide to long-term treatment. Am J Respir Crit Care Med 1999; 159:1043–1051.

36. Lim S, Jatakanan A, John M, Gilbey T, O'Conner BJ, Fan K, Barnes PJ. Effect of inhaled budesonide on lung function and airway inflammation. Am J Respir Crit Care Med 1999; 159:22–30.

37. Reddel HK, Jenkins CR, Marks GB, Ware SI, Xuan W, Salome CM, Badcock CA, Woolcock AJ. Optimal asthma control, starting with high doses of inhaled budesonide. Eur Respir J 2000; 16:226–235.

38. Hofstra WB, Neijens HJ, Duiverman EJ, Kouwenberg JM, Mulder PG, Kuethe MC, Sterk PJ. Dose–response over time to inhaled fluticasone propionate: treatment of exercise- and methacholine-induced bronchoconstriction in children with asthma. Pediatr Pulmonol 2000; 29:415–423.

39. Anderson SD, Brannan J, Trevillion L, Young IH. Lung function and bronchial provocation tests for intending divers with a history of asthma. SPUMS J 1995; 25:233–248.

40. Sinclair DG, Sims MM, Hoad NA, Winfield CR. Exercise-induced airway narrowing in army recruits with a history of childhood asthma. Eur Respir J 1995; 8:1314–1317.

41. Freed R, Anderson SD, Wyndham J. The use of bronchial provocation tests for identifying asthma. A review of the problems for occupational assessment and a proposal for a new direction. ADF Health 2002; 3:77–85.

42. Anderson SD, Silverman M, Konig P, Godfrey S. Exercise-induced asthma. A review. Br J Dis Chest 1975; 69:1–39.

43. Anderson SD, McEvoy JDS, Bianco S. Changes in lung volumes and airway resistance after exercise in asthmatic subjects. Am Rev Respir Dis 1972; 106:30–37.

44. Anderson SD, Silverman M, Walker SR. Metabolic and ventilatory changes in asthmatic patients during and after exercise. Thorax 1972; 27:718–725.

45. Anderson SD, Seale JP, Ferris L, Schoeffel RE, Lindsay DA. An evaluation of pharmacotherapy for exercise-induced asthma. J Allergy Clin Immunol 1979; 64:612–624.

46. Silverman M, Konig P, Godfrey S. The use of serial exercise test to assess the efficacy and duration of action of drugs in asthma. Thorax 1973; 28:574–578.

47. Godfrey S, Konig P. Inhibition of exercise-induced asthma by different pharmacological pathways. Thorax 1976; 31:137–143.

48. Silverman M, Anderson SD. Standardization of exercise tests in asthmatic children. Arch Dis Childhealth 1972; 47:882–889.

49. Godfrey S, Silverman M, Anderson SD. The use of the treadmill for assessing exercise-induced asthma and the effect of varying the severity and the duration of exercise. Pediatrics 1975; 56:893S–898S.

50. Godfrey S, Konig P. Suppression of exercise-induced asthma by salbutamol, theophylline, atropine, cromolyn, and placebo in a group of asthmatic children. Pediatrics 1975; 56:930–934.

51. Henriksen JM. Effect of inhalation of corticosteroids on exercise induced asthma: randomised double blind crossover study of budesonide in asthmatic children. Br Med J 1985; 291:248–249.

52. Henriksen JM, Dahl R. Effects of inhaled budesonide alone and in combination with low-dose terbutaline in children with exercise-induced asthma. Am Rev Respir Dis 1983; 128:993–997.

53. Pedersen S, Hansen OR. Budesonide treatment of moderate and severe asthma in children: a dose–response study. J Allergy Clin Immunol 1995; 95:29–33.

54. Yoshikawa T, Shoji S, Fujii T, Kanazawa H, Kudoh S, Hirata K, Yoshikawa J. Severity of exercise-induced bronchoconstriction is related to airway eosinophilic inflammation in patients with asthma. Eur Respir J 1998; 12:879–884.

55. Kivity S, Argaman A, Onn A, Shwartz Y, Man A, Greif J, Fireman E. Eosinophil influx into the airways in patients with exercise-induced asthma. Respir Med 2000; 94:1200–1205.

56. Anderson SD, Seale JP, Rozea P, Bandler L, Theobald G, Lindsay DA. Inhaled and oral salbutamol in exercise-induced asthma. Am Rev Respir Dis 1976; 114:493–500.

57. Anderson SD, Rodwell LT, Du Toit J, Young IH. Duration of protection by inhaled salmeterol in exercise-induced asthma. Chest 1991; 100:1254–1260.

58. Henriksen JM, Agertoft L, Pedersen S. Protective effect and duration of action of inhaled formoterol and salbutamol on exercise-induced asthma in children. J Allergy Clin Immunol 1992; 89:1176–1182.

59. Hancox RJ, Subbarao P, Kamada D, Watson RM, Hargreave FE, Inman MD. B_2-agonist tolerance and exercise-induced bronchospasm. Am J Respir Crit Care Med 2002; 165:1068–1070.

60. Simons FE, Gerstner TV, Cheang MS. Tolerance to the bronchoprotective effect of salmeterol in adolescents with exercise-induced asthma using concurrent inhaled glucocorticoid treatment. Pediatrics 1997; 99:655–659.

61. Ramage L, Lipworth BJ, Ingram CG, Cree IA, Dhillon DP. Reduced protection against exercise induced bronchoconstriction after chronic dosing with salmeterol. Respir Med 1994; 88:363–368.

62. Nelson JA, Strauss L, Skowronski M, Ciufo R, Novak R, McFadden ER. Effect of long-term salmeterol treatment on exercise-induced asthma. N Engl J Med 1998; 339:141–146.

63. Spooner C, Rowe BH, Saunders LD. Nedocromil sodium in the treatment of exercise-induced asthma: a meta-analysis. Eur Respir J 2000; 16:30–37.

64. Kemp JP, Dockhorn RJ, Shapiro GG, Nguyen HH, Reiss TF, Seidenberg BC, Knorr B. Montelukast once daily inhibits exercise-induced bronchoconstriction in 6- to 14-year-old children with asthma. J Pediatr 1998; 133:424–428.

65. Leff JA, Busse WW, Pearlman D, Bronsky EA, Kemp J, Hendeles L, Dockhorn R, Kundu S, Zhang J, Seidenberg BC, Reiss TF. Montelukast, a leukotriene-receptor antagonist, for the treatment of mild asthma and exercise-induced bronchoconstriction. N Engl J Med 1998; 339:147–152.

66. Crapo RO, Casaburi R, Coates AL, Enright PL, Hankinson JL, Irvin CG, MacIntyre NR, McKay RT, Wanger JS, Anderson SD, Cockcroft DW, Fish JE, Sterk PJ. Guidelines for methacholine and exercise challenge testing— 1999. Am J Respir Crit Care Med 2000; 161:309–329.

67. Roca J, Whipp BJ, Agustí AGN, Anderson SD, Casaburi R, Cotes JE, Donner CF, Estenne M, Folgering H, Higenbottam TW, Killian KJ, Palange P, Patessio A, Prefault C, Sergysels R, Wagner PD, Weisman IM. Clinical exercise testing with reference to lung diseases: indications, standardization and interpretation strategies. Position document of the European Respiratory Society. Eur Respir J 1997; 10:2662–2689.

68. Anderson SD, Lambert S, Brannan JD, Wood RJ, Koskela H, Morton AR, Fitch KD. Laboratory protocol for exercise asthma to evaluate salbutamol given by two devices. Med Sci Sports Exer 2001; 33:893–900.

69. Rosenthal RR. Simplified eucapnic voluntary hyperventilation. J Allergy Clin Immunol 1984; 73:676–685.

70. Phillips YY, Jaeger JJ, Laube BL, Rosenthal RR. Eucapnic voluntary hyperventilation of compressed gas mixture. A simple system for bronchial challenge by respiratory heat loss. Am Rev Respir Dis 1985; 131:31–35.

71. Argyros GJ, Roach JM, Hurwitz KM, Eliasson AH, Phillips YY. Eucapnic voluntary hyperventilation as a bronchoprovocation technique. Development of a standardized dosing schedule in asthmatics. Chest 1996; 109:1520–1524.

72. Anderson SD, Argyros GJ, Magnussen H, Holzer K. Provocation by eucapnic voluntary hyperpnoea to identify exercise induced bronchoconstriction. Br J Sports Med 2001; 35:344–347.

73. Rundell KW, Anderson SD, Spiering BA, Judelson DA. Field exercise versus laboratory test using eucapnic voluntary hyperpnea to identify airway hyperesponsiveness in elite cold weather athletes. Chest 2004; 125:909–915.

74. Smith CM, Anderson SD, Seale JP. The duration of action of the combination of fenoterol hydrobromide and ipratropium bromide in protecting against asthma provoked by hyperpnea. Chest 1988; 94:709–717.

75. Israel E, Dermarkarian R, Rosenberg M, Sperling R, Taylor G, Rubin P, Drazen JM. The effects of a 5-lipoxygenase inhibitor on asthma induced by cold, dry air. N Engl J Med 1990; 323:1740–1744.

76. Bisgaard H, Nielsen KG. Bronchoprotection with a leukotriene receptor antagonist in asthmatic preschool children. Am J Respir Crit Care Med 2000; 162:187–190.

77. Koskela H, Hyvärinen L, Brannan JD, Chan HK, Anderson SD. Sensitivity and validity of three bronchial provocation tests to demonstrate the effect of inhaled corticosteroids in asthma. Chest 2003; 124:1341–1349.

78. Nielsen KG, Bisgaard H. The effect of inhaled budesonide on symptoms, lung function, and cold air and methacholine responsiveness in 2- to 5-year-old asthmatic children. Am J Respir Crit Care Med 2000; 162:1500–1506.

79. Anderson SD. Is there a unifying hypothesis for exercise-induced asthma? J Allergy Clin Immunol 1984; 73:660–665

80. Smith CM, Anderson SD. Hyperosmolarity as the stimulus to asthma induced by hyperventilation? J Allergy Clin Immunol 1986; 77:729–736

81. Smith CM, Anderson SD. A comparison between the airway response to isocapnic hyperventilation and hypertonic saline in subjects with asthma. Eur Respir J 1989; 2:36–43.

82. Smith CM, Anderson SD. Inhalational challenge using hypertonic saline in asthmatic subjects: a comparison with responses to hyperpnoea, methacholine and water. Eur Respir J 1990; 3:144–151.

83. Smith CM, Anderson SD. An investigation of the hyperosmolar stimulus to exercise-induced asthma. Aust N Z J Med 1987; 17:S513.

84. Sterk PJ, Fabbri LM, Quanjer PH, Cockcroft DW, O'Byrne PM, Anderson SD, Juniper EF, Malo JL. Airway responsiveness: standardized challenge testing with pharmacological, physical and sensitizing stimuli in adults. Eur Respir J 1993; 6:53–83.

85. Gibson PG, Saltos N, Borgas T. Airway mast cells and eosinophils correlate with clinical severity and airway hyperresponsiveness in corticosteroid-treated asthma. J Allergy Clin Immunol 2000; 105:752–759.

86. Rodwell LT, Anderson SD, du Toit J, Seale JP. Nedocromil sodium inhibits the airway response to hyperosmolar challenge in patients with asthma. Am Rev Respir Dis 1992; 146:1149–1155.

87. Brannan JD, Anderson SD, Freed R, Leuppi JD, Koskela H, Chan HK. Nedocromil sodium inhibits responsiveness to inhaled mannitol in asthmatic subjects. Am J Respir Crit Care Med 2000; 161:2096–2099.

88. Aldridge RE, Hancox RJ, Robin Taylor D, Cowan JO, Winn MC, Frampton CM, Town GI. Effects of terbutaline and budesonide on sputum cells and bronchial hyperresponsiveness in asthma. Am J Respir Crit Care Med 2000; 161:1459–1464.

89. Gibson PG, Saltos N, Fakes K. Acute anti-inflammatory effects of inhaled budesonide in asthma. A randomized controlled trial. Am J Respir Crit Care Med 2001; 163:32–36.

90. Rabone S, Phoon WO, Anderson SD, Wan KC, Seneviratne M, Gutierrez L, Brannan J. Hypertonic saline challenge in an adult epidemiological field survey. Occup Med 1996; 46:177–185.

91. Briffa P, Perry C, Camps J, West SN, Lumby G, Ridler P, Mayrhofer P, Serwach N, Anderson SD. Bronchial responsiveness in applications to the NSW Police Force with a history or symptoms suggestive of asthma. Available from URL http://www.anzsrs.org.au/2003asm.pdf [accessed 2003 Sept 09], 2003.

92. Anderson SD, Spring J, Moore B, Rodwell LT, Spalding N, Gonda I, Chan K, Walsh A, Clark AR. The effect of inhaling a dry powder of sodium chloride on the airways of asthmatic subjects. Eur Respir J 1997; 10:2465–2473.

93. Anderson SD, Brannan J, Spring J, Spalding N, Rodwell LT, Chan K, Gonda I, Walsh A, Clark AR. A new method for bronchial-provocation testing in asthmatic subjects using a dry powder of mannitol. Am J Respir Crit Care Med 1997; 156:758–765.

94. Brannan JD, Koskela H, Anderson SD, Chew N. Responsiveness to mannitol in asthmatic subjects with exercise- and hyperventilation-induced asthma. Am J Respir Crit Care Med 1998; 158:1120–1126.

95. Brannan JD, Anderson SD, Gomes K, King GG, Chan HK, Seale JP. Fexofenadine decreases sensitivity to and montelukast improves recovery from inhaled mannitol. Am J Respir Crit Care Med 2001; 163:1420–1425.

96. Currie GP, Haggart K, Lee DKC, Fowler SJ, Wilson AM, Brannan JD, Anderson SD, Lipworth BJ. Effects of mediator antagonism on mannitol and adenosine monophosphate challenges. Clin Exp Allergy 2003; 33:783–788.

97. Leuppi JD, Salome CM, Jenkins CR, Anderson SD, Xuan W, Marks GB, Koskela H, Brannan JD, Freed R, Andersson M, Chan HK, Woolcock AJ. Predictive markers of asthma exacerbations during stepwise dose-reduction of inhaled corticosteroids. Am J Respir Crit Care Med 2001; 163:406–412.

98. Leuppi JD, Salome CM, Jenkins CR, Koskela H, Anderson SD, Andersson M, Chan HK, Woolcock AJ. Markers of airway inflammation and airway hyperresponsiveness in patients with well-controlled asthma. Eur Respir J 2001; 18:444–450.

99. Holzer K, Anderson SD, Chan HK, Douglass J. Mannitol as a challenge test to identify exercise-induced bronchoconstriction in elite athletes. Am J Respir Crit Care Med 2003; 167:534–547.

100. Currie GP. Relationship between airway hyperesponsiveness to mannitol and adenosine monophophate. Allergy 2003; 58:762–766.

101. Backer V, Dirksen A, Bach-Mortensen N, Hansen KK, Laursen EM, Wendelboe D. The distribution of bronchial responsiveness to histamine and exercise in 527 children and adolescents. J Allergy Clin Immunol 1991; 88:68–76.

102. Weiss JW, Rossing TH, McFadden ER, Ingram RH. Relationship between bronchial responsiveness to hyperventilation with cold air and methacholine in asthma. J Allergy Clin Immunol 1983; 72:140–144.

103. Holzer K, Anderson SD, Douglass J. Exercise in elite summer athletes: challenges for diagnosis. J Allergy Clin Immunol 2002; 110:374–380.

104. O'Byrne PM. Why does airway inflammation persist? Is it leukotrienes? Am J Respir Crit Care Med 2000; 161:S186–S187

105. Moloney ED, Griffin S, Burke CM, Poulter LW, O'Sullivan S. Release of inflammatory mediators from eosinophils following a hyperosmolar stimulus. Respir Med 2003; 97:1–5.

106. Pliss LB, Ingenito EP, Ingram RH, Pichurko B. Assessment of bronchoalveolar cell and mediator response to isocapnic hyperpnea in asthma. Am Rev Respir Dis 1990; 142:73–78.

107. Anderson SD, Bye PTP, Schoeffel RE, Seale JP, Taylor KM, Ferris L. Arterial plasma histamine levels at rest, during and after exercise in patients with asthma: effects of terbutaline aerosol. Thorax 1981; 36:259–267.

108. Hartley JPR, Charles TJ, Monie RDG, Seaton A, Taylor WH, Westood A, William JD. Arterial plasma histamine after exercise in normal individuals and in patients with exercise induced asthma. Clin Sci 1981; 61:151–157.

109. Koskela H, Di Sciascio M, Anderson SD, Andersson M, Chan HK, Gadalla S, Katelaris C. Nasal hyperosmolar challenge with a dry powder of mannitol in patients with allergic rhinitis. Evidence for epithelial cell involvement. Clin Exp Allergy 2000; 30:1627–1636.

110. Kemp JP, Dockhorn RJ, Busse WW, Bleecker ER. Prolonged effect of inhaled salmeterol against exercise-induced bronchospasm. Am J Respir Crit Care Med 1994; 150:1612–1615.

111. Argyros GJ, Roach JM, Hurwitz KM, Eliasson AH, Phillips YY. The refractory period after eucapnic voluntary hyperventilation challenge and its effect on challenge technique. Chest 1995; 108:419–424.

112. Bar-Yishay E, Ben-Dov I, Godfrey S. Refractory period after hyperventilation-induced asthma. Am Rev Respir Dis 1983; 127:572–574.

113. Daxun Z, Rafferty P, Richards R, Summerell S, Holgate ST. Airway refractoriness to adenosine 5'-monophosphate after repeated inhalation. J Allergy Clin Immunol 1989; 83:152–158.

114. Edmunds A, Tooley M, Godfrey S. The refractory period after exercise-induced asthma: its duration and relation to the severity of exercise. Am Rev Respir Dis 1978; 117:247–254.

115. Belcher NG, Rees PJ, Clark TJM, Lee TH. A comparison of the refractory periods induced by hypertonic airway challenge and exercise in bronchial asthma. Am Rev Respir Dis 1987; 135:822–825.

116. Crapo RO, Hankinson JL, Irvin C, MacIntyre NR, Voter KZ, Wise RA, Graham B, O'Donnell C, Paoletti P, Roca J, Viegi G. Standardization of

spirometry. 1994 Update. The Official Statement of the American Thoracic Society. Am J Respir Crit Care Med 1994; 152:1107–1136.

117. Crapo RO, Morris AH, Gardner RM. Reference spirometric values using techniques and equipment that meet ATS recommendations. Am Rev Respir Dis 1981; 123:659–664.

118. Johns DP, Pierce R. Pocket Guide to Spirometry (ISBN 0–07–471331-0). Australia: McGraw-Hill, 2003.

119. Rundell KW, Im J, Mayers LB, Wilber RL, Szmedra L, Schmitz HR. Self-reported symptoms and exercise-induced asthma in the elite athlete. Med Sci Sports Exerc 2001; 33.:208–213.

120. Godfrey S, Springer C, Bar-Yishay E, Avital A. Cut-off points defining normal and asthmatic bronchial reactivity to exercise and inhalation challenges in children and young adults. Eur Respir J 1999; 14:659–668.

121. Carlsen KH, Engh G, Mørk M. Exercise induced bronchoconstriction depends on exercise load. Respir Med 2000; 94:750–755.

122. Eliasson AH, Phillips YY, Rajagopal KR, Howard RS. Sensitivity and specificity of bronchial provocation testing. An evaluation of four techniques in exercise-induced bronchospasm. Chest 1992; 102:347–355.

123. Rodwell LT, Anderson SD, du Toit J, Seale JP. Different effects of inhaled amiloride and furosemide on airway responsiveness to dry air challenge in asthmatic subjects. Eur Respir J 1993; 6:855–861.

124. Koskela HO, Räsänen SH, Tukiainen HO. The diagnostic value of cold air hyperventilation in adults with suspected asthma. Respir Med 1997; 91: 470–478.

125. Modl M, Eber E, Steinbrugger B, Weinhandl E, Zach MS. Comparing methods for assessing bronchial responsiveness in children: single step cold air challenge, multiple step cold air challenge, and histamine provocation. Eur Respir J 1995; 8:1742–1747.

126. Assoufi BK, Dally MB, Newman-Taylor AJ, Denison DM. Cold air test: a simplified standard method for airway reactivity. Bull Eur Physiopathol Respir 1986; 22:349–357.

127. Zach M, Polgar G, Kump H, Kroisel P. Cold air challenge of airway hyperreactivity in children: practical application and theoretical aspects. Pediatr Res 1984; 18:469–478.

128. McFadden ER, Nelson JA, Skowronski ME, Lenner KA. Thermally induced asthma and airway drying. Am J Respir Crit Care Med 1999; 160:221–226.

129. Jones PD, Hankin R, Simpson J, Gibson PG, Henry RL. The tolerability, safety, and success of sputum induction and combined hypertonic saline challenge in children. Am J Respir Crit Care Med 2001; 164:1146–1149.

130. Rodwell LT, Anderson SD. Hyperosmolar saline aerosol challenge: a useful tool in the management of subjects with cystic fibrosis. Paediatr Pulmonol 1996; 21:282–289.

131. Anderson SD, Gibson P. The use of aerosols of hypertonic saline and distilled water (fog) for the patient with asthma. In: Barnes PJ, Grunstein MM, Leff A, Woolcock AJ, eds. Asthma. New York: Raven Press, 1997:1135–1150.

132. Anderson SD, Smith CM, Rodwell LT, du Toit JI, Riedler J, Robertson CF. The use of non-isotonic aerosols for evaluating bronchial hyperresponsive-

ness. In: Spector S, ed. Provocation Challenge Procedures. New York: Marcel Dekker, 1995:249–278.

133. Subbarao P, Brannan JD, Ho B, Anderson SD, Chan HK, Coates AL. Inhaled mannitol identifies methacholine-responsive children with active asthma. Pediatr Pulmonol 2000; 29:291–298.

134. Barben J, Roberts M, Carlin JB, Robertson CF. Repeatability of bronchial responsiveness to mannitol dry powder in children with asthma. Eur Respir J 2001; 18:493s.

135. Chan W, Cushley MJ, Holgate ST. The effect of inhaled adenosine 5'-monophosphate (AMP) on airway calibre in normal and asthmatic subjects. Clin Sci 1986; 70:65P–66P.

136. Polosa R, Holgate ST. Adenosine bronchoprovocation: a promising marker of allergic inflammation in asthma?. Thorax 1997; 52:919–923.

137. Polosa R. Adenosine-receptor subtypes: their relevance to adenosine-mediated responses in asthma and chronic obstructive pulmonary disease. Eur Respir J 2002; 20:488–496.

138. Polosa R, Ng WH, Crimi N, Vancheri C, Holgate ST, Church MK, Mistretta A. Release of mast-cell-derived mediators after endobronchial adenosine challenge in asthma. Am J Respir Crit Care Med 1995; 151:624–629.

139. Dahlén B, Roquet A, Inman MD, Karlsson Ö, Naya I, Anstrén G, O'Byrne PM, Dahlén SE. Influence of zafirlukast and loratadine on exercise-induced bronchoconstriction. J Allergy Clin Immunol 2002; 109:789–793.

140. Rutgers SR, Koeter GH, van der Mark TW, Postma DS. Short-term treatment with budesonide does not improve hyperresponsiveness to adenosine 5'-monophosphate in COPD. Am J Respir Crit Care Med 1998; 157:880–886.

141. Polosa R, Ciamarra I, Prosperini G, Pagano C, Vancheri C, Mistretta A, Crimi N. Sputum eosinophilia correlates with bronchial responsiveness to AMP in patients with rhinitis. Am J Respir Crit Care Med 1997; 155:A978.

142. Lorentzson S, Boe J, Eriksson G, Persson G. Use of inhaled corticosteroids in patients with mild asthma. Thorax 1990; 45:733–735.

143. Haahtela T, Jarvinen M, Kava T, Kiviranta K, Koskinen S, Lehtonen K, Nikander K, Persson T, Reinikainen K, Selroos O, Sovijarvi A, Stenius-Aarniala B, Svahn T, Tammivaara R, Laitinen LA. Comparison of a beta 2-agonist, terbutaline, with an inhaled corticosteroid, budesonide, in newly detected asthma. N Engl J Med 1991; 325:388–392.

144. Djukanovic R, Wilson JW, Britten KM, Wilson SJ, Walls AF, Roche WR, Howarth PH, Holgate ST. Effect of an inhaled corticosteroid on airway inflammation and symptoms in asthma. Am Rev Respir Dis 1992; 145:669–674.

145. Godfrey S. Monitoring asthma severity and response to treatment. Respiration 2001; 68:637–648.

146. Fuller RW, Choudry NB, Eriksson G. Action of budesonide on asthmatic bronchial hyperresponsiveness. Effects on directly and indirectly acting bronchoconstrictors. Chest 1991; 100:670–674.

147. Groot CA, Lammers JW, Molema J, Festen J, van Herwaarden CL. Effect of inhaled beclomethasone and nedocromil sodium on bronchial hyperresponsiveness to histamine and distilled water. Eur Respir J 1992; 5:1075–1082.

148. O'Connor BJ, Ridge SM, Barnes PJ, Fuller RW. Greater effect of inhaled budesonide on adenosine 5′-monophosphate-induced than on sodium-metabisulfite-induced bronchoconstriction in asthma. Am Rev Respir Dis 1992; 146:560–564.

149. Prosperini G, Rajakulasingam K, Cacciola RR, Spicuzza L, Rorke S, Holgate ST, Di Maria GU, Polosa R. Changes in sputum counts and airway hyperresponsiveness after budesonide: monitoring anti-inflammatory response on the basis of surrogate markers of airway inflammation. J Allergy Clin Immunol 2002; 110:855–861.

150. Reynolds CJ, Togias A, Proud D. Airways hyper-responsiveness to bradykinin and methacholine: effects of inhaled fluticasone. Clin Exp Allergy 2002; 32:1174–1179.

151. Waalkans HJ, van Essen-Zandvliet EEM, Gerritsen J, Duiverman EJ, Kerrebijn KF, Knol K, the Dutch CNSLD Study Group. The effect of an inhaled corticosteroid (budesonide) on exercise-induced asthma in children. Eur Respir J 1993; 6:652–656.

152. Jonasson G, Carlsen KH, Blomqvist P. Clinical efficacy of low-dose inhaled budesonide once or twice daily in children with mild asthma not previously treated with steroids. Eur Respir J 1998; 12:1099–1104.

153. Pennings HJ, Wouters EF. Effect of inhaled beclomethasone dipropionate on isocapnic hyperventilation with cold air in asthmatics, measured with forced oscillation technique. Eur Respir J 1997; 10:665–671.

154. Nielsen KG, Bisgaard H. Lung function response to cold air challenge in asthmatic and healthy children of 2–5 years of age. Am J Respir Crit Care Med 2000; 161:1805–1809.

155. Ketchell RI, Jensen MW, Lumley P, Wright AM, Allenby MI, O'Conner BJ. Rapid effect of inhaled fluticasone propionate on airway responsiveness to adenosine 5′-monophosphate in mild asthma. J Allergy Clin Immunol 2002; 110:603–606.

156. Thio BJ, Slingerland GLM, Nagelkerke AF, Roord JJ, Mulder PGH, Dankert-Roelse JE. Effects of single-dose fluticasone on exercise-induced asthma in asthmatic children: a pilot study. Pediatr Pulmonol 2001; 32: 115–121.

157. The National Asthma Council. Asthma Management Handbook. Melbourne: National Asthma Council Australia Ltd, 2002.

158. Van Essen-Zandvliet EE, Hughes MD, Waalkens HJ, Duiverman EJ, Pocock SJ, Kerrebijn KF, the Dutch Chronic Non-Specific Lung Disease Study Group. Effects of 22 months of treatment with inhaled corticosteroids and/or beta-2-agonists on lung function, airway responsiveness, and symptoms in children with asthma. Am Rev Respir Dis 1992; 146:547–554.

159. Ward C, Pais M, Bish R, Reid D, Feltis B, Johns D, Walters EH. Airway inflammation, basement membrane thickening and bronchial hyperresponsiveness in asthma. Thorax 2002; 57:309–316.

160. Wilson AM, Lipworth BJ. Dose–response evaluation of the therapeutic index for inhaled budesonide in patients with mild-to-moderate asthma. Am J Med 2000; 108:269–275.

161. Bousquet J, Jeffery PK, Busse WW, Johnson M, Vignola AM. Asthma. From bronchoconstriction to airways inflammation and remodeling. Am J Respir Crit Care Med 2000; 161:1720–1745.

162. Jones SL, Herbison P, Cowan JO, Flannery EM, Hancox RJ, McLachlan CR, Taylor DR. Exhaled NO and assessment of anti-inflammatory effects of inhaled steroid: dose–response relationship. Eur Respir J 2002; 20:601–608.

163. Kraft M, Martin RJ, Lazarus SC, Fahy JV, Boushey HA, Lemanske RFJ, Szefler SJ. Airway tissue mast cells in persistent asthma: predictor of treatment failure when patients discontinue inhaled corticosteroids. Chest 2003; 124:42–50.

164. Jenkins C. An update on asthma management. Intern Med J 2003; 33:365–371.

165. Holt S, Suder A, Weatherall M, Cheng S, Shirtcliffe P, Beasley R. Dose–response relation of inhaled fluticasone propionate in adolescents and adults with asthma: meta-analysis. Br Med J 2001; 323:253–256.

166. Chanez P, Karlstrom R, Godard P. High or standard initial dose of budesonide to control mild-to-moderate asthma? Eur Respir J 2001; 17:856–862

167. Boulet LP, Cournoyer I, Deschesnes F, Leblanc P, Nouwen A. Perception of airflow obstruction and associated breathlessness in normal and asthmatic subjects: correlation with anxiety and bronchodilator needs. Thorax 1994; 49:965–970.

168. Sont JK, Han J, van Krieken JM, Evertse CE, Hooijer R, Willems LN, Sterk PJ. Relationship between the inflammatory infiltrate in bronchial biopsy specimens and clinical severity of asthma in patients treated with inhaled steroids. Thorax 1996; 51:496–502.

169. Frank TL, Adisesh A, Pickering AC, Morrison JF, Wright T, Francis H, Fletcher A, Frank PI, Hannaford P. Relationship between exhaled nitric oxide and childhood asthma. Am J Respir Crit Care Med 1998; 158:1032–1036.

170. Salome CM, Roberts AM, Brown NJ, Dermand J, Marks GB, Woolcock AJ. Exhaled nitric oxide measurements in a population sample of young adults. Am J Respir Crit Care Med 1999; 159:911–916.

171. Leuppi JD, Downs SH, Downie SR, Marks GB, Salome CM. Exhaled nitric oxide levels in atopic children: relation to specific allergic sensitisation, AHR and respiratory symptoms. Thorax 2002; 57:518–523.

172. Baraldi E, Azzolin NM, Zanconato S, Dario C, Zacchello F. Corticosteroids decrease exhaled nitric oxide in children with acute asthma. J Pediatr 1997; 131:381–385.

173. Lim S, Jatakanon A, Meah S, Oates TK, Chung KF, Barnes PJ. Relationship between exhaled nitric oxide and mucosal eosinophilic inflammation in mild to moderately severe asthma. Thorax 2000; 55:184–188.

174. Powell H, Gibson PG. Inhaled corticosteroid doses in asthma: an evidence-based approach. Med J Aust 2003; 178:223–225.

175. Gibson PG, Simpson JL, Hankin R, Powell H, Henry RL. Relationship between induced sputum eosinophils and the clinical pattern of childhood asthma. Thorax 2000; 58:116–121.

176. Wark PA, Simpson J, Hensley MJ, Gibson PG. Airway inflammation in thunderstorm asthma. Clin Exp Allergy 2002; 32:1750–1756.

177. Green RH, Brightling CE, McKenna S, Hargadon B, Parker D, Bradding P, Wardlow AJ, Pavord ID. Asthma exacerbations and sputum eosinophil counts: a randomised controlled trial. Lancet 2002; 3360:1715–1721.

178. The British Thoracic Society, The National Asthma Campaign, The Royal College of Physicians of London in association with the General Practitioner in Asthma Group, the British Association of Accident and Emergency Medicine, the British Paediatric Respiratory Society, the Royal College of Paediatrics and Child Health. The British Guidelines on Asthma Management 1995 Review and Position Statement. Thorax 1997; 52:S1–S20.

179. Jatakanon A, Lim S, Kharitonov SA, Chung KF, Barnes PJ. Correlation between exhaled nitric oxide, sputum eosinophils, and methacholine responsiveness in patients with mild asthma. Thorax 1998; 53:91–95.

180. Boulet LP, Turcotte H, Brochu A. Persistence of airway obstruction and hyperresponsiveness in subjects with asthma remission. Chest 1994; 105: 1024–1031.

181. van Den Berge M, Meijer RJ, Kerstjens HA, de Reus DM, Koeter GH, Kauffman HF, Postma DS. PC_{20} adenosine 5′-monophosphate is more closely associated with airway inflammation in asthma than PC_{20} methacholine. Am J Respir Crit Care Med 2001; 163:1546–1550.

182. Barnes PJ. Inhaled glucocorticoids for asthma. N Engl J Med 1995; 332: 868–875.

183. Lipworth BJ. Systemic adverse effects of inhaled corticosteroid therapy: a systematic review and meta-analysis. Arch Intern Med 1999; 159:941–955.

184. Gibson PG, Wong BJ, Hepperle MJ, Kline PA, Girgis-Gabardo A, Guyatt G, Dolovich J, Denburg JA, Ramsdale EH, Hargreave FE. A research method to induce and examine a mild exacerbation of asthma by withdrawal of inhaled corticosteroid. Clin Exp Allergy 1992; 22:525–532.

185. Marabini A, Cardinalini G, Severini C, Ripandelli A, Siracusa A. Is normal bronchial responsiveness in asthmatics a reliable index for withdrawing inhaled corticosteroid treatment? Chest 1998; 113:964–967

186. Hawkins G, McMahon AD, Twaddle S, Wood SF, Ford I, Thomson NC. Stepping down inhaled corticosteroids in asthma: randomised controlled trial. Br Med J 2003; 326:1115–1117.

187. Mussaffi H, Springer C, Godfrey S. Increased bronchial responsiveness to exercise and histamine after allergen challenge in children with asthma. J Allergy Clin Immunol 1986; 77:48–52.

188. Aalbers R, Kauffman HF, Koeter GH, Postma DS, De Vries K, De Monchy JGR. Dissimilarity in methacholine and adenosine 5′-monophosphate responsiveness 3 and 24 h after allergen challenge. Am Rev Respir Dis 1991; 144:352–357.

189. Crimi E, Chiaramondia M, Milanese M, Rossi G, Brusasco V. Increased numbers of mast cells in bronchial mucosa after the late-phase asthmatic response to allergen. Am Rev Respir Dis 1991; 144:1282–1286.

190. Gauvreau GM, Ronnen GM, Watson RM, O'Byrne PM. Exercise-induced bronchoconstriction does not cause eosinophilic airway inflammation or airway hyperresponsiveness in subjects with asthma. Am J Respir Crit Care Med 2000; 162:1302–1307.

191. Murray AB, Ferguson AC. Dust-free bedrooms in the treatment of asthmatic children with house dust mite allergy: a controlled trial. Pediatrics 1983; 71:418–422.

192. Peroni DG, Boner AL, Vallone G, Antolini I, Warner JO. Effective allergen avoidance at high altitude reduces allergen-induced bronchial hyperresponsiveness. Am J Respir Crit Care Med 1994; 149:1442–1446.

193. Grootendorst DC, Dahlen SE, Van Den Bos JW, Duiverman EJ, Veselic-Charvat M, Vrijlandt EJ, O'Sullivan S, Kumlin M, Sterk PJ, Roldaan AC. Benefits of high altitude allergen avoidance in atopic adolescents with moderate to severe asthma, over and above treatment with high dose inhaled steroids. Clin Exp Allergy 2001; 31:400–408.

194. Platts-Mills TAE, Tovey ER, Mitchell EB, Moszoro H, Nock P, Wilkins SR. Reduction of bronchial hyperreactivity during prolonged allergen avoidance. Lancet 1982; 2(8300):675–678.

195. Vervloet D, Penaud A, Razzouk H, Senft M, Arnaud A, Boutin C, Charpin J. Altitude and house dust mites. J Allergy Clin Immunol 1982; 69:290–296.

196. Charpin D, Kleisbauer JP, Lanteaume A, Razzouk H, Vervloet D, Toumi M, Faraj F, Charpin J. Asthma and allergy to house-dust mites in populations living in high altitudes. Chest 1988; 93:758–761.

197. Fiorina A, Legnani D, Fasano V, Cogo A, Basnyat B, Passalacqua G, Scordamaglia A. Pollen, mite and mould samplings by a personal collector at high altitude in Nepal. J Invest Allergol Clin Immunol 1998; 8:85–88.

12

Induced Sputum in Asthma

D. E. SHAW, M. A. BERRY, R. H. GREEN, and I. D. PAVORD

Department of Respiratory Medicine and Thoracic Surgery, Institute for Lung Health,
   Glenfield Hospital,
Leicester, U.K.

Introduction

The goals of asthma management are the accurate diagnosis and effective control of symptoms, including nocturnal symptoms and exercise induced asthma, prevention of exacerbations, and the achievement of best pulmonary function with minimal side effects (1). Whilst this is achieved in the majority of patients, there remains a significant number who are misdiagnosed (2) or who suffer from troublesome symptoms and frequent exacerbations (3). The routine diagnosis and treatment of asthma in primary-care and most secondary care settings involves evaluating variable airflow obstruction with spirometry and peak flow measurement, and assessing symptom control, but does not normally assess the two cardinal features of asthma: airway inflammation and airway hyper-responsiveness. The question arises as to whether extending the goal of management to include these features may lead to better outcomes. Current treatment guidelines for asthma involve a concept of a stepwise increase in medication based on symptom control and peak flow measurements (1). However, patients who appear clinically well controlled on inhaled corticosteroids can still have evidence of airway inflammation and airway hyper-responsiveness (4,5) and be vulnerable to exacerbations, airway remodeling and possibly fixed airways obstruction (6,7). A treatment strategy based on an attempt to return airway responsiveness towards normal has been shown to reduce exacerbations and reduce sub-epithelial reticular basement thickening (8). The development of feasible and valid non-invasive methods to assess airway inflammation has made it possible to examine whether assessment of airway inflammation improves outcomes in patients with asthma. Assessment of airway inflammation may lead to more accurate diagnosis as well as better identification of vulnerable patients who need more intensive anti-inflammatory treatment. However, in order to be useful, the method used to assess airway inflammation needs to be feasible in a clinical setting and the results need to inform the physician about clinically important aspects of the disease that cannot be discerned by a simpler method. In this chapter, we discuss to what extent assessment of airway inflammation using induced sputum fulfills these criteria.

Feasibility of Measuring Airway Inflammation

Various methods exist to measure markers of airway inflammation. These include the measurement of cells and biomarkers found in induced sputum, blood eosinophil count, eosinophilic cationic protein (ECP) (in blood and sputum), assessment of exhaled gases (including exhaled nitric oxide and carbon monoxide), breath condensate, broncho alveolar lavage, and bronchial biopsy.

Table 1 summarizes the feasibility and what is known about the influence on patient outcomes of the various approaches to assessing airway inflammation. Sputum induction has been shown to be easy and safe and sputum differential cell counts and mediator concentrations have been demonstrated to be repeatable and responsive in a variety of clinical situations (9,10). It has the advantage of providing measurements of the type of airway inflammation (eosinophilic vs. neutrophilic) as well as its severity. The technique is inexpensive, although labor intensive and does require training and experience to obtain reliable results. There are now wellvalidated methods for induction and processing of induced sputum (Boxes 1 and 2). Our view is that these advantages of induced sputum make it the most useful non-invasive technique to measure airway inflammation in a secondary care setting. Exhaled nitric oxide has the advantage of being simple to measure and provides an immediate result, but it cannot provide information on the nature of the inflammatory response. Currently exhaled nitric oxide is most likely to find a role in primary care as an aid to diagnosis and to facilitate titration of anti-inflammatory treatment.

Table 1 Comparison of Methods Measuring Airway Inflammation

	Safety and ease of performing technique	Ease of analyzing result	Time to result	Cost	Influence on outcome proved	Potential use
Induced sputum	+++	++	3–4 hr	Moderate	Yes	Secondary care
Blood eosinophil count	++++	++++	30 min	Inexpensive	Possible (79)	Secondary care
Eosinophil cationic protein	++++	++++	3–4 hr	Moderate	Not proven conclusively	Research
Exhaled nitric oxide	++++	++++	Immediate	Expensive	Not proven	Research
Carbon monoxide	+++	+++	Immediate	Inexpensive	Studies awaited	Research
Breath condensate (hydrocarbons)	++	+	Moderate	Inexpensive	Studies awaited	Research
BAL, bronchial wash and biopsy	+	+	2 days	Moderate	Not proven	Tertiary care

Box 1 Protocol for Ssputum Induction
A doctor must be nearby during each procedure:

1. Measure baseline FEV_1 on three occasions as per the ERS guidelines.
2. Give 200 μg of salbutamol by MDI and via a spacer.
3. After 20 min, measure post-bronchodilator FEV_1 3 times. Use the best post-bronchodilator FEV_1 value to calculate any subsequent fall in FEV_1 during the procedure.
4. Do not proceed if the FEV_1 after inhalation of the short-acting β-agonist is less than 1.0 L.
5. Fill the nebulizer cup with 5 mL of 3% pyrogen-free hypertonic saline. Hold the nebulizer upright and do not adjust from the default maximum output setting. Ask the patient to breath tidally, whilst taking a slightly deeper breath every minute. Do not use a nose clip. Discontinue if significant symptoms occur or if the patient experiences undue discomfort. (A discard vessel should be available for the patient to spit out any excessive saliva generated during the induction).
6. After 5 min, ask the patient to rinse their mouth and throat with water and to blow their nose in order to reduce squamous cell contamination and post-nasal drip.
7. Ask the patient to cough any sputum into a plastic sputum pot using a deep cough. Several attempts at coughing should be made until the sound of the cough becomes dry and unproductive.
8. Measure FEV_1 [three measurements will be made if FEV_1 falls by greater than 10% or 200 mLs (whichever is greater) compared with the best post-bronchodilator FEV_1].
9. Steps 5–8 should be repeated again on two occasions with 4% and 5% pyrogen-free hypertonic saline, respectively, if the FEV_1 has not fallen by more than 10% or 200 mL (which ever is greater) of the best post-bronchodilator value. If the FEV_1 falls by more than 10% or 200 mL (whichever is greater) but less than 20% or 400 mL (whichever is greater), repeat steps 5–8 with the same concentration of saline. Patients should not breathe saline for > 15 min in total.
10. If the FEV_1 falls by more than 20% or 400 mL (which ever is greater) of the best post-bronchodilator value, or if significant symptoms occur, stop nebulization and administer repeat short-acting β-agonist.

Box 2 Preparation of Cytospins
Sputum is collected on ice and processed at 4°C within 2 hr of expectoration. Procedures 1–6 below must be performed on ice:

1. Select sputum plugs from saliva and transfer to Petri dish. Transfer sputum free from salivary contamination into an empty (pre-weighed) polypropylene centrifuge tube (opaque) with screw top.
2. Subtract the weight of the empty centrifuge tube from the weight of the centrifuge tube plus selected sputum to obtain the weight of sputum portion to be processed.
3. Add dithiothrietol (DTT) freshly diluted from a stock solution of 1–0.1% using phosphate buffered saline using 4× weight/volume (e.g., 4 mL DTT per gram of selected sputum).
4. Disperse sputum by repeated gentle aspiration into a plastic pipette, 15 sec vortex and 15 min rocking on a bench rocker on ice.
5. Add an equal volume of Dulbecco's phosphate buffered saline (D-PBS). Vortex for a further 15 sec, filter the sputum suspension through a 48 μm nylon gauze pre-wet flat with D-PBS, shake off excess and centrifuge at 2000 rpm (790 g) for 10 min. Aliquot all of the supernatant in 0.5 mL portions into 2 mL microtubes, leaving behind a covering of fluid and the undisturbed pellet. There should be sufficient supernatant for 2–4 microtubes of supernatant.
6. Resuspend the cell pellet in 0.5–1 mL of D-PBS (depending on size of cell pellet) and mix gently with a wide bore plastic pipette.
7. Assess total cell count and cell viability using a Neubauer hemocytometer and the trypan blue exclusion method:

   - Flood hemocytometer with 10 μl of cell suspension mixed thoroughly with 10 μl of 0.4% trypan blue (dilution = 2).
   - Count all cells in the center square and in the four 1 mm corner squares of chamber 1 of the hemocytometer. Cells should be classified as viable, non-viable and squamous (whether viable or not).
   - Calculate the mean number of cells per square and the portion of viable and squamous cells.
   - Calculate the total number of cells and the total cell count (cells/ml sputum).
   - Total number of cells = mean number of cells/square × 2 × 10,000 × volume cells resuspended in (mL).
   - Total cell count (cells/g sputum) = mean number of cells/square × 2 × 10,000 × volume cells resuspended in (ml)/weight of selected sputum (g).

8. Adjust the cell suspension to 0.5–0.75×10^6 cells/ml with D-PBS.

9. Use 50 µl to prepare two cytospins, and centrifuge at 450 rpm (18.1g) for 6 min using a Shandon III cytocentrifuge
10. Air dry four slides for at least 15 min at room temperature, then fix with methanol for 10 min.

Perform a 400 cell count (non-squamous cells), differentiating between eosinophils, neutrophils, macrophages, epithelial cells, and lymphocytes.

Methodology

Sputum induction using nebulized hypertonic saline is used to collect respiratory secretions from the airways of patients who do not expectorate spontaneously. It is generally agreed that the central airways are sampled with induced sputum; this view is supported by studies showing a greater proportion of granulocytes in both sputum and bronchial samples compared with bronchoalveolar lavage (11–13) and by the demonstration that sputum induction results in greater clearance of radiolabeled aerosol from the central airways than the peripheral airway (14). There is evidence that increasing the duration of sputum induction leads to sampling of more distal airways (15) although, as yet, the clinical utility of this technique has not been explored. The precise mechanism leading to production of secretions is not known, but it may involve both direct and indirect mechanisms. The increased osmolarity of the airway lining fluid during induction is thought to precipitate production of mucous by the submucosal glands and also increase the vascular permeability of the bronchial mucosa. It may also result in release of pro-inflammatory mediators and increased mucous production.

A variety of protocols for sputum induction have been published and shown to be safe provided patients are pre-treated with bronchodilators and monitored carefully (16). Risk factors for bronchoconstriction include a low baseline FEV_1% predicted (17), overuse of short-acting β_2-agonists (18), and poor asthma control (19). Theoretically, higher nebulizer output, higher concentration of inhaled saline, a longer duration of saline inhalation and reduced frequency and timing of safety assessment by forced expiratory volume in 1 sec or peak expiratory flow might also influence safety. The use of higher output nebulizers have also been associated with the development of a sputum neutrophilia 24 hr after sputum induction. Whether this is seen with the low output nebulizers is unknown. Our practise is to use a relatively low output ultrasonic nebulizer (output 0.7–0.9 mL/min) since there is wide experience with this method and it has been shown to be successful in various settings (9,20). Furthermore, there are theoretical reasons to suggest that that the risk of bronchoconstriction and the effect of sputum induction on neutrophil counts might be less (21).

Table 2 Cell Types and Molecular Markers that have been Successfully Measured in Induced Sputum

Cells	Effector mediators	Cellular markers	Cytokines
Eosinophils	Leukotrienes C/D/ E_4	Eosinophilic cationic protein	Interleukin-8
Neutrophils	Prostaglandin D_2	Neutrophil elastase	
Macrophages	Histamine		
Lymphocytes			
Epithelial Cells			

Once expectorated sputum should be processed within 2 hr. There is evidence that sputum can be stored for up to 9 hr in a refrigerator at 4°C or that sputum can be snap frozen for longer without affecting cell counts (22), although experience with these techniques is limited. The whole expectorate or selected sputum plugs can be processed. The latter approach has the advantage of producing better quality cytospins, which may result in more repeatable counts (23,24). Sputum plugs are selected and centrifuged with dithiothrietol. The total cell count, cell viability, and squamous cell contamination are assessed using a hemocytometer. Differential cell counts are determined by counting 400 leucocytes on an appropriately stained cytospin. Other biomarkers can also be measured in the sputum supernatant. Some of the molecular markers of airway inflammation that have been successfully measured in sputum are shown in Table 2.

Measurement Characteristics of Induced Sputum

Induced sputum is well validated (10) and normal ranges have been published for large adult populations (25,26). Age has been shown to influence differential sputum neutrophil counts, with the higher values occurring in the older age groups (Table 3). Up to 80% of corticosteroid-naïve patients (27) and 50% of corticosteroid treated patients (28) with current asthmatic symptoms have a sputum eosinophil count above the normal range. There is good evidence that the sputum differential eosinophils, macrophage and neutrophil counts, and the sputum supernatant concentration of ECP, cysteinyl-leukotrienes, prostanoids, and IL-8 can be measured repeatably in asthma (23,27,29) and COPD (30). The differential lymphocyte and epithelial cell count and the total cell count are less repeatable. The sputum eosinophil count is responsive in that it increases when asthma worsens [e.g., after allergen challenge and following relevant occupational exposures (31–33)], and decreases when asthma improves with inhaled corticosteroid treatment (20). There is a suggestion that the sputum eosinophil count is more responsive to change following treatment with corticosteroids

Table 3 Mean (SD) Differential Cell Counts (%) and Total Cell Count ($\times 10^6$/ml sputum) for All Subjects and When Subgrouped by Age. *Source:* From Thomas et al. (80) and in two other studies—Belda et al. (25) and Spanevello et al. (26).

	Data from Thomas et al. (80)						Belda et al. (25)	Spanevello et al. (26)
	Total population	0–29 years	30–39 years	40–49 years	50–59 years	60+ years		
Number (male)	66 (24)	17 (9)	12 (4)	13 (3)	13 (2)	11 (6)	96 (53)	90 (46)
Neutrophil	47.0 (27.0)	26.9 (19.8)	38.4 (19.2)	40.4 (25.2)	69.3 (20.8)	68.5 (20.6)	37.5 (64.0)	27.3 (13)
Lymphocyte	1.0 (1.4)	1.0 (1.0)	1.1 (1.3)	0.8 (1.1)	0.6 (0.7)	1.5 (2.8)	1.0 (2.6)	1.0 (1.2)
Eosinophil	0.3 (0.6)	0.5 (0.8)	0.2 (0.5)	0.3 (0.3)	0.2 (0.3)	0.3 (0.6)	0.4 (1.1)	0.6 (0.8)
Macrophage	49.0 (25.2)	65.6 (17.8)	59.5 (16.7)	56.6 (25.2)	27.6 (20.2)	28.5 (18.5)	58.8 (86.1)	69.2 (13)
Epithelial	2.5 (3.2)	3.3 (3.2)	1.5 (1.6)	2.3 (1.6)	2.5 (4.4)	2.4 (4.4)	1.6 (4.4)	1.5 (1.8)
Total cell count $\times 10^6$/ml	2.1 (2.36)	2.9 (2.5)	2.1 (1.5)	1.5 (1.0)	1.6 (1.5)	2.3 (4.1)	4.1 (9.7)	2.7 (2.5)

(20,34) or anti-IL-5 (35,36) than tissue eosinophil counts. Currently, no intervention has been consistently shown to decrease the sputum differential neutrophil count. There are theoretical reasons to suggest that the total neutrophil count may be a more responsive measure than the differential count when the sputum differential neutrophil count is high, since the relationship between them becomes relatively flat above a differential neutrophil count of 80% (37).

Findings in Asthma

Asthma has been traditionally viewed as a condition where eosinophilic airway inflammation causes airway hyper-responsiveness, which in turn leads to variable airflow obstruction and symptoms. This hypothesis is deeply embedded, to the point where it is incorporated into recent definitions of asthma (1). However cross-sectional and longitudinal studies of airway inflammation using sputum induction in large populations with a diverse range of presentations suggest that this hypothesis requires modification.

Our view of the importance of eosinophilic airway inflammation in the pathogenesis of asthma has been heavily influenced by bronchoscopy studies performed over the last 20 years (38). These, by necessity, were largely limited to young volunteers with mild disease. The development of a non-invasive technique to assess airway inflammation has made it possible to relate the presence of airway inflammation to objective measures of disordered airway function in larger and more heterogeneous populations than was possible with bronchoscopy studies. In general, these studies have contradicted findings in the earlier bronchoscopy studies in that they have not found a correlation between the sputum eosinophil count and various markers of airway dysfunction (39–43).

One surprising observation has been that a subset of symptomatic asthmatics do not have sputum evidence of eosinophilic airway inflammation (20,41–43). Many have a sputum neutrophilia. This sputum profile is evident in corticosteroid-naïve (42) as well as corticosteroid-treated subjects (43–45) suggesting it is not always an artifact related to treatment. Importantly, patients with non-eosinophilic asthma respond less well to inhaled budesonide than a group with more typical sputum features (20,42). Similar sputum findings have been reported in more severe asthmatics (43,44), and Wenzel (45) has identified a subgroup of patients with refractory asthma who have bronchoscopic evidence of neutrophilic airway inflammation, normal eosinophil counts, and a normal basement membrane thickness. These findings suggest the presence of a distinct asthma phenotype characterized by a predominantly neutrophilic airway inflammatory response and relative corticosteroid resistance across the range of asthma severity. However, they are based on single observations, and in a variable disease there is a clear need to establish whether this asthma phenotype and the associated impaired response to corticosteroid treatment persists in the longer term.

Thus, cross-sectional studies suggest that to a large extent disordered airway function and eosinophilic airway inflammation appear to be independently regulated, suggesting that our earlier paradigm of a simple causal relationship between them needs to be modified. The real patient examples shown in Figures 1 and 2 illustrate this point well.

Within patients, there is a relationship between change in airway function and eosinophilic airway inflammation following interventions such as allergen challenge (31) and treatment with corticosteroids (20), suggesting that the relationship between changes in these markers within patients might be closer than that between patients. However, whether changes in eosinophilic airway inflammation are causally linked to changes in airway function has been called into question by recent findings with humanized monoclonal antibodies to IL-5. One study has shown that the antibody causes a profound and long lasting reduction in blood and induced sputum eosinophil counts but has no effect on airway responsiveness, lung function,

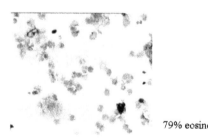

79% eosinophils

Week 2 date	12/10	13/10	14/10	15/10	16/10	17/10	18/10
Daytime asthma	0	0	0	0	0	0	0
Night time wakening	0	0	0	0	0	0	0
Peak flow AM/PM	440/500	440/490	440/470	440/470	430/470	430/470	430/460
No. of puffs of ventolin	2	2	2	2	2	2	2

Figure 1 Induced sputum cytospin preparation (*top*) and diary card recordings (*bottom*) from a 42-year old asthmatic with severe corticosteroid-dependent but currently stable asthma who had three severe exacerbations requiring ventilation in the past 3 years. Despite apparently good clinical control at the time of study, this patient has markedly raised numbers of eosinophils in the sputum (note the eosinophilic staining of the cytoplasm and characteristic bi-lobed nucleus).

0% eosinophils

Week 2 date	22/11	23	24	26	27	28	29
Daytime asthma	2	2	2	2	3	1	1
Night time wakening	3	3	2	3	3	2	3
Peak flow AM/PM	290/300	210/250	200/230	300/250	280/200	350/350	400/350
No. of puffs of ventolin	11	15	13	12	16	8	6

Figure 2 Induced sputum cytospin preparation (*top*) and diary card recordings (*bottom*) from a 22-year-old female asthmatic with unstable asthma despite use of inhaled corticosteroids. The majority of cells seen are macrophages. Although this patient does not here sputum eosinophilia, she has unstable asthma.

or symptoms before or after allergen challenge (36). In another study, there was no evidence of improvement in traditional markers of asthma control in a cohort of patients with more severe asthma who were symptomatic and had disordered airway function despite treatment with high dose inhaled corticosteroids (44). One problem in interpreting these studies is that the anti-IL-5 antibody only partially reduces the tissue eosinophilia (36), although the effects seen were significant, and probably equivalent to the effects of inhaled and oral corticosteroids on tissue eosinophilia. Our view is that the findings with anti-IL-5 monoclonal antibodies strongly suggest that changes in airway function and eosinophilic airway inflammation are independent and that the abnormalities of airway function seen in asthma are causally linked to other aspects of the inflammatory response that, although closely linked to eosinophilic airway inflammation, can be disassociated from it (46).

What Features of the Inflammatory Response Contribute to Disordered Airway Function?

A dissociation between eosinophilic airway inflammation and airway hyper-responsiveness can be clearly observed in patients with eosinophilic bronchitis; a condition characterised by corticosteroid-responsive cough and the presence of a sputum eosinophilia occurring in the absence of variable airflow obstruction or airway hyper-responsiveness (47–50). Closer study of this condition may be particularly informative since any difference in pathology between the two conditions is likely to give important clues to the features that are relevant to the different functional associations. In a recent study, we found that several of the traditional characteristics of the immunopathology of asthma, including a submucosal eosinophilia and thickening of the basement membrane and lamina reticularis, are also features of eosinophilic bronchitis and are therefore unlikely to be critical factors causing airway hyper-responsiveness or variable airflow obstruction. Indeed, the only difference that we observed in our detailed comparison of the two conditions was increased mast cells within the airway smooth muscle in asthma (51). These findings suggest that localization of mast cells within the airway wall, rather than the presence of eosinophils in the airway mucosa, is the crucial determinant of the functional associations of airway inflammation (46,51,52).

How Does Eosinophilic Airway Inflammation Contribute to the Pathophysiology of Asthma?

Both eosinophilic bronchitis and asthma are associated with cough, and it is possible that eosinophilic airway inflammation is directly responsible for this aspect of the asthmatic process. Our previous demonstration of a significant correlation between the improvement in cough reflex sensitivity and fall in induced sputum eosinophil count following treatment of subjects with eosinophilic bronchitis with inhaled corticosteroids would be consistent with a causal association (53). We have reported an increased rate of decline in FEV_1 and the development of fixed airflow obstruction in a patient with eosinophilic bronchitis (54) and it is possible that this important complication of chronic asthma is also related to eosinophilic airway inflammation.

Exacerbations are an important feature of asthma and exacerbation frequency is increasingly seen as an important outcome measure in clinical trials (55). The pathophysiology of exacerbations is complex, but likely includes airway mucosal edema, mucous hypersecretion, and decrease of the airway lumen by impaction with cellular debris, as well as airway smooth muscle contraction. Recent studies have shown that the exacerbation frequency does not relate closely to symptoms and measures of disordered airway function suggesting that the mechanisms responsible for these features of asthma are different (40,56,57). This view is supported by the findings of the FACET study, which showed that higher dose inhaled corticosteroids had a marked beneficial effect on exacerbation frequency, but relatively less effect on symptoms and peak expiratory flow, whereas with the addition of long-acting β_2-agonists the opposite was true (3). The beneficial effect of corticosteroids on exacerbation frequency would be consistent with the view that eosinophilic airway inflammation is particularly important in the genesis of exacerbations. In keeping with this, several recent studies have shown that the sputum eosinophil count is an independent variable predicting the occurrence of an asthma exacerbation after inhaled corticosteroid withdrawal (58–60). Moreover, significant increases in the sputum eosinophil count occur well before the onset of exacerbations (61).

Clinical Role for Monitoring Airway Inflammation

Role in Diagnosis

None of the currently available diagnostic tests are sufficiently sensitive to rule out asthma (62), with the result that treatment trials are often instigated without good evidence of variable airflow obstruction, airway hyper-responsiveness or airway inflammation. One study has shown that out of 263 subjects referred to a tertiary referral center with suspected asthma, 160 received an alternative diagnosis (63). Many of these had received prolonged treatment with potentially toxic therapy before the correct diagnosis was reached. Even in tertiary referral centers the diagnosis of refractory asthma can be difficult to make with certainty (2). The presence of a sputum eosinophilia in asthma is sufficiently common to suggest that it may have a role in the diagnosis of asthma. Two studies have directly addressed this question. Hunter et al. (62) showed that the validity of a sputum eosinophil count outside the normal range in identifying asthma (defined as consistent symptoms with objective evidence of abnormal variable airflow obstruction) was better than PEF amplitude % mean and the acute bronchodilator response and approached the sensitivity and specificity of measurement of airway responsiveness. Smith et al. (64) have reported similar findings, although in this study a high exhaled nitric oxide concentration achieved a similarly high diagnostic accuracy Table 4.

There is evidence that incorporation of induced sputum into the routine diagnostic workup of patients with asthma might identify patients with a high risk of adverse outcomes more reliably since a high sputum eosinophil count has been associated with exacerbation risk (58). It might also facilitate the recognition of patients with non-eosinophilic asthma allowing the clinician to avoid the unnecessary use of high dose corticosteroids.

Identification of Corticosteroid-Responsive Disease

There is increasing evidence that the presence of a sputum eosinophilia may predict corticosteroid responsiveness. This was first clearly demonstrated in the 1950s by Morrow-Brown (65) who showed that asthmatic patients with

Table 4 Sensitivity and Specificity of Spirometry, Methacholine PC20 and Peak Expiratory Flow Amplitude % of Mean, and Sputum and Blood Eosinophilia in the Diagnosis of Asthma.
Spirometry values are given as mean (SEM). PEF values recorded as amplitude percent of mean (A%M). This is the difference between the highest and lowest PEF over 14 days as a percentage of the mean PEF, and is expressed as the mean. Blood and sputum eosinophil counts, and PC_{20} are given as geometric mean (log SEM).

Test	Normal value	Sensitivity (%)	Specificity (%)	Positive predictive value	Negative predictive value
FEV_1/FVC	> 76.6	61	60	84	31
BD response	< 2.9%	49	70	85	29
PEF A%M	< 21.6%	43	75	86	28
PC_{20}	> 8 mg/mL	91	90	97	75
Sputum eosinophils	< 1%	72	80	93	46
Blood eosinophils	< 6.3%	21	100	100	27

BD, Bronchodilator.
Source: Reproduced from Hunter et al. (62).

an eosinophilia improved with systemic corticosteroids, whereas those without a sputum eosinophilia did not. We have also found that patients with non-eosinophilic asthma respond less well to inhaled budesonide than a group with more typical sputum features (20,42). This is also the case with longer-term corticosteroid treatment in patients with more severe asthma (9). A sputum eosinophilia is a predictor of a steroid response irrespective of the clinical context: patients with chronic cough and a sputum eosinophilia respond well to inhaled corticosteroids compared to those without an eosinophilia, and similarly patients with COPD with a sputum eosinophilia respond better to corticosteroids than those without (53,66–68).

Role in Monitoring Asthma

The clear implication of the studies discussed above is that eosinophilic airway inflammation is more closely related to the genesis of asthma exacerbations than day-to-day symptoms and airway caliber. Thus, the clinician who relies on an assessment of symptoms and simple tests of lung function might have a limited ability to predict the extent of eosinophilic airway inflammation and, by implication, the exacerbation risk (69). There might also be a danger of unnecessary use of high dose inhaled and oral corticosteroids in a patient who has non-eosinophilic, corticosteroid resistant disease. A recent study has directly tested the hypothesis that a management approach that measures and attempts to normalize eosinophilic airway inflammation, as well as minimize symptoms and maximize lung function, might be particularly effective in preventing exacerbations.

We have recently reported a randomized controlled trial of 74 subjects attending outpatients with moderate-to-severe asthma (9). Subjects were randomized to treatment either according to the British Thoracic Society guidelines or to a management strategy where treatment was adjusted according to the sputum eosinophil counts. In the sputum management group, decisions about anti-inflammatory treatment were made in accordance with an algorithm based on control of symptoms and maintenance of the sputum eosinophil count at or below 3% with a minimum dose of anti-inflammatory treatment. The 3% cut-off was chosen because this was previously shown to identify individuals with corticosteroid-responsive asthma (20). If the sputum eosinophil count was less than 1%, anti-inflammatory treatment was reduced irrespective of asthma control. If the eosinophil count was 1–3%, no changes to anti-inflammatory treatment were made, and if eosinophil count was greater than 3%, anti-inflammatory treatment was increased. Decisions about changes in bronchodilator treatment were based on individual patients' symptoms, peak expiratory flow readings, and use of rescue β_2-agonists compared with baseline using the same criteria as in the BTS management group. Management decisions were made by an independent individual who was unaware of the clinical characteristics of the patient, and who recorded separate treatment plans to be followed depending on whether the patients' asthma was poorly or well controlled. The strategy based on sputum eosinophil counts achieved significantly better control of eosinophilic related airway inflammation over the 12 months of the trial (Fig. 3). There was also an improvement in methacholine PC_{20}. Both management strategies achieved equivalent control of symptoms, quality of life, and disordered airway function (Fig. 3). However, in the sputum management group, there was a marked reduction in severe asthma exacerbations and significantly fewer hospital admissions with asthma exacerbations (Fig. 4). This study therefore supports the view that assessment of eosinophilic airway inflammation provides additional important information, necessary for the optimum management of more severe asthmatics. It also supports the view that there is a causal association between eosinophilic airway inflammation and asthma exacerbations, although it remains possible that airway eosinophilia is a surrogate marker of another airway abnormality, and that these other corticosteroid-responsive abnormalities are more important in the pathogenesis of asthma exacerbations. A key remaining question is whether anti-IL-5 therapy, which has a more selective effect on eosinophilic airway inflammation, has any effect on exacerbation frequency.

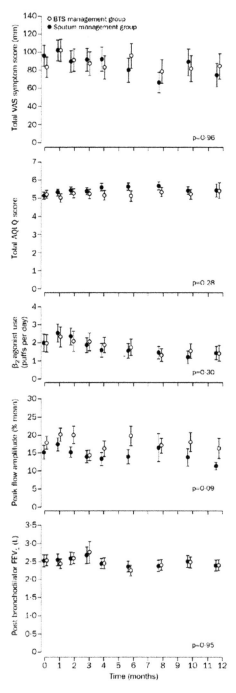

Figure 3   *(Caption on facing page)*

Results: Severe Exacerbartions

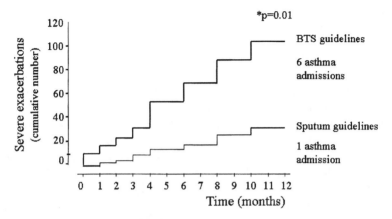

Figure 4 Comparison of effects of two treatment strategies on rates of severe exacerbations of asthma. One strategy (BTS guidelines) utilized standard guidelines of the British Thoracic Society (BTS) and the other (sputum guidelines) adjusted the anti-inflammatory treatment with corticosteroids based on the eosinophil counts (see text for criteria). *Source:* Reproduced from Green et al. (9).

Future Directions

Sputum induction may shed more light on the complex relationship between asthma and COPD, as it can be used to easily quantify and qualify the different cell types present. The presence of a sputum eosinophilia in COPD is related to corticosteroid responsive disease (66). Further work is required to determine whether the presence of a sputum eosinophilia in COPD is related to other clinically important outcomes such as exacerbation frequency or long-term decline in FEV_1. Analysis of sputum cells may also provide insight into novel cellular mechanisms. For example, a recent study by Duncan et al. (70) suggested that asthma severity inversely correlates with the induced sputum eosinophil apoptotic ratio. This study

---

Figure 3 *(facing page)* Comparison of effects of two treatment strategies on symptoms score [assessed by visual analog score (VAS)]. Asthma quality of life questionnaire (AQLQ), β_2-agonist use to relieve asthma symptoms, peak expiratory flow, and post-bronchodilator FEV_1. One strategy (BTS management group) utilizsed standard guidelines of the British Thoracic Society (BTS) and the other (sputum management group) adjusted the anti-inflammatory treatment with corticosteroids based on the eosinophil counts (see text for criteria). Source: Reproduced from Green et al. (9).

provides additional evidence that eosinophil apoptosis may be important in the resolution of eosinophilic airway inflammation in asthma and raises the possibility that asthma severity may be related to a lower turn over of eosinophils.

One of the major limitations of sputum induction is that the induction and processing are labor intensive and need to be done relatively quickly. New advances in the preservation of sputum may help circumvent this problem (71). A further problem is that it is not possible to get an immediate result, limiting the clinical utility of the technique. There is an important need for simpler measures that might be applicable in primary care settings. Blood eosinophilic cationic protein (ECP) concentration is a potential marker. A small study of 31 patients showed that blood eosinophil counts of $> 0.4 \times 10^9$/L, blood ECP of $>20 \,\mu$/L, and ECP in the sputum supernatant of $> 40 \,\mu$/L all predicted mild exacerbations in patients with mild and well-controlled asthma (72). However, another study has shown that ECP concentration in blood or sputum supernatant was not predictive of a favorable response to steroids in a mixed group of asthmatics whereas the sputum eosinophil count was (73). Exhaled nitric oxide has the advantages of being simple to measure and providing an immediate result. Exhaled nitric oxide has been shown to be related to sputum eosinophil counts (74) and may provide a non-invasive method for measuring eosinophilic airway inflammation. It also offers the possibility of relating asthma severity to the area of lung affected, since it is feasible to derive a measure of alveolar nitric oxide by analyzing the nitric oxide output at different flow rates (75). Lehtimaki et al., have used exhaled nitric oxide to demonstrate that patients with nocturnal symptoms have elevated alveolar nitric oxide concentrations (76) and that alveolar nitric oxide concentration does not fall in response to treatment with inhaled corticosteroids (77). Further work is required to evaluate the role of exhaled nitric oxide in monitoring asthma and other airways diseases.

Summary

Induced sputum is safe in both children (78) and adults (16), repeatable and inexpensive. It provides a clinically important marker of airway inflammation in the diagnosis of asthma. It can help guide treatment dosing and response and can reliably predict exacerbations. It can also be used to measure a variety of cells, effector mediators, cellular markers, and cytokines leading to new insights into the pathophysiology and management of asthma and airways disease. The development of this technique has been a significant advance in asthma management and has lead to important new insights into the disease.

References

1. British guideline on the management of asthma. Thorax 2003; 58(suppl 1): il–i94.
2. Robinson DS, Campbell DA, Durham SR, Pfeffer J, Barnes PJ, Chung KF. Systematic assessment of dtfficult-to-treat asthma. Eur Respir J 2003; 22(3): 478–483.
3. Tattersfield AE, Postma DS, Barnes PJ, Svensson K, Bauer CA, O'Byrne PM, et al. Exacerbations of asthma: a descriptive study of 425 severe exacerbations. The FACET International Study Group. Am J Respir Crit Care Med 1999; 160(2):594–599 .
4. Sont JK, Han J, van Krieken JM, Evertse CE, Hooijer R, Willems LN, et al. Relationship between the inflammatory infiltrate in bronchial biopsy specimens and clinical severity of asthma in patients treated with inhaled steroids. Thorax 1996; 51(5):496–502.
5. Boulet LP, Turcotte H, Brochu A. Persistence of airway obstruction and hyperresponsiveness in subjects with asthma remission. Chest 1994; 105(4): 1024–1031.
6. Beckett PA, Howarth PH. Pharmacotherapy and airway remodelling in asthma? Thorax 2003; 58(2):163–174.
7. Lange P, Parner J, Vestbo J, Schnohr P, Jensen G. A 15-year follow-up study of ventilatory function in adults with asthma. N Engl J Med 1998; 339(17): 1194–1200.
8. Sont JK, Willems LN, Bel EH, van Krieken JH, Vandenbroucke JP, Sterk PJ. Clinical control and histopathologic outcome of asthma when using airway hyperresponsiveness as an additional guide to long-term treatment. The AMPUL Study Group. Am J Respir Crit Care Med 1999; 159(4 Pt 1):1043–1051.
9. Green RH, Brightling CE, McKenna S, Hargadon B, Parker D, Bradding P, et al. Asthma exacerbations and sputum eosinophil counts: a randomised controlled trial. Lancet 2002; 360(9347):1715 (NLM-MEDLINE).
10. Pavord ID, Pizzichini MM, Pizzichini E, Hargreave FE. The use of induced sputum to investigate airway inflammation. Thorax 1997; 52(6):498–501.
11. Alexis N, Soukup J, Ghio A, Becker S. Sputum phagocytes from healthy individuals are functional and activated: a flow cytometric comparison with cells in bronchoalveolar lavage and peripheral blood. Clin Immunol 2000; 97(l):21–32.
12. In't Veen JC, Grootendorst DC, Bel EH, Smits HH, Van Der KM, Sterk PJ, et al. CD1 lb and L-selectin expression on eosinophils and neutrophils in blood and induced sputum of patients with asthma compared with normal subjects. Clin Exp Allergy 1998; 28(5):606–615.
13. Moodley YP, Krishnan V, Lalloo UG. Neutrophils in induced sputum arise from central airways. Eur Respir J 2000; 15(l):36–40.
14. Alexis NE, Hu SC, Zeman K, Alter T, Bennett WD. Induced sputum derives from the central airways: confirmation using a radiolabeled aerosol bolus delivery technique. Am J Respir Crit Care Med 2001; 164(10 Pt 1):1964–1970.
15. Gershman NH, Liu H, Wong HH, Liu JT, Fahy JV. Fractional analysis of sequential induced sputum samples during sputum induction: evidence that

different lung compartments are sampled at different time points. J Allergy Clin Immunol 1999; 104(2 Pt l):322–328.

16. Paggiaro PL, Chanez P, Holz O, Ind PW, Djukanovic R, Maestrelli P, et al. Sputum induction. Eur Respir J 2002; 37(suppl):3s–8s.

17. de la Fuente PT, Romagnoli M, Godard P, Bousquet J, Chanez P. Safety of inducing sputum in patients with asthma of varying severity. Am J Respir Crit Care Med 1998; 157(4 Pt 1):1127–1130.

18. Pizzichini E, Pizzichini MM, Leigh R, Djukanovic R, Sterk PJ. Safety of sputum induction. Eur Respir J 2002; 37(suppl):9s–18s.

19. ten Brinke A, de Lange C, Zwinderman AH, Rabe KF, Sterk PJ, Bel EH. Sputum induction in severe asthma by a standardized protocol: predictors of excessive bronchoconstriction. Am J Respir Crit Care Med 2001; 164(5):749–753.

20. Pavord ID, Brightling CE, Woltmann G, Wardlaw AJ. Non-eosinophilic corticosteroid unresponsive asthma. Lancet 1999; 353(9171):2213–2214.

21. Pavord ID. Sputum induction to assess airway inflammation: is it an inflammatory stimulus? Thorax 1998; 53(2):79–80.

22. Efthimiadis A, Jayaram L, Weston S, Carruthers S, Hargreave FE. Induced sputum: time from expectoration to processing. Eur Respir J 2002; 19(4): 706–708.

23. Gershman NH, Wong HH, Liu JT, Mahlmeister MJ, Fahy JV. Comparison of two methods of collecting induced sputum in asthmatic subjects. Eur Respir J 1996; 9(12):2448–2453.

24. Ward R, Woltmann G, Wardlaw AJ, Pavord ID. Between-observer repeatability of sputum differential cell counts. Influence of cell viability and squamous cell contamination. Clin Exp Allergy 1999; 29(2):248–252.

25. Belda J, Leigh R, Parameswaran K, O'Byrne PM, Sears MR, Hargreave FE. Induced sputum cell counts in healthy adults. Am J Respir Crit Care Med 2000; 161(2 Pt l):475–478.

26. Spanevello A, Confalonieri M, Sulotto F, Romano F, Balzano G, Migliori GB, et al. Induced sputum cellularity. Reference values and distribution in normal volunteers. Am J Respir Crit Care Med 2000; 162(3 Pt 1):1172–1174.

27. Pizzichini E, Pizzichini MM, Efthimiadis A, Evans S, Morris MM, Squillace D, et al. Indices of airway inflammation in induced sputum: reproducibility and validity of cell and fluid-phase measurements. Am J Respir Crit Care Med 1996; 154(2 Pt l):308–317.

28. Louis R, Lau LC, Bron AO, Roldaan AC, Radermecker M, Djukanovic R. The relationship between airways inflammation and asthma severity. Am J Respir Crit Care Med 2000; 161(1):9–16.

29. In't Veen JC, de Gouw HW, Smits HH, Sont JK, Hiemstra PS, Sterk PJ, et al. Repeatability of cellular and soluble markers of inflammation in induced sputum from patients with asthma. Eur Respir J 1996; 9(12):2441–2447.

30. Brightling CE, Monterio W, Green RH, Parker D, Morgan MD, Wardlaw AJ, et al. Induced sputum and other outcome measures in chronic obstructive pulmonary disease: safety and repeatability. Respir Med 2001; 95(12):999–1002.

31. Pin I, Freitag AP, O'Byrne PM, Girgis-Gabardo A, Watson RM, Dolovich J, et al. Changes in the cellular profile of induced sputum after allergen-induced asthmatic responses. Am Rev Respir Dis 1992; 145(6):1265–1269.

32. Wark PA, Simpson J, Hensley MJ, Gibson PG. Airway inflammation in thunderstorm asthma. Clin Exp Allergy 2002; 32(l2):1750–1756.

33. Lemiere C, Pizzichini MM, Balkissoon R, Clelland L, Efthimiadis A, O'Shaughnessy D, et al. Diagnosing occupational asthma: use of induced sputum. Eur Respir J 1999; 13(3):482–488.

34. Bentley AM, Hamid Q, Robinson DS, Schotman E, Meng Q, Assoufi B, et al. Prednisolone treatment in asthma. Reduction in the numbers of eosinophils, T cells, tryptase-only positive mast cells, and modulation of IL-4, IL-5, and interferon-gamma cytokine gene expression within the bronchial mucosa. Am J Respir Crit Care Med 1996; 153(2):551–556.

35. Flood-Page P, Menzies-Gow A, Phipps S, Ying S, Wangoo A, Ludwig MS, et al. Anti-IL-5 treatment reduces deposition of ECM proteins in the bronchial subepithelial basement membrane of mild atopic asthmatics. J Clin Invest 2003; 112(7):1029–1036.

36. Leckie MJ, ten Brinke A, Khan J, Diamant Z, O'Connor BJ, Walls CM, et al. Effects of an interleukin-5 blocking monoclonal antibody on eosinophils, airway hyper-responsiveness, and the late asthmatic response. Lancet 2000; 356(9248):2144–2148.

37. Neale N. The relationship between total and differential cell counts in induced sputum. Eur Respir J 2002; 20(3):274s.

38. Djukanovic R, Roche WR, Wilson JW, Beasley CR, Twentyman OP, Howarth RH, et al. Mucosal inflammation in asthma. Am Rev Respir Dis 1990; 142(2):434–457.

39. Crimi E, Spanevello A, Neri M, Ind PW, Rossi GA, Brusasco V. Dissociation between airway inflammation and airway hyperresponsiveness in allergic asthma. Am J Respir Crit Care Med 1998; 157(l):4–9.

40. Rosi E, Ronchi MC, Grazzini M, Duranti R, Scano G. Sputum analysis, bronchial hyperresponsiveness, and airway function in asthma: results of a factor analysis. J Allergy Clin Immunol 1999; 103(2 Pt l):232–237.

41. Gibson PG, Simpson JL, Saltos N. Heterogeneity of airway inflammation in persistent asthma : evidence of neutrophilic inflammation and increased sputum interleukin-8. Chest 2001; 119(5):1329–1336.

42. Green RH, Brightling CE, Woltmann G, Parker D, Wardlaw AJ, Pavord ID. Analysis of induced sputum in adults with asthma: identification of subgroup with isolated sputum neutrophilia and poor response to inhaled corticosteroids. Thorax 2002; 57(10):875–879.

43. Jatakanon A, Uasuf C, Maziak W, Lim S, Chung KF, Barnes PJ. Neutrophilic inflammation in severe persistent asthma. Am J Respir Crit Care Med 1999; 160(5 Pt l):1532–1539.

44. The ENFUMOSA cross-sectional European multicentre study of the clinical phenotype of chronic severe asthma. Eur Respir J 2003; 22(3):470–477.

45. Wenzel SE. A different disease, many diseases or mild asthma gone bad? Challenges of severe asthma. Eur Respir J 2003; 22(3):397–398.

46. Brightling CE, Symon FA, Birring SS, Bradding P, Wardlaw AJ, Pavord ID. Comparison of airway immunopathology of eosinophilic bronchitis and asthma. Thorax 2003; 58(6):528–532.

47. Carney IK, Gibson PG, Murree-Allen K, Saltos N, Olson LG, Hensley MJ. A systematic evaluation of mechanisms in chronic cough. Am J Respir Crit Care Med 1997; 156(l):211–216.

48. Brightling CE, Ward R, Goh KL, Wardlaw AJ, Pavord ID. Eosinophilic bronchitis is an important cause of chronic cough. Am J Respir Crit Care Med 1999; 160(2):406–410.

49. Birring SS, Berry M, Brightling CE, Pavord ID. Eosinophilic bronchitis: clinical features, management and pathogenesis. Am J Respir Med 2003; 2(2): 169–173.

50. Gibson PG, Dolovich J, Denburg J, Ramsdale EH, Hargreave FE. Chronic cough: eosinophilic bronchitis without asthma. Lancet 1989; l(8651): 1346–1348.

51. Brightling CE, Bradding P, Symon FA, Holgate ST, Wardlaw AJ, Pavord ID. Mast-cell infiltration of airway smooth muscle in asthma. N Engl J Med 2002; 346(22):1699–1705.

52. Brightling CE, Bradding P, Pavord ID, Wardlaw AJ. New insights into the role of the mast cell in asthma. Clin Exp Allergy 2003; 33(5):550–556.

53. Brightling CE, Ward R, Wardlaw AJ, Pavord ID. Airway inflammation, airway responsiveness and cough before and after inhaled budesonide in patients with eosinophilic bronchitis. Eur Respir J 2000; 15(4):682–686.

54. Brightling CE, Woltmann G, Wardlaw AJ, Pavord ID. Development of irreversible airflow obstruction in a patient with eosinophilic bronchitis without asthma. Eur Respir J 1999; 14(5):1228–1230.

55. Cockcroft DW, Swystun VA. Asthma control versus asthma severity. J Allergy Clin Immunol 1996; 98(6 Pt 1):1016–1018.

56. Reddel H, Ware S, Marks G, Salome C, Jenkins C, Woolcock A. Differences between asthma exacerbations and poor asthma control. Lancet 1999; 353(9150):364–369.

57. Kips JC. Treating asthma, or is simple too simple? Am J Respir Crit Care Med 2001; 164(8 Pt 1):1336–1338.

58. Jatakanon A, Lim S, Barnes PJ. Changes in sputum eosinophils predict loss of asthma control. Am J Respir Crit Care Med 2000; 161(l):64–72.

59. Jones SL, Kittelson J, Cowan JO, Flannery EM, Hancox RJ, McLachlan CR, et al. The predictive value of exhaled nitric oxide measurements in assessing changes in asthma control. Am J Respir Crit Care Med 2001; 164(5):738–743.

60. Leuppi JD, Salome CM, Jenkins CR, Anderson SD, Xuan W, Marks GB, et al. Predictive markers of asthma exacerbation during stepwise dose reduction of inhaled corticosteroids. Am J Respir Crit Care Med 2001; 163(2):406–412.

61. Pizzichini MM, Pizzichini E, Clelland L, Efthimiadis A, Pavord I, Dolovich J, et al. Prednisone-dependent asthma: inflammatory indices in induced sputum. Eur Respir J 1999; 13(1):15–21.

62. Hunter CJ, Brightling CE, Woltmann G, Wardlaw AJ, Pavord ID. A comparison of the validity of different diagnostic tests in adults with asthma. Chest 2002; 121(4):1051–1057.

63. Joyce DP, Chapman KR, Kesten S. Prior diagnosis and treatment of patients with normal results of methacholine challenge and unexplained respiratory symptoms. Chest 1996; 109(3):697–701.

64. Smith AD, Cowan JO, Filsell S, McLachlan C, Monti-Sheehan G, Jackson P, et al. Diagnosing asthma: comparisons between exhaled nitric oxide measurements and conventional tests. Am J Respir Crit Care Med 2004; 169(4): 473–478.

65. Brown HM. Treatment of chronic asthma with prednisolone; significance of eosinophils in the sputum. Lancet 1958; 2(7059):1245–1247.

66. Brightling CE, Monteiro W, Ward R, Parker D, Morgan MD, Wardlaw AJ, et al. Sputum eosinophilia and short-term response to prednisolone in chronic obstructive pulmonary disease: a randomised controlled trial. Lancet 2000; 356(9240):1480–1485.

67. Pizzichini E, Pizzichini MM, Gibson P, Parameswaran K, Gleich GJ, Berman L, et al. Sputum eosinophilia predicts benefit from prednisone in smokers with chronic obstructive bronchitis. Am J Respir Crit Care Med 1998; 158(5 Pt 1): 1511–1517.

68. Pizzichini MM, Pizzichini E, Parameswaran K, Clelland L, Efthimiadis A, Dolovich J, et al. Nonasthmatic chronic cough: no effect of treatment with an inhaled corticosteroid in patients without sputum eosinophilia. Can Respir J 1999; 6(4):323–330.

69. Parameswaran K, Pizzichini E, Pizzichini MM, Hussack P, Efthimiadis A, Hargreave FE. Clinical judgement of airway inflammation versus sputum cell counts in patients with asthma. Eur Respir J 2000; 15(3):486–490.

70. Duncan CJ, Lawrie A, Blaylock MG, Douglas JG, Walsh GM. Reduced eosinophil apoptosis in induced sputum correlates with asthma severity. Eur Respir J 2003; 22(3):484–490.

71. Kelly MM, Hargreave FE, Cox G. A method to preserve sputum for delayed examination. Eur Respir J 2003; 22(3):996–1000.

72. Belda J, Giner J, Casan P, Sanchis J. Mild exacerbations and eosinophilic inflammation in patients with stable, well-controlled asthma after 1 year of follow-up. Chest 2001; 119(4):1011–1017.

73. Meijer RJ, Postma DS, Kauffman HF, Arends LR, Koeter GH, Kerstjens HA. Accuracy of eosinophils and eosinophil cationic protein to predict steroid improvement in asthma. Clin Exp Allergy 2002; 32(7):1096–1103.

74. Jatakanon A, Lim S, Kharitonov SA, Chung KF, Barnes PJ. Correlation between exhaled nitric oxide, sputum eosinophils, and methacholine responsiveness in patients with mild asthma. Thorax 1998; 53(3):91–95.

75. Hogman M, Drca N, Ehrstedt C, Merilainen P. Exhaled nitric oxide partitioned into alveolar, lower airways and nasal contributions. Respir Med 2000; 94(10):985–991.

76. Lehtimaki L, Kankaanranta H, Saarelainen S, Turjanmaa V, Moilanen E. Increased alveolar nitric oxide concentration in asthmatic patients with nocturnal symptoms. Eur Respir J 2002; 20(4):841–845.

77. Lehtimaki L, Kankaanranta H, Saarelainen S, Turjanmaa V, Moilanen E. Inhaled fluticasone decreases bronchial but not alveolar nitric oxide output in asthma. Eur Respir J 2001; 18(4):635–639.

78. Gibson PG, Grootendor DC, Henry RL, Pin I, Rytila PH, Wark P, et al. Sputum induction in children. Eur Respir J 2002; 37(suppl):44s–46s.

79. Horn BR, Robin ED, Theodore J, Van Kessel A. Total eosinophil counts in the management of bronchial asthma. N Engl J Med 1975; 292(22):1152–1155.
80. Thomas RA, Green RH, Brightling CE, Birring S, Pavord ID. The influence of age on induced sputum differential cell counts in normal subjects. Thorax 2001; 56:iii79.

13

Exhaled Biomarkers in Monitoring Asthma

ILDIKO HORVATH

Department of Pathophysiology, National Koranyi Institute for Pulmonology, Budapest, Hungary

Introduction

Variable airway obstruction, typical symptoms, bronchial hyper-responsiveness, and airway inflammation form the current definition of asthma and international guidelines place central attention of the treatment of inflammation in this condition (1). Although currently the assessment of disease severity and progression is based on clinical symptoms and lung function tests, it is widely agreed that monitoring the nature, extent, and intensity of inflammation has central importance. Currently, available options to monitor the inflammatory processes and their response to therapy are limited. Symptoms and their perception vary widely between individuals and do not reflect accurately the extent of airway inflammation. Lung function measurements are used in most centers to monitor disease activity; however, it has been recognized that changes in lung function tests are not closely related to the degree of inflammation and intensive inflammatory processes may well precede changes in lung function (2,3). On the other hand, a recently published study demonstrated that when markers of inflammation (sputum eosinophils and exhaled nitric oxide) are used to guide

349

asthma treatment instead of traditional methods (lung function), better control and lower exacerbation rate could be achieved (4). Therefore, there is a growing need to include an "inflammometer" into our tests for monitoring asthma. The "gold standard" to obtain samples directly from the airways is bronchoscopy. However, this technique is limited because it is invasive. Its use is limited in small children and also in severely ill patients, and it cannot be repeated often. Therefore, the routine clinical use of bronchoscopy for monitoring airway inflammation/oxidative stress is limited. Sputum induction is another way of obtaining samples from the lower airways; however, it requires an inhalation of a hypertonic salt solution, which may provoke bronchoconstriction in asthmatic patients. Furthermore, it cannot be repeated too often, as the procedure by itself induces inflammatory changes in the airways. Along these lines, the least invasive technique is the collection of exhaled breath samples. Several mediators are present in the exhaled breath (Table 1) (5). Some of them, including nitric oxide (NO) and carbon monoxide (CO) can be measured in the gas phase, while others such as hydrogen peroxide, adenosine, and prostaglandins can be determined in the cooled exhalate called "exhaled breath condensate."

This chapter will focus on the use of breath biomarkers to monitor airway inflammation in asthmatic patients. The field of exhaled biomarkers advances with an enormous speed and may have profound clinical implications.

Table 1   Exhaled Biomarkers Measured in Asthmatic Patients

Exhaled gases
  Nitric oxide
  Carbon monoxide
  Ethane
  Penthane
Mediators in exhaled breath condensate
  Adenosine
  Ammonia
  Hydrogen peroxide
  Interferon-γ
  Interleukin-4
  Ions (hydrogen, etc.)
  8-Isoprostane
  Leukotrienes
  Nitrite/nitrate
  Nitrosothiol
  Nitrotyrosine
  Prostaglandins
  Thromboxane

Exhaled Gases

Exhaled NO

Endogenously formed NO is derived from L-arginine by the NO synthase (NOS) enzymes, which have at least three distinct isoforms; constitutive NOS, inducible NOS (iNOS), and neural NOS (6). The cellular source of NO in the lower respiratory tract is not completely known. It is accepted that airway epithelial cells and inflammatory cells, mainly eosinophils, produce NO. In asthmatic airway inflammation, iNOS is upregulated in several cell types and this is likely to be the main reason for increases in exhaled NO in the disease (7,8). Increase in iNOS expression in airway epithelial cells was demonstrated from asthmatic subjects and this was inhibited by corticosteroid treatment (8). A recent study further confirmed that exhaled NO largely originates from iNOS in asthma by showing that inhibition of iNOS by a specific NOS inhibitor greatly reduced exhaled NO (9). It must be mentioned that NO may also originate from non-enzymatic sources, i.e., from nitrite protonation forming nitrous acid, which releases NO gas under acidic conditions and therefore these processes may have an influence on its exhaled level.

Measurement of Exhaled NO

Measurements of exhaled NO concentration are usually performed by using a chemiluminescence method (Fig. 1). There are internationally accepted guidelines for exhaled NO measurement both for adults (10,11) and

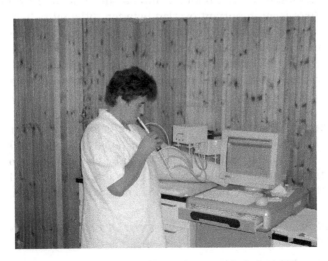

Figure 1 Measurement of exhaled NO requires an exhalation with controlled flow against resistance. It is a non-line measurement providing immediate result.

children (12). One of the most important recommendations from these guidelines is to exclude NO originating from the upper airway by using exhalation against a resistance sufficient to close the soft palate. This is necessary because there are considerable amounts of NO formed in the nose and paranasal sinuses, which could have a great influence on readings of exhaled NO (13). Furthermore, the level of environmental NO must be monitored since high ambient levels may influence exhaled NO readings (14).

Measurement of Exhaled NO for Early Diagnosis of Asthma

The level of exhaled NO is elevated in atopic subjects who exhibit airway hyper-responsiveness, where sub-clinical airway inflammation is likely to be already present (15).

Elevated NO is also found in approximately one-third of patients with allergic rhinitis, which may also indicate ongoing inflammatory changes in the lower airways (16). Furthermore, adolescents with history of childhood asthma have increased exhaled NO levels without having asthma symptoms (3). In a recent study, Malmberg et al. (17) demonstrated that exhaled NO was superior to baseline respiratory function and bronchodilator respon-siveness in identifying pre-school children with probable asthma (17).

Differential Diagnosis

In asthma, levels of exhaled NO can be increased several fold compared to healthy subjects (18–20), while in other inflammatory diseases of the air-ways this elevation—if there is an elevation at all—is a lot less pronounced, although there is an important overlap between different patients (21–23). The usefulness of exhaled NO measurement in differential diagnosis of air-way diseases was analyzed in patients with dry cough (24). In this study, ele-vation in exhaled NO differentiated between asthmatic and non-asthmatic cough with good sensitivity and specificity. It is important to mention, how-ever, that the typical high increase in exhaled NO is mostly seen in atopic asthmatic patients, and some studies showed that in non-atopic asthmatic subjects normal levels of exhaled NO can be detected (25). This observa-tion may be explained by the fact that in non-atopic asthma sometimes neutrophilic inflammation is seen instead of the characteristic eosinophilic inflammation in atopic asthma (26), and elevation in exhaled NO is closely linked with eosinophil cell count (27), but not with neutrophilia.

Relation between Exhaled NO Levels and Other Markers of Airway Inflammation

Levels of exhaled NO are associated with airway hyper-responsiveness (27–29), the number of eosinophil cells in blood (29) and induced sputum

(27,30,31), and also with the concentration of eosinophilic cationic protein (32). This strong relation between eosinophil cell number and exhaled NO levels suggests that exhaled NO is a marker of eosinophilic inflammation. In asthma exacerbations and also during the late phase of allergen-induced airway responses, exhaled NO increases (33–35). Furthermore, increases in exhaled NO levels can be observed during natural allergen exposure (36,37) further confirming that changes in exhaled NO level reflect changes in asthmatic airway inflammation.

Effect of Medication on Exhaled NO

Inhalation of methacholine or salbutamol does not alter exhaled NO (38–40). Anti-inflammatory treatment either with corticosteroids or with leukotriene antagonists causes a decrease in exhaled NO (40–47), proving that elevation in exhaled NO levels in steroid-naïve asthmatics is due to NO overproduction linked with inflammation. Treatment with inhaled and/or oral corticosteroids causes a dose-dependent reduction in exhaled NO (42,43). In the study of Bisgaard et al. (46), exhaled NO decreased significantly after the use of a leukotriene receptor antagonist and this was followed by a further decrease with the addition of low dose (200 µg) of inhaled corticosteroids (46). The reduction in exhaled NO by anti-inflammatory treatment is explained by suppressing inflammation resulting in reduced levels of inflammatory cytokines and therefore decreasing the signal for NO overproduction by iNOS. These observations suggest that measurement of exhaled NO can be used to monitor the efficacy of anti-inflammatory treatment. Regarding other drugs used for asthma, theophylline has no effect on exhaled NO level (48). Exhaled NO levels are in the normal range in well-controlled patients with asthma. In corticosteroid-treated patients with stable asthma, reduction of the dose of corticosteroids causes an increase in exhaled NO levels, which precedes the worsening of symptoms, lung function, and also precedes the increase in sputum eosinophils (42,49). Based on the relation between changes in clinical measures of asthma control and exhaled NO level, measurement of exhaled NO seems to be a useful marker for monitoring the efficacy of asthma control (50–52).

Advantages of Exhaled NO Measurement for Monitoring Asthma

Measurement of exhaled NO is a simple, non-invasive way of monitoring asthma, which can be performed in all patient groups including young children and patients with severe disease. The measurement has been standardized and therefore results from different centers are comparable, providing opportunity for its use in multicenter studies and wider clinical practice. Exhaled NO is useful for monitoring not only disease but also to establish the effectiveness of and compliance with asthma treatment, and will possibly lead to better individual adjustment of treatment dosage, an especially desirable aspect in children. These advantages were all taken into account when this test became officially accepted in the United States to measure asthmatic airway inflammation in clinical practice at the beginning of 2003.

Exhaled Carbon Monoxide

Heme-oxygenase (HO) is considered to be an antioxidant enzyme, which catabolizes heme to produce carbon monoxide (CO) and biliverdin (53). The exhaled CO concentrations are higher in asthmatic patients not receiving inhaled corticosteroids and similar in asthmatic patients receiving inhaled corticosteroids compared with those in non-smoking healthy control subjects both in adults and in children (54–56). Patients with symptomatic asthma have reductions in exhaled CO concentration after inhaled corticosteroid treatment (57). The source of exhaled CO is likely to be the HO enzyme family. Evidence for this is that HO-1 expression is increased in airway macrophages and bilirubin levels are elevated in induced sputum of asthmatic patients, who present elevated exhaled CO level (55). Furthermore, exhaled CO increases after inhalation of the HO substrate hemin in normal subjects (55). Exhaled CO levels are increased after allergen exposure during the late response, and also during the early response within minutes of allergen challenge (35).

Exhaled CO measurements are easy to make and are reproducible. The CO analyzers are relatively simple and cheap so that this measurement may be widely available. The measurement of exhaled CO is not complicated by nasal contamination, which is a major issue with exhaled NO measurements. On the other hand, exhaled CO levels are markedly affected by environmental CO, which may fluctuate considerably during the course of the day, particularly in cities. Previous exposure to high environmental CO levels may also result in subsequently increases in exhaled CO, as CO dissociates from carboxyhemoglobin. Active and passive smoking markedly affect exhaled CO levels and it may be important to check smoking status by measuring urinary cotinine.

Other Gases

The volatile gases ethane and pentane can also be detected in the breath and have been used to measure lipid peroxidation to reflect oxidative stress (58). Exhaled pentane is increased in asthma exacerbations and decreases during recovery (59). Exhaled ethane is also increased in asthma, and the levels are lower in patients treated with inhaled corticosteroids (60). A disadvantage of this measurement is that it is expensive and time consuming, and avoidance of contamination with environmental ethane is important. However, it is useful as way of validating other and easier measurements of oxidative stress, such as exhaled CO.

Mediators in Exhaled Breath Condensate

Expired airway droplets can be collected by cooling the exhaled air resulting in a sample most frequently called "exhaled breath condensate" (EBC). EBC mainly consists of water vapor, but it also contains large number of mediators. EBC collection is simple: exhaled breath is led through a cooling system resulting in a fluid or "snow" from its water vapor content depending on the cooling temperature. During collection, the subject breathes through a mouthpiece and a two-way non-rebreathing valve, which also serves as a saliva trap. In the collected sample, several mediators can be measured including hydrogen peroxide, adenosine, 8-isoprostane, prostaglandins, interleukins, and other cytokines, etc. (61–63).

In asthma, levels of exhaled H_2O_2 are elevated in steroid-naïve patients with mild asthma compared to normal controls and are related to the eosinophil differential counts in induced sputum and also to airway responsiveness (30,64–67). In patients with an exacerbation of asthma, higher levels have been reported than in patients with stable disease (66,67). Exhaled H_2O_2 holds promise as a guide of anti-inflammatory treatment in asthma, because its level is lowered by treatment with corticosteroids.

NO may be oxidized to nitrite (NO_2) and nitrate (NO_3). Concentrations of nitrite and/or $NO_2 + NO_3$ were significantly higher in asthma compared to healthy controls (68–71). In patients with exacerbation, higher nitrite level was observed than in stable patient and EBC nitrite measurement was suggested as a marker for acute asthma, which could be determined by the patients at home (68). Treatment with inhaled corticosteroid caused a significant decrease in expired nitrite levels in patients with asthma further confirming that its EBC level is related to disease activity (70). Nitrotyrosine concentrations were increased in patients with mild asthma compared to healthy controls and there was a significant association between exhaled nitrotyrosine and NO levels in these patients (72). Nitrosothiols (RS-NOs) are detectable in EBC of healthy subjects and are increased in patients with inflammatory airway diseases including asthma (73).

Some lines of evidence suggest that adenosine may be produced in asthmatic airway inflammation and may be involved in allergen- and exercise-induced bronchospasm in asthma (74–76). EBC adenosine concentration is elevated in steroid-naïve asthmatic patients and its level is related with worsening of asthma symptoms and elevation in exhaled NO (77). Leukotrienes, products of the lipoxygenase pathway, are implicated in the pathogenesis of obstructive airway diseases. In EBC, cysteinyl-leukotrienes were elevated in asthmatic patients as compared to normal subjects (78–80). Leukotriene measurement in EBC may be a useful method to assess the effect of leukotriene antagonists in the airways. 8-Isoprostane, a suggested marker of lipid peroxidation, is also elevated in EBC in asthmatic patients (78,80). Interestingly, a marked decrease in EBC pH can be detected in patients with acute asthma and EBC pH raises back to normal after successful treatment with steroids (81,82), suggesting that airway acidification may be an important process in the asthmatic airway inflammation and EBC pH measurement may be a simple and robust marker of the inflammatory processes. Changes in interleukin-4 (IL-4) and interferon- γ were also described in EBC in asthma (83). Hence, these measurements in EBC could play a role in non-invasive monitoring of airway inflammation and optimizing the dose of prescribed inhaled corticosteroids in asthmatic patients.

Because EBC sampling is completely non-invasive, simple, and can be performed not only in health-care units but even at home, it is reasonable to think that analysis of EBC may become a way of assessing airway inflammation and oxidative stress not only in research but also in clinical settings and help clinicians to monitor airway diseases non-invasively in the near future. Before there is wider clinical application of this way of disease monitoring, better understanding of the sampling technique is required as well as further studies involving large patient populations and investigation of the relationship between exhaled biomarkers and other markers of airway inflammation.

Summary

Asthma is defined as an inflammatory disorder of the airways. Therefore, it is reasonable to add an "inflammometer" to our methods of disease monitoring. In this respect, several biomarkers have been tested from different samples including blood, urine, and exhaled breath. Breath tests offer great opportunities for disease monitoring as they are simple, completely non-invasive, can be performed in children and also in severe patients, and can be repeated even within short intervals. From now, longitudinal studies are needed to establish their potential use as a guide to treatment of asthma.

Acknowledgment

I wish to acknowledge our many clinical colleagues who have collaborated with our laboratory during the course of studies on exhaled biomarkers. The work on exhaled biomarkers at the National Koranyi Institute is supported by grants from the Hungarian Research Foundation (OTKA T43396) and by the Hungarian Ministry of Health (160/2001).

References

1. American Thoracic Society. Standards for the diagnosis and care of patients with chronic obstructive pulmonary disease (COPD) and asthma Am Rev Respir Dis 1987; 136:225–244.
2. Rytila P, Metso T, Heikkinen K, Saarelainen P, Helenius IJ, Haahtela T. Airway inflammation in patients with symptoms suggestive to asthma but with normal lung function. Eur Respir J 2000; 16:824–830.
3. Toorn LM, Prins J, Overbeek SE, de Jongste JC, Leman K, Hoogsteden HC, Prins JB. Airway inflammation is present during clinical remission of atopic asthma. Am J Respir Crit Care Med 2001; 164:2107–2113.
4. Green RH, Brightling CE, McKenna S, Hargadon B, Parker D, Bradding P, Wardlaw AJ, Pavord ID. Asthma exacerbations and sputum eosinophil counts: a randomised controlled trial. Lancet 2002; 360:1715–1721.
5. Kharitonov SA, Barnes PJ. Exhaled markers of pulmonary disease. Am J Respir Crit Care Med 2001; 163:1693–1722.
6. Stuehr DJ, Griffith OW. Mammalian nitric oxide synthases. Adv Enzymol Relat Areas Mol Biol 1992; 65:287–346.
7. Guo FH, Comhair SAA, Zheng S, Dweik RA, Eissa NT, Thomassen MJ, Calhoun W, Erzurum SC. Molecular mechanism of increased nitric oxide (NO) in asthma: evidence for transcriptional and posttranslational regulation of NO synthesis. J Immunol 2000; 164:5970–5980.
8. Massaro AF, Mehta S, Lilly CM, Kobzik L, Reilly JJ, Drazen JM. Elevated nitric oxide concentrations in isolated lower airway gas of asthmatic subjects. Am J Respir Crit Care Med 1996; 153:1510–1514.
9. Hansel TT, Kharitonov SA, Donnelly LE, Erin EM, Currie MG, Moore WM, Manning PT, Recker DP, Barnes PJ. A selective inhibitor of inducible nitric oxide synthase inhibits exhaled breath nitric oxide in healthy volunteers and asthmatics. FASEB J 2003; 17:1298–1300. Epub May 08, 2003.
10. Kharitonov SA, Alving K, Barnes PJ. Exhaled and nasal nitric oxide measurements: recommendations. Eur Respir J 1997; 10:1683–1693.
11. American Thoracic Society. Recommendations for standardized procedures for the online and offline measurement of exhaled lower respiratory nitric oxide and nasal nitric oxide in adults and children. Am J Respir Crit Care Med 1999; 160:2104–2117.
12. Baraldi E, de Jongste JC. European Respiratory Society, American Thoracic Society. Measurement of exhaled nitric oxide in children, 2001. Eur Respir J 2002; 20:223–237.
13. Lundberg JON, Farkas-Szallasi T, Weitzberg E, Rinder J, Lidholm J, Anggaard A, Hokfelt T, Lundberg JM, Alving K. High nitric oxide production in human paranasal sinuses. Nat Med 1995; 1:370–373.
14. Binding N, Müller W, Czeschinski PA, Witting U. NO chemiluminescence in exhaled air: interference of compounds from endogenous and exogenous sources. Eur Respir J 2000; 16:499–503.
15. Horváth I, Barnes PJ. Exhaled monoxides in asymptomatic atopic subjects. Clin Exp Allergy 1999; 29:1276–1280.

16. Martin U, Bryden K, Devoy M, Howarth P. Increased level of exhaled nitric oxide during nasal and oral breathing in subjects with seasonal rhinitis. J Allergy Clin Immunol 1996; 97:768–773.
17. Malmberg LP, Pelkonen AS, Haahtela T, Turpeinen M. Exhaled nitric oxide rather than lung function distinguishes preschool children with probable asthma. Thorax 2003; 58:494–499.
18. Alving K, Weitzberg E, Lundberg JM. Increased amount of nitric oxide in exhaled air of asthmatics. Eur Respir J 1993; 6:1368–1370.
19. Kharitonov SA, Yates D, Robbins RA, Logan-Sinclair R, Shinebourne EA, Barnes PJ. Increased nitric oxide in exhaled air of asthmatics. Lancet 1994; 343:133–135.
20. Persson MG, Zetterstrom O, Argenius V, Ihre E, Gustaffson LE. Single breath nitric oxide measurements in asthmatic patients and smokers. Lancet 1994; 343:146–147.
21. Horvath I, Loukides S, Wodehouse T, Csiszer E, Cole PJ, Kharitonov SA, Barnes PJ. Comparison of exhaled and nasal nitric oxide and exhaled carbon monoxide levels in bronchiectatic patients with and without primary ciliary dyskinesia. Thorax 2003; 58:68–72.
22. Narang I, Ersu R, Wilson NM, Bush A. Nitric oxide in chronic airway inflammation in children: diagnostic use and pathophysiological significance. Thorax 2002; 57:586–589.
23. Machado RF, Stoller JK, Laskowski D, Zheng S, Lupica JA, Dweik RA, Erzurum SC. Low levels of nitric oxide and carbon monoxide in alpha 1-antitrypsin deficiency. J Appl Physiol 2002; 93:2038–2043. Epub Aug 30, 2002.
24. Chatkin JM, Ansarin K, Silkoff PE, McClean P, Gutierrez C, Zamel N, Chapman KR. Exhaled nitric oxide as a non-invasive assessment of chronic cough. Am J Respir Crit Care Med 1999; 159:1810–1815.
25. Gratziou C, Lignos M, Dassiou M, Roussos C. The influence of atopy on exhaled nitric oxide in patients with asthma and/or rhinitis. Eur Respir J 1999; 14:897–901.
26. Busse WW, Vrtis RF, Dick EC. The role of viral infections in intrinsic asthma: activation of neutrophil inflammation. Agents Actions Suppl 1989; 28:41–56.
27. Jatakanon A, Lim S, Kharitonov SA, Chung KF, Barnes PJ. Correlation between exhaled nitric oxide, sputum eosinophils, and methacholine responsiveness in patients with mild asthma. Thorax 1998; 53:91–95.
28. Dupont LJ, Rochette F, Demedts MG, Verleden GM. Exhaled nitric oxide correlates with airway hyperresponsiveness in steroid-naive asthmatic patients. Am J Crit Care Med 1998; 157:894–898.
29. Steerenberg PA, Janssen NAH, de Meer G, Fisher PH, Nierkens S, van Loveren H, Opperhuizen A, Brunekreef B, van Amsterdam JGC. Relationship between exhaled NO, respiratory symptoms, bronchial hyperresponsiveness, and blood eosinophilia in school children. Thorax 2003; 58:242–245.
30. Horváth I, Donnelly LE, Kiss A, Kharitonov SA, Lim S, Fan Chung K, Barnes PJ. Combined use of exhaled hydrogen peroxide and nitric oxide in monitoring asthma. Am J Resp Crit Care Med 1998; 158:1042–1046.

31. Brightling CE, Symon FA, Birring SS, Bradding P, Wardlaw AJ, Pavord ID. Comparison of airway immunopathology of eosinophilic bronchitis and asthma. Thorax 2003; 58:528–532.

32. Meijer RJ, Postma DS, Kauffman HF, Arends LR, Koeter GH, Kerstjens HA. Accuracy of eosinophils and eosinophil cationic protein to predict steroid improvement in asthma. Clin Exp Allergy 2002; 32:1096–1103.

33. Massaro AF, Gaston B, Kita D, Fanta C, Stamler J, Drazen JM. Expired nitric oxide levels during treatment of acute asthma. Am J Respir Crit Care Med 1995; 152:800–803.

34. Kharitonov SA, O'Conner BJ, Evans DJ, Barnes PJ. Allergen-induced late asthmatic reactions are associated with elevation of exhaled nitric oxide. Am J Respir Crit Care Med 1995; 151:1894–1899.

35. Paredi P, Leckie MJ, Horváth I, Allegra L, Kharitonov SA, Barnes PJ. Changes in exhaled carbon monoxide and nitric oxide levels following allergen challenge in patients with asthma. Eur Respir J 1999; 13:48–53.

36. Simpson A, Custovic A, Pipis S, Adisesh A, Faragher B, Woodcock A. Exhaled nitric oxide, sensitization, and exposure to allergens in patients with asthma who are not taking inhaled steroids. Am Respir Crit Care Med 1999; 160: 45–49.

37. Baraldi E, Carra S, Dario C, Azzolin N, Ongaro R, Marcer G, Zacchello F. Effect of natural grass pollen exposure on exhaled nitric oxide in asthmatic children. Am J Respir Crit Care Med 1999; 159:262–266.

38. Yates DH, Kharitonov SA, Barnes PJ. Effect of short- and long-acting inhaled β2-agonist on exhaled nitric oxide in asthmatic patients. Eur Respir J 1997; 10:1483–1488.

39. Deykin A, Belostotsky O, Hong C, Massaro AF, Lilly CM, Israel E. Exhaled nitric oxide following leukotriene E4 and methacholine inhalation in patients with asthma. Am J Respir Crit Care Med 2000; 162:1685–1689.

40. Baraldi E, Azzolin NM, Zanconato S, Dario C, Zaccbello F. Corticosteroids decrease nitric oxide in children with acute asthma. J Pediatr 1997; 131:381–385.

41. Yates DH, Kharitonov SA, Robbins RA, Thomas PS, Barnes PJ. Effect of nitric oxide synthase inhibitor and a glucocorticosteroid on exhaled nitric oxide. Am J Respir Crit Care Med 1995; 52:892–896.

42. Kharitonov SA, Yates DH, Chung KF, Barnes PJ. Changes in the dose of inhaled steroid affect exhaled nitric oxide levels in asthmatic patients. Eur Respir J 1996; 9:196–201.

43. Jatakanon A, Kharitonov SA, Lim S, Chung KF, Barnes PJ. Effect of differing doses of budenoside on markers of airway inflammation in patients with mild asthma. Thorax 1999; 54:108–114.

44. Little SA, Chalmers GW, MacLeod KJ, McSharry C, Thomson NC. Non-invasive markers of airway inflammation as predictors of oral responsiveness in asthma. Thorax 2000; 55:232–234.

45. Nelson BV, Sears S, Woods J, Ling CY, Hunt J, Clapper LM, Gaston B. Expired nitric oxide as a marker for childhood asthma. J Pediatr 1997; 130:423–427.

46. Bisgaard H, Loland L, Anhol J. NO in exhaled air of asthmatic children is reduced by the leukotriene receptor antagonist montelukast. Am J Respir Crit Care Med 1999; 160:1227–1231.

47. Tamaoki J, Kondo M, Sakai N, Nakata J, Takemura H, Nagai A, Takizawa T, Konno K. Leukotriene antagonist prevents exacerbation of asthma during reduction of high-dose inhaled corticosteroid. Am J Respir Crit Care Med 1997; 155:1235–1240.

48. Lim S, Tomita K, Carramori G, Jatakanon A, Oliver B, Keller A, Adcock I, Chung KF, Barnes PJ. Low-dose theophylline reduces eosinophilic inflammation but not exhaled nitric oxide in mild asthma. Am J Respir Crit Care Med 2001; 164:273–276.

49. Jatakanon A, Lim S, Barnes PJ. Changes in sputum eosinophils predict loss of asthma control. Am J Respir Crit Care Med 2000; 161:64–72.

50. Stirling RG, Kharitonov SA, Campbell D, Robinson D, Durham SR, Chung KF, Barnes PJ. Increase in exhaled nitric oxide levels in patients with difficult asthma and correlation with symptoms and disease severity despite treatment with oral and inhaled and corticosteroids. Thorax 1998; 53:1030–1034.

51. Jones SL, Kittelson J, Cowan JO, Flannery EM, Hancox RJ, McLachlan CR, Taylor DR. The predictive value of exhaled nitric oxide measurements in assessing changes in asthma control. Am J Respir Crit Care Med 2001; 164:738–743.

52. Sippel JM, Holden WE, Tilles SA, O'hollaren M, Cook J, Thukkani N, Priest J, Nelson B, Osborne ML. Exhaled nitric oxide levels correlates with measures of disease control in asthma. J Allergy Clin Immunol 2000; 106:645–650.

53. Maines MD. Heme oxygenase: function, multiplicity, regulatory mechanisms, and clinical applications. FASEB J 1988; 2:2557–2568.

54. Zayasu K, Sekizawa K, Okinaga S, Yamaya M, Ohrui T, Sasaki H. Increased carbon monoxide in exhaled air of asthmatic patients. Am J Respir Crit Care Med 1997; 156:1140–1143.

55. Horváth I, Donnelly LE, Kiss A, Paredi P, Kharitonov SA, Barnes PJ. Raised levels of exhaled carbon monoxide are associated with an increased expression of heme oxygenase-1 in airway macrophages in asthma: a new marker of oxidative stress. Thorax 1998; 53:668–672.

56. Uasaf C, Jatakanon A, James A, Kharitonov SA, Wilson NM, Barnes PJ. Exhaled carbon monoxide in childhood asthma. J Pediatr 1999; 135:569–574.

57. Yamaya M, Sekizawa K, Ishizuka S, Monma M, Sasaki H. Exhaled carbon monoxide levels during treatment of acute asthma. Eur Respir J 1999; 13:757–760.

58. Horváth I, MacNee W, Kelly FJ, Dekhuijzen PN, Phillips M, Doring G, Choi AM, Yamaya M, Bach FH, Willis D, Donnelly LE, Chung KF, Barnes PJ. "Haemoxygenase-1 induction exhaled markers of oxidative stress in lung diseases," summary of the ERS Research Seminar in Budapest, Hungary, September 1999. Eur Respir J 2001; 18:420–430.

59. Olopade CO, Zakkar M, Swedler WI, Rubinstein I. Exhaled pentane levels in acute asthma. Chest 1997; 111:862–865.

60. Paredi P, Kharitonov SA, Barnes PJ. Elevation of exhaled ethane concentration in asthma. Am J Respir Crit Care Med 2000; 162:1450–1454.

61. Hunt J. Exhaled breath condensate: an evolving tool for noninvasive evaluation of lung disease. J Allergy Clin Immunol 2002; 110:28–34.

62. Mutlu GM, Garey KW, Robbins RA, Danziger LH, Rubinstein I. Collection and analysis of exhaled breath condensate in humans. Am J Respir Crit Care Med 2001; 164:731–737.

63. Horváth I. Exhaled breath condensate for disease monitoring. Clin Pulmonol Med 2003; 10:195–200.

64. Antczak A, Nowak D, Shariati B, Krol M, Piasecka G, Kurmanowska Z. Increased hydrogen peroxide and thiobarbituric acid-reactive products in expired breath condensate of asthmatic patients. Eur Respir 1997; 10:1231–1241.

65. Jöbsis Q, Raatgeep HC, Hermans PW, de Jongste JC. Hydrogen peroxide in exhaled air is increased in stable asthmatic children. Eur Respir J 1997; 10:519–521.

66. Dohlman AW, Black HR, Royall JA. Expired breath hydrogen peroxide is a marker of acute airway inflammation in pediatric patients with asthma. Am Rev Respir Dis 1993; 148:955–960.

67. Antczak A, Kurmanowska Z, Kasielski M, Nowak D. Inhaled glucocorticosteroids decrease hydrogen peroxide in expired air condensate in asthmatic children. Respir Med 2000; 94:416–421.

68. Hunt J, Byrns RE, Ignarro LJ, Gaston B. Condensed expirate nitrite as a home marker for acute asthma. Lancet 1995; 346:1235–1236.

69. Ganas K, Loukides S, Papatheodorou G, Panagou P, Kalogeropoulos N. Total nitrite/nitrate in expired breath condensate of patients with asthma. Respir Med 2001; 95:649–654.

70. Kharitonov SA, Donnelly LE, Montuschi P, Corradi M, Collins JV, Barnes PJ. Dose-dependent onset and cessation of action of inhaled budenoside on exhaled nitric oxide and symptoms in mild asthma. Thorax 2002; 57:889–896.

71. Formanek W, Inci D, Lauener RP, Wildhaber JH, Frey U, Hall GL. Elevated nitrite in breath condensates of children with respiratory disease. Eur Respir J 2002; 19:487–491.

72. Hanazawa T, Kharitonov SA, Barnes PJ. Increased nitrotyrosine in exhaled breath condensate of patients with asthma. Am J Respir Crit Care Med 2000; 162:1273–1276.

73. Corradi M, Montuschi P, Donnelly LE, Pesci A, Kharitonov SA, Barnes PJ. Increased nitrosothiols in exhaled breath condensate in inflammatory airway diseases. Am J Respir Crit Care Med 2001; 163:854–858.

74. Driver AG, Kukoly CA, Ali A, Mustafa SJ. Adenosine in bronchoalveolar lavage fluid in asthma. Am Rev Respir Dis 1993; 15:161–165.

75. Mann JS, Holgate ST, Renwich AG, Cushley MJ. Airway effects of purine nucleosides and nucleotides and release with bronchial provocation in asthma. J Appl Physiol 1986; 61:1667–1676.

76. Vizi É, Huszár É, Csoma ZS, Boszormenyi-Nagy G, Barat E, Horvath I, Herjavecz I, Kollai M. Plasma adenosine concentration increases during exercise: a possible contributing factor to exercise-induced bronchoconstriction in asthma. J Allergy Clin Immunol 2002; 109:446–448.

77. Huszár É, Vass G, Vizi É, Csoma Z, Barat E, Molnar Vilagos G, Herjavecz I, Horvath I. Adenosine in exhaled breath condensate in healthy volunteers and in patients with asthma. Eur Respir J 2002; 20:1–6.
78. Antczak A, Montuschi P, Kharitonov S, Gorski P, Barnes PJ. Increased exhaled cysteinyl-leukotrienes and 8-isoprostane in aspirin-induced asthma. Am J Respir Crit Care Med 2002; 166:301–306.
79. Montuschi P, Barnes PJ. Exhaled lekotrienes and prostaglandins in asthma. J Allergy Clin Immunol 2002; 109:615–620.
80. Montuschi P, Corradi M, Ciabattoni G, Corradi M, van Rensen L, Geddes DM, Hodson ME, Barnes PJ. Increased 8-isoprostane, a marker of oxidative stress, in exhaled condensate of asthma patients. Am J Respir Crit Care Med 1999; 160:216–220.
81. Hunt JF, Fang K, Malik R, Snyder A, Malhotra N, Platts-Mills TA, Gaston B. Endogenous airway acidification: implications for asthma pathophysiology. Am J Respir Crit Care Med 2000; 161:694–699.
82. Kostikas K, Papatheodorou G, Ganas K, Psathakis K, Panagou P, Loukides S. pH in expired breath condensate of patients with inflammatory airway diseases. Am J Respir Crit Care Med 2002; 165:1364–1370.
83. Shahid SK, Kharitonov SA, Wilson NM, Bush A, Barnes PJ. Increased inter-leukin-4 and decreased interferon- γ in exhaled breath condensate of children with asthma. Am J Respir Crit Care Med 2002; 165:1290–1293.

14

Monitoring Childhood Asthma

PETER D. SLY and FELICITY S. FLACK

Telethon Institute for Child Health Research and
    Centre for Child Health Research, University of Western Australia,
Perth, Western Australia

Introduction

Asthma is a chronic condition for which there is no cure. With adequate treatment children with asthma can live normal lives and participate in the same activities as their peers. The aim of modern asthma treatment is symptom control, with adequate attention to reducing underlying inflammation. This requires appropriate treatment, with the use of the lowest doses of medication possible. Written asthma management plans have been shown to improve asthma control in both adults and children (1). These plans usually include some asthma education and monitoring of either peak expiratory flow (PEF) or symptoms. Most studies show a reduction in hospitalization, emergency room visits, visits to the doctor, days off work, or school and nocturnal asthma. In children symptom monitoring has been successful in a number of studies. Although symptoms can be used effectively to monitor asthma there still may be a role for objective measurements of lung function and inflammatory parameters in children. Children are not necessarily good at perceiving airway obstruction (2). This may complicate the monitoring of asthma in children. In addition, parents and caregivers are not always reliable witnesses, as they do not spend all day with children.

What Is Childhood Asthma?

Pediatric asthma incorporates a variety of clinical patterns and is more appropriately thought of as a syndrome. Wheezing at different ages may have different implications. In this chapter, the essence of asthma in children will first be briefly reviewed and the monitoring of asthma will be divided into three age groups, infants, pre-school children and older children as different monitoring techniques are required.

There is a growing recognition that what pediatricians call asthma may not be the same condition that their adult colleagues treat. A recent book titled "Childhood Asthma and Other Wheezing Disorders" (3) has highlighted the issues by declaring, "that we are not facing a single disorder in children but a number of asthmas." This is further outlined by the fact that the definition of asthma accepted by the majority of pediatricians and general practitioners is that "three or more wheezing episodes, occurring after the first year of life" constitutes asthma. There is no "test" or battery of investigations that can positively confirm or exclude the diagnosis of asthma in young children.

Clinically, at least three distinct wheezing phenotypes are recognized in children, i.e., transient infantile wheeze, viral-associated wheeze, and atopic asthma (Fig. 1). Whether these phenotypes represent different parts of a single clinical spectrum or are different conditions is not clear (Fig. 2). While these conditions appear distinct from an epidemiological point of view (4,5) determining which syndrome an individual child fits into is much more difficult.

Wheeze is a symptom and not a diagnosis. Physiologically, wheeze simply indicates the presence of flow-limitation (6), a condition that occurs when the desired flow exceeds the maximal flow that can be carried by the airway at the particular lung volume. Clinically, wheeze occurs most commonly during expiration due to the normal tendency for intra-thoracic airways to narrow during expiration. Once flow-limitation occurs flow is independent of the driving force and the excess energy is dissipated in airway wall vibrations, which are heard as wheezes (6). Wheezing can be produced by airways that are too small, too compliant or narrowed by airway smooth muscle shortening or by mucosal swelling and edema. The presence of wheeze does not give any information about the cause!

Transient Infantile Wheeze

While wheezing in infancy is very common, the true prevalence is not known. Silverman (3) reports that the cumulative prevalence of wheezing

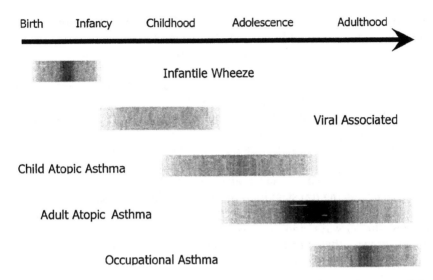

Figure 1 A schematic representation of the different wheezing syndromes and the ages at which they are commonly seen.

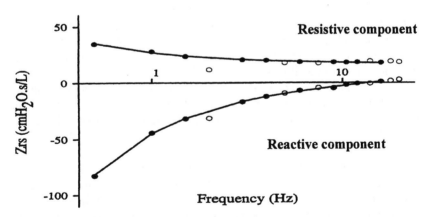

Figure 2 A representative impedance spectrum of the respiratory system (Zrs) recorded from a healthy infant. The symbols represent the data measured at each frequency contained in the measurement signal and the lines represent the model fit to the data. The resistive component of the impedance spectrum represents airway resistance at higher frequencies (>5–10 Hz) and tissue resistance at lower frequencies (<2–4 Hz). The reactive component represents lung elastance (or stiffness) at lower frequencies and airway inertance at higher frequencies. The frequency where the reactive component is known as the resonant frequency and occurs where the elastance and inertance are equal and opposite, hence they cancel each other.

over the first year of life varies between 25% and 60%, depending on the population and the definition used. Most wheezing in infants is episodic and associated with viral infections, with the majority of infants ceasing to wheeze by age 3 (5). The major risk factors for this type of wheezing are maternal smoking, especially during pregnancy (7–10) low birth weight (10), male sex (8), and younger mothers (11).

While the mechanism(s) predisposing to transient infantile wheeze is not known, several studies have shown that (a) pre-morbid lung function is lower (on a group basis) in infants who wheeze (5,12) and (b) that lung function is lower at birth in infants born to mothers who smoked during pregnancy (7,13). Thus smaller airways may be the important common factor in producing transient infantile wheeze. Mucosal swelling and edema, as would occur during a viral lower respiratory infection, would further narrow the airways and increase the likelihood of wheezing. As the infant grows, their lung volume and airway calibre would increase, decreasing the likelihood of wheezing with viral infections.

Viral-Associated Wheeze

Episodic wheeze, associated with viral infections, are very common in young children. The age at which children contract viral infections depends, to a large degree, on their social situation. Children with older siblings, those who attend day care and those who live in crowded conditions are likely to have viral respiratory infections at a younger age (14). Up to 30% of all children have one or more wheezing episodes during lower respiratory infections (LRIs), however, most do not go on to have typical atopic asthma in later life (4,5).

The mechanism(s) of viral-associated wheeze are not known with certainty. Acutely, one would expect mucosal swelling and edema narrowing airways and predisposing to wheeze. Epidemiological studies have suggested that airway responsiveness is increased for several weeks following viral infections (15,16). These data have been confirmed by studies deliberately inoculating adult volunteers with respiratory viruses and measuring airway responsiveness (17–19). While the mechanisms involved in humans have not been determined, animal studies suggest that certain viruses, e.g., parainfluenza and influenza that contain a neuraminidase, result in an exaggerated release of acetylcholine following vagal stimulation. This is thought to occur by the neuraminidase cleaving a sialic acid residue in the pre-junctional M_2 muscarinic receptor (responsible for feedback inhibition of acetylcholine release) decreasing the affinity for muscarinic agonist for the receptor (20). This effect should be relatively shortlived as the damaged M_2 receptors are replaced. RSV does not have a neuraminidase, although animal studies do suggest a short-lived imbalance in cholinergic discharge similar to that seen with parainfluenza (21).

The long-term association between RSV infection in early life and recurrent wheeze at the age of 6 but not at the age of 13 years reported by Stein et al. requires a different explanation. Stein et al. (4) did show that these children had lower baseline lung function (FEV_1), which was normalized by inhaled bronchodilator, suggesting some abnormality of airway function but not structure. Again data from animal studies suggest a long-term abnormality in the control of airway smooth muscle tone occurs when RSV infection occurs in early life (4). Whether these same mechanisms occur in humans is not known.

Atopic Asthma

The prevalence of atopic sensitization increases through childhood and the contribution of atopy and allergic factors to asthma is also thought to increase (4). At age 6 years, atopy is a less important factor contributing to current asthma than viral infections, yet by age 13 years, atopy is the most important factor (4). As most adult asthmatics are atopic (22), there is a view that it is predominantly atopic asthma that persists from childhood into adult life (23). Unfortunately this has lead to an over-emphasis on atopic asthma at the expense of the other wheezing syndrome seen in children and resulted in a tendency to treat all wheezing in children as atopic asthma.

What Are the Characteristics of a "Good Monitor?"

When determining whether a technique is likely to be useful for monitoring, a number of questions should be addressed, including:

- Does the technique detect/track change in lung function and/or disease activity?
- Does the technique predict the onset of exacerbations in disease activity?
- Does use of the technique improve disease control?
- Will patients use the technique to monitor their disease?

Unfortunately, very few systematic studies have been conducted to determine how well the various techniques suggested for use in monitoring asthma actually perform. The best-studied technique is home monitoring of PEF in children with asthma and this will be discussed in detail later in this chapter.

Monitoring Asthma in Infants

Monitoring the progress of infants with asthma is largely based on clinical history and examination. The most important feature in the history that indicates troublesome asthma is wheeze interfering with feeding and/or sleep. Parents are frequently concerned about respiratory noises made by their infants and symptoms are likely to be reported early. A careful history about the association of wheeze with feeding and with changes in posture may give indications that investigations to exclude gastro-esophageal reflux are required. A chest x-ray of the first presentation of wheeze is justified to exclude uncommon structural abnormalities that may present with airway obstruction (24).

Clinically, the most reliable parameter for determining the severity of asthma, the need for treatment and treatment response is the infant's growth pattern. An infant who is growing (and developing) normally is unlikely to require aggressive treatment and frequently parents are happy to withhold treatment, provided they can be reassured that there is nothing seriously wrong with their child. Poor growth that improves following the introduction of therapy is a good indication that the treatment is successful and should be continued. A child who is symptomatic during the night and disturbing the parent's sleep also warrants treatment.

Objective monitoring of asthma in infants is difficult as they are unable to cooperate with most tests used in older children and adults. There are no standard, well-validated tests available to monitor asthma in infants. However, there are several experimental techniques that are being investigated.

Lung Function Tests in Infants

A variety of techniques have been used to measure lung function tests in infants. Standard protocols have been developed and published by a task force from the European Respiratory and American Thoracic societies (23–33).

One particularly promising technique is the forced oscillation technique (FOT). This technique has the advantage of being able to separately determine the mechanical properties of the airways and pulmonary parenchyma. FOT is generally performed by measuring the impedance to the input of pressure waves to the respiratory system (34). The infant is sedated and a computer controlled pump and solenoid valves are used to inflate a supine infant through a facemask to a transrespiratory pressure of 20 cm H_2O. This causes an end-inspiratory occlusion and invokes the Hering–Breuer reflex, which gives an apneic period in which to take measurements. A loudspeaker is connected to the mask through a side arm that generates small-amplitude, pseudorandom oscillations of between 0.5 and 20.75 Hz. This allows the collection of low frequency respiratory impedance spectra (Zrs) from which frequency independent resistence (Raw), inertance (Iaw), viscous damping (G), and elastance (H) can be determined (34).

Studies in infants have shown that FOT may be a useful tool for monitoring lung function in infants. It has been used successfully to measure both bronchodilator and bronchoconstrictor responses in infants. Hayden et al. (35) measured lung function in infants using FOT before and after administration of an aerosol of 500 μg of salbutamol or a placebo. They showed a significant fall in Raw (13%) following administration of salbutamol but not placebo ($p < 0.01$). In this study, while the bronchodilator response measured in infants with recurrent wheeze was greater than that seen in normal infants ($17.6 \pm 8.7\%$ vs. $7.7 \pm 5.5\%$), this difference failed to reach statistical significance—most likely due to the small number of infants studied.

While measurements of bronchial responsiveness are possible in infants, most studies do not find substantial differences between healthy infants and those with recurrent wheeze (36), regardless of what technique is used. This may be because the tests are not sufficiently sensitive or because infants are studied when they are asymptomatic.

It is difficult to predict whether a wheezy infant will have transient or persistent wheezing. Asymptomatic infants with a history of recurrent wheezing persisting into the second year of life have been shown to have abnormal parenchymal mechanics, assessed by FOT (37). However, the predictive value of this finding has not yet been tested in a longitudinal study.

The current methods for measuring lung function in infants require the infant to be sedated and, as such, are largely restricted to specialist centers. New techniques that do not require the infant will need to be developed before it is practical to include measurements of lung function in the routine clinical management of infants with asthma.

Exhaled Nitric Oxide (ENO)

Measurement of ENO or the fractional concentration of exhaled NO (FE_{NO}) is a marker of airway inflammation. Its use in monitoring asthma in adults has been discussed in Chapter? ENO is measured in adults and older children by exhaling at a constant flow against a resistance and obtaining a plateau in the FE_{NO} signal. Infants are unable to perform this maneuver so other techniques have been assessed to measure FE_{NO} in infants. Techniques for measuring FE_{NO} in infants should be:

1. Simple to apply
2. Non-invasive
3. Should not alter the infants' breathing pattern
4. Should take into account the flow dependence of FE_{NO}
5. Should exclude contamination with nasal NO

Several techniques are described in the ERS/ATS guidelines (25,26).

Tidal Breathing Offline Collection

Exhaled air can be collected from infants without the use of sedation during tidal breathing. The infant breathes NO-free air through a facemask connected to a non-rebreathing valve. When a stable breathing pattern is achieved, exhaled breath is collected into an NO-inert bag fitted to an expiratory port. The respiratory port provides an expiratory resistance of 2 cm H_2O. Baraldi et al. (38) investigated FE_{NO} levels in infants with recurrent wheezing using this method. They found that the wheezing infants had higher levels of FE_{NO} than normal infants during an exacerbation. These levels decreased after steroid therapy.

Single Breath Technique

The level of FE_{NO} is influenced by expiratory flow (39) and the amount of nasal NO. A method to overcome the effects of these two methods has been tested. The single-breath technique with positive expiratory pressure has been adapted for use in infants. A modification of the raised volume rapid thoracic compression technique with expiration against a flow resistor can be used to measure FE_{NO} at a constant expiratory flow. The vellum closes during this technique and it is therefore unlikely that there is contamination with nasal NO (40).

Tidal Breathing Online Collection

Recently Hall et al. (41) described a technique for measuring FE_{NO} in infants, online during tidal breathing. They showed that tidal FE_{NO} and the nitric oxide flow (V'NO) could be measured during quiet sleep. They used CO_2 washout to identify airway and alveolar emptying. They measured FE_{NO} and V' simultaneously. This method was used to compare FE_{NO} in infants exposed to environmental tobacco smoke and infants not exposed. Infants exposed to prenatal cigarette smoke had significantly lower FE_{NO} and V_{NO}.

Is FE_{NO} a Good Monitor of Asthma in Infants?

While it is technically possible to measure FEno in infants in specialized laboratories, no systematic studies have been performed to determine whether this aids in the clinical management of asthma in infants. This technique can be included in epidemiological studies, e.g., those investigating the environmental influences on the development of and triggering of asthma in infants, but will not be suitable for use as a home monitor.

Monitoring Asthma in Pre-School Children

Monitoring asthma in pre-school children relies primarily on the history given by the parents. The clinical pattern of the symptoms, particularly the presence of nocturnal and early morning symptoms, symptoms induced by exercise and the length of symptom-free periods give the best indication of disease severity and treatment efficacy.

Pre-school children present a special problem with objective monitoring. They are too old to be sedated for "infant" lung function tests yet unable to co-operate with the tests used in older, co-operative children. As discussed by the ATS/ERS Working Group on Infant and Young Children Pulmonary Function Testing in their discussion paper, the ideal lung function test for use in preschool children should be:

1. Applicable to any age so the longitudinal studies can be conducted.
2. Safe.
3. Simple to perform.
4. Reproducible.
5. Sensitive enough to detect changes with growth and distinguish clearly between health and disease.
6. Acceptable to both subject and parent.

Considerable research is currently underway to determine the optimal method for measuring lung function in children aged 2–6 years.

Spirometry has been a standard method of monitoring lung function in adults and older children for many years. Until recently it has been considered too difficult for pre-school children to perform the forced expiratory maneuvers reliably. Several studies have now been completed which show that children aged between 3 and 6 years are capable of performing spirometry. Eigen (42) tested 259 healthy 3–6 year-old-children and found that 82.6% could perform technically acceptable maneuvers after 15 min of training. Crenesse et al. (43) tested 355 children aged between 3–6 years who had been referred to their pulmonary function test laboratory. They found that 75.3% of children could perform 2 or 3 acceptable maneuvers. Nystad et al. (44) tested 603 children aged 3–6 years recruited from a day care center. They found that 92% of children could complete two acceptable tests. All of these studies found that the younger children were less likely to perform acceptable tests.

Bronchial provocation tests have also been investigated in this age group. We have recently performed a methacholine challenge using a modified Yan technique (45) in a random sample of 711 5–7 year-old-children taking part in longitudinal birth cohort study (46). Of these, 34 were unable to perform the repeated forced expiratory maneuvers required and 112 (seven with current asthma) were excluded with a low baseline FEV_1 (< 80% predicted) leaving a test sample of 565. The challenge was successfully completed in 537 (95% of the test sample), with 28 unable to finish for technical reasons. Of those completing the challenge, FEV_1 fell by at least

20% in 420 (78%), by at least 15% in 457 (85%) and by at least 10% in 495 (92%) children. There were no differences in methacholine responsiveness between males and females, regardless of which index was examined.

Children with current asthma were also more sensitive to methacholine than those without asthma. When children with current asthma were sub-divided by asthma severity there was a progressive decrease in lung function and increase in methacholine responsiveness as asthma severity increased (Table 1) with significant decrements in FVC, FEV_1, FEF_{25-75}, DRS, $PC_{15}FEV_1$, and in $PC_{10}FEV_1$.

No systematic studies have been performed to date to show whether methacholine challenge tests could play a useful role in monitoring asthma in pre-school children.

One of the major problems with spirometry in this age group is that healthy children essentially empty their lungs within 1 sec. As shown in the table above, the FEV_1/FVC ratio was 94% for healthy children and 93% for those with asthma. The utility of FEV_1 as a measure of lung function in adults and older children is that flow is limited during the forced expiratory maneuver, provided a reasonable effort is made, which means that FEV_1 reflects the mechanical properties of the lungs and airways. Elegant physiological studies performed in adults have shown that flow-limitation is likely to be maintained during the forced expiration until approximately 85% of the vital capacity has been exhaled (47). Studies of forced expiration, performed with inflatable jackets in sedated infants have cast doubt on the ability to maintain flow-limitation to low lung volumes (48–50). Thus it is unlikely that pre-school children will be able to maintain expiratory flow-limitation until greater than 90% of their vital capacity has been exhaled. Despite this realization, no systematic studies have yet been performed to determine whether the forced expiratory volume exhaled in 0.5 or 0.75 sec would be a more physiologically reliable variable to report from forced expiration in preschool children.

Plethysmography is a standard method for measuring Raw in adults and older children. This technique, as used in adults, is not suitable for pre-school children, as it requires the child to be alone inside the plethysmograph. For measurements of alveolar pressure and thoracic gas volume to be made the child needs to perform a breathing maneuver against a closed shutter, something they are unlikely to do reliably. Klug and Bisgaard (51) have described a method for measuring a "specific resistance" in which an adult accompanies the child during measurements. They did not measure thoracic gas volume, thus avoiding the need for the child to perform a breathing manoeuvre. Satisfactory measurements were achieved in 83% of children aged between 2–8 years. This method has been used as a diagnostic tool to measure bronchodilator responses in preschool children and compared with the interrupter technique and the impulse oscillation

Table 1 Lung Function and Methacholine Responsiveness Related to Asthma Status

	Nonasthma	Current asthma	p^{*}	Mild asthma	Moderate asthma	Severe asthma	p^{**}
Spirometry	$n = 1365$	$n = 308$		$n=149$	$n = 74$	$n = 97$	
FVC(l) mean (SD)	1.17 (0.22)	1.16 (0.23)	0.530	1.19 (0.25)	1.13 (0.21)	1.12 (0.21)	0.033
FEV_1(l) mean (SD)	1.09 (0.19)	1.06 (0.20)	0.023	1.09 (0.19)	1.04 (0.20)	1.03 (0.20)	0.023
FEF_{25-75}(L/sec) mean (SD)	1.52 (0.46)	1.42 (0.44)	0.001	1.48 (0.44)	1.34 (0.45)	1.38 (0.43)	0.042
FEV_1/F VCmean (SD)	0.94 (0.07)	0.93 (0.08)	0.002	0.93 (0.08)	0.93 (0.07)	0.93 (0.10)	0.78
Methacholine challenge	$n = 440$	$n = 80$		$n = 39$	$n = 22$	$n = 19$	
DRS mean (SD)	0.19 (0.59)	0.34 (0.42)	0.034	0.19 (0.12)	0.38 (0.57)	0.58 (0.47)	< 0.001
$PC_{10}FE$ V_1(mg/ mL) mean SD	1.44 (1.49)	0.94 (1.32)	0.003	1.34 (1.69)	0.79 (0.840)	0.34 (0.43)	0.009
$PC_{15}FE$ V_1(mg/ mL) mean(SD)	1.93 (1.71)	1.27 (1.48)	0.001	1.54 (1.70)	1.45 (1.41)	0.54 (0.70)	0.028
$PC_{20}FE$ V_1(mg/ mL) mean (SD)	2.18 (1.65)	1.37 (1.23)	O.001	1.56 (1.22)	1.59 (1.38)	0.86 (1.00)	0.070

*p values from t-tests between non-asthma and current asthma.
**p values for ANOVA between severity categories.

technique (52). It was found to have the highest discriminatory capacity of the three techniques and to be the most sensitive method for assessing bronchodilator responsiveness.

The FOT is gaining popularity as a measure of lung function in this age group. While the basics of the technique are the same as described earlier in this chapter, it is an attractive technique for this age group as it can be performed during gentle tidal breathing. The report from an ERS task force on this technique has been published recently and the interested reader is recommended to consult this for more details and for normative data. This technique has been found to be useful in following the progress of asthma in preschool children and for measuring response to bronchodilators (53,54).

The interrupter technique has also been used to measure resistance (Rint) in this age group (55–58). Measurements are made during quiet tidal breathing by a shutter closing and briefly (100 ms) occluding the child's breathing. Rint is calculated from measurements of the pressure change following the occlusion and the flow occurring at the time of the occlusion. Rint approximates the Newtonian resistance of the airways, lung tissues and chest wall. This technique has been found to be useful in determining the presence of airway obstruction in asthmatic children and in determining the response to bronchodilators.

Monitoring Asthma in Older Children

Spirometry

Measurement of lung function with standard spirometry is a recognized part of asthma management in older children (59). Achieving and maintaining best lung function are important goals of optimal asthma management in Australian asthma management guidelines since their inception. One of the best demonstrations of the importance of achieving normal lung function comes from the U.S. 6 Cities study (60), in which they clearly demonstrated that children with low lung function, as judged by a low FEV_1 were

Table 2 FEV_1 and Risk of Asthma Attach Over a 1 Year Period

FEV_1 (% predicted), measured when well	Risk (odds ratio, 95% CI) of asthma attack in next 12 months
> 80%	1
60–80%	1.4, 1.2–1.7
< 60%	5.3, 2.2–12.9

more likely to report asthma exacerbations. The risk increased progressively with lower lung function (Table 2).

Measurement of lung function is a routine part of the assessment in many pediatric asthma specialist clinics. In our own clinic, standard spirometry is measured on each visit, with a bronchodilator response measured periodically and certainly if the child's lung function is abnormal.

Peak Expiratory Flow

The role of PEF monitoring in the management of asthma in older children has been reviewed extensively (61,62). The routine daily use of a PEF meter can not be justified in children with asthma, as PEF monitoring: frequently does not accurately track changes in lung function measured with a spirometer (63,64) does not predict the onset of asthma attacks in the majority of childrens (65), does not match other measures of asthma control (66) and has no benefit over monitoring symptoms for improving asthma control (67). Recent studies using covert monitoring techniques also question whether children with asthma will use PEF meters reliably enough to give useful information about disease control (68).

Measurements of Bronchial Responsiveness

Effective management of asthma with inhaled corticosteroids does lead to a reduction in bronchial responsiveness in children (66,69) and as current theories suggest that heightened bronchial responsiveness is an expression of poorly controlled airway inflammation, using measurements of bronchial responsiveness to monitor disease control is theoretically appealing. At least one study in adults (70) has investigated the possibility of using regular measurements of methacholine responsiveness to guide asthma management. They randomized 75 asthmatic adults to have their asthma management guided by measurements by regular measurements of methacholine PC_{20} in addition to standard assessments of symptoms and lung function or to standard assessments alone. Patients were followed over a 2-year period. The "methacholine" group were prescribed more inhaled steroids and had a greater improvement in asthma control, as evidenced by fewer exacerbations per year (0.23 vs. 0.43 per patient per year), fewer symptoms and a greater improvement in airway histology. Similar studies would need to be performed in children before such an approach could be advocated.

Exhaled Nitric Oxide

Measuring the fractional content of nitric oxide in exhaled breath (FE_{NO}) has been mooted as a non-invasive method of detecting the presence of airway inflammation. This suggestion has come from the finding that the largest source of NO in the airways comes from airway epithelial cells and inflammatory cells in the airway lumen. This NO is produced when the expression of the inducible for of the nitric oxide synthetase enzyme is upregulated in response to inflammatory stimuli (71,72). FEno has been shown to be higher in asthmatics, at least in adults. In children the situation is not as clear, with atopic children showing increased FEno, even in the absence of any history of respiratory symptoms (73). Furthermore, atopic asthmatics have higher FEno than non-atopic asthmatics (74–78), raising the possibility that atopy is the primary signal in children and that airway inflammation may be less important.

There are data showing that FEno does have some relationship with active disease in children, at least in atopic asthmatics (79). When FEno was measured in children completing the Childhood Asthma Management Program (CAMP) (79) at the Denver site, it was shown to correlate with other markers of inflammation (total eosinophil count, serum ECP), atopy (number of positive skin prick tests, serum IgE) and bronchial responsiveness (bronchodilator response and sensitivity to inhaled methacholine) (79). However, studies tracking response to initiation of treatment with inhaled corticosteroids generally show that FEno falls before symptom control is achieved, pulmonary function improves or bronchial responsiveness decreases (80), severely limiting the value of measuring FE_{NO} as a marker of disease activity in the short term.

Sputum Eosinophils

While many children with asthma do not freely produce sputum, assessment of inflammatory cell in induced sputum samples is feasible in older children, even during acute exacerbations (81). One recent study has investigated the usefulness of using assessment of sputum eosinophils to guide asthma management in adults (82). Seventy four patients were randomized to have their asthma managed according to British Thoracic Society guidelines or to management aimed to keep their sputum eosinophil count below 3%. Over the 12-month follow-up period, those in the "sputum" group had lower sputum eosinophil counts, had significantly fewer severe asthma exacerbations (35 vs. 109, $p = 0.01$) and fewer patients were admitted to hospital (1 vs. 6, $p = 0.047$). Whether monitoring sputum eosinophils in children with asthma would produce the same benefits is debatable, but would need to be tested before adopted.

References

1. Gibson PG, Coughlan J, Wilson AJ, et al. Self-management education and regular practitioner review for adults with asthma. Cochrane Database Syst Rev 2002 (3):CD001117.

2. Sly PD, Landau LI, Weymouth R. Home recording of peak expiratory flow rates and perception of asthma. Am J Dis Children 1985; 139:479–182.
3. Silverman M. Wheezing disorders in infants and young children. In: Silverman M, ed. Childhood Asthma and Other Wheezing Disorders. London: Arnold, 2002:307–332.
4. Stein RT, Sherrill D, Morgan WJ, et al. Respiratory syncytial virus in early life and risk of wheeze and allergy by age 13 years (see comments). Lancet 1999; 354:541–545.
5. Martinez FD, Wright AL, Taussig LM, Holberg CJ, Halonen M, Morgan WJ. Asthma and wheezing in the first six years of life. The Group Health Medical Associates (see comments). N Eng J Med 1995; 332:133–138.
6. Gavriely N, Kelly KB, Grotberg JB, Loring SH. Forced expiratory wheezes are a manifestation of airway flow limitation. J Appl Physiol 1987; 62(6):2398–2403.
7. Dezateux C, Stocks J, Dundas I, Fletcher ME. Impaired airway function and wheezing in infancy: the influence of maternal smoking and a genetic predisposition to asthma. Am J Respir Crit Care Med 1999; 159:403–410.
8. Young S, Sherrill DL, Arnott J, Diepeveen D, LeSouef PN, Landau LI. Parental factors affecting respiratory function during the first year of life. Pediatr Pulmonol 2000; 29:331–340.
9. Baker D, Henderson J. Differences between infants and adults in the social aetiology of wheeze. J Epidemiol Community Health 1999; 53:636–642.
10. Gold DR, Burge HA, Carey V, Milton DK, Platts-Mills T, Weiss ST. Predictors of repeated wheeze in the first year of life: the relative roles of cockroach, birth weight, acute lower respiratory illness, and maternal smoking. Am J Respir Crit Care Med 1999; 160:227–236.
11. Infante-Rivard C. Young maternal age: a risk factor for childhood asthma? Epidemiology 1995; 6:178–180.
12. Young S, Le Souef PN, Geelhoed GC, Stick SM, Turner KJ, Landau LI. The influence of a family history of asthma and parental smoking on airway responsiveness in early infancy. N Eng J Med 1991; 324:1168–1173.
13. Stick SM, Burton PR, Gurrin L, Sly PD, LeSouef PN. Effects of maternal smoking during pregnancy and a family history of asthma on respiratory function in newborn infants. Lancet 1996; 348:1060–1064.
14. Ball TM, Castro-Rodriguez JA, Griffith KA, Holberg CJ, Martinez FD, Wright AL. Siblings, day-care attendance, and the risk of asthma and wheezing during childhood. N Eng J Med 2000; 343:538–543.
15. Sterk PJ. Virus-induced airway hyperresponsiveness in man. Eur Respir J 1993; 6:894–902.
16. Empey DW, Laitinen LA, Jacobs L, Gold WM, Nadel JA. Mechanisms of bronchial hyperreactivity in normal subjects after upper respiratory tract infection. Am Rev Respir Dis 1976; 113:131–139.
17. Cheung D, Dick EC, Timmers MC, de Klerk EP, Spaan WJ, Sterk PJ. Rhinovirus inhalation causes long-lasting excessive airway narrowing in response to methacholine in asthmatic subjects in vivo. Am J Respir Crit Care Med 1995; 152:1490–1496.

18. Gern JE, Calhoun W, Swenson C, Shen G, Busse WW. Rhinovirus infection preferentially increases lower airway responsiveness in allergic subjects. Am J Respir Crit Care Med 1997; 155:1872–1876.
19. Bardin PG, Sanderson G, Robinson BS, Holgate ST, Tyrrell DA. Experimental rhinovirus infection in volunteers. Eur Respir J 1996; 9:2250–2255.
20. Jacoby DB, Fryer AD. Interaction of viral infections with muscarinic receptors. Clin Experimental Allergy 1999; 29:59–64.
21. Larsen GL, Colasurdo MD. Neural control mechanisms within airways: disruption by respiratory syncytial virus. J Pediatr 1999; 135:s21–s27.
22. Woolcock AJ, Peat JK, Trevillion LM. Is the increase in asthma prevalence linked to increase in allergen load? Allergy 1995; 50:935–940.
23. Holt PG, Macaubas PA, Stumbles, Sly PD. The role of allergy in the development of asthma. Nature 1999; 402:B12–B17.
24. Sly PD, Stokes KB, Campbell PE. Congenital lobar emphysema due to a pre-eparterial tracheal bronchus. Pediatr Surg Int 1989; 4:124–126.
25. Anonymous. Recommendations for standardized procedures for the on-line and off-line measurement of exhaled lower respiratory nitric oxide and nasal nitric oxide in adults and children-1999. This official statement of the American Thoracic Society was adopted by the ATS Board of Directors, July 1999. (comment). Am J Respir Crit Care Med 1999; 160:2104–2117.
26. Baraldi E, de Jongste JC, Gaston B, Alving K, Barnes PJ, Bisgaard H, Bush A, Gaultier C, Grasemann H, Hunt JF, Kissoon N, Piacentini GL, Ratjen F, Silkoff P, Stick S. European Respiratory S, American Thoraic S. Measurement of exhaled nitric oxide in children, 2001. Eur Respir J 2002; 20:223–237.
27. Morris MG, Gustafsson P, Tepper R, Gappa M, Stocks J, Testing EAT-FoSflRF. The bias flow nitrogen washout technique for measuring the functional residual capacity in infants. ERS/ATS Task Force on Standards for Infant Respiratory Function Testing. Eur Respir J 2001; 17:529–36.
28. Stocks J, Godfrey S, Beardsmore C, Bar-Yishay E, Castile R, Society EAT-FoSflRFTERSAT. Plethysmographic measurements of lung volume and airway resistance. ERS/ATS Task Force on Standards for Infant Respiratory Function Testing. European Respiratory Society/ American Thoracic Society. Eur Respir J 2001; 17:302–312.
29. Gappa M, Colin AA, Goetz I, Stocks J, Society EATFoSflRFTERSAT. Passive respiratory mechanics: the occlusion techniques. Eur Respir J. 2001; 17: 141–148.
30. Bates JH, Schmalisch G, Filbrun D, Stocks J. Tidal breath analysis for infant pulmonary function testing. ERS/ATS Task Force on Standards for Infant Respiratory Function Testing. European Respiratory Society/American Thoracic Society. Eur Respir J 2000; 16:1180–1192.
31. Frey U, Stocks J, Sly P, Bates J. Specification for signal processing and data handling used for infant pulmonary function testing. ERS/ATS Task Force on Standards for Infant Respiratory Function Testing. European Respiratory Society/American Thoracic Society. Eur Respir J 2000; 16:1016–1022.
32. Sly PD, Tepper R, Henschen M, Gappa M, Stocks J. Tidal forced expirations. ERS/ATS Task Force on Standards for Infant Respiratory Function Testing.

European Respiratory Society/American Thoracic Society. (comment). Eur Respir J 2000; 16:741–748.

33. Frey U, Stocks J, Coates A, Sly P, Bates J. Specifications for equipment used for infant pulmonary function testing. ERS/ATS Task Force on Standards for Infant Respiratory Function Testing. European Respiratory Society/ American Thoracic Society. (comment). Eur Respir J 2000; 16:731–740.

34. Sly PD, Hayden MJ, Petak F, Hantos Z. Measurement of low-frequency respiratory impedance in infants. Am J Respir Crit Care Med 1996; 154:161–166.

35. Hayden MJ, Petak F, Hantos Z, Hall G, Sly PD. Using low-frequency oscillation to detect bronchodilator responsiveness in infants. Am J Respir Crit Care Med 1998; 157:574–579.

36. Hall GL, Hantos Z, Wildhaber JH, Petak F, Sly PD. Methacholine responsiveness in infants assessed with low frequency forced oscillation and forced expiration techniques. Thorax 2001; 56:42–47.

37. Hall GL, Hantos Z, Sly PD. Altered respiratory tissue mechanics in asymptomatic wheezy infants. Am J Respir Crit Care Med 2001; 164:1387–1391.

38. Baraldi E, Dario C, Ongaro R, et al. Exhaled nitric oxide concentrations during treatment of wheezing exacerbation in infants and young children. Am J Respir Crit Care Med 1999; 159:1284–1288.

39. Silkoff PE, McClean PA, Slutsky AS, et al. Marked flow-dependence of exhaled nitric oxide using a new technique to exclude nasal nitric oxide. Am J Respir Crit Care Med 1997; 155:260–267.

40. Wildhaber JH, Hall GL, Stick SM. Measurements of exhaled nitric oxide with the single-breath technique and positive expiratory pressure in infants. Am J Respir Crit Care Med 1999; 159:74–78.

41. Hall GL, Reinmann B, Wildhaber JH, Frey U. Tidal exhaled nitric oxide in healthy, unsedated newborn infants with prenatal tobacco exposure. J Appl Physiol 2002; 92:59–66.

42. Eigen H, Bieler H, Grant D, et al. Spirometric pulmonary function in healthy preschool children. Am J Respir Crit Care Med 2001; 163:619–623.

43. Crenesse D, Berlioz M, Bourrier T, Albertini M. Spirometry in children aged 3 to 5 years: reliability of forced expiratory maneuvers. Pediatric Pulmonol 2001; 32:56–61.

44. Nystad W, Samuelsen SO, Nafstad P, Edvardsen E, Stensrud T, Jaakkola JJ. Feasibility of measuring lung function in preschool children. Thorax 2002; 57:1021–1027.

45. Yan K, Salome C, Woolcock AJ. Rapid method for measurement of bronchial responsiveness. Thorax 1983; 38:760–765.

46. Joseph-Bowen J, de Klerk NH, Firth MJ, Kendall GE, Holt PG, Sly PD. Lung function, bronchial responsiveness, and asthma in a community cohort of 6-year-old children. Am J Respir Crit Care Med 2004; 169:850–854.

47. Hyatt RE. Forced expiration. In: Fishman AP, ed. The Respiratory System: Mechanics of Breathing. Vol. III. Baltimore: American Physiological Society, 1986:295–314.

48. Feher A, Castile R, Kisling J, et al. Flow limitation in normal infants: a new method for forced expiratory maneuvers from raised lung volumes. J Appl Physiol 1996; 80:2019–25.

49. Tepper RS, Jones M, Davis S, Kisling J, Castile R. Rate constant for forced expiration decreases with lung growth during infancy. Am J Respir Crit Care Med 1999; 160:835–838.

50. Jones M, Castile R, Davis S, et al. Forced expiratory flows and volumes in infants. Normative data and lung growth. Am J Respir Crit Care Med 2000; 161:353–359.

51. Klug B, Bisgaard H. Measurement of the specific airway resistance by plethysmography in young children accompanied by an adult. Eur Respir J 1997; 10:1599–605.

52. Nielsen KG, Bisgaard H. Discriminative capacity of bronchodilator response measured with three different lung function techniques in asthmatic and healthy children aged 2 to 5 years (see comment). Am J Respir Crit Care Med 2001; 164:554–559.

53. Delacourt C, Lorino H, Herve-Guillot M, Reinert P, Harf A, Housset B. Use of the forced oscillation technique to assess airway obstruction and reversibility in children. Am J Respir Crit Care Med 2000; 161:730–736.

54. Ducharme FM, Davis GM. Measurement of respiratory resistance in the emergency department: feasibility in young children with acute asthma. Chest 1997; 111:1519–1525.

55. Beelen RM, Smit HA, van Strien RT, et al. Short and long term variability of the interrupter technique under field and standardised conditions in 3-6 year old children (see comment). Thorax 2003; 58:761–764.

56. Lombardi E, Sly PD, Concutelli G, et al. Reference values of interrupter respiratory resistance in healthy preschool white children. Thorax 2001; 56:691–695.

57. Oswald-Mammosser M, Llerena C, Speich JP, Donata L, Lonsdorfer. Measurements of respiratory system resistance by the interrupter technique in healthy and asthmatic children. Pediatr Pulmonol 1997; 24:78–85.

58. Bridge PD, Ranganathan S, McKenzie SA. Measurement of airway resistance using the interrupter technique in preschool children in the ambulatory setting (see comment). Eur Respir J 1999; 13:792–796.

59. Anonymous. Asthma Management Handbook. Melbourne: National Asthma Council Australia, 2002.

60. Fuhlbrigge AL, Kitch BT, Paltiel AD, et al. FEV(l) is associated with risk of asthma attacks in a pediatric population. J Allergy Clin Immunol 2001; 107:61–67.

61. Brand PL, Roorda RJ. Usefulness of monitoring lung function in asthma. Arch Dis Childhood 2003; 88:1021–1025.

62. Sly PD, Flack F. Is home monitoring of lung function worthwhile for children with asthma? (letter; comment). Thorax 2001; 56:164–165.

63. Sly PD, Cahill P, Willet K, Burton P. Accuracy of mini peak flow meters in indicating changes in lung function in children with asthma (see comments). BMJ 1994; 308:572–574.

64. Eid N, Yandell B, Howell L, Eddy M, Sheikh S. Can peak expiratory flow predict airflow obstruction in children with asthma? Pediatrics 2000; 105: 354–358.

65. Clough JB, Sly PD. Association between lower respiratory tract symptoms and falls in peak expiratory flow in children. Eur Respir J 1995; 8:718–22.

66. Brand PLP, Duiverman EJ, Waalkens HJ, van Essen-Zandvliet EEM, Kerrebijn KF. Peak flow variation in childhood asthma: correlation with symptoms, airways obstruction, and hyperresponsiveness during long term treatment with inhaled corticosteroids. Thorax 1999; 54:103–107.

67. Uwyyed K. Home recording of PEF in young asthmatics: does it contribute to management? Eur Respir J 1996; 9:872–879.

68. Kamps AW, Reorda RJ, Brand PL. Peak flow diaries in childhood asthma are unreliable (comment). Thorax 2001; 56:180–182.

69. Hofstra WB, Neijens HJ, Duiverman EJ, et al. Dose–responses over time to inhaled fluticasone propionate treatment of exercise- and methacholine-induced bronchoconstriction in children with asthma. Pediatr Pulmonol 2000; 29:415–423.

70. Sont JK. Clinical control and histopathologic outcome of asthma when using airway hyperresponsiveness as an additional guide to long-term treatment. Am J Respir Crit Care Med 1999; 159:1043–1051.

71. Hamid Q, Springall DR, Riveros-Moreno V, et al. Induction of nitric oxide synthase in asthma. Lancet 1993; 342:1510–1513.

72. Kharitonov SA, Yates D, Robbins RA, Logan-Sinclair R, Shinebourne EA, Barnes PJ. Increased nitric oxide in exhaled air of asthmatic patients. Lancet 1994; 343:133–135.

73. Franklin PJ, Taplin R, Stick SM. A community study of exhaled nitric oxide in healthy children. Am J Respir Crit Care Med 1999; 159:69–73.

74. Ludviksdottir D, Janson C, Hogman M, Hedenstrom H, Bjornsson E, Boman G. Exhaled nitric oxide and its relationship to airway responsiveness and atopy in asthma. BHR-Study Group. Respir Med 1999; 93:552–556.

75. Henriksen AH, Lingaas-Holmen T, Sue-Chu M, Bjermer L. Combined use of exhaled nitric oxide and airway hyperresponsiveness in characterizing asthma in a large population survey. Eur Respir J 2000; 15:849–855.

76. Silvestri M, Sabatini F, Sale R, et al. Correlations between exhaled nitric oxide levels, blood eosinophilia, and airway obstruction reversibility in childhood asthma are detectable only in atopic individuals. Pediatr Pulmonol 2003; 35:358–363.

77. Silvestri M, Sabatini F, Spallarossa D, et al. Exhaled nitric oxide levels in non-allergic and allergic mono- or polysensitised children with asthma. Thorax 2001; 56:857–862.

78. Ho LP, Wood FT, Robson A, Innes JA, Greening AP. Atopy influences exhaled nitric oxide levels in adult asthmatics. Chest 2000; 118:1327–1331.

79. Covar RA, Szefler SJ, Martin RJ, et al. Relations between exhaled nitric oxide and measures of disease activity among children with mild-to-moderate asthma (see comment). J Pediatr 2003; 142:469–475.

80. Bates CA, Silkoff PE. Exhaled nitric oxide in asthma: from bench to bedside. J Allergy Clin Immunol 2003; 111:256–262.

81. Gibson PG, Simpson JL, Hankin R, Powell H, Henry RL. Relationship between induced sputum eosinophils and the clinical pattern of childhood asthma. Thorax 2003; 58:116–121.

82. Green RH, Brightling CE, McKenna S, et al. Asthma exacerbations and sputum eosinophil counts: a randomized controlled trial (see comment). Lancet 2002; 360:1715–1721.

15

Asthma Epidemics, Monitoring Mortality

NEIL PEARCE

Centre for Public Health Research, Massey University Wellington Campus, Wellington, New Zealand

Introduction

The epidemics of asthma deaths in the 1960s and 1970s have provided the main motivation for monitoring asthma mortality. In this chapter, the author briefly reviews the background to these studies, before proceeding to discuss the methodological issues and approaches involved. These include (i) assessing possible artifactual explanations for an increase in mortality; (ii) assessing possible explanations for a real increase in mortality including considering whether an increase is due to a change in prevalence or incidence (or whether there has been an increase in the case fatality rate), considering whether some demographic groups are particularly affected by an increase in mortality, and using this information to consider possible causal explanations for an increase in mortality; and (iii) conducting cohort or case–control studies of asthma deaths to test these causal explanations.

It was once held that "the asthmatic pants into old age" and that asthmatics rarely died of their disease (1). This is now known to be incorrect, but asthma deaths were certainly very rare in the first-half of the 20th

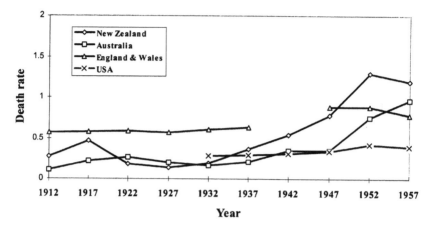

Figure 1   Asthma mortality in persons aged 5–34 years in New Zealand, Australia, and England and Wales, 1910–1960. *Source*: From Ref. 7.

century (2–4). Since that time, the patterns of asthma mortality have become considerably more complex (5–7). In contrast to the relatively stable asthma death rates during the first-half of the 20th century (Fig. 1), asthma mortality increased dramatically in at least six developed countries in the 1960s: England and Wales, Scotland, Ireland, New Zealand, Australia, and Norway. The time trends are shown in Fig. 2 for three of the epidemic countries (England and Wales, Australia, and New Zealand) and for three countries that did not experience epidemics (the United States, Canada, and West Germany). In the 1970s and 1980s, a second asthma mortality epidemic occurred in New Zealand but not in other countries.

   In recent years, attention has also focused on the possible causes of the gradual increase in mortality (Fig. 3) that appears to have occurred in a number of countries during the 1970s and 1980s (8–14,82). However, recent data suggest that mortality may now be declining again in some countries since about 1988 (15–24).

   It should be stressed that studies of time trends, particularly gradual (rather than epidemic) time trends, suffer from the same limitations as other ecologic analyses and provide relatively weak evidence as to causal associations (25). Many factors may change over time (asthma prevalence, sales of asthma drugs, sales of television sets, etc.), and there are, therefore, major difficulties in establishing causality on the basis of time trends alone, particularly if only a gradual increase in mortality has occurred. However, analyses of such trends may still provide important descriptive information. The author's emphasis here will be on considering epidemic increases in asthma mortality (particularly the 1960s epidemics and the

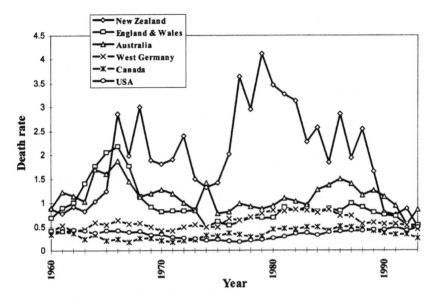

Figure 2   International patterns of asthma mortality in persons aged 5–34 years, 1960–1990. *Source*: From Ref. 6.

1970s epidemic in New Zealand), and the author will stress that in this context, analyses of time trends should primarily be used as part of a process of generating hypotheses as to the possible causes of the epidemic increases. These hypotheses should then be tested in more formal epidemiological studies.

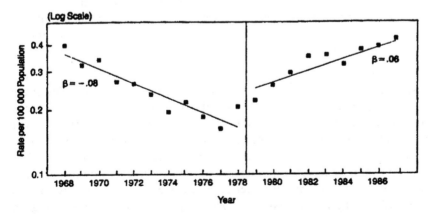

Figure 3   Trends in U.S. asthma mortality among person aged 5–34 years in the United States during 1968–1986. *Source*: From Ref. 14.

As Stolley and Lasky (26) note, any explanation for the 1960s epidemics must account for several key features of the epidemics including (i) that the epidemic of deaths among asthmatics began abruptly; (ii) that the epidemic affected only some countries and spared others; and (iii) that asthma mortality had been remarkably constant in most countries until the epidemic began. Stolley and Lasky (26) list nine questions that should be considered by an epidemiologist attempting to ascertain the causes of such an increase in mortality:

1. Is the increase in death rates real or an artifact of reporting practices or nosologic changes? Has there been a change in nosology, nomenclature, or coding practices over the course of the presumed epidemic and what is the possible effect of such changes?
2. Has there been a change in the denominator so that the population at risk in calculation of the rate is either undercounted or overcounted?
3. Has a new diagnostic tool been introduced that could lead to improved diagnosis or detection of the disease of interest, thus artifactually elevating death rates compared with earlier periods?
4. Has there been a change in the incidence or prevalence of the disease that could account for the change in the death rates?
5. Is the increase in death rates uniform in all groups at risk or concentrated among particular groups?
6. If the deaths are plotted on a "spot map," do they cluster geographically?
7. If deaths are examined month by month, do they cluster or concentrate seasonally or temporally in any pattern?
8. Has a new treatment been introduced that could lead to an improved or worsened outcome for affected persons?
9. If the death rate increases are real and represent the true picture of mortality, what working hypotheses can explain this unusual phenomenon?

These questions naturally fall into two groups. Questions 1–3 involve assessing the validity of the reported the increase in mortality. The subsequent questions involve assessing possible explanations for a real increase in mortality, including considering whether the increase is due to a change in prevalence or incidence (prevalence is the most relevant measure in this instance because it provides the "denominator" population at risk of asthma death) or whether an increase in the case fatality rate has occurred (question 4), considering whether some demographic groups are particularly affected by the increase in mortality (questions 5–7), and using this information to consider possible causal explanations for the increase in mortality (questions 8 and 9).

Assessing the Validity of Time Trends

Of the possible types of bias listed by Stolley and Lasky (26), an undetected change in the denominator is not a plausible explanation for the asthma mortality epidemics because the time trends are based on national census data and national death data. However, the other possible biases are relevant to time trends in asthma mortality. In particular, the key methodological issues in assessing the validity of such time trends are (i) the accuracy of death certificates; (ii) changes in disease classification; and (iii) changes in diagnostic fashion (27). In each instance, these factors could account for gradual changes in death rates over time but could not account for epidemic increases. In particular, Speizer et al. (28) conducted a detailed examination of the mortality trends in the 5–34 year age-group in England and Wales and concluded that the epidemic was real and was not due to changes in death certification, disease classification, or diagnostic practice, and similar conclusions were reached by Jackson et al. (29) with regard to the second epidemic in New Zealand.

Accuracy of Death Certificates

The first consideration in assessing time trends in asthma mortality is the accuracy of the death certificate information on asthma deaths (16). Almost all comparative studies of asthma mortality have been confined to the 5–34 year age-group, because the diagnosis of asthma mortality is more firmly established in this group (29–31). For example, Sears et al. (32) studied asthma deaths in New Zealand during 1981–1983 and found that in patients aged <35 years, the recorded information was considered accurate in 98% of all certified deaths, and in 100% of deaths coded as asthma in national mortality data; the corresponding estimates for those aged ≥65 years were 44% and 55%, respectively (Fig. 4).

Similarly, the Research Committee of the British Thoracic Association conducted an enquiry into death from asthma in adults aged 15–64 years in the West Midland and Mersey regions during 1979 (30). Death certificates recording the word "asthma" were received for 153 persons. The panel was unable to agree about the role of asthma in five deaths, and there was one other death for which insufficient information was available. For the other 147 deaths, Table 1 compares the panel's assessment of cause of death with that coded by the national Office of Population Censuses and Surveys (OPCS). Overall, 89 patients were considered by the panel to have died from asthma; in 77 (87%) of these cases, the death certificates were considered to have been correctly coded, whereas in 12 (13%), death was considered to have been wrongly attributed to asthma (i.e., false positives); as with other similar studies, the agreement was much greater in the younger age-groups (90% in the 15–44 year age-group, 76% in the 45–54

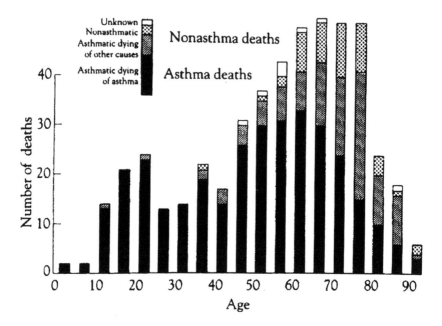

Figure 4 Accuracy of certification of asthma deaths, as judged by a review panel of physicians, of 492 cases with "asthma" in part I of the death certificate or on the coroner's report of cause of death. *Source*: From Ref. 72.

year age-group and 61% in the 55–64 year age-group). On the other hand, 24 of the 58 deaths that were not considered by the panel to have been due to asthma were coded as asthma by the OPCS. Thus, the total number of 101 deaths coded as being due to asthma represented a net overestimate of 13% when compared with the panel's coding of 89 deaths as being due to asthma.

Table 1 Comparability of ICD Coding by the Office of Population Censuses and Surveys (OPCS) and Panel Classification of Asthma Deaths

OPCS coding	Panel's assessment		
	Asthma was cause of death	Other cause of death	Total
Asthma death	77	24	101
Other cause of death	12	34	46
Total	89	58	147

Source: From Ref. 30.

Most studies of this type have only examined the possibility of false-positive reporting (i.e., deaths from other causes being falsely attributed to asthma). A New Zealand study (29) found that false-negative reporting (i.e., asthma deaths being falsely assigned to other categories) appeared to be very rare; in 66 cases in which death was attributed to disorders which could have been confused with asthma, only one case was considered to have died with asthma, but even in this case, death could not be confidently attributed to asthma. However, a more recent study in the United Kingdom (33) found that four of 22 asthma deaths had been incorrectly certified as non-asthma deaths (two as deaths from chronic obstructive pulmonary disease and two as deaths from cardiovascular disease). A recent study in Minnesota (34) also found significant false-negative reporting. However, in this population, the median age at death was 74 years, with an interquartile range of 63–82 years. Considerably lower rates of misclassification have been found in studies of younger asthmatics (32). Thus, given the accuracy of death rates in the 5–34 year age-group, it is clear that inaccuracies in death certificates could not explain epidemic increases occurring over a period of just a few years.

Changes in Disease Classification

Changes in disease classification are also of concern when examining time trends in asthma mortality. The International Classification of Diseases has gone through several major changes in coding practices for asthma deaths since the early 1900s. These largely involved changes in the coding of deaths due to "asthma and bronchitis" that were assigned to bronchitis during some periods and to asthma during others (Table 2). However, these changes have primarily affected the data for the older age-groups, and they appear to have had little effect on the key trends in the 5–34 year age-group (27). For example, the most important revision occurred with the change from ICD-4 to ICD-5 when the method of coding the underlying cause of death was changed, but no major changes in mortality rates occurred. A further significant change occurred with the change from ICD-8 to ICD-9. However, an analysis of death registrations in New Zealand (10) found that the maximum possible increase that could be attributed to the change was ~5%, and a similar estimate was obtained in the United Kingdom (35). Thus, changes in disease classification could account for modest changes in death rates but could not account for epidemic increases.

Changes in Diagnostic Fashion

The effects of changes in diagnostic fashion over time are more difficult to quantify, although several attempts have been made by simultaneously examining time trends in other respiratory diseases that could be confused with asthma (27). In general, these have found that changes in diagnostic

Table 2 Changes to Coding of Asthma Deaths During this Century and Years of Use of Each Code

Classification	Years	Comments
ICD-1	1900–1909	"Asthma and bronchitis" coded according to which was judged to be underlying cause of death
ICD-2	1910–1920	"Asthma and bronchitis" coded according to which was judged to be underlying cause of death
ICD-3	1921–1929	"Asthma and bronchitis" coded according to which was judged to be underlying cause of death
ICD-4	1930–1938	"Asthma and bronchitis" coded according to which was judged to be underlying cause of death
ICD-5	1939–1948	"Asthma and bronchitis" coded as bronchitis "Asthmatic bronchitis" coded as asthma
ICD-6	1949–1957	"Asthma and bronchitis" coded as asthma
ICD-7	1958–1967	"Asthma and bronchitis" coded as bronchitis, unless the asthma was specified as allergic
ICD-8	1968–1978	"Asthma due to bronchitis" coded as bronchitis
ICD-9	1979–1998	"Asthma due to bronchitis" coded as bronchitis "Bronchitis due to asthma" coded as asthma
ICD-10	1999–till to date	"Asthma due to bronchitis" coded as bronchitis "Bronchitis due to asthma" coded as asthma

fashion could not account for the asthma mortality epidemics. For example, Speizer et al. (28) examined possible explanations for the sudden epidemics of asthma mortality that commenced in England and Wales, as well as in five other countries, in the early 1960s. One possible explanation for the increased mortality was a change in diagnostic criteria used by physicians certifying the cause of death. They examined this possibility by comparing the trends in asthma deaths and those for a variety of other respiratory diseases; the latter included bronchitis, bronchiectasis, emphysema without mention of bronchitis, and pneumonias during 1959–1965 (Table 3). They found that no appreciable change took place in the death rates from bronchitis and other chronic respiratory diseases; some decrease occurred for pneumonias, but this was less than half of the increase in asthma deaths over the same period. Moreover, the number of deaths attributed to bronchitis for which asthma was mentioned on the death certificate did not

Table 3 Death Rates from Respiratory Diseases in the 5–34 Year Age-Group in England and Wales 1959–1965

Diagnostic category	Year						
	1959	1960	1961	1962	1963	1964	1965
Bronchitis	0.65	0.57	0.66	0.67	0.65	0.62	0.66
Chronic respiratory disease	0.45	0.49	0.39	0.40	0.38	0.39	0.40
Pneumonias	2.61	2.15	2.24	2.47	2.15	2.04	1.93
Asthma	0.66	0.68	0.89	1.00	1.40	1.76	2.05

Source: From Ref. 28.

decrease, as would have been expected if doctors had tended to attribute the underlying cause to asthma alone rather than to asthma and bronchitis. Furthermore, the number of asthma deaths that were certified by coroners increased more rapidly than asthma deaths in general. They argued that if the increase were an artifact, then one would have to postulate that there had been a greater diagnostic change among pathologists than among clinicians or that there had been a change in the type of case referred to coroners, and both these possibilities appeared most unlikely. Speizer et al (28), therefore, concluded that the increase in mortality from asthma in the 5–34 year age-group was largely real and was not due to changes in diagnostic fashion.

However, it is not possible to exclude changes in diagnostic fashion as an explanation for more gradual changes in asthma mortality. Diagnostic fashion may be a more important source of bias in international comparisons than in comparisons of time trends within a single country. For example, asthma deaths may be underestimated in some populations in the United States, and Burney (36) found major differences in the certification of two ambivalent case histories by physicians from eight European countries.

Assessing Possible Explanations for Time Trends

If it is assumed that an increase in asthma deaths is real, then attention shifts to assessing the possible explanations for the increase.

Has there been a Change in Asthma Prevalence or Incidence?

The first issue to consider is whether the increase in mortality is due to an increase in asthma prevalence (or in the prevalence of severe asthma) or whether there has been a change in the case fatality rate. In both epidemics (28,29), there was little evidence available on whether or not asthma prevalence had changed (and virtually no information on asthma incidence).

However, in both instances, it was considered highly unlikely that the epidemics could be due to changes in asthma prevalence because the evidence that was available did not indicate any dramatic increase in prevalence, the epidemics had commenced so abruptly after a long period of stable asthma death rates, and the epidemic countries were scattered around the world while some neighboring countries had not experienced epidemics. Therefore, although direct information on changes in asthma prevalence was not available, this was considered to be a highly unlikely explanation for the epidemics, and attention, therefore, shifted to considering possible explanations for a change in the case fatality rate.

More recent evidence has shown that asthma prevalence has increased gradually in a number of Western countries since the 1950s (7), but although these increases could certainly account for gradual changes in mortality over time, it could not account for epidemic increases.

Does the Increase in Mortality Affect Particular Groups?

The first step in considering possible explanations for an increase in case fatality is to examine whether the increase in mortality is concentrated in particular demographic groups. This is the standard "descriptive epidemiology" approach of considering variations in mortality by person, place, or time (Stolley and Lasky's questions 5–7). For example, as noted earlier, the 1960s epidemics occurred in some countries and not others, and occurred after a long period of relatively stable asthma death rates. There was less information available on characteristics of the patients who died, but Speizer et al. (28) noted that the increase in mortality was greatest in the 10–19 year age-group and that "at these ages, children have begun to act independently and may be particularly prone to misuse a self-administered form of treatment." Similarly, the 1970s epidemic in New Zealand particularly affected young Maori males, and two U.S. studies (37,38) found that asthma mortality had particularly increased in below-income households and in African-Americans.

A related issue is when the epidemic deaths occurred. For example, in the 1970s epidemic in New Zealand, most deaths occurred at night or in the weekends when there may have been greater problems of access to medical care (39). Several studies have found seasonal patterns with peaks in asthma mortality during the summer months while peaks in asthma hospitalizations occur during the winter (40–43). A number of reasons for these different patterns have been proposed including seasonal changes precipitating the "triggering" of an asthma attack, or an altered routine, perhaps associated with holidays when there may be reduced access to health services.

What Hypotheses Might Explain These Changes in the Case Fatality Rate?

Thus, in both the 1960s and 1970s epidemics, it appeared that the increases in mortality were real and were due to an increase in the case fatality rate and had particularly affected groups that were likely to overuse medication and/or delay seeking treatment for an acute asthma attack. This was consistent with the hypothesis that there had been some change in medical management that had occurred relatively suddenly in some countries, but not in others.

The 1960s Epidemics

With regard to the 1960s epidemics, it was noted that the sudden increase in deaths had followed the introduction of pressurized beta-agonist aerosols in 1961 and that the increase in mortality paralleled the increase in sales (44). These initial observations were complemented by a number of case series reports (45–50). For example, Fraser et al. (51) examined the circumstances preceding death in asthma deaths in the 5–34 year age-group in Greater London and the South-East Lancashire conurbation in the period 1 February 1968 to 31 January 1969. Copies of death certificates were provided by local Registrars of Births and Deaths, and 43 asthma deaths were identified; further 9 deaths were subsequently identified from the General Register Office in London. Interviews were conducted with general practitioners for 51 of the deaths and with next-of-kin for 42 of the deaths, and necropsy reports were obtained in 45 cases. They found that 59% of patients died during a new attack of episodic asthma, 29% after an acute exacerbation of chronic wheeziness, and 10% after a period of steady deterioration. Death was sudden and "unexpected" in 84% of patients. They concluded that excessive inhalation of bronchodilators might have been a factor in approximately one-third of the deaths. The duration of the terminal episode in the patients who used drugs excessively was longer than in other patients, and it was possible that the excessive users found an effective dose for a time but then reached and failed to recognize a state in which they were unable to respond to bronchodilators.

Similar case series reports have been conducted in the United States (52), Australia (53,54) and New Zealand (39,55). Case reports cannot in themselves establish the cause of an increase in mortality, but they can suggest possible hypotheses or identify phenomena that need to be explained. In the 1960s mortality epidemics, it was known that the deaths were often sudden and unexplained, most occurred outside hospital (56), direct information on drug usage was scanty, and the likely mechanism of death was unknown. However, it was noted that the relief of symptoms could enable a patient to tolerate worsening hypoxia and to unduly delay seeking medical help (47). It was also argued that both chronic and acute side effects of inhaled beta-agonists could occur, and that direct toxicity could occur in certain circumstances, as isoprenaline (one of the most commonly used beta-agonists at the time) is a non-selective beta-agonist (57), Thus, the case reports, as well as other available information, were consistent with a possible role of beta-agonist aerosols in the epidemics (44).

However, although the time trends seemed to be consistent with the hypothesis that the epidemics were due to the introduction of beta-agonist aerosols, the geographic patterns were inconsistent with this hypothesis as the epidemics did not occur in some countries, including the United States, in which beta-agonist aerosol sales were relatively high. These anomalies were eventually clarified by Stolley (58) who noted that a high-dose formulation of isoprenaline (isoprenaline forte), that contained five times the dose per administration of other isoprenaline aerosols, had only been licensed in eight countries (Table 4). Six of these (England and Wales, Ireland, Scotland, Australia, New Zealand, and Norway) had mortality epidemics that coincided with the introduction of the drug, and in the other two countries (the Netherlands and Belgium), the preparation was introduced relatively late and sales volumes were low. Overall, there was a strong positive correlation internationally between the asthma mortality rate and isoprenaline forte sales in these eight countries, whereas no mortality epidemics occurred in countries in which isoprenaline forte was not licensed, such as Sweden, Canada, West Germany, and the United States (58). Thus, the time trend evidence was inconsistent with a general effect of beta-agonist aerosols, but was highly consistent with the hypothesis that the epidemic was due to the high-dose beta-agonist aerosol isoprenaline forte.

Some anomalies still remained in the time trend data, but these were generally minor. For example, Gandevia (59) found no correlation between beta-agonist aerosol sales and asthma mortality in Australia when sales were examined on a state-by-state basis. However, Campbell (60) subsequently reanalyzed the same data and found that there was a remarkably

Table 4 Cross-Classification of Countries by Presence or Absence of an Epidemic of Asthma Mortality and Presence or Absence of Sales of Isoprenaline Forte Aerosols

Epidemic of asthma mortality in the 1960s	Isoprenaline forte aerosols		
	Available	Not available	Total
Present	6	0	6
Absent	2	6	6
Total	8	6	14

Source: From Ref. 66.

high correlation in each of the four most populated states until 1966. After that time, widespread publicity about the mortality epidemic, as well as the elimination of non-prescription availability of beta-agonist aerosols, was followed by a decrease in the death rate independently of isoprenaline forte sales. Similar phenomena had been noted in other epidemic countries (5). Formal analytical epidemiological studies were never mounted because the epidemic declined before there was time to conduct them. Nevertheless, the weight of evidence was highly consistent with the isoprenaline forte hypothesis, and death from bronchodilator aerosols was designated one of the most important adverse drug reactions since thalidomide (61).

The potential hazards of beta-agonist aerosols were disputed in many subsequent texts and reviews (62–65). However, very little new evidence has appeared since 1972, with the exception of further analyses conducted by Stolley and Schinnar (66) that strengthened Stolley's original conclusions. They carried out a multiple regression analysis of time trends in drug sales and asthma mortality, using data from six countries during 1962–1974. These showed a strong correlation between sales of isoprenaline forte and asthma deaths in the countries in which the high-dose preparation had been marketed; there was no significant correlation between asthma deaths and sales of regular isoprenaline, orciprenaline, or other beta-agonist aerosols. Figure 5 shows the time trends in drug sales and asthma mortality in England and Wales (which experienced a mortality epidemic) and Fig. 6 shows the corresponding data for the United States (which did not experience an epidemic). In England and Wales, there was a strong parallel in sales of regular isoprenaline and those of isoprenaline forte, and it was therefore not possible to separate their relative contributions to the mortality epidemic; the death rate strongly paralleled the rise and fall in sales of both formulations. In the United States, isoprenaline forte was not available, and the death rate remained stable and then fell slightly during the period that other six countries were experiencing mortality epidemics.

The Second New Zealand Epidemic

Similar issues and controversies accompanied the analyses of second New Zealand asthma mortality epidemic. The initial case report (55) involved 22 asthma deaths in Auckland, including 16 patients in whom death was seen to be sudden and unexpected.

Keating et al. (67) analyzed trends in sales of asthma drugs in Australia, New Zealand, and the United Kingdom during 1975–1981 and found that there had been a striking increase in per capita sales of beta-agonist aerosols and oral theophyllines in all three countries, with the greatest increase occurring in New Zealand. However, the striking increase in beta-agonist sales in New Zealand (Fig. 7) commenced in 1979, whereas the epidemic of deaths commenced in 1976. Furthermore, appreciable

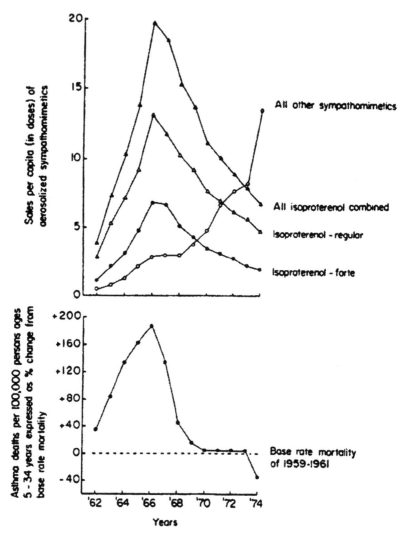

Figure 5 Asthma mortality per 100,000 persons aged 5–34 years in relation to per capita sales of beta-agonist aerosols in England and Wales during 1962–1974. *Source*: From Ref. 66.

increases in sales had also occurred in Australia and the United Kingdom, and no epidemics of deaths had occurred. Thus, it seemed most unlikely that the general increase in beta-agonist sales (as a class) was the cause of the New Zealand epidemic.

However, Crane et al. (68) examined the New Zealand time trend data and found that one particular beta-agonist, fenoterol, was introduced to New Zealand in April 1976 and that the epidemic began in the same year,

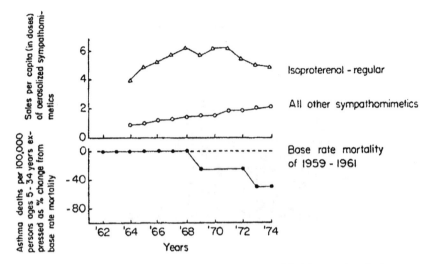

Figure 6 Asthma mortality per 100,000 persons aged 5–34 years in relation to per capita sales of beta-agonist aerosols in the United States during 1962–1974. *Source*: From Ref. 66.

with a close parallel between fenoterol sales and asthma deaths in the early years of the epidemic; by 1979, fenoterol accounted for a market share of nearly 30%, and mortality had increased threefold. After 1979, the fenoterol market share remained relatively constant, but mortality fell gradually

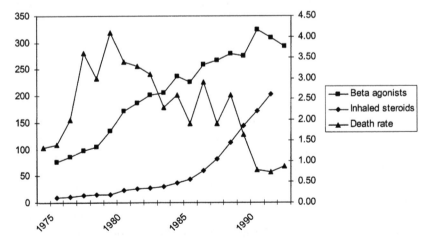

Figure 7 Time trends in asthma mortality aged 5–34 years in New Zealand during 1974–1990 and total sales of inhaled beta-agonists (doses) and inhaled corticosteroids (100 μg equivalents). *Source*: Pearce (1995).

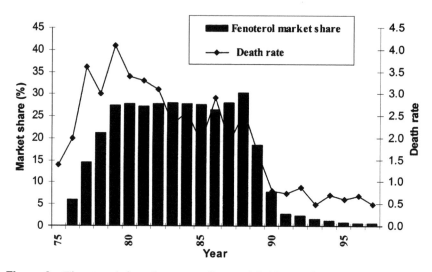

Figure 8   Time trends in asthma mortality aged 5–34 years in New Zealand during 1974–1992 and fenoterol market share. *Source*: Ref. 69.

(Fig. 8). The reasons for this are unclear, but it is likely that management may have changed in other ways during this period. In particular, the epidemic was first publicized in 1981 (55), and it was possible that concerns about the safety of asthma drugs may have lead to greater care in their use and a resulting decline in mortality. Pearce et al. (69) subsequently found that mortality fell by one-half after warnings was issued about the safety of fenoterol in mid- 1989 and remained low in subsequent years (Fig. 8).

Cohort and Case–Control Studies of Asthma Deaths

Time trend analyses provide relatively weak evidence as to the causes of asthma deaths, and a major problem with case series reports is the lack of a control group. Thus, if a certain proportion of patients are reported to have been prescribed a particular asthma drug, the lack of a control group means that it is very difficult to determine whether the patients who died had been prescribed the drug more or less often than might have been "expected." Similarly, it is very difficult to determine whether other factors such as overuse of medication, delays in seeking medical help, psychosocial factors, or underuse of corticosteroids occurred more often than expected.

   In this section, the author considers the various formal epidemiological study design options theoretically available for studying the causes of asthma deaths and the links between them. Most cohort and case–control studies of asthma deaths, have focused on pharmacological risk factors, and the author therefore gives emphasis to methodological issues in studies of such factors. In particular, the author discusses the various study design options in the context of investigating the hypothesis that prescription of a particular drug increases the risk of asthma mortality (in comparison with other drugs within the same class).

The ideal approach to testing such a hypothesis would be a randomized controlled trial, but this is usually impractical and unethical. However, the randomized controlled trial remains the "gold standard" for epidemiological studies of asthma deaths (7). The author, therefore, first discusses the design of a hypothetical randomized trial to compare the death rate in patients prescribed a drug that is suspected to increase the risk of asthma death (Drug A) with that in patients prescribed the standard treatment (Drug B); next, the author designs a hypothetical cohort study to achieve the same objective; finally, he designs a hypothetical case–control study to achieve the same objective more efficiently than the full cohort study.

Randomized Trial of Asthma Mortality

In a randomized trial of asthma medication and asthma mortality, it would be most appropriate to study the effects of the asthma drugs in the clinical setting in which they are most commonly used (70). In any case, there would be major practical problems with mounting a study involving randomization of medication at the time of acute attacks, and asthma patients tend to also use their regular prescribed medication for relief in acute attacks. Thus, the most reasonable approach would be to randomize patients to receive either Drug A or Drug B as their regular prescribed therapy. This approach is most feasible and appropriate irrespective of whether the hypothesis under study involves chronic or acute effects. As asthma deaths are a rare event, it would also be important to base the randomized trial on a group of "high risk" asthmatics, rather than asthmatics in general. Patients recently hospitalized for asthma would be one suitable population for study, because it is known that such patients are at increased risk of asthma death during the subsequent year (71).

Figure 9 shows the design of a hypothetical study of this type. Patients would be identified at the time of hospitalization for asthma and would be randomized to receive either Drug A or Drug B. They would then be followed over time, and any subsequent deaths from asthma would be identified from national death registrations (some deaths would be identified directly because they occurred in hospital but most would occur outside of hospital). There would be two major methodological issues.

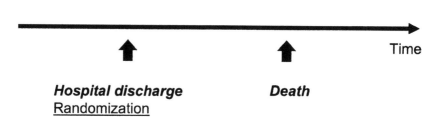

Figure 9   A hypothetical clinical trial or cohort study of asthma mortality.

First, for a variety of reasons, some patients would have changes to their therapy after they had been randomized. In particular, patients who were experiencing acute attacks with an increasing frequency or severity might have changes to their medication. However, in analyzing such a study, it would be incorrect to take such changes into account, as these might result in serious bias if the increasing severity was caused by the drug to which they had been randomized. The correct approach would be to analyze the data according to the "intention to treat" principle, i.e., the study subjects would be classified according to the regular prescribed medication that they were originally randomized to, and subsequent changes to their medication would be ignored.

The second methodological problem is that although randomization should generally ensure that the two groups under study are similar with respect to their chronic asthma severity, this cannot be guaranteed in every instance. Thus, it would be important to gather information on recognized markers of chronic asthma severity at the time of randomization, such as frequency of previous hospital admissions for asthma, and on recent prescription of oral corticosteroids. The two groups would then be compared with respect to their average chronic asthma severity. If they were found to differ in this respect, then the analysis would be controlled for, or stratified on, chronic asthma severity. For example, the study might be split into two groups: those that had chronically severe asthma according to a particular severity marker and those that did not; the comparison between Drug A and Drug B would then be conducted within each of these two subgroups, and an overall effect estimate adjusted for chronic severity would also be derived if this were appropriate. It is important to note that only the baseline severity at the time of randomization would be relevant in this regard. It would be incorrect to consider subsequent changes in acute or chronic severity, as these could be a result of treatment. Thus, only the baseline severity (at time of randomization) should be used when considering the potential for confounding by severity.

Table 5 shows data from such a hypothetical randomized trial. This involved enrolling 80,000 patients aged 5–34 years who had been admitted to hospital with asthma over a 5-year period. The study subjects were

Table 5 Findings from a Hypothetical Randomized Trial or Cohort Study of Asthma Mortality

	Drug A	Drug B
Deaths	70	35
Survivors	39,930	39,965
Total	40,000	40,000
Risk	70/40,000	35/40,000
Relative risk (95% CI)	2.0 (1.3–3.0)	

randomized to receive either Drug A or Drug B in equal numbers, and each study subject was followed for a period of 1 year after randomization. There were 70 deaths in Group B and 35 deaths in Group B, yielding a relative risk of 2.0 (95% confidence interval (CI) 1.3–3.0). However, there would be considerable problems with conducting a randomized trial of this type, particularly because of the large numbers of patients required. Thus, although some notable randomized trials have been conducted of beta-agonists and non-fatal hazardous outcomes (72), it is usually impractical and sometimes unethical to conduct such a trial involving a fatal outcome both because of ethical issues and because of the large numbers required. For example, Castle et al. (73) conducted a double-blind randomized clinical trial to assess the safety of salmeterol, a new long-acting beta-agonist. The study involved 25,180 patients followed for 16 weeks, but there were only 14 asthma-related deaths in the study, and it was not possible to draw firm conclusions.

Cohort Study of Asthma Mortality

Thus, a randomized trial of asthma deaths is usually impractical, and an epidemiological (observational) approach is required. One obvious option would be to conduct a cohort study. The design of such a hypothetical cohort study would be identical to that of the hypothetical randomized trial shown in Fig. 9, except that the subjects would not be randomized into treatment groups. Instead, their regular prescribed medication (either Drug A or Drug B) would be ascertained (rather than randomly allocated) at time of discharge. Once again, they would be followed for 1 year (or until their next admission) to ascertain subsequent asthma deaths.

The two major methodological concerns of the hypothetical randomized trial would also apply to this hypothetical cohort study. First, some patients would change their medication after leaving hospital, particularly if their asthma subsequently became more troublesome or severe, but it would be inappropriate to take such changes into account in the analysis. Although the "intention to treat" principle does not apply as a general rule in non-randomized studies, the specific biases discussed earlier in the context of clinical trials would also apply to a cohort study, and it would once again be necessary to analyze the data according to the regular prescribed medication at time of discharge.

Second, Group A and Group B might differ according to their chronic asthma severity at time of discharge. This problem would be of potentially greater concern in the cohort study (than in the clinical trial), because patients had not been randomized to treatments. However, the solution would be the same: to gather information on various markers of chronic asthma severity at time of hospitalization and to conduct analyses of subgroups defined by these severity markers. Once again, only the baseline chronic asthma severity at the time of commencement of follow-up (at time of hospitalization) would be relevant, and it would be incorrect to consider subsequent changes in severity. In particular, subsequent changes in acute or chronic asthma severity could well be a result of treatment, and it would be incorrect to control for this. Assuming that there was little difference in the baseline chronic asthma severity of those prescribed Drug A and those prescribed Drug B, then the findings of the hypothetical cohort study would be similar to those of the hypothetical clinical trial shown in Table 5; if there were differences in baseline chronic severity between Group A and Group B, then this could be controlled for with the severity subgroup analyses described earlier.

Thus, a hypothetical cohort study might involve enrolling 80,000 patients aged 5–34 years who had been admitted to hospital with asthma over a given period and recording their regular prescribed medication from hospital notes at the time of discharge. Assume for simplicity that when this was done, it was found that 50% of patients had been prescribed Drug A and 50% prescribed Drug B. Each study subject was followed for a period of 1 year after randomization. Once again, there were 70 deaths in the Group A and 35 deaths in Group B, and the relative risk was 2.0 (95% CI 1.3–3.0).

Such a hypothetical cohort study would have two major advantages over a randomized trial: it would not have the same ethical problems and it could be conducted historically rather than prospectively. However, it would still have one major problem: the need to enroll a large number of patients and to collect information on prescribed medication for all of them. Although this is occasionally possible (74), it is rare to have historical records available in sufficient numbers for a historical cohort study to be conducted.

Case–Control Study of Asthma Mortality

When a disease outcome is rare, as is the case with asthma deaths, the case–control approach is usually more efficient than a cohort study (7). In a case–control study, a group of persons with a disease (or an event, such as asthma death) is compared to a control group of persons without the disease (or event) with respect to their past exposure to a particular factor. The first modern case–control study was published in 1926 and this method is now perhaps the predominant form of epidemiological research (7). It is thus surprising that the first case–control study of asthma deaths was not published until 1985 (75), and the first case–control study of the role of specific asthma drugs in asthma deaths was not published until 1989 (68).

Figure 10 shows the design of a case–control study intended to achieve the same results as the cohort study in a more efficient manner. This would involve studying all of the cases of asthma mortality generated by the cohort, and a control group sampled at random from the same cohort. Once again, the same major methodological considerations would apply as in the clinical trial and cohort study.

First, the data would be analyzed according to the regular prescribed medication at time of discharge, and changes in medication that occurred after discharge from hospital would not be considered (70). Information on the quantity of medication used in the fatal attack is particularly problematic because it is almost impossible to determine whether high medication use caused the fatality or merely reflected the severity of the final attach (76).

Second, the potential for bias due to differences in baseline chronic asthma severity would be exactly the same as in the full cohort study. The solution would also be exactly the same: to collect information on chronic asthma severity at time of hospitalization (i.e., at baseline). Once again, it

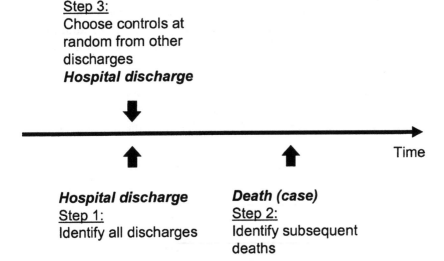

Figure 10 A hypothetical case–control study of asthma mortality.

would be incorrect to control for subsequent changes in acute or chronic severity, as these might be a result of treatment. It should also be noted that the subsequent acute severity of the controls would, by design, be different from that of the cases, as the cases died and the controls did not. In this context, it should be emphasized that the controls are, in general, intended to be representative of the cohort (source population) that generated the cases and are not required to be identical with the cases in every respect. It is also important to note the appropriate approach to assessing whether a drug (e.g., Drug A) was selectively prescribed to patients with more severe asthma. In a full cohort study, this would be assessed by examining the full cohort (not just those who died) and comparing the baseline chronic severity of Group A and Group B. Because the control group (in the case–control study) is a sample of the full cohort, the same conclusions can be drawn (as would have been drawn from examining the full cohort) by comparing the average chronic severity of the controls prescribed Drug A to the average chronic severity of the controls prescribed Drug B. The cases are not relevant in this context, and incorrect results may be obtained if they are considered.

Table 6 shows the data from a hypothetical case–control study, that involved studying the 105 asthma deaths that would have been identified in the full cohort study, and from a sample of 420 controls (four for each case). As before, there were 70 deaths in Group A and 35 deaths in Group B. The controls were distributed in the same proportions as the cohort from which they were sampled: 210 (50%) were on Drug A and 210 (50%) were on Drug B. In fact, the proportion will not be exactly 50:50 if the controls were sampled from the survivors, but this minor bias is trivial as asthma deaths are so rare, and is avoided if controls are selected by density sampling rather than cumulative incidence sampling (77). In addition, the proportion of controls on Drug A may be different from 50% merely by chance, but on the average the control distribution will be similar to that shown in Table 6.

The odds ratio is then the ratio of the odds of being a case in Group A (70/210) to the odds of being a case in Group B (35/210). This, once again, yields a relative risk of 2.0 (95% CI 1.3–3.2); exactly the same answer can be

Table 6 Findings from a Hypothetical Case–control Study of Asthma Mortality

	Drug A	Drug B	Odds
Deaths (cases)	70	35	70/35
Controls	210	210	210/210
Odds	70/210	35/210	
Odds ratio (95% CI)			2.0(1.3–3.2)

obtained by taking the ratio of the odds of being prescribed Drug A in the case group (70/35) to that of being prescribed Drug A in the control group (210/210). Thus, such a case–control study would achieve the same findings as the full cohort study but would be considerably more efficient, because it would involve ascertaining the prescribed medication of 525 patients (105 cases and 420 controls) rather than 80,000. This remarkable gain in efficiency is achieved with only a very minimal reduction in the precision of the relative risk estimate (reflected in the slightly wider CI for the odds ratio estimate).

A case–control study of the type shown in Fig. 10 could be nested within a formal cohort, created by listing all hospital admissions for asthma in a country or region over a period of time. However, the same result could be achieved more efficiently in the manner illustrated in Fig. 11. This shows a study in which the first step is to identify asthma deaths from national death registration records. For each death, the records of hospitals to which the patient was likely to have been admitted in an acute attack were then searched to identify any admission for asthma in the previous 12 months. If such an admission were identified, the death was included in the study, and the admission closest to death was used. For each death, one or more controls was then selected at random from patients discharged from the same hospital with the diagnosis of asthma at the time that the case's discharge occurred. The prescribed medication at discharge was then ascertained for cases and controls from hospital records (for the admission

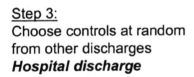

Step 3:
Choose controls at random
from other discharges
Hospital discharge

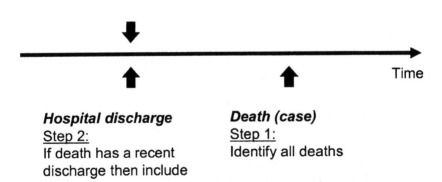

Time

Hospital discharge
Step 2:
If death has a recent
discharge then include

Death (case)
Step 1:
Identify all deaths

Figure 11 Alternative design for a hypothetical case–control study of asthma mortality.

prior to death for the cases and for the corresponding admission for the controls). This would yield the same findings as the case–control design shown in Fig. 10 and the cohort/clinical trial design shown in Fig. 9), but would have the advantage that it would not be necessary to enumerate the entire cohort before selecting controls.

It should also be noted that in some situations, the control group might not be chosen as a completely random sample of the source population. For example, it is common to ensure that the control group has a similar age-distribution to the cases (i.e., age matching) in order to make it easier to control for potential confounding by age. Similarly, it might be considered desirable to ensure that the control group had a similar average chronic severity to the cases at the time of hospitalization (it would be impossible for the controls to have the same acute severity at the time of the final attack, as the cases died and the controls did not). This would not be necessary if there were, in fact, no tendency for Drug A to be selectively prescribed to more severe asthmatics. However, if this were not known with certainty, then it might be considered appropriate to match for chronic asthma severity, either directly or indirectly. A direct match for severity ("pair matching") would involve taking each case and ensuring that the matched controls were identical to the case with respect to certain markers of chronic asthma severity. An indirect approach (analogous to frequency matching) might involve requiring potential controls to have had a further hospital admission within a 1-year period, so that the cases had had an admission followed by death within 1 year and the controls had had an admission followed by another admission within 1 year (Fig. 12).

Studies of Fenoterol and Asthma Deaths

These different study designs can be illustrated with regards to case–control studies of fenoterol and asthma deaths. Table 7 summarizes the study designs and Table 8 summarizes the findings of key case–control studies of this issue (68,95,78,98).

Grainger et al. (1992) conducted a case–control study of asthma deaths in the 5–45 year age-group in New Zealand during August 1981–December 1987. The study design was similar to that depicted in Fig. 10. The study was based on 32 hospitals throughout New Zealand, and the potential cases comprised all patients aged 5–45 years who died from asthma during that period and who had been admitted to one of these hospitals during the 12 months before death. A total of 112 such deaths were identified and were included as cases in the study. Controls (referred to as control group B in the original publication) were selected at random from all asthma admissions to these major hospitals in this age-group and time period. For each case, four controls were selected from all patients discharged from the same hospital with the diagnosis of asthma in the

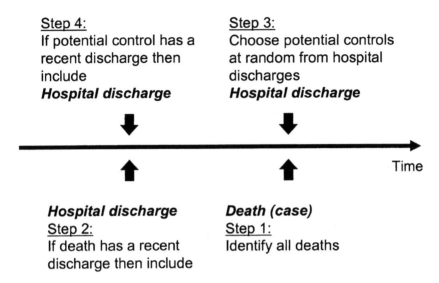

Figure 12 A further alternative design for a hypothetical case–control study of asthma mortality.

calendar year in which the case occurred. Prescribed medication at discharge was recorded from hospital notes for the index admission (the admission in the 12 months before death for the cases and the admission for the controls). Table 8 shows that the death rate in those prescribed fenoterol was 2.5 times that in those prescribed salbutamol.

Grainger et al. (78) also included a further control group (control group A), which was selected from the same group of asthma hospital admissions on which the study was based, but which involved an additional restriction. For each case, controls were selected from patients discharged from the same hospital, with the diagnosis of asthma, in the calendar year in which the death occurred, and who had also had a previous hospital admission during the 12 months prior to the admission under consideration. This control selection procedure, which is similar to that in Fig. 12, was adopted to achieve an indirect match for asthma severity. Once again, four controls were selected for each case, with the exception of 17 cases for whom sufficient controls could not be obtained. The study thus involved a total of 112 cases and 427 Group A controls. For both groups, information on prescribed asthma medication was obtained from hospital records (for the admission prior to death for the cases and for the corresponding admission for the controls). The findings for fenoterol and salbutamol are summarized in Table 8. Once again, the death rate in the fenoterol group was about twice that in the salbutamol group, but the odds ratio (2.0) was slightly lower than that obtained with the "unmatched" control group (2.5),

Table 7 Studies of Fenoterol and Asthma Deaths

	First New Zealand study	Second New Zealand study	Third New Zealand study	Saskatchewan study
Study period	1981–1983	1977–1981	1981–1987	1980–1987
Age-group	5–45 years	5–45 years	5–45 years	5–54 years
Source population	Asthmatics	Patients with a hospital admission for asthma in previous year	Patients with a hospital admission for asthma in previous year	Patients with 10 different asthma prescriptions during 1978–1987
Study design	Case–control study	Case–control study	Case–control study	Nested case–control study
Matching for severity?	Yes	Yes	Yes	No
Source of drug information	General practitioner (cases) Hospital records (controls)	Hospital records	Hospital records	Pharmacy records
Main exposure information	Prescribed[a] medication	Prescribed[a] medication	Prescribed[a] medication	Dispensed medication
Additional information	Nil	Nil	Nil	Number of units per month
Information on use?	No	No	No	No
Severity markers	Hospital admissions, oral steroids, three or more categories	Hospital admissions, oral steroids, three or more categories	Hospital admissions, oral steroids, three or more categories	Hospital admissions, oral steroids

[a]Prescribed beta-agonists were free during the study period.

Table 8 Findings from Studies of Fenoterol and Asthma Deaths: Odds Ratio (95% CI)

	First New Zealand study	Second New Zealand study	Third New Zealand study With control Group A	Third New Zealand study With control Group B	Saskatchewan study
Fenoterol	1.6 (1.0–2.3)	2.0 (1.1–3.6)	2.1 (1.4–3.2)	2.7 (1.7–4.1)	4.8 (2.5–9.3)
Salbutamol	0.7 (0.5–1.1)	0.7 (0.4–1.2)	0.6 (0.4–1.0)	0.5 (0.4–0.8)	0.9 (0.4–1.7)
Fenoterol only	1.6 (1.0–2.5)	1.9 (1.0–3.7)	2.0 (1.3–3.2)	2.5 (1.6–3.9)	3.7 (1.7–8.0)
Salbutamol only[a]	1.0	1.0	1.0	1.0	1.0

[a]Reference category.

indicating that there had been weak confounding in the analysis based on the "unmatched" controls.

Overall, this series of studies in New Zealand and Saskatchewan using a variety of study designs, together with the supporting evidence from Germany (79) and Japan (80), suggests that the prescription of fenoterol (in the high-dose formulation in which it was marketed) increases the risk of asthma death in comparison with the prescription of other beta-agonists (81). The most persistent criticism of these studies relates to the potential for confounding by severity (82–86). It has been suggested that fenoterol was marketed for more severe asthmatics and selectively prescribed to this group or that as fenoterol was the newer drug, then asthmatics might be switched to fenoterol as a result of deteriorating asthma (82). In fact, there is little or no evidence that fenoterol was selectively prescribed to more severe asthmatics in the population of recently hospitalized asthmatics on which the New Zealand studies were based (87). Furthermore, the findings from the three New Zealand studies show that the fenoterol relative risk did not decrease markedly, and in fact tended to increase, when the analysis was restricted to more severe asthmatics (Table 9). This is the most important piece of evidence that the case–control findings are not due to confounding by severity (Elwood, 1990) (88,89). Further support for this interpretation comes from Cox and Elwood (90), who reported that the results observed in the New Zealand case–control studies could not be produced by random misclassification in the severity markers used. Thus, the fenoterol studies illustrate how carefully designed epidemiological studies can investigate the role of specific drug therapy in asthma mortality, addressing the major potential problem of confounding by severity and obtaining similar findings in both cohort and case–control studies in several different countries.

Table 9 Subgroup Findings [for Fenoterol Odds Ratios (and 95% CIs)] from Studies of Fenoterol and Asthma Deaths

Subgroup	First New Zealand study	Second New Zealand study	Third New Zealand study	
			Group A	Group B
Total	1.6 (1.0–2.3)	2.0 (1.1–3.6)	2.1 (1.4–3.2)	2.7 (1.7–4.1)
Three or more categories of asthma drugs	2.2 (1.3–3.9)	3.0 (1.2–7.7)	2.2 (1.3–3.9)	2.8 (1.6–4.9)
Hospital admission in last year	2.2 (1.1–4.1)	3.9 (1.8–8.5)	2.5 (1.4–4.2)	2.7 (1.5–4.8)
Prescribed oral corticosteroids	6.5 (2.7–15.3)	5.8 (1.6–21.0)	3.2 (1.5–6.8)	3.8 (1.7–8.5)
Hospital admission in last year and prescribed oral corticosteroids	13.3 (3.5–51.2)	9.8 (2.2–43.4)	2.8 (1.1–6.9)	4.0 (1.5–11.0)

Summary

Until recently, epidemiological studies of asthma deaths had mostly involved analyses of time trends, supplemented by case series reports. Studies of time trends, particularly non-epidemic time trends, suffer from the same limitations as other ecologic analyses and provide relatively weak evidence of causal associations. Thus, analyses of time trends should primarily be used as part of a process of generating hypotheses as to the possible causes of the epidemic increases. The stages in this process include (i) assessing possible artifactual explanations for an increase in mortality and (ii) assessing possible explanations for a real increase in mortality including considering whether an increase is due to a change in prevalence or incidence (or whether there has been an increase in the case fatality rate), considering whether some demographic groups are particularly affected by an increase in mortality, and using this information to consider possible causal explanations for an increase in mortality.

More formal epidemiological studies are, therefore, needed to test specific hypotheses as to the causes of asthma deaths. The ideal approach would be a randomized controlled trial, but this is usually impractical and unethical. Similarly, cohort studies are usually impractical because of the large numbers involved, and case–control studies are the method of choice. Nevertheless, in designing a cohort or case–control study of the causes of asthma deaths, it is important to keep in mind the clinical trial that ideally would have been done and to design the cohort or case–control study with the aim of obtaining the same findings that would have been obtained in a randomized trial. In this context, it should be emphasized that different research questions involve very different methodological issues and require different methodological approaches. For example, studies of non-pharmacological risk factors usually involve sampling controls at random from the source population, whereas studies of pharmacological risk factors usually require some form of matching for non-pharmacological risk factors. Similarly, studying a class effect is generally more difficult and involves different study design and analysis issues than involved in comparing drugs within the same class. Although epidemiology has a role to play in investigating class effects, the findings should be regarded with considerable caution and interpreted carefully together with other available information. The emphasis should be on using "appropriate technology" to address the question under consideration and on using all of the available evidence when interpreting the study findings.

Acknowledgment

The Center for Public Health Research is funded by a Programme Grant from the Health Research Council of New Zealand.

References

1. Osler W. The Principles and Practice of Medicine. 4th ed. Edinburgh: Pentland, 1901.
2. Speizer FE, Doll R. A century of asthma deaths in young people. Br Med J 1968; iii:245–246.
3. Beasley R, Smith K, Pearce NE, et al. Trends in asthma mortality in New Zealand, 1908–1986. Med J Aust 1990; 152:570–573.
4. Baumann A, Lee S. Trends in asthma mortality in Australia, 1911–1986. Med J Aust 1990; 153:366. Letter.
5. Pearce NE, Crane J, Burgess C, et al. Beta agonists and asthma mortality: déjà vu. Clin Exp Allergy 1991; 21:401–410.
6. Pearce NE, Beasley R, Crane J, Burgess C. Epidemiology of asthma mortality. In: Busse W, Holgate S, eds. Asthma and Rhinitis. Oxford: Blackwell Scientific, 1994:58–69.
7. Pearce N, Beasley R, Burgess C, Crane J. Asthma Epidemiology: Principles and Methods. New York: Oxford University Press, 1998.
8. Burney PGJ. Asthma mortality in England and Wales: evidence for a further increase, 1974–1984. Lancet 1986; ii:323–326.
9. Sly RM. Mortality from asthma, 1979–1984. J Allergy Clin Immunol 1988; 82:705–717.
10. Jackson R, Sears MR, Beaglehole R, et al. International trends in asthma mortality: 1970–1985. Chest 1988; 94:914–918.

11. La Vecchia C, Fasoli M, Negri E, Tognoni G. Fall and rise in asthma mortality in Italy, 1968–1984. Int J Epidemiol 1992; 21:998–999. Letter.

12. Foucard T, Graff-Lonnevig V. Asthma mortality rate in Swedish children and young adults 1973–88. Allergy 1994; 49:616–619.

13. Ito Y, Tamakoshi A, Wakai K, et al. Trends in asthma mortality in Japan. J Asthma 2002; 39:633–639.

14. Weiss KB, Wagener DK. Changing patterns of asthma mortality: identifying populations at high risk. JAMA 1990; 264:1683–1687.

15. Beasley R, Pearce N, Crane J. International trends in asthma mortality. The Rising Trends in Asthma. Ciba Foundation Symposium 206. Chichester: Wiley, 1997:140–156.

16. Jorgensen IM, Bulow S, Jensen VB, et al. Asthma mortality in Danish children and young adults, 1973–1994: epidemiology and validity of death certificates. Eur Respir J 2000; 15:844–848.

17. Sly RM. Decreases in asthma mortality in the United States. Ann Asthma Allergy Immunol 2000; 85:121–127.

18. Romano F, Recchia G, Staniscia T, et al. Rise and fall of asthma-related mortality in Italy and sales of beta-2 agonists. Eur J Epidemiol 2000; 16:783–787.

19. Moorman JE, Mannino DM. Increasing asthma mortality rates: who is really dying? J Asthma 2001; 38:65–71.

20. Baluga JC, Sueta A, Ceni M. Asthma mortality in Uruguay. Ann Allergy Asthma Immunol 2001; 87:124–128.

21. Soler M, Chatenoud L, Negri E, La Vecchia C. Trends in Asthma Mortality in Italy and Spain, 1980–1996. Eur J Epidemiol 2001; 17:545–549.

22. Tanihara S, Nakamura Y, Oki J, et al. Trends in asthma morbidity and mortality in Japan between 1984 and 1996. J Epidemiol 2002:12:217–222.

23. Zar HJ, Stickells D, Toerien A, et al. Changes in fatal and near-fatal asthma in an urban area of South Africa from 1980–1997. Eur Respir J 2001; 18:33–37.

24. Matsui T. Did childhood asthma deaths in Japan really decrease in recent years? Jpn J Clin Med 2001; 59:1931–1937.

25. Greenland S, Robins J. Ecologic studies—biases, misconceptions, and counterexamples. Am J Epidemiol 1994; 139:747–760.

26. Stolley P, Lasky T. Asthma mortality epidemics: the problem approached epidemiologically. In: Beasley R, Pearce NE, eds. The Role of Beta Agonist Therapy in Asthma Mortality. New York: CRC Press, 1993:49–63.

27. Jackson R. A century of asthma mortality. In: Beasley R, Pearce NE, eds. The Role of Beta-Agonist Therapy in Asthma Mortality. New York: CRC Press, 1993:29–47.

28. Speizer FE, Doll R, Heaf P. Observations on recent increase in mortality from asthma. Br Med J 1968; i:335–339.

29. Jackson RT, Beaglehole R, Rea HH, et al. Mortality from asthma: a new epidemic in New Zealand. Br Med J 1982; 285:771–774.

30. British Thoracic Association (BTA). Accuracy of death certificates in bronchial asthma. Thorax 1982; 39:505–509.

31. Sirken MG, Rosenberg HM, Chevarley FM, Curtin LR. The quality of cause-of-death statistics. Am J Publ Health 1987; 77:137–139.

32. Sears MR, Rea HH, de Boer G, et al. Accuracy of certification of deaths due to asthma: a national study. Am J Epidemiol 1986; 124:1004–1011.

33. Guite HF, Burney PGJ. Accuracy of recording of deaths from asthma in the UK: the false negative rate. Thorax 1996; 51:924–928.

34. Hunt LW, Silverstein MD, Reed C, et al. Accuracy of the death certificate in a population-based study of asthmatic patients. JAMA 1993; 269:1947–1952.

35. Lambert PM. Oral theophylline and fatal asthma. Lancet 1981; ii:200–201. Letter.

36. Burney PGJ. The effect of death certification practice on recorded national asthma mortality rates. Rev Epidem Santé Publ 1989; 37:385–389.

37. Schleicher NC, Koziol JA, Christiansen SC. Asthma mortality rates among California youths. J Asthma 2000; 37:259–265.

38. Grant EN, Lyttle CS, Weiss KB. The relation of socioeconomic factors and racial/ethnic differences in US asthma mortality. Am J Publ Health 2000; 90:1923–1925.

39. Sears MR, Rea HH, Beaglehole R, et al. Asthma mortality in New Zealand: a two year national study. N Z Med J 1985; 98:271–275.

40. Khot A, Burn R. Seasonal variation and time trends of deaths from asthma in England and Wales 1960–1982. Br Med J 1984; 289:233–234.

41. Weiss KB. Seasonal trends in US asthma hospitalisations and mortality. JAMA 1990; 263:2323–2328.

42. Kimbell-Dunn M, Pearce N, Beasley R. Seasonal variation in asthma hospitalisations and death rates in New Zealand. Respirology 2000; 5:241–246.

43. Ellison-Loschmann L, Cheng S, Pearce N. Time trends and seasonal patterns of asthma deaths and hospitalisations among Maori and non-Maori. N Z Med J 2002; 115:6–9.

44. Inman WHW, Adelstein AM. Rise and fall of asthma mortality in England and Wales in relation to use of pressurized aerosols. Lancet 1969; ii:279–285.

45. MacDonald JB, Seaton A, Williams DA. Asthma deaths in Cardiff 1963–1974: 90 deaths outside hospital. Br Med J 1976a; ii:1493–1495.

46. MacDonald JB, MacDonald ET, Seaton A, Williams DA. Asthma deaths in Cardiff 1963–1974: 53 deaths in hospital. Br Med J 1976b; ii:721–723.

47. Speizer FE, Doll R, Heaf P, et al. Investigation into use of drugs preceding death from asthma. Br Med J 1968b; i:339–343.

48. Cochrane GM, Clark TJH. A survey of asthma mortality in patients between ages 35 and 64 in the Greater London hospitals in 1971. Thorax 1975; 30:300–305.

49. Ormerod LP, Stableforth DE. Asthma mortality in Birmingham 1975–1977: 53 deaths. Br Med J 1980; i:687–690.

50. British Thoracic Association (BTA). Deaths from asthma in two regions of England. Br Med J 1982; 285:1251–1255.

51. Fraser PM, Speizer FE, Waters DM, et al. The circumstances preceding death from asthma in young people in 1968 to 1969. Br J Dis Chest 1971; 65:71–84.

52. Barger LW, Vollmer WM, Felt RW, Buist AS. Further investigation into the recent increase in asthma death rates: a review of 41 asthma deaths in Oregon in 1982. Ann Allergy 1988; 60:31–39.

53. Campbell DA, MacLennan G, Coates JR, et al. A comparison of asthma deaths and near-fatal asthma attacks in South Australia. Eur Respir J 1994; 7:490–497.

54. Robertson CF, Rubinfeld AR, Bowes G. Deaths from asthma in Victoria: a 12 month survey. Med J Aust 1990; 152:511–517.

55. Wilson JD, Sutherland DC, Thomas AC. Has the change to beta-agonists combined with oral theophylline increased cases of fatal asthma? Lancet 1981; i:1235–1237.

56. Anon. Asthma deaths: a question answered. Br Med J 1972; ii:443–444. Editorial.

57. Beasley R, Pearce NE, Crane J, et al. Asthma mortality and inhaled beta-agonist therapy. Aust N Z J Med 1991; 21:753–763.

58. Stolley PD. Why the United States was spared an epidemic of deaths due to asthma. Am Rev Resp Dis 1972; 105:883–890.

59. Gandevia B. Pressurized sympathomimetic aerosols and their lack of relationship to asthma mortality in Australia. Med J Aust 1973; 1:273–277.

60. Campbell AH. Mortality from asthma and bronchodilator aerosols. Med J Aust 1976; i:386–391.

61. Venning GR. Identification of adverse reactions to new drugs. I. What have been the important adverse reactions since thalidomide? Br Med J 1983; 286:199–202.

62. Anon. Fatal asthma. Lancet 1979; ii:337–338. Editorial.

63. Benatar SR. Fatal asthma. New Engl J Med 1986; 314:423–429.

64. Buist AS. Is asthma mortality increasing? Chest 1988; 93:449–450. Editorial.

65. Paterson JW, Musk AW. Death in patients with asthma. Med J Aust 1987; 147:53–55.

66. Stolley PD, Schinnar R. Association between asthma mortality and isoproterenol aerosols: a review. Prev Med 1978; 7:319–338.

67. Keating G, Mitchell EA, Jackson R, et al. Trends in sales of drugs for asthma in New Zealand, Australia and the United Kingdom, 1975–1981. Br Med J 1984; 289:348–351.

68. Crane J, Pearce N, Flatt A, et al. Prescribed fenoterol and death from asthma in New Zealand, 1981–1983: a case–control study. Lancet 1989; i:917–922.

69. Pearce N, Beasley R, Crane J, et al. End of the New Zealand asthma mortality epidemic. Lancet 1995; 345:41–44.

70. Elwood JM. Review of studies relating prescribed fenoterol to deaths from asthma in New Zealand. In: Beasley R, Pearce NE, eds. The role of beta-agonist therapy in asthma mortality. New York: CRC Press, 1993:85–123.

71. Crane J, Pearce NE, Burgess C, et al. Markers of risk of asthma death or readmission in the 12 months following a hospital admission for asthma. Int J Epidemiol 1992; 21:737–744.

72. Sears MR. Trends in asthma mortality—New Zealand and international experience. In: Ruffin RE, ed. Asthma Mortality: Proceedings of the Second National Asthma Mortality Workshop. Sydney: Excerpta Medica, 1990:1–3.

73. Castle W, Fuller R, Hall J, Palmer J. Serevent nationwide surveillance study: comparison of salmeterol with salbutamol in asthmatic patients who require regular, bronchodilator treatment. Br Med J 1993; 306:1034–1037.

74. Suissa S, Ernst P, Boivin J-F, et al. A cohort analysis of excess mortality in asthma and the use of inhaled β-agonists. Am J Respir Crit Care Med 1994; 149:604–610.

75. Strunk RC, Mrazek DA, Wolfson Fuhrmann GS, LaBrecque JF. Physiologic and psychological characteristics associated with deaths due to asthma in childhood. JAMA 1985; 254:1193–1198.

76. Abramson MJ, Bailey MJ, Couper FJ, et al. Are asthma medications and management related to deaths from asthma?. Am J Respir Crit Care Med 2001; 163:12–18.

77. Checkoway H, Pearce N, Dement JM. Design and conduct of occupational epidemiology studies: I. Design aspects of cohort studies. Am J Ind Med 1989; 15:363–373.

78. Grainger J, Woodman K, Pearce NE, et al. Prescribed fenoterol and death from asthma in New Zealand, 1981–1987: a further case–control study. Thorax 1991; 46:105–111.

79. Crieé CP, Quast CH, Ludtke R, et al. Use of beta-agonists and mortality in patients with stable COPD [abstr]. Eur Respir J 1993; 6:426S.

80. Matsui T. Asthma death and β$_2$-agonists. In: Shimomiya K (ed). Current Advances in Paediatric Allergy and Clinical Epidemiology Selected proceedings from the 32nd Annual Meeting of the Japanese Society of Paediatric Allergy and Clinical Immunology. Tokyo: Churchill Livingstone, 1996; pp. 161–4.

81. Pearce N, Hensley ML. Beta–agonists and asthma deaths. Epidemiol Rev 1998; 20:173–186.

82. Buist AS, Burney PGJ, Feinstein AR, et al. Fenoterol and fatal asthma. Lancet 1989; i:1071. Letter.

83. O'Donnell TV, Hoest P, Rea HH, Sears MR. Fenoterol and fatal asthma. Lancet 1989; i:1070–1071. Letter.

84. Blais L, Ernst P, Suissa S. Confounding by indication and channeling over time: the risks of β$_2$-agonists. Am J Epidemiol 1996; 144:1161–1169.

85. Garrett JE, Lanes SF, Kolbe J, Rea HH. Risk of severe life threatening asthma and β agonist type: an example of confounding by severity. Thorax 1996; 51:1093–1099.

86. Rea HH, Garrett JE, Lanes SF, et al. The association between asthma drugs and severe life-threatening attacks. Chest 1996; 110:1446–1451.

87. Beasley R, Pearce NE, Burgess C, et al. Confounding by severity does not explain the association between fenoterol and asthma death. Clin Exp Allergy 1994; 24:660–668.

88. Sackett DL, Shannon HS, Browman GW. Fenoterol and fatal asthma. Lancet 1990; i:46. Letter.

89. Hensley MJ. Fenoterol and death from asthma. Med J Aust 1992; 156:882. Letter.

90. Cox B, Elwood JM. The effect on the stratum-specific odds ratios of non-differential misclassification of a confounder measured at two levels. Am J Epidemiol 1991; 133:202–207.

91. Esdaile JM, Feinstein AR, Horwitz RI. A reappraisal of the United Kingdom epidemic of fatal asthma. Arch Intern Med 1987; 147:543–549.

92. Jackson R. Undertreatment and asthma deaths. Lancet 1985; ii:500. Letter.
93. Korsgaard J. Mite asthma and residency: a case–control study on the impact of exposure to house-dust mites in dwellings. Am Rev Respir Dis 1983; 128: 231–235.
94. Lanes SF, Walker AM. Do pressurized bronchodilator aerosols cause death among asthmatics? Am J Epidemiol 1987; 125:755–760.
95. Pearce NE, Grainger J, Atkinson M, et al. Case–control study of prescribed fenoterol and death from asthma in New Zealand, 1977–1981. Thorax 1990; 45:170–175.
96. Read J. The reported increase in mortality from asthma: a clinico-fiinctional analysis. Med J Aust 1968; i:879–891.
97. Sears MR, Rea HH, Fenwick J, et al. 75 deaths in asthmatics prescribed home nebulisers. Br Med J 1987; 294:477–480.
98. Spitzer WO, Suissa S, Ernst P, et al. Beta agonists and the risk of asthma death and near fatal asthma. N Engl J Med 1992; 326:501–506.
99. Weiss KB, Gergen PJ, Wagener DK. Breathing better or wheezing worse? The changing epidemiology of asthma morbidity and mortality. Annu Rev Publ Health 1993; 14:491–513.

16

Monitoring Asthma in Populations

**GUY B. MARKS and
MARGARET WILLIAMSON**

Australian Centre for Asthma Monitoring,
    Woolcock Institute of Medical Research,
Sydney, Australia

DEBORAH F. BAKER

Centre for Epidemiology and Research,
    NSW Health Department,
North Sydney, Australia

Introduction

Asthma is a complex disease of largely unknown etiology but with a relatively well-defined and effective clinical management strategy (1,2). The high, but variable, prevalence of asthma in many countries (3,4), together with substantial impacts of the disease on quality of life (5,6), health-care costs, (7) and mortality (8–11), have led to substantial public interest in the disease. There is evidence that a range of environmental factors influence the course of asthma, by triggering exacerbations (12–16), and possibly by inducing longer-term changes (17,18). Clinical management has a major impact on the course of the disease: usually beneficial, but occasionally adverse (19–21). There is evidence that utilization of beneficial clinical management strategies for asthma (22,23) is sub-optimal.

In this chapter, we first set the context for considering methods of monitoring asthma in populations by reviewing the purposes for undertaking this monitoring. In the next section, we review the problem of identifying and classifying asthma, an important pre-requisite for monitoring the disease. Finally, in the main body of this chapter, we consider a range of aspects of asthma and asthma care that are commonly monitored in populations: prevalence, mortality, hospitalization rates, primary care utilization rates, drug therapy, and impact on quality of life. For each of these, we discuss the rationale for measurement at a population level, review the various approaches to measuring each indicator and discuss, in general terms, some of the issues in relation to data sources.

Purposes of Monitoring Asthma in Populations

The large burden of illness, observed variability between populations, potential environmental triggers, and inadequately implemented effective treatments point to substantial opportunities for health gain from public health action. Identifying these opportunities and assessing progress in realizing them requires monitoring of populations. A number of specific purposes for monitoring asthma in populations can be identified.

Resource Allocation Based on Current and Future Disease Burden

Although there are many factors that influence the allocation of resources among health priorities (24), the relative burden of disease is one influential factor. Hence, measurement of current burden of asthma, relative to other diseases, is relevant to resource allocation. Furthermore, prediction of future burden is also important for estimating future needs. This has not been attempted in relation to asthma.

Resources applied to the prevention and management of asthma are allocated from limited health-care budgets and compete with other health priorities for available resources. Population data have been used to quantify the existing allocation of resources (7,25–28).

Not all patients with asthma require equal health-care resources for management of their illness. Requirements for hospital care and other urgent medical care are greater in patients with persistent disease (29) and with poorly controlled disease (30). Population monitoring data have been used to demonstrate the resource savings that could follow from the optimization of medical management leading to improved asthma control (31).

Potential for Improved Prevention and Control, Based on Prevalence of Modifiable Risk Factors and Current Management Practices

Clinical Management

International and national guidelines for the management of asthma, initially based on consensus (32–35), but increasingly based on higher levels of evidence (1,22,23,36,37), now clearly show a path towards improved outcomes for patients with asthma. From the population health perspective, there is value in identifying the extent of current implementation of the key elements of the effective interventions. This highlights the potential for health gain. For example, in New South Wales, Australia, a population-based health survey of adults, conducted in 1997 (38), demonstrated that a majority of patients with asthma who would be expected to derive benefit from using preventer medications for asthma, were not doing so (Fig. 1). Similar observations about under-utilization of effective management for asthma have been made in other population surveys (39–41) and also among patients with asthma seeking urgent medical care (42–47).

Population monitoring may also lead to the identification of subgroups of the population in whom asthma management is particularly sub-optimal. A multi-center study of patients presenting to the Emergency Department with an exacerbation of asthma found that the risk of poor asthma management skills was greater in those with low income and lower educational attainment and that poor asthma management skills was correlated with continued smoking and lower likelihood of using inhaled corticosteroids (45). Lack of a sense of self-efficacy (48,49), poor literacy (50), and mood disturbance (42,51) have also been identified as predictors of poor asthma management skills. Further information on demographic and geographic variation in adherence to, or availability of, effective asthma management and self-management would enable the most efficient targeting of public health interventions directed at these processes.

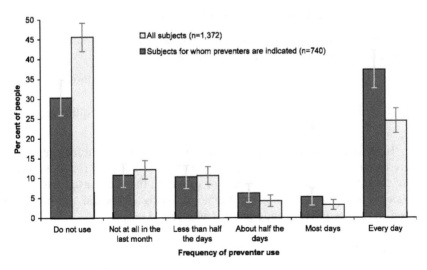

Figure 1 Frequency of preventer use in people with asthma, age 16–54 years, New South Wales, Australia, 1997. *Source*: From Ref. 229.

Environmental Risk Factors

Similar strategies could potentially be implemented to control exposure to environmental risk factors for asthma. Unfortunately, definitive identification of the causes of asthma is not currently possible. However, a number of potentially modifiable environmental factors have been implicated either in the etiology of the disease or in triggering exacerbations requiring hospitalization.

A detailed discussion of these risk factors is beyond the scope of this chapter. However, some key exposures are worth highlighting. It is clear that maternal smoking during pregnancy increases the risk of wheezing illness during early life (52,53). Environmental tobacco smoke exposure probably also causes more symptoms and exacerbations of asthma among children with the disease (54,55). Among adults, occupational exposures are the most clearly defined environmental inducers of asthma (and other allergic diseases) and they may also aggravate existing asthma (56). Other airborne exposures including aerobiological (18,57), gaseous, and particulate agents (58,59) also have effects on human airways and influence the course of asthma either through allergic or non-allergic mechanisms. The relation between these exposures and the various airway effects has not, as yet, been clearly defined.

From the population health perspective, there is value in monitoring the levels of exposure to these environmental risk factors, both to assess the magnitude of risk and to identify areas in which specific risk factor reduction interventions are likely to be most beneficial.

Tracking Change and Identifying Clusters

Monitoring change over time in the outcomes of asthma has value as a public health information tool from two standpoints:

1. contributing to the evaluation of programs for asthma prevention and control and
2. identification of adverse trends or clusters that require investigation and, where possible, intervention.

In theory, monitoring trends over time should be useful for predicting future trends. However, past trends have not proved to be a reliable indicator of future trends in this disease. For example, the substantial rise in the prevalence of asthma during the 1980s and early 1990s did not continue during the subsequent decade in Australia (60,61).

Evaluation

Randomized controlled trials are the principal, and definitive, tool for evaluation purposes (62). However, while public policy initiatives may be based upon interventions that have been evaluated in this way, the effect of their implementation at a population level is rarely subject to such evaluation. Similarly, the impact of trends in clinical management that is not the subject of deliberate public policy, but may result, for example, from the marketing of a new drug or class of drugs, cannot be directly evaluated in an experimental design. As these interventions are distributed in the population outside an experimental setting, evaluation of their impact requires an observational design.

Trend analysis, that is, examining change in outcomes during the course of implementing the policy or management strategy, is one component of a strategy to evaluate the impact of public policy and other interventions for the prevention and control of disease.

The impact of rising sales of anti-inflammatory medications for asthma (inhaled corticosteroids and leukotriene receptor antagonists) on deaths due to asthma was evaluated in Japan, where these drugs have been relatively recently introduced (63). A significant negative correlation between sales of these anti-inflammatory medications and deaths from asthma was observed.

The interpretation of this study, and other similar studies in which trends are interpreted for evaluation purposes, must be cautious. Other time variable factors, such as environmental change, use of other medications, health promotion campaigns, or even change in death certification, may influence the observed trends and can be difficult to adequately adjust for in analysis. Nevertheless, trend analysis such as this may contribute towards assessment of the impact of interventions at a population level.

Identification of Adverse Trends or Clusters

Surveillance for disease clusters is a well-established tool in communicable disease epidemiology but has been less widely utilized in chronic disease control.

Trends in mortality due to asthma have been monitored for decades in many countries. It was the observation of rising trends in deaths due to asthma in young adults in several countries during the 1960s that alerted clinicians and scientists to the possible adverse effect of high-dose, nonselective beta-agonists (11,19,64,65). A similar observation in New Zealand in the late 1980s stimulated a series of case–control studies that implicated another potent inhaled beta-agonist, fenoterol, as a probable cause of the rising trend (21,66,67). However, subsequent events highlight the difficulty in ascribing causality on the basis of trend analysis. Although there was a decline in sales of fenoterol that was accompanied by a substantial decline in mortality in New Zealand, a similar decline in mortality was observed in other countries, including Australia, where fenoterol was never sold in substantial quantities (68). The subject remains controversial. Other interventions, including public campaigns to promote effective asthma management, may have contributed to these observed improvements in death rates due to asthma.

Local epidemics or clusters of cases have led to the discovery of important environmental causes of exacerbations of asthma. Perhaps the most famous of these is the epidemics of hospitalization for asthma that occurred in relation to unloading of soybeans in Barcelona port (69). Thunderstorm-related epidemics have also been noted in several countries and have been ascribed to high-dose exposure to allergen-containing starch particles derived from pollen grains (57,70–72).

While deaths and exacerbations requiring hospitalization for asthma are the outcomes of asthma most amenable to routine surveillance, clusters or trends in new incident cases of asthma are also informative. Information on incidence of asthma is not routinely available. However, in the occupational setting, the identification of an outbreak of new cases of asthma may lead to the identification of novel occupational sensitizers or allergens (e.g., 73).

Surveillance or monitoring of trends in asthma outcomes has an important role in the early identification and investigation of adverse environmental and therapeutic factors.

Identification of Asthma for Monitoring Purposes

The Absence of a Criterion or "Gold Standard" for Asthma

It is self-evident that monitoring asthma in populations requires the identification of individuals with asthma, both for the enumeration of cases of asthma and for the assessment of factors associated with asthma. There are two phases to this identification: establishment of a criterion (or "gold standard") and assessment of various tools for reliability and for validity as measures of the criterion. Ideally, these measurement tools will enable the classification of all individuals within a population as having, or not having, asthma based on the presence or absence of necessary and sufficient conditions for asthma. However, it is apparent that the first stage of this process, establishment of a criterion, presents substantial problems.

The Global Initiative for Asthma workshop report advocates the following "operational definition" of asthma, which might form the basis of a criterion:

> Asthma is a chronic inflammatory disorder of the airways in which many cells and cellular elements play a role. The chronic inflammation causes an associated increase in airway hyperresponsiveness that leads to recurrent episodes of wheezing, breathlessness, chest tightness and coughing, particularly at night or in the early morning. These episodes are usually associated with widespread

but variable airflow obstruction that is often reversible either spontaneously or with treatment (1).

Unfortunately, this definition, while describing some of the features of asthma, does not lend itself to interpretation as a necessary and sufficient condition, or criterion, for the identification of individuals with asthma. Indeed, current understanding of the nature of asthma does not allow any criterion for this disease. Examination of some of the elements of the above definition supports this view. For example, the symptoms of asthma are not unique to this disease but are shared by other cardio-respiratory diseases including chronic obstructive pulmonary disease, left ventricular failure, and bronchiolitis. These symptoms may also occur occasionally in people who would not generally be regarded as having any chronic respiratory illness. The lung function abnormalities that are characteristic of asthma, reversible airflow obstruction and airway hyper-responsiveness, exist in a continuum with no clear distinction between normal and abnormal levels. Furthermore, the nature of this continuum varies among different stimuli used to elicit airway hyper-responsiveness. Finally, it can readily be appreciated that the nature and extent of airway inflammation also varies in a continuous manner and, while some features of airway inflammation are characteristic of asthma, there is no clear threshold which distinguishes asthma from either the normal state or other airway diseases. Hence, there are no attributes that can be considered both necessary and sufficient for the diagnosis of asthma.

In the absence of a universally applicable criterion, it is appropriate to select pragmatic criteria that are relevant to the purpose of the investigation. Reported diagnoses, symptoms, and physiological measures, including bronchodilator response, airway hyper-responsiveness, and peak expiratory flow rate variability over time, have all been used to identify cases of asthma within the population for monitoring purposes. These are discussed further in Section Monitoring Key Specific Indicators.

Heterogeneity in Asthma: Different Types of Asthma

The identification of asthma for monitoring purposes is further complicated by the fact that asthma is not a homogeneous disease entity. Several patterns have emerged. Historically, the methods of classifying asthma have reflected the existing disease paradigms.

An early distinction between intrinsic (non-allergic) and extrinsic (allergic or atopic) asthma found acceptance in the International Classification of Diseases and the terms allergic and non-allergic asthma are still used (74). However, the demonstration that patients with intrinsic asthma shared many of the pathological features observed in extrinsic asthmatics (75) has led to a waning in the use of this distinction.

Most existing guidelines classify patients with asthma as having intermittent or persistent asthma (35,76,77). It is not clear whether this distinction represents a fundamental characteristic of the illness, a marker of disease severity or, possibly, a marker of the periodicity of exposure to triggers. The latter may be partially true since intermittent asthma seems to be more common in children, where it is associated with viral infections (78) and in regions where seasonal allergens play an important role as triggers for asthma (79). Nevertheless, the distinction between intermittent and persistent asthma does appear to have long-term prognostic significance, as does the distinction between frequent and infrequent intermittent asthma (80).

Studies of the natural history of asthma have led to the elucidation of several longitudinal patterns of asthma. For example, the Tuscon birth cohort study has identified "transient early wheeze," which presents with symptoms before age three that remit before age six, "late onset wheeze," in which children develop wheeze after age three years, and "persistent wheeze," a group of children who have wheeze before age three that persists at least until age six years (81).

Asthma is also classified according to severity. However, many of the features of asthma are responsive to therapy, particularly with corticosteroids, and, hence, most "severity" classifications are actually better described as assessments of disease control. Distinctions are necessarily arbitrary, but most classifications are based on the presence and frequency of daytime and nocturnal symptoms, the frequency of need for bronchodilator, and the level and variability of lung function (77,82). Some classifications also incorporate information on the frequency and severity of disease exacerbations.

Information about asthma in populations is enhanced by measurements that accommodate the heterogeneity in the disease. However, as there are several dimensions to this heterogeneity, the specific classifications that are appropriate are usually best selected on the basis of relevance to the purpose or intention of the measurements. For example, in monitoring the uptake of various treatment modalities for asthma, it is relevant to classify people with asthma in accordance with asthma management guidelines (1).

Monitoring Key Specific Indicators

Prevalence of Asthma

Counting the number of people with asthma is of fundamental importance from the population monitoring perspective. It is relevant to the assessment of disease burden and the appropriate allocation and distribution of resources. Geographical and temporal variation in prevalence may provide insights into the nature of environmental risk factors for this disease

(72,83–86). In theory, it may also be used to assess the impact of policy initiatives aimed at preventing asthma at a population level.

Incidence vs. Prevalence

Ideally, the assessment of risk factors for the onset of asthma and the effectiveness of interventions to prevent asthma would be better served by measurement of the incidence of asthma, that is, the occurrence of new cases of the disease over a defined period of time, rather than the number of prevalent cases at any particular time. The latter represents the combined effects of cumulative (lifetime) incidence, remissions, and premature mortality, all of which may have different risk factors or causes. Incidence may be measured in cohort studies: for example, cohorts of infants recruited at birth (87,88), cohorts of older children and adults (89,90), and disease-free cohorts recruited in an occupational setting (91,92). Unfortunately, cohort studies are expensive and time consuming to conduct and are not commonly implemented for the purpose of monitoring asthma in populations.

Cross-sectional studies, in which a population is surveyed at a single point in time to count the number of cases of asthma and, if relevant, the occurrence of risk factors or exposures, are more feasible to implement and have been used extensively to assess the burden of asthma and to investigate risk factors for the disease. There are difficulties in estimating the incidence of asthma in cross-sectional studies. The often ill-defined nature of the incident event and its remote past occurrence for most adults, both mean that there are major problems in measuring the timing of the onset, and hence the incidence, of this disease. Furthermore, there may be incomplete recollection of childhood symptoms among adults and this may influence the attribution of adult-onset symptoms to relapse, as opposed to incidence, of asthma. Hence, prevalence is usually measured for the purposes of asthma monitoring, and information about changes in incidence is usually inferred from cross-sectional prevalence estimates.

Questionnaires for Measuring the Prevalence of Asthma

The difficulties inherent in defining asthma for epidemiological purposes have been discussed in Section Identification of Asthma for Monitoring Purposes. Despite these difficulties, a number of questionnaires have been used extensively in epidemiological studies measuring the prevalence of asthma in adults and children (93–99). Newer questionnaires have also been proposed (100–102). Each of these questionnaires is comprised of items or elements about asthma symptoms and diagnoses.

In this section, we describe the evaluation of some of the elements that have been used alone, or in combination, as tools for assessing the prevalence of asthma. The evaluation includes information on the feasibility, reliability, and validity of the available measures. While reliability and feasibility are relatively independent of the purpose of the measurement and, hence, can readily be assessed, validity is a more complex attribute. The validity of the measure is usually expressed as sensitivity and specificity. It can only be assessed by reference to a specific criterion. Since there is no universal criterion for asthma, validity cannot be assessed in a universally applicable manner. In interpreting the reports on the validity of individual measurement tools, it is important to be cognizant of this limitation.

The most commonly used question to identify asthma in populations simply asks "Have you ever had asthma?" (93). In the American Thoracic Society/Division of Lung Diseases 1978 (ATS-DLD-78) adult questionnaire, this item is followed by "Do you still have it?" and "Was it confirmed by a doctor?". Wheeze, cough, chest tightness, and shortness of breath are common symptoms of asthma but may also occur in other diseases or, under some circumstances, in the absence of disease.

Questions about asthma symptoms and about asthma diagnosis have been shown to be moderately or highly repeatable in several populations of adults [Table 1, (95)] and children [Table 2, (96,103)]. The reliability of these elements has been further assessed in adolescents by comparing responses to a written questionnaire with responses to a video questionnaire. The latter required subjects to respond to questions about video images of actors demonstrating wheezing and other respiratory symptoms [Table 3, (105–109)]. Overall, agreement between these two forms of administration was only moderate. Similarly, agreement between parent-completed written questionnaires and subject-completed versions of the same questionnaire was also moderate [kappa = 0.48 for current wheeze, (104)]. Test–retest repeatability was slightly better in this same population (kappa = 0.59).

Table 1 Repeatability of Questions[a] About Asthma and Asthma Symptoms in Adults and their Relation to a Measure of Non-specific Airway Hyper-responsiveness.

Question	Kappa[b]	Sensitivity[b,c]	Specificity[b,c]
Wheeze	0.73–0.95	0.59–0.95	0.62–0.80
Morning tightness	0.46–0.67	0.33–0.79	0.57–0.93
Attacks of shortness of breath	0.40–0.56	0.11–0.74	0.67–0.80
Waking with shortness of breath	0.63–0.85	0.37–0.74	0.77–0.97
Asthma ever	0.70–1.0	0.33–0.80	0.74–1.00
Asthma in last 12 months	0.59–0.94	0.26–0.68	0.76–1.00

[a]Questions for the IUATLD Bronchial Symptoms Questionnaire.
[b]Range of values observed in four centres (Finland, Germany, France, England). Note that the sensitivity of questions for AHR was lower in Germany than in other countries.
[c]As predictors of airway hyperresponsiveness ($PD_{20}FEV_1$ (histamine) $< 8\,\mu mol$).
Source: Ref. 95.

Table 2 Repeatability of Selected Questions About Asthma and Asthma Symptoms Administered to the Parents of Children

Question	Kappa
Dutch children aged 6–12 years (n = 411) (103)	
Wheeze in last 12 months	0.73
Asthma attacks in the last 12 months	0.96
Shortness of breath	0.75
Doctor diagnosed asthma	0.76
Asthma attacks last year	0.66
Asthma medication	0.66
Australian children aged 8–10 years (n = 312)[a] (96)	
Diagnosed asthma	0.78
Wheeze ever	0.67
Wheeze last 12 months	0.65
Night cough ever	0.48
Night cough last 12 months	0.41
Any respiratory symptom ever	0.51

[a]Self-completed compared with interviewer-administered

The validity of questions about asthma symptoms and reported diagnoses has been assessed by examining their relation to an objective measure, usually airway hyper-responsiveness (AHR), or to an independently ascertained clinical diagnosis of asthma.

Table 3 Agreement (kappa) Between ISAAC Written Questionnaire and Video Questionnaire for Assessing Current Wheeze Among 13–14 year Old Subjects in Various Settings. (Adapted from (105)).

Country	Center	Kappa	Ref.
Germany	Bochum	0.35	(107)
England	W. Sussex	0.46	(107)
New Zealand	Wellington	0.52	(107)
Australia	Adelaide	0.68	(107)
Australia	Sydney	0.44	(107)
Finland	Kuopio	0.41	(108)
Finland	Helsinki	0.40	(108)
Finland	Turku	0.45	(108)
Finland	Lapland	0.41	(108)
China	Hong Kong	0.30	(109)
China	Hong Kong	0.44	(112)
Canada	Hamilton	0.47	(105)
Canada	Saskatoon	0.49	(105)
Australia	Western Sydney	0.41	(106)

Although asthma symptoms and reported diagnoses of asthma are clearly associated with the presence of AHR, overall they are not good predictors of this outcome in adults [(Table 1) (95,110,111)] or in children (106,112) and Burney et al. were unable to identify any specific question or combination of questions which performed well in this regard. While some authors have claimed better sensitivity than specificity and others the reverse, this is probably mainly due to differences in the threshold for defining the presence of AHR.

Since a reported diagnosis of asthma is based upon a clinical diagnosis of asthma it is expected to agree well with an independent clinical assessment. In fact, self-reported ever diagnosed asthma in adults has a variable sensitivity ranging from 48% to 100% against a diagnosis confirmed by a doctor (95,113,114). Specificity is higher: ranging from 77% to 100%. One study, conducted among children, found that parent-reported asthma had a sensitivity of 55% and a specificity of 94% for asthma confirmed by a doctor (115). These differences are presumably attributable to recall error on the part of questionnaire respondents.

In adults, asthma symptoms in the last 12 months have a sensitivity ranging from 26% to 83% and a specificity ranging from 76% to 100% for asthma diagnosis (95,113,114,116). de Marco et al. (113) examined the sensitivity and specificity of single questions on symptoms in the last year, and combinations of these questions, for predicting a doctor's verification of current asthma. Individually, each question (wheeze, shortness of breath, asthma attack, and ever asthma) had a high specificity (91–99%) but low sensitivity (32–68%), particularly for shortness of breath and asthma attack. Wheeze was the most sensitive but least specific marker. The combination of asthma attack, and current use of medication did not improve sensitivity but specificity remained high (99.7%). However, the combination of wheeze, and/or shortness of breath or self-reported current asthma improved sensitivity (82.9%) but specificity dropped substantially (86.7%). In contrast, Jenkins et al. (116) report sensitivity of 80% and high specificity of 97% for a question about having "suffered attacks of asthma or wheezy breathing" within the last 12 months for predicting an expert clinical diagnosis of asthma. Grassi et al. (117) also found that calculation of a score based on the number of positive responses to a series of questions from the European Community Respiratory Health Survey screening questionnaire (recent wheeze, shortness of breath with wheeze, wheeze without colds, waking with tightness in the chest, being woken by an attack of breathlessness, having had an attack of asthma, and taking treatment for asthma) was a good predictor of expert clinician diagnosis of asthma.

Among children, parental responses to questions on various symptoms within the last 12 months have a sensitivity ranging from 55% to 85% and specificity 81–99% for a physician-verified diagnosis of asthma (115,116,118,119). Individually, no symptom stands out as being more sensitive or specific for a clinical verification of asthma, although nocturnal cough is usually least specific (118,119). The International Study of Asthma and Allergies in Childhood (ISAAC) questionnaire defines current "asthma symptoms" as a positive response to the question "Have you had wheezing or whistling in the chest in the last 12 months?" (3). Among Tasmanian school children this question had a sensitivity of 85% and a specificity of 81% for physician-verified diagnosis of asthma (116). Among school-age children in Ohio, United States of America, the presence of cough and/ or breathing problems had a sensitivity of 80% and a specificity of 75% for an expert diagnosis of asthma (100). Among Finnish school children reporting symptoms, in the last 12 months, of "wheezing apart from colds," "attacks of shortness of breath with wheezing" and "shortness of breath when playing or walking up stairs," each had a high specificity (97–98%) but only moderate sensitivity (66–78%) for clinical asthma defined by an allergist on the basis of symptoms, spirometry, and a challenge test (119). Among children attending primary care clinics in Hartford, Connecticut, a question about persistent cough with colds had the highest specificity (86%) but lowest sensitivity (63%) for a clinician diagnosis of asthma (118). Wheezing (83%) and exercise-induced symptoms (81%) were also relatively specific. A positive response to any one of four symptoms increased sensitivity to 94% but at substantial cost to specificity (55%). Similarly, addition of subjects whose parents report wheezing with colds to those with parent-reported asthma increases sensitivity for a physician confirmed diagnosis, but at a cost to specificity (115).

This agreement between symptom responses and a clinical diagnosis of asthma is to be expected because, in the interval-phase (that is, between acute episodes or exacerbations), the clinical diagnosis of asthma is most commonly established on the basis of reports of asthma-like symptoms and response to asthma treatment. Enthusiasm for questionnaire-based identification of asthma cases on the basis of this validation should be tempered by the limitations of the clinical diagnosis of asthma that are alluded to above. The validity of symptoms alone as a basis for measuring the prevalence of asthma has particular limitations in the young (120–122) and the elderly (123), where a number of competing diagnoses [virus-associated wheeze, bronchiolitis, cardiac failure, and chronic obstructive pulmonary disease (COPD)] have similar predominant symptoms.

In summary, there is conflicting information on the validity of symptom-based questions for measuring the prevalence of asthma. This highlights the difficulties inherent in measuring an illness for which there is no "gold standard." However, there is consistent evidence that response to a combination of questions yields findings that agree more closely with an expert clinical diagnosis of asthma, than response to individual questions.

Physiological Measures for Identifying Cases of Asthma

Airway Hyper-responsiveness

AHR is a physiological hallmark of asthma and has been shown to be closely associated with asthma symptoms (124–128) and outcomes of asthma (129–131). A significant relationship between response to various nonspecific bronchial challenge agents and a range of asthma symptoms, diagnosis of asthma, and use of asthma medications has also been reported (125,127). Use of AHR as a tool for epidemiological surveillance is complicated by the range of agents used to elicit the airway response and the continuous distribution of the response, which must be arbitrarily dichotomized to estimate the prevalence of AHR. Furthermore, there are many people who have symptoms of asthma, particularly children, who do not have AHR (124,132–134) and AHR is not found solely in people with asthma symptoms (125,133,135). The meaning of these discordant states remains unclear.

The measurement of AHR can be performed on a population scale (136). As noted above, it provides information that is distinct from that provided by measures of symptoms and diagnoses. Unlike reported diagnoses and symptoms, the finding of AHR is independent of diagnostic or labeling fashion. Changes in the prevalence of AHR over time represent the most solid evidence of true changes in the prevalence of asthma (86).

Peak Flow Variability

Portable peak expiratory flow meters are used in clinical practice for serial home monitoring to assist in the assessment of management of patients with asthma. Although they have been used in population studies (137,138), there are practical limitations that apply to the use of serial peak flow monitoring for population surveillance. It requires monitoring over a (variable) period of time and the quality of data may be poor in the absence of supervision. This may be a particular problem in a general population sample.

Spirometry

Measurement of spirometric function, and the response to bronchodilator, is used in clinical practice in the diagnosis of asthma in individuals who present with airflow obstruction. However, this measurement lacks sensitivity for the diagnosis of asthma in a general population setting since most people with asthma have near normal lung function most of the time.

Combined Measure: Recent Wheeze and AHR

The presence of both recent wheeze and AHR (i.e., symptomatic airway hyper-responsiveness) identifies a subgroup of subjects with more morbidity due to asthma (129,130), with evidence of significant airway inflammation (139) and with a worse prognosis (131). This has been recommended as an operational definition of current asthma for epidemiological purposes (129) and may be regarded as identifying "asthma that matters."

Conclusion

No single question, questionnaire, test, or combination of these can lay claim to being the universally applicable best measure of asthma in populations. Each has strengths and weaknesses, as outlined above. Decisions on appropriate methods depend on the purpose of monitoring, the scale of the monitoring task, the need for longitudinal or cross-sectional comparisons, and the resources available. Where it is feasible to do so, there are advantages in monitoring a range of subjective and objective measures that are relevant to the prevalence of asthma. When these yield consistent findings, the conclusions are strengthened. When the findings are inconsistent, investigation of the basis for the observed discrepancies may be illuminating (60).

Mortality Attributable to Asthma

Fortunately, death is a rare event in the population with asthma and there is evidence that asthma mortality rates are declining (2,140,141), However, some deaths attributable to asthma are potentially avoidable (142) and increases in asthma mortality rates, especially those that persist over long periods, often generate concerns about the effects of changes in treatment (143,144) as well as increases in prevalence, or changes in disease severity (145). Changes in mortality may also reflect changes in diagnostic and labeling fashion.

For these reasons, monitoring of asthma mortality is considered to be a key indicator in any asthma surveillance system. It contributes to the evaluation of health care and clinical service delivery aimed at preventing and managing severe asthma and exacerbations of asthma. Death in patients with asthma is the ultimate measure of management failure. Mortality data are also relevant to adverse event monitoring and reflect the impact and costs of asthma for the individual and for the community.

Reliability and Validity of Asthma Mortality Data

Information on asthma mortality is obtained exclusively from death certificates, completed by medical practitioners at the time of the patient's death and assigned to International Classification of Diseases (ICD) codes by trained clerical staff.

The reliability and validity of mortality data are influenced by variation in the propensity of attending medical practitioners to diagnose and label patients as dying from asthma. A number of validation studies examining the accuracy of death certification for asthma have demonstrated that the diagnosis and certification of asthma is variable, with adult deaths from asthma either under-enumerated (146–148) or over-enumerated (149–151). It has also been reported that hospital doctors and non-family doctors are less likely to diagnose asthma accurately than coroners and family doctors (149).

Certification of asthma death is considered to be relatively accurate for people aged 5–34 years, although a recent study has also demonstrated under-enumeration of asthma deaths in children and young adults (152). Accuracy declines with increasing age (149,151) and certification of asthma deaths is most unreliable in people aged 65 years and over (146,149,150). In this age range, there is substantial misclassification between chronic obstructive pulmonary disease (COPD) and asthma (146,148,150,153).

Revisions in the World Health Organization's International Classification of Diseases (ICD) coding occur periodically to account for new diseases or new disease classification. Changes in the classification, and in the associated coding rules, often result in artifactual changes in the time series of cause-specific mortality rates. The effect of these changes may be quantified by dual coding a sample of death records according to both old (outgoing) and new (incoming) coding systems (154). Recently many countries have switched from using ICD version 9 to the ICD version 10. In the United States, the conversion rate for deaths from asthma under ICD9 to deaths from asthma under ICD10 was 0.89 (140). In Australia, the conversion rate from ICD9 to ICD10 was 0.75 (155). Further investigation revealed that this conversion rate was substantially age-dependent, with a conversion factor of 1.0 (i.e., no conversion) for all ages less than 35 years; 0.84 for ages 35–64 years; and 0.68 for ages 65 years and over (156).

The greater reliability and validity of asthma death certification in the age range 5–34 years has led to recommendations that data for this age range be used as the basis for monitoring time trends and observing geographical variation in asthma mortality rates (63,157). However, this approach excludes the monitoring of the majority of deaths attributable to asthma, since most of these deaths occur in the elderly.

Data Availability

In many jurisdictions, death data are routinely collected and reported to a central registering authority. Often the reporting of a death is a legal requirement and, under these circumstances, the mortality data set could be considered to be near complete. In some settings these data are the only accessible data for population monitoring purposes.

However, even in countries where there is a legal requirement to notify all deaths, there may still be under-enumeration of specific population or minority groups due to poor identification. For example, Aboriginal and Torres Strait Islander people are often under-enumerated in Australian mortality data, due to the lack of a clear, routinely applied definition of Aboriginal status (158).

Examples of Interpretation of Mortality Data

Variation in asthma mortality between population groups and over time may reflect variation in the prevalence of asthma or variation in case fatality rates. Factors that have been linked to increased risk of death from asthma are: more severe disease, requirement for more than three medications, extensive use of health services, a previous life-threatening asthma attack, and non-compliance with medication or medical follow-up (142,145). Interventions to improve asthma control and reduce severity can be expected to reduce death rates from asthma.

Increases in asthma deaths that are sustained over a period of time may also raise concerns about changes in medical management. At various times in the past, investigators have proposed that the introduction of therapeutic agents for asthma were responsible for "epidemics" of asthma deaths. For example, the marked increase in asthma deaths among young people in the 1960s was attributed to over-reliance on high dose isoproteronol aerosols, which were available over the counter (144). Legislation restricting the use of such medications coincided with a drop in mortality.

There may be variation in mortality rates between population groups based on ethnicity, social status, or geographical location (140,159–161). However, caution is required when interpreting these analyses as they are dependent not only on the accuracy of cause of death data but also the accuracy of these other socio-demographic indicators in the mortality dataset. For example, the identifier for race may not be reliable and definitions used are not always standardized. This may result in under-reporting of race in some instances (158,162), which, in turn, will affect the reporting of mortality for asthma by racial background.

Studies from the United Kingdom, Australia, and the United States have shown seasonal variation in rates of death from asthma, which varies between age groups (2,163,164). In the United States and the United Kingdom there is a peak in mortality amongst 5–34 year olds in late summer (163,164). Most deaths from asthma in the older age group occur in the winter months.

Conclusions

Death from asthma is a readily observable and widely recorded event. At least in young adults it is reliably and validly measured in a range of different settings and, hence, it provides a robust and feasible basis for examining trends over time and comparisons between populations. However, the consequences for public policy of monitoring mortality due to asthma are less clear. It is a rare event. The relative importance of the prevention, chronic care, and acute care sectors in responding to changes in asthma mortality is uncertain. It remains a key global indicator of the burden of asthma.

Hospital Utilization for Asthma

In contrast to asthma deaths, hospital separations for asthma are a much more common event. However, the majority of health care for asthma still occurs in other settings, such as primary care or Emergency Departments. In general, hospital admission signifies intervention for a more severe adverse event in the course of asthma.

Despite this limitation, hospital utilization is a convenient, well-defined event to monitor for surveillance purposes. Hospitalization data have been shown to reflect variation and changes in disease severity, the effectiveness of disease management, and the quality of primary health-care services (165,166). Information on hospital utilization includes the occurrence of hospital admission as well as length of stay, cost and use of services. Therefore, it is also an important input into assessments of expenditure on asthma for both the individual and the community (167). Hospital utilization may also reflect the accessibility of hospital care for patients with exacerbations of asthma and the extent to which alternative community-based care for exacerbations, for example, after hours care, is available and supported (168). Finally, hospital readmission rates are considered to be an indicator of quality of care (169). In relation to asthma care, prevention of re-admission depends on effective management of the exacerbation and effective implementation of a longer-term asthma management plan. Hence, re-admission rates for asthma probably reflect the quality of three health-care system components: hospital care for the exacerbation, communication between the hospital and the primary care system, and the primary care system itself.

Measures of Hospital Utilization

There are several inter-related measures of hospital utilization. These are:

- hospital separation rate for asthma;
- hospital patient-days for asthma (total patient-days);
- length of stay for asthma; and
- hospital re-admission-rate for asthma (within a specified time frame).

Rate of Hospital Separations for Asthma

The term "separations" refers to episodes of hospital care. For administrative purposes, these are counted at the time of hospital discharge (or death). However, the separation rate is effectively the same as the admission rate, offset by a few days. The rate of hospital separations for asthma is an indicator of occurrence of exacerbations requiring hospital care.

There are limitations to the interpretation of these data as an indicator of exacerbations of asthma. In isolation from additional information, for example on length of stay or clinical characteristics at presentation, this rate does not allow assessment of the severity of the episodes. Hospitalization rates may be substantially influenced by variation in policies on the admission of patients with relatively mild exacerbations (170) and also by variation in administrative policies on the classification of patients who spend several hours in the Emergency Department.

Routinely available data simply enumerate episodes of hospital separation. In these data, an individual who has several episodes of hospitalization over the observation period contributes several units to the total count. Perhaps, a more intuitively meaningful indicator is the number of individuals who have been admitted to hospital over a defined observation period. This rate can be directly compared with the estimated prevalence of asthma to give an indication of the proportion of people with asthma who require hospital care. In most data systems, which lack a universal patient identifier, the estimation of the number of individuals with hospital separations for asthma requires the development of a linkage key to identify repeated separations attributable to the same individual.

When presenting data on hospital separation, rates are usually expressed as population-based rates. However, the accurate estimation of population-based rates requires knowledge of the extent of the population serviced by the hospitals whose separation rates have been enumerated. This is feasible for large administrative areas (cities, regions, or countries) but for smaller areas or for individual hospitals, it may be more difficult to define because of unknown patterns of patient referral or travel across boundaries.

Length of Stay for Asthma

This measure reflects the severity of exacerbations, the existence of complicating co-morbidities, and the efficiency of hospital care. However, it is also influenced, in an inverse direction, by variation in admission and administrative policies referred to above. Hence, a more stringent admission policy leading to a reduction in admissions of patients with mild exacerbations will usually result in an increase in average length of stay (unless other factors also change). This can lead to erroneous interpretation of changes in average length of stay.

Rate of Hospital Patient-days for Asthma

As alluded to above, changes in administrative policies and practices may have spurious effects on hospital utilization data. For example, a more stringent admission policy may reduce admission rates but increase average length of stay. A more aggressive discharge policy may result in shorter length of stay but may increase re-admission rates. Calculation of the total hospital patient-days for asthma overcomes the problems in interpreting the individual components of the hospital utilization data. Spurious, inverse changes in separation rates and average length of stay will cancel each other out in the estimate of total patient-days for asthma as this reflects both the number of hospital admissions (separations) and the average length of stay.

The rate of total patient-days for asthma is simply the sum of all the bed-days occupied by people with asthma divided by the population covered by the included hospital(s). It is directly relevant to the cost of hospital care for asthma. On the other hand, as it combines information on number of separations with length of stay, it cannot be taken as a direct measure of the rate of exacerbations requiring hospital care. However, the inclusion of length of stay in the measure does mean that it reflects information on the severity of exacerbations.

The total number of hospital-bed days for asthma is influenced by the prevalence of asthma, the rate and severity of exacerbations of asthma, the efficiency of hospital care for exacerbations of asthma, and the range of community-based alternatives for initial or early follow-up of patients with exacerbations of asthma.

Rate of Hospital Re-admissions for Asthma

Rates of re-admission to hospital, after initial discharge, are considered to be an indicator of the effectiveness and quality of care. For conditions such as asthma, where there are recommended guidelines for care that have been shown to improve patient outcomes, admission to hospital provides an important point of contact with the health-care system and an opportunity for assessment, care planning, and establishing an ongoing therapeutic relationship. There is evidence that effective asthma management does result in a reduction in the risk of re-admission (171–175). Factors influencing the likelihood of re-admission include the quality of care in hospital (176), quality of discharge planning and communication with primary care, and quality of care in the community (171). A failure at any point in this continuum of care may result in re-admission to hospital. Hence, re-admission rates can be regarded as an indicator of the effectiveness of the asthma care across this continuum.

The time span over which re-admission is assessed is variably defined, but one month (28 days) is often chosen as there is evidence that most preventable admissions occur within this time frame (177). The indicator may be expressed as either a population-based rate or as a proportion of all asthma-related separations. The latter method may be spuriously influenced by hospital admission policies. For example, a hospital that admits patients with relatively mild asthma will have a large denominator and, because patients with mild disease are less likely to be re-admitted, a small numerator on this indicator, compared with an otherwise similar hospital in which admissions are limited to patients with severe asthma. While the re-admission rate expressed as a population-based rate is not influenced by variable admission policies, it has the disadvantage of being more difficult to measure because re-admission must be linked to area of residence, rather than hospital of admission.

It may not be possible to accurately identify, on a routine basis, cases that are re-admitted to hospital if the patient unique identifier does not extend beyond the admitting hospital. This may result in an under-estimate of the re-admission rate, as the people who are re-admitted to a different hospital will not be counted. Strategies to overcome this include limiting the analysis to large, geographically distinct areas covered by a unique patient identifier (178), or creating a linkage key from the available information using probabilistic methods (179).

Data Availability

In some countries, there is a process for reporting of all hospital separations data obtained at the service level to a national body, which is responsible for collation of, and reporting on, these data (180). However, in other jurisdictions, such as the United States, there is no complete national record of hospital separations. Alternative sources of information include sample surveys, such as the National Hospital Discharge Survey, which is conducted annually using a sample of around 275,000 patient records in approximately 500 non-federal general and specialist hospitals (140). Non-random samples may also provide valuable information including individual hospitals or health services, administrative regions, or health maintenance organizations (181).

Examples of Interpretation of Hospital Utilization Data

While death from asthma is an unequivocally bad outcome, hospital admission may be interpreted as an adverse outcome or a beneficial outcome. Insofar as it reflects the occurrence of a severe exacerbation that medical management has failed to prevent, it is an adverse outcome. The cost and inconvenience of hospital admission also represent deleterious consequences. However, among patients with severe exacerbations, having access to hospital care is advantageous. The alternative, lack of access to hospital care, may be associated with more severe suffering and even risk of death.

Many of the factors affecting mortality also impact on hospital utilization measures. Periodic changes to International Classification of Diseases (ICD) have had an impact on hospital utilization measures, as they have for mortality data. In Australia, the recent change from ICD version 9 to ICD version 10 resulted in fewer hospital separations being attributed to asthma. The effect of this change was strongly related to age, with no effect on coding in persons aged less than 35 years but a 0.64 fold reduction in deaths coded as asthma under ICD 10 for 35–64 year olds and a 0.53 fold reduction for persons aged 65 years and over (2).

The issue of variation in diagnostic and labeling practices also applies to the interpretation of hospital utilization data. There has been limited work on validation of the coding of diagnoses during hospital admissions. The available evidence suggests that a diagnosis of asthma is most accurate in younger ages but accuracy decreases with age (182). In particular, there is overlap with chronic obstructive pulmonary disease (COPD), especially in people aged over 55, and with other respiratory conditions in infants. Interpretation of trends and differentials in hospital utilization data for asthma should take into account the potential for lack of reliability of the data in these age ranges.

Variation in the prevalence of asthma may explain some variation in the rate of hospital bed utilization for asthma. In order to be able to attribute changes in this indicator to changes in the level of control of asthma (and, hence, changes in the effectiveness of disease management), it would be important to adjust for confounding due to variation in the prevalence of asthma. This could also be achieved by monitoring a case-based rate (i.e., using the prevalence of asthma as the denominator population).

Use of hospital care for the management of exacerbations may be influenced by the accessibility of hospital services and the accessibility of alternative services such as primary care physicians, especially after hours (168). Hence, for the purpose of assessing exacerbation rate it would be more meaningful to use an index combining hospital separations, Emergency Department attendances, and primary care visits for acute care. However, if there has been no change in accessibility of components of the health system, changes in hospital separation rates for asthma probably do reflect changes in the rate of severe exacerbations of asthma.

Changing patterns of management in the Emergency Department and changes to hospital admission criteria will affect hospital separation rates for asthma. Similarly, interventions in both hospital and community settings that aim to improve asthma control and reduce severity will impact on hospital separations and patient days.

Seasonal variation in hospitalization rates has been observed, with higher rates in winter months amongst older age groups, and higher rates in summer and autumn amongst children and young adults (2,183–185). Annual and monthly rates should be examined to investigate seasonal variation.

Use of hospital utilization data as an indicator of racial differences in the burden of asthma may be limited by under-reporting or inaccurate reporting of race or ethnic group in administrative data, such as hospital separation data (158,162).

Conclusion

Hospital bed utilization for asthma is a major component of the cost of asthma care. In most cases, hospital admission for asthma reflects a failure of chronic care for the condition. However, lack of access to hospital care, when required, equally reflects a failure of acute care. This complicates the interpretation of hospitalization rates as an indicator of the effectiveness of health policy in relation to asthma.

Appropriate Asthma Medication Use

Drug therapy is the mainstay of asthma management, and is aimed at improving lung function and symptom control, and preventing exacerbations without undesirable adverse effects. The drugs used to treat asthma can be broadly grouped into short-acting bronchodilators (including short-acting beta agonists and anti-cholinergics), long-acting bronchodilators (long-acting beta agonists), inhaled corticosteroids, cromones, and leukotriene receptor antagonists. Medications that combine long-acting beta agonists with inhaled corticosteroids are also available.

Based on substantial evidence, inhaled corticosteroids are the preferred treatment for moderate and severe asthma (22). There is growing evidence that they also have a role in mild asthma (186–188). Short-acting beta agonists and anti-cholinergics are mainly used to relieve symptoms when they occur, or can be used to prevent expected exacerbations (exercise induced asthma). More recently, long-acting beta agonists have been prescribed, mainly in combination with inhaled corticosteroids, to improve asthma control while reducing or maintaining inhaled corticosteroid dose (189,190). Leukotriene receptor antagonists are a more recently available alternative or adjunct to inhaled corticosteroid therapy (191,192). Due to their common role in the management of asthma, inhaled corticosteroids, combined medications, cromones, and leukotriene receptor antagonists are colloquially referred to as "preventers".

People with poorly controlled asthma who rely on short-acting reliever medication are more likely to have exacerbations of asthma requiring attendance at an Emergency Department or admission to hospital, while treatment with inhaled corticosteroids reduces the likelihood of hospitalization (193–197). There is substantial evidence that many people, for whom preventers are indicated, are not receiving them (198–201). Recent reports suggest that excess doses of newer, stronger inhaled corticosteroids in some patients are being prescribed with serious adverse effects (202,203). Asthma medication data reflect prescribing practice, adherence to asthma management guidelines and, ultimately, the quality of clinical management of asthma. Data provided by consumers give some insight into patient compliance with medical advice.

Reliability of Asthma Medication Data

Data about the prescription, wholesaling, and use of asthma medication may be collected from a range of sources, each with its own advantages and limitations. Information on the wholesaling of medications to pharmacies and hospitals is available from IMS Health. Where they exist, primary care data collections may provide prescription data. Data on the purchase of medications may be available through pharmacy surveys or government-based or insurance-based drug databases. Information about the actual use of drugs must be collected directly via consumer health surveys.

Drug utilization data derived from wholesale suppliers cannot be linked to the reason for medication use or to the characteristics of the purchaser. In many countries, including Australia, this is also true of data from government-based databases. As many drugs prescribed for the management of asthma can also be used in the management of other respiratory conditions, including COPD, this limits the specificity of these data as an indicator of drug therapy for asthma.

Measures of the Quality of Drug Therapy for Asthma

Ratio of Inhaled Corticosteroid to Bronchodilator

On an individual clinical level, people who are treated according to guidelines will use inhaled corticosteroids regularly and should only need to use inhaled short-acting bronchodilators sparingly. Hence, they will have a higher ratio of inhaled corticosteroid use to bronchodilator use. The validity of this measure, as an indicator of quality of care, is dependent on the availability of comprehensive data on reliever use (which can be bought without prescription in some countries) and diagnosis in the pharmaceutical data sources. To test the validity of this measure for population monitoring of the quality of asthma prescribing, Shelley et al. (204) linked hospital admission data for asthma with dispensed prescription data and found no significant correlation. Although theoretically an attractive index, there is no empirical evidence that this ratio is a good indicator of quality or effectiveness of asthma care.

Prescription Rate of Bronchodilators

Bronchodilator prescription or wholesale data has been used to evaluate the impact of asthma treatment guidelines on trends in bronchodilator prescribing (205). Monitoring this measure is also dependent on the availability of data about all bronchodilator use and asthma diagnosis; otherwise the indicator lacks accuracy and specificity for asthma. Its specificity, as an asthma-related measure, may be improved by limiting the age group for which prescription data are analyzed to 5–34 years in order to largely exclude people with COPD from the study population. Prescription data does not provide any information on the appropriateness of medication use. Furthermore, large volumes of bronchodilator usage by a small number of individuals may influence population-based data on this measure.

Prescription Rate of Corticosteroids

Like the measure above, it has been widely used but has many of the same limitations.

Proportion of People with Asthma for Whom Preventers are Indicated and Who Use Preventers Regularly

Marks et al. (38) showed that 30% of people for whom preventers were indicated were not using them appropriately. Monitoring this measure requires survey data about an individual's asthma control and frequency of their preventer use. Although this proportion may more validly reflect the use of appropriate asthma management in the target group, measuring the "proportion of people with asthma for whom preventers are indicated" via survey questions may introduce substantial imprecision into the measurement of this measure.

Proportion of People with Asthma Who Use Preventers Regularly

Although less specific than the previous measure, it does not require the identification of a sub-group of people with asthma for whom preventers are indicated and has the advantage of being more readily and reliably measured than the indicator described above.

Conclusion

Regular use of preventer medications is the cornerstone of effective asthma management, leading to improved quality of life and reduced risk of exacerbations. The extent to which preventer medications are utilized by the people with asthma who have the potential to benefit from them is a key indicator of the effectiveness of asthma policy. Unfortunately, as described above, it is a difficult indicator to measure at a population level.

Primary Care Visits for Asthma

Primary care physicians (PCPs) diagnose, maintain, and manage acute care for most people with asthma in the community. Therefore, it is crucial to monitor the utilization of primary care encounters related to asthma in order to better understand the impact of asthma on community resources and the level of accessibility to primary asthma care. Variations in resource utilization and accessibility across different groups and geographical areas provide important information for policy and planning purposes, including the development and evaluation of community interventions. Previous studies have shown that socio-economically disadvantaged adults and children have higher rates of overall primary care consultations than those less disadvantaged (206–208). Saxena et al. (207) showed that children from these groups also had poorer health and lower rates of preventive primary care visits.

People with asthma visit PCPs for a variety of reasons, including: the acute or reactive management of a severe exacerbation or increased symptom frequency (this may include the initial diagnosis); a review visit during or following an acute episode; or a visit for maintenance activities such as obtaining prescriptions. Recent, convincing evidence that self-management education for people with asthma combined with written asthma action plans, self-monitoring, and regular medical review improve patient outcomes (209), has led to professional and government groups encouraging PCPs to initiate an opportunistic review when the patient visits for another condition or to schedule a structured planned review. In Australia, this is being encouraged through a Practice Incentive Program (PIP), the Asthma 3+ Visit Plan, which supports planned review encounters by PCPs, and encourages patients to seek regular planned care to maintain asthma control and prevent acute exacerbations. Such interventions, if effective, will ultimately lead to decreased rates of asthma-related primary care encounters.

Ideally, it would be useful to have indicators that can measure the rates for all asthma-related primary care encounters, acute management visits for exacerbations, and structured review visits.

Although the rate of primary care visits is an imprecise measure of the effects of interventions, it may be the only measure currently available. This measure also provides information on access to primary care services for asthma, especially when interpreted with data on rates of Emergency Department visits and hospitalizations. Information on utilization of primary care for the management of asthma also contributes to knowledge about the level of health resources used to provide asthma care in the community and costs for individuals.

Quality of Primary Care Data

There are four potential sources of information on primary care visits: Government, Health Maintenance Organization (HMO) or insurance databases used mainly to reimburse patients or primary care practitioners for the costs of primary care visits; primary care research databases; primary care practice surveys and population surveys.

Only primary care reimbursement databases with information on diagnosis would be useful for this purpose. The databases of HMOs in the United States usually hold information about diagnosis linked with all health service episodes of care. These data, if available, provide the most valid information.

General Practice (GP) research databases, which are based on regional groupings of GPs who volunteer to collect information, usually about primary care management of asthma and other chronic or acute conditions, include the General Practice Research Database (GPRD) in the United Kingdom (210), and University Family Practice Network in Australia (211). The generalizability of these data may be limited due to volunteer bias. However, the validity of the GPRD, which represents a large network of participating GPs, was supported by evidence of good agreement with data collected in the fourth Morbidity Survey in General Practice (212).

General Practice surveys gather data from a random sample of GPs about reasons for consultations, medications prescribed, referrals, and other management activities. Most surveys are carried out irregularly, e.g., the UK Morbidity Surveys in General Practice. However, others are continuous surveys targeting a rolling random sample of practitioners. Examples include the Australian "Bettering the Evaluation and Care of Health" (BEACH) primary care surveys (213) and the USA National Disease and Therapeutic Index (NDTI) physician survey conducted by IMS HEALTH (Plymouth Meeting, Pennsylvania, USA) (214). Although these surveys use random sampling techniques, where participation rates are low, data validity and generalizability remain problematic.

Population-based surveys allow respondents to be asked about how frequently they visited the PCP for asthma in a given time period. Further information on the reason for, nature of, and outcome of the encounter may also be obtained. While self-reported data may be an over- or under-estimation of the actual number of visits, the consumer or patient perspective on primary care activity derived from these surveys is a useful complement to data derived from the providers, as described above.

Measures of Primary Care Management of Asthma

Four possible measures of rates for asthma-related primary care visits might be useful. Depending on the data available, a range of denominators could be used: total encounters, total population or total number of people with asthma in the practices. Total encounters would reflect the relative burden of asthma in primary care compared with other conditions. Total population would signify the burden of asthma in the community, possibly be a crude measure of changes due to interventions in the primary care of asthma, and provide some indication of access to primary care. Use of "people with asthma" as the denominator population would more accurately reflect changing patterns of primary care service utilization for asthma and provide information about access to and quality of primary care services for asthma.

All these measures are dependent on the completeness and accuracy of the available data source and will be influenced by diagnostic fashion and patient health care seeking behavior (215). These limitations need to be kept in mind when interpreting the data.

As foreshadowed by the previous discussion, there are three potential numerators for measures of primary care activity in relation to asthma.

Asthma-related Primary Care Visit Rate

Potentially, this indicator could be measured in many countries either using primary care research databases or surveys.

Primary Care Visit Rate for Exacerbations of Asthma

Routinely available data sources do not allow the separate identification of visits for acute or reactive care, as opposed to health maintenance or review visits. For this reason, data collection for this indicator is more problematic. It may have to rely on specific questions being asked in general practice surveys or the utilization of an "acute visit" field in primary care research databases. If it is possible to measure this indicator, it provides more useful information about outcomes of asthma care.

Primary Care Asthma Review Visit Rate

Similar to the measure above, new questions or fields may need to be added to data sources. This indicator will provide feedback on the quality of care based on current recommendations about regularly reviewing patients with asthma.

Conclusion

Primary care is the major setting in which patients with asthma seek medical care. From the population monitoring standpoint, this sector generates a substantial component of expenditure on asthma. It is also the major setting in which effective interventions, such as assessment, education and review, are implemented. Finally, consultation with PCPs is an important indicator of the occurrences of exacerbations of asthma. It is difficult to measure disease-specific activities within this sector. However, a range of routine and research-based data sources are being developed to enhance the value of data that will be relevant to asthma monitoring.

Health-related Quality of Life

Traditional measures of disease impact such as those discussed above, prevalence, mortality, and health-care utilization rates, provide an incomplete indication of the impact of asthma. They measure an incomplete range of the impacts of the disease. Furthermore, they are influenced by non-disease outcome-related factors, in particular, accessibility of the health care whose utilization is being measured. Clinical measures of asthma, including measures of symptoms, lung function, and medication requirement, are also regarded as indicators of asthma status. However, these clinical measures also provide only a limited range of information about asthma outcomes and impact and there is only a weak-to-moderate correlation between these clinical indices and measures of health-related quality of life (HRQoL) (216–218).

HRQoL measures complement traditional health and clinical measures and capture the broader impacts that asthma has in the physical, psychological, and social domains. HRQoL is a more holistic measure of health outcome than the traditional measures cited above. The development of valid and standardized HRQoL measures is challenging because of the uniqueness inherent in an individual's perception of their quality of life. Nonetheless, to ignore HRQoL as an outcome of asthma will result in an incomplete appreciation of its impact. People with chronic diseases, such as asthma, are generally most concerned about the impact of their condition on functional capacity and well-being. It is for this reason that standardized methods of assessment of HRQoL have been developed and validated so that comparisons can be made between populations and various groups (219).

Purposes of HRQoL Measures

HRQoL can be used to describe health outcomes and functional status, guide clinical management, predict health outcomes, formulate clinical policy, and assist in the allocation of resources. The context and purposes for which HRQoL measures are used may be classified as discrimination, evaluation, and prediction (219).

Discriminative Measures

One of the purposes of population monitoring is to discern sub-groups of the population who have greater or lesser impacts attributable to asthma (219). High burden sub-groups identified in this way may then be targeted for specific interventions. A discriminative instrument is required for this purpose. Important attributes of discriminative HRQoL measures for use in asthma population monitoring are that they are reliable and valid measures of the attributes of HRQoL relevant to asthma and that they are sensitive enough to detect differences between groups.

Evaluative Measures

Perhaps the most common context for health research is evaluating the effect of an intervention. Many HRQoL measurement instruments have been designed as evaluative instruments, particularly asthma-specific HRQoL measures. The key attributes of these measurement instruments are that they are valid measures of change in HRQoL and that they are responsive to within-subject change in the HRQoL attributes.

Predictive Measures

Predictive instruments are used in HRQoL measurement to either predict the result in another measure or to forecast an outcome at a future time (219). These can be useful for assisting in decision making processes, classifying individuals entering a study or identifying those who are likely to develop a particular outcome.

Types of HRQoL Measures

HRQoL measures have been developed from a number of disciplines resulting in diversity in the approaches to HRQoL measurement (220). A range of formats and content domains have been used in population health surveys including single item measures and more sophisticated multidimensional HRQoL profile measurement instruments. There is no universally accepted framework for classifying HRQoL measurement instruments. However, a number of characteristics can be used to describe HRQoL measures including: the scope or range of domains and dimensions measured, the number of items, the degree of disease specificity of the content, and the scaling method used (e.g., psychometric, utility or other method). This section provides an overview of the different types of HRQoL measures and compares their strengths and weaknesses.

Single Item and Brief Measures

Single item or very brief measures may attempt to address the global domain of HRQoL or may focus on a single domain or even a single dimension. The broadest and simplest class of HRQoL measures is that which addresses the "global" domain of HRQoL or self-perceived health status with a single item or a very small number of items (or questions). The question, "In general, would you say your health is excellent, very good, good, fair or poor?", is an example of a single item health status measure.

Brief global measures such as this have the advantage of being simple to use with low respondent burden (the effort and time required for a respondent to answer) and this can be particularly attractive in large-scale population surveys where there are many issues competing for space in the survey. The main disadvantage of any single item (or very brief) instrument, as opposed to multi-item, multi-dimensional profiles, is that the content, although it may be broad ranging or global in intent, does not adequately sample from a comprehensive range of HRQoL dimensions and may not adequately reflect all the relevant domains. Furthermore, it provides no information on the relative impact on physical, psychological, and social domains of health (221), and this limits their usefulness in terms of planning an appropriate response. Furthermore, since they usually have only a small number of possible response options, the measurement range is limited in relation to the actual range that is likely to be present in the general population. This reduces the sensitivity of the instrument. Hence, due to problems with both validity and sensitivity, studies using these single item or very brief global instruments as the sole tool for assessing HRQoL should be interpreted with caution (222).

Some single item measurement instruments only focus on a single HRQoL domain rather than HRQoL globally. This focus on a single domain may be an advantage for a single item measure, as long as the interpretation of the findings does not extend beyond that domain. Sick days due to asthma, that is the number of days away from work or school or the number of reduced activity days due to asthma, and symptom-free days, that is, the number of days in which the subject does not experience asthma symptoms, are both examples of this form of disease-specific, single domain, single item measures for the impact of asthma (223). These single item, single domain measures may be more valid and sensitive, for their intended purpose, than the single item global measures, as long as their interpretation does not extend beyond the single domain or dimension that has been measured. They should *not* be interpreted as global measures of HRQoL.

As asthma is an episodic disease, it can be difficult to adequately capture the time-variable impacts in a single measure. Some of the single-item, single dimension measures referred to above, such as sick days, unhealthy days, or healthy days, in which the number of affected days over a defined period are counted, represent a useful way to address this issue of time variability.

Multi-element and Multi-dimensional Profiles

To address the limitations of single item or very brief HRQoL measures, instruments have been developed to measure the core physical, psychological, and social domains of HRQoL more comprehensively [e.g., the Short Form (SF)-36, 224]. In most instances several dimensions within each domain are measured. The dimensions are the issue, factor or experience that is the object of assessment, such as general health perceptions, functional status, or impairment and limitations on lifestyle. These are measured in elements such as tiredness, degree of distress, and so on. These are usually scored, using a psychometric approach, as an overall summary score and/or as a profile of scores for the various dimensions that were measured (225).

Psychometric measures provide quantitative information but can only be used to compare data collected using the same scale. An alternative scoring approach is to quantify information about health status on a scale between perfect health and death, using a utility-based approach (226).

Generic and Specific HRQoL Measures

The focus of the content within HRQoL instruments may be on impacts that are relevant to a specific disease or, alternatively, on impacts that are relevant to a broad range of health conditions. Both generic and disease-specific instruments have a role in the evaluation of HRQoL. Generic questionnaires aim to assess the impact of any and all adverse health states on HRQoL, without reference to the impacts of any specific disease. Disease-specific HRQoL instruments measure the specific impacts of the target disease.

Generic HRQoL measurement instruments, such as the SF-36 questionnaire, can be used to assess overall HRQoL in all individuals in the study population. The strength of these instruments is that all members of the population, including those with no illness and those with a range of different illnesses, are measured on the same scale. Reference values, based on the scores in healthy individuals, have been derived for some generic HRQoL questionnaires (227). This facilitates the assessment of the HRQoL of sub-groups, such as those with asthma, relative to other members of the population or relative to reference values. It also allows comparison of HRQoL outcomes between population groups with different diseases. The limitation of these questionnaires is that they may not adequately focus on those aspects of HRQoL that are particularly relevant to the people with a particular disease and, hence, may lack sensitivity in relation to the impacts of a specific disease.

Specific measurement instruments are designed for specific diagnostic or population groups, such as people diagnosed with asthma. The rationale for the use of these questionnaires is that they will be more relevant, and also more sensitive, to differences between population sub-groups and responsive to changes over time. Disease-specific profiles or health indexes are widely recognized as useful tools for assessing the impact of asthma and, particularly, for evaluating the impact of interventions to ameliorate the condition. However, for population-based monitoring the important limitation of disease-specific instruments is that they are only applicable to people with that condition in the population and, unlike generic instruments, cannot be used to compare HRQoL with the general population or with other disease or population groups.

Another possible limitation of some disease-specific measures is that they may not be accurate in attributing impacts to the specific disease in question. This is not an issue when the impact is unique to a specific disease (e.g., wheeze or embarrassment about inhaler use, for people with asthma) but may be a problem when the adverse outcome could have many possible causes (such as tiredness or time away from work or school). Respondents may inadvertently under-estimate or over-estimate the importance of a specific cause for these non-specific adverse outcomes. This is demonstrated in the Australian National Health Survey 2001, in which the number of people who reported time away from work or study due to asthma was fewer than the excess number of people with asthma, compared to people without asthma, who reported any time away from work or study (2).

Conclusion

Health-related quality of life is a broad-ranging outcome that encompasses many, but not all, of the outcomes of illness that are relevant to patients. The importance of the domains of quality of life to patients with asthma was first recognized by clinical scientists, who developed disease-specific quality of life measures as evaluative tools for use in clinical trials. The application of quality of life measures to data monitoring is a more recent development, reflecting recognition of the need for a broad view of the impact of the disease on society. However, there are theoretical and pragmatic issues to solve before a robust and feasible method for monitoring quality of life in populations can be recommended (228).

Conclusions

In this chapter we have considered the topic of "monitoring" from beyond the individual patient perspective. Monitoring populations is an unfamiliar concept to clinicians but is very familiar to public health practitioners. It forms the basis of planning and evaluating preventive health and health service delivery strategies.

The purpose of this chapter has been to draw a link between clinicians' and public health practitioners' understanding of monitoring. We have shown that the complex nature of the disease makes simplistic evaluations of the burden of the disease unreliable. A more robust approach entails simultaneous measurement of a number of different indicators with careful interpretation of findings.

Acknowledgments

The authors wish to acknowledge the contribution of Patricia Correll to the section on quality of life and the assistance provided by Leanne Poulos in editing the manuscript.

This manuscript draws on work undertaken by the authors on behalf of Australian Centre for Asthma Monitoring (2,156,228). The Australian Centre for Asthma Monitoring is a collaborating unit of the Australian Institute of Health and Welfare funded as part of the Australian Government's initiative to establish and maintain the Australian System for Monitoring Asthma.

References

1. Global strategy for asthma management and prevention (updated 2003). 2003. (Accessed 27th April, 2004, at www.einasthma.com.).
2. Australian Centre for Asthma Monitoring. Asthma in Australia 2003. Canberra: Australian Institute of Health and Welfare; 2003. Report No.: AIHW Cat. no. ACM1.
3. International Study of Asthma and Allergies in Childhood (ISAAC) Steering Committee. Worldwide variation in the prevalence of symptoms of asthma,

allergic rhinoconjunctivitis, and atopic eczema: ISAAC. Lancet 1998; 351: 1225–1232.

4. Janson C, Anto J, Burney P, et al. The European Community Respiratory Health Survey: what are the main results so far? European Community Respiratory Health Survey II. Eur Respir J 2001; 18(3):598–611.

5. Ford ES, Mannino DM, Homa DM, et al. Self-reported asthma and health-related quality of life: findings from the behavioral risk factor surveillance system. Chest 2003; 123(1):119–127.

6. Goldney R, Ruffin R, Fisher L, Wilson D. Asthma symptoms associated with depression and lower quality of life: a population survey. Med J Aust 2003; 178(9):437–441.

7. Smith D, Malone D, Lawson K, Okamoto L, Battista C, Saunders W. National estimates of the economic costs of asthma. Am J Respir Crit Care Med 1997; 156:787–793.

8. So S, Ng M, Ip M, Lam W. Rising asthma mortality in young males in Hong Kong, 1976–85. Respir Med 1990; 84:457–461.

9. Mitchell E, Jackson R. Recent trends in asthma mortality, morbidity and management in New Zealand. J Asthma 1989; 26:349–354.

10. Bates D, Baker-Anderson M. Asthma mortality and morbidity in Canada. J Allergy Clin Immunol 1987; 80:395–397.

11. Burney P. Asthma deaths in England and Wales 1931–85: evidence for a true increase in asthma mortality. J Epidemiol Comm Health 1988; 42:316–320.

12. Tarlo S, Broder I, Corey P, et al. The role of symptomatic colds in asthma exacerbations: influence of outdoor allergens and air pollutants. J Allergy Clin Immunol 2001; 108:52–58.

13. Green RM, Custovic A, Sanderson G, Hunter J, Johnston SL, Woodcock A. Synergism between allergens and viruses and risk of hospital admission with asthma; case–control study. Br Med J 2002; 324(7340):763–766.

14. Almqvist C, Wickman M, Perfetti L, et al. Worsening of asthma in children allergic to cats, after indirect exposure to cat at school. Am J Respir Crit Care Med 2001; 163(3 Pt 1):694–698.

15. Atkinson RW, Strachan DP. Role of outdoor aeroallergens in asthma exacerbations: epidemiological evidence. Thorax 2004; 59(4):277–278.

16. Chew F, Goh D, Ooi B, Saharom R, Hui J, Lee B. Association of ambient air-pollution levels with acute asthma exacerbation among children in Singapore. Allergy 1999; 54:320–329.

17. Zureik M, Neukirch C, Leynaert B, Liard R, Bousquet J, Neukirch F. Sensitisation to airborne moulds and severity of asthma: cross sectional study from European Community respiratory health survey. Br Med J 2002; 325(7361): 411–414.

18. Downs S, Mitakakis T, Marks G, et al. Clinical importance of Alternaria exposure in children. Am J Respir Crit Care Med 2001; 164:455–459.

19. Inman W, Adelstein A. Rise and fall of asthma mortality in England and Wales in relation to use of pressurised aerosols. Lancet 1969; ii:279–284.

20. Sears M, Taylor D, Print C, et al. Regular inhaled beta-agonist treatment in bronchial asthma. Lancet 1990; 336:1391–1396.

21. Pearce N, Grainger J, Atkinson M, et al. Case–control study of prescribed fenoterol and death from asthma in New Zealand, 1977–81. Thorax 1990; 45:170–175.

22. Adams N, Bestall J, Jones P. Inhaled beclomethasone versus placebo for chronic asthma (Cochrane Review). In: The Cochrane Library. Chichester, UK: John Wiley & Sons, Ltd, 2004.

23. Gibson PG, Powell H, Coughlan J, Wilson AJ, Abramson M, Haywood P, Bauman A, Hensley MJ, Walters EH. Self-management education and regular practitioner review for adults with asthma. The Cochrane Database of Systematic Reviews 2002, Issue 3. Art. No.: CD001117. DOI: 10.1002/14651858.CD001117.

24. Shickle D. Public preferences for health care: prioritisation in the United Kingdom. Bioethics 1997; 11(3–4):277–290.

25. Valovirta E, Kocevar VS, Kaila M, et al. Inpatient resource utilisation in younger (2–5 yrs) and older (6–14 yrs) asthmatic children in Finland. Eur Respir J 2002; 20(2):397–402.

26. Mellis C, Peat J, Bauman A, Woolcock A. The cost of asthma in New South Wales. Med J Aust 1991; 155:522–528.

27. Szucs T, Anderhub H, Rutishauser M. The economic burden of asthma: direct and indirect costs in Switzerland. Eur Respir J 1999; 13:281–286.

28. Lozano P, Sullivan SD, Smith DH, Weiss KB. The economic burden of asthma in US children: estimates from the National Medical Expenditure Survey. J Allergy Clin Immunol 1999; 104(5):957–963.

29. Fuhlbrigge AL, Adams RJ, Guilbert TW, et al. The burden of asthma in the United States: level and distribution are dependent on interpretation of the National Asthma Education and Prevention Program guidelines. Am J Respir Crit Care Med 2002; 166(8):1044–1049.

30. Dolan CM, Fraher KE, Bleecker ER, et al. Design and baseline characteristics of the epidemiology and natural history of asthma: Outcomes and Treatment Regimens (TENOR) study: a large cohort of patients with severe or difficult-to-treat asthma. Ann Allergy Asthma Immunol 2004; 92(1):32–39.

31. Van Ganse E, Laforest L, Pietri G, et al. Persistent asthma: disease control, resource utilisation and direct costs. Eur Respir J 2002; 20(2):260–267.

32. Woolcock A, Rubinfeld AR, Seale JP, et al. Thoracic society of Australia and New Zealand. Asthma management plan, 1989. Med J Aust 1989; 151 (11–12):650–653.

33. British Thoracic Society, Research Unit of the Royal College of Physicians of London, King's Fund Centre, National Asthma Campaign. Guidelines for management of asthma. I. Chronic persistent asthma. Br Med J 1990; 301:651–653.

34. National Heart Lung and Blood Institute of National Institutes for Health. International consensus report on diagnosis and treatment of asthma. Eur Respir J 1992; 5:601–641.

35. Warner J, Naspitz C, Cropp G. Third International Pediatric Consensus Statement on the Management of Childhood Asthma. Pediatr Pulmonol 1998; 25:1–17.

36. Adams N, Bestall J, Jones P. Budesonide for chronic asthma in children and adults (Cochrane Review). In: The Cochrane Libary, Issue 4. Chichester, UK: John Wiley & Sons, Ltd, 2003.

37. Guevara JP, Wolf FM, Grum CM, Clark NM. Effects of educational interventions for self management of asthma in children and adolescents: systematic review and meta-analysis. Br Med J 2003; 326(7402):1308–1309.

38. Marks G, Jalaludin B, Williamson M, Atkin N, Bauman A. Use of "preventer" medications and written asthma management plans among adults with asthma in New South Wales. Med J Aust 2000; 173:407–410.

39. Rabe KF, Vermeire PA, Soriano JB, Maier WC. Clinical management of asthma in 1999: the Asthma Insights and Reality in Europe (AIRE) study. Eur Respir J 2000; 16(5):802–807.

40. Beilby J, Wakefield M, Ruffin R. Reported use of asthma management plans in South Australia. Med J Aust 1997; 166:298–301.

41. Adams R, Fuhlbrigge A, Guilbert T, Lozano P, Martinez F. Inadequate use of asthma medication in the United States: results of the asthma in America national population survey. J Allergy Clin Immunol 2002; 110(1):58–64.

42. Marks G, Heslop W, Yates D. Prehospital management of exacerbations of asthma: relation to patient and disease characteristics. Respirology 2000; 5:45–50.

43. Hanania N, David-Wang A, Kesten S, Chapman K. Factors associated with emergency department dependence of patients with asthma. Chest 1997; 111:290–295.

44. Goeman DP, Aroni RA, Sawyer SM, et al. Back for more: a qualitative study of emergency department reattendance for asthma. Med J Aust 2004; 180(3):113–117.

45. Radeos MS, Leak LV, Lugo BP, et al. Risk factors for lack of asthma self-management knowledge among ED patients not on inhaled steroids. Am J Emerg Med 2001; 19(4):253–259.

46. Taylor DM, Auble TE, Calhoun WJ, Mosesso VN, Jr. Current outpatient management of asthma shows poor compliance with International Consensus Guidelines.[see comment]. Chest 1999; 116(6):1638–1645.

47. Kolbe J, Vamos M, James F, Elkind G, Garrett J. Assessment of practical knowledge of self-management of acute asthma. Chest 1996; 109(1):86–90.

48. Hanson J. Parental self-efficacy and asthma self-management skills. J Soc Pediat Nurses 1998; 3(4):146–154.

49. Scherer Y, Bruce S. Knowledge, attitudes, and self-efficacy and compliance with medical regimen, number of emergency department visits, and hospitalizations in adults with asthma. Heart Lung 2001; 30(4):250–257.

50. Williams MV, Baker DW, Honig EG, Lee TM, Nowlan A. Inadequate literacy is a barrier to asthma knowledge and self-care. Chest 1998; 114(4):1008–1015.

51. Bosely C, Fosbury J, Cochrane G. The psychological factors associated with poor compliance with treatment in asthma. Eur Respir J 1995; 8:899–904.

52. Ehrlich R, Du Toit D, Jordaan E, et al. Risk factors for childhood asthma and wheezing: importance of maternal and household smoking. Am J Respir Crit Care Med 1996; 154:681–688.

53. Lewis S, Butland B, Strachan D, et al. Study of the aetiology of wheezing illness at age 16 in two national British birth cohorts. Thorax 1996; 51:670–676.

54. Strachan DP, Cook DG. Health effects of passive smoking. 6. Parental smoking and childhood asthma: longitudinal and case–control studies. Thorax 1998; 53(3):204–212.

55. Jaakkola J, Jaakkola M. Effects of environmental tobacco smoke on the respiratory health of children. Scand J Work Environ Health 2002; 28(suppl 2):71–83.

56. Malo JL, Chan-Yeung M. Occupational asthma. J Allergy Clin Immunol 2001; 108(3):317–328.

57. Bellomo R, Gigliotti P, Treloar A, et al. Two consecutive thunderstorm associated epidemics of asthma in the city of Melbourne. The possible role of rye grass pollen. Med J Aust 1992; 156:834–837.

58. Lin M, Chen Y, Burnett RT, Villeneuve PJ, Krewski D. Effect of short-term exposure to gaseous pollution on asthma hospitalisation in children: a bi-directional case-crossover analysis. J Epidemiol Community Health 2003; 57(1):50–55.

59. Gent JF, Triche EW, Holford TR, et al. Association of low-level ozone and fine particles with respiratory symptoms in children with asthma. JAMA 2003; 290(14):1859–1867.

60. Toelle BG, Ng K, Belousova EG, Salome CM, Peat JK, Marks GB. The prevalence of asthma and allergy in schoolchildren in Belmont, Australia: three cross sectional surveys over 20 years. Br Med J 2004; 328:386–387.

61. Robertson CF, Roberts MF, Kappers JH. Asthma prevalence in Melbourne schoolchildren: have we reached the peak? Med J Aust 2004; 180(6):273–276

62. Eccles M, Grimshaw J, Campbell M, Ramsay C. Research designs for studies evaluating the effectiveness of change and improvement strategies. Qual Saf Health Care 2003; 12(1):47–52.

63. Suissa S, Ernst P. Use of anti-inflammatory therapy and asthma mortality in Japan. Eur Respir J 2003; 21(1):101–104.

64. Beasley R, Smith K, Pearce N, Crane J, Burgess C, Culling C. Trends in asthma mortality in New Zealand, 1908–1986. Med J Aust 1990; 152(11):570.

65. Sears M, Rea H, Rothwell R, et al. Asthma mortality comparison between New Zealand and England. Br Med J 1986; 293:1342–1345.

66. Grainger J, Woodman K, Pearce N, et al. Prescribed fenoterol and death from asthma in New Zealand, 1981–7: a further case control study. Thorax 1991; 46:105–111.

67. Pearce N, Crane J, Burgess C, Jackson R, Beasley R. Beta agonists and asthma mortality: deja vu. Clin Exp Allergy 1991; 21:401–410.

68. Lanes SF, Birmann B, Raiford D, Walker AM. International trends in sales of inhaled fenoterol, all inhaled beta-agonists, and asthma mortality, 1970–1992. J Clin Epidemiol 1997; 50(3):321–328.

69. Anto J, Sunyer J, Reed C, et al. Preventing asthma epidemics due to soybeans by dust-control measures. N Engl J Med 1993; 329:1760–1763.

70. Newson R, Strachan D, Archibald E, Emberlin J, Hardaker P, Collier C. Effect of thunderstorms and airborne grass pollen on the incidence of acute asthma in England, 1990–94. Thorax 1997; 52:680–685.

71. Girgis S, Marks G, Downs S, Kolbe A, Car N, Paton R. Thunderstorm-associated asthma in an inland town in south eastern Australia. Who is at risk? Eur Respir J 2000; 16:3–8.

72. Marks G, Colquhoun J, Girgis S, et al. Thunderstorm outflows preceding epidemics of asthma during spring and summer. Thorax 2001; 56:468–471.

73. Tarlo S, Wong L, Roos J, Booth N. Occupational asthma caused by latex in a surgical glove manufacturing plant. J Allergy Clin Immunol 1990; 85: 626–631.

74. Johansson SGO, Hourihane JOB, Bousquet J, et al. A revised nomenclature for allergy: an EAACI position statement from the EAACI nomenclature task force. Allergy 2001; 56(9):813–824.

75. Humbert M, Durham SR, Ying S, et al. IL-4 and IL-5 mRNA and protein in bronchial biopsies from patients with atopic and nonatopic asthma: evidence against "intrinsic" asthma being a distinct immunopathologic entity. Am J Respir Crit Care Med 1996; 154(5):1497–1504.

76. National Asthma Education and Prevention Program. Expert Panel Report 2: Guidelines for the Diagnosis and Management of Asthma. Bethesda, MD: National Institutes of Health. National Heart, Lung, and Blood Institute; 1997.

77. Asthma Management Handbook 2002. National Asthma Council Australia Ltd, 2002. (Accessed 14th July 2003, at http://www.National Asthma. org.au/publications/amh/amhcont.htm.).

78. Johnston S, Pattemore P, Sanderson G, et al. Community study of the role of viral infections in exacerbations of asthma in 9–11 year old children. Br Med J 1995; 310:1225–1228.

79. Boulet LP, Cartier A, Thomson NC, Roberts RS, Dolovich J, Hargreave FE. Asthma and increases in nonallergic bronchial responsiveness from seasonal pollen exposure. J Allergy Clin Immunol 1983; 71(4):399–406.

80. Phelan P, Robertson C, Olinsky A. The Melbourne Asthma Study: 1964–1999. J Allergy Clin Immunol 2002; 109(2):189–194.

81. Martinez F, Stern D, Wright A, Taussig L, Halonen M. Differential immune responses to acute lower respiratory illness in early life and subsequent development of persistent wheezing and asthma. J Allergy Clin Immunol 1998; 102:915–920.

82. Reddel H, Jenkins C, Marks G, et al. Optimal asthma control, starting with high doses of inhaled budesonide. Eur Respir J 2000; 16:226–235.

83. Anto J, Sunyer J, Rodriguez-Roisin R, Suarez-Cevera M, Vazquez L. Community outbreaks of asthma associated with inhalation of soybean dust. New Engl J Med 1989; 320:1097–1102.

84. Leung R, Ho P. Asthma, allergy, and atopy in three south-east Asian populations. Thorax 1994; 49:1205–1210.

85. von Mutius E, Martinez F, Fritzsch C, Nicolai T, Roell G, Thiemann HH. Prevalence of asthma and atopy in two areas of West and East Germany. Am J Respir Crit Care Med 1994; 149:358–364.

86. Peat JK, van den Berg RH, Green WF, Mellis CM, Leeder SR, Woolcock AJ. Changing prevalence of asthma in Australian children. Br Med J 1994; 308(6944):1591–1596.

87. Gissler M, Jarvelin MR, Louhiala P, Hemminki E. Boys have more health problems in childhood than girls: follow up of the 1987 Finnish birth cohort. Acta Paediatrica 1999; 88:310–314.

88. Anderson HR, Pottier AC, Strachan DP. Asthma from birth to age 23: incidence and relation to prior and concurrent atopic disease. Thorax 1992; 47:537–542.

89. Gilliland FD, Berhane K, Islam T, et al. Obesity and the risk of newly diagnosed asthma in school-age children. Am J Epidemiol 2003; 158(5):406–415.
90. Shima M, Nitta Y, Ando M, Adachi M. Effects of air pollution on the prevalence and incidence of asthma in children. Arch Environ Health 2002; 57(6):529–535.
91. Fuortes LJ, Weih L, Pomrehn P, et al. Prospective epidemiologic evaluation of laboratory animal allergy among university employees. Am J Ind Med 1997; 32(6):665–669.
92. Archambault S, Malo JL, Infante-Rivard C, Ghezzo H, Gautrin D. Incidence of sensitization, symptoms, and probably occupational rhinoconjunctivitis and asthma in apprentices starting exposure to latex. J Allergy Clin Immunol 2001; 107:921–923.
93. Ferris BG. Epidemiology Standardization Project (American Thoracic Society). Am Rev Respir Dis 1978; 118(6 Pt 2):1–120.
94. Burney P, Chinn S. Developing a new questionnaire for measuring the prevalence and distribution of asthma. Chest 1987; 91:79s–83s.
95. Burney PG, Laitinen LA, Perdrizet S, et al. Validity and repeatability of the IUATLD (1984) Bronchial Symptoms Questionnaire: an international comparison. Eur Respir J 1989; 2(10):940–945.
96. Peat J, Salome CM, Wachinger S, Toelle B, Bauman A, Woolcock A. Reliability of a respiratory history questionnaire and the effect of mode of administration on classification of asthma in children. Chest 1992; 102:153–157.
97. Burney P, Luczynska C, Chinn S, Jarvis D, for the European Community Respiratory Health Survey. The European Community Respiratory Health Survey. Eur Respir J 1994; 7:954–960.
98. Asher M, Keil U, Anderson H. International study of asthma and allergies in childhood (ISAAC): rationale and methods. Eur Respir J 1995; 8:483–491.
99. Asher M, Pattemore P, Harrison A, et al. International comparison of the prevalence of asthma symptoms and bronchial hyperresponsiveness. Am Rev Respir Dis 1988; 138:524–529.
100. Redline S, Larkin EK, Kercsmar C, Berger M, Siminoff LA. Development and validation of school-based asthma and allergy screening instruments for parents and students. Ann Allergy Asthma Immunol 2003; 90(5):516–528.
101. Wolf RL, Berry CA, Quinn K. Development and validation of a brief pediatric screen for asthma and allergies among children.(see comment). Ann Allergy Asthma Immunol 2003; 90(5):500–507.
102. Kilpelainen M, Terho EO, Helenius H, Koskenvuo M. Validation of a new questionnaire on asthma, allergic rhinitis, and conjunctivitis in young adults. Allergy 2001; 56(5):377–384.
103. Brunekreef B, Groot B, Rijcken B, Hoek G, Steenbekkers A, de Boer A. Reproducibility of childhood respiratory symptom questions. Eur Respir J 1992; 5(8):930–935.
104. Fuso L, de Rosa M, Corbo GM, et al. Repeatability of the ISAAC video questionnaire and its accuracy against a clinical diagnosis of asthma. Respir Med 2000; 94(4):397–403.
105. Pizzichini MM, Rennie D, Senthilselvan A, Taylor B, Habbick BF, Sears MR. Limited agreement between written and video asthma symptom questionnaires. Pediatr Pulmonol 2000; 30(4):307–312.

106. Gibson PG, Henry R, Shah S, et al. Validation of the ISAAC video questionnaire (AVQ3.0) in adolescents from a mixed ethnic background. Clin Exp Allergy 2000; 30(8):1181–1187.

107. Pearce N, Weiland S, Keil U, et al. Self-reported prevalence of asthma symptoms in children in Australia, England, Germany and New Zealand: an international comparison using the ISAAC protocol. Eur Respir J 1993; 6: 1455–1461.

108. Pekkanen J, Remes ST, Husman T, et al. Prevalence of asthma symptoms in video and written questionnaires among children in four regions of Finland. Eur Respir J 1997; 10(8):1787–1794.

109. Leung R, Wong G, Lau J, et al. Prevalence of asthma and allergy in Hong Kong schoolchildren: an ISAAC study. Eur Respir J 1997; 10:354–360.

110. Venables KM, Farrer N, Sharp L, Graneek BJ, Newman Taylor AJ. Respiratory symptoms questionnaire for asthma epidemiology: validity and reproducibility. Thorax 1993; 48(3):214–219.

111. Dales R, Ernst P, Hanley J, Battista R, Becklake M. Prediction of airway reactivity from responses to a standardized respiratory symptom questionnaire. Am Rev Respir Dis 1987; 135:817–821.

112. Lai CK, Chan JK, Chan A, et al. Comparison of the ISAAC video questionnaire (AVQ3.0) with the ISAAC written questionnaire for estimating asthma associated with bronchial hyperreactivity. Clin Exp Allergy 1997; 27(5): 540–545.

113. dc Marco R, Cerveri I, Bugiani M, Ferrari M, Verlato G. An undetected burden of asthma in Italy: the relationship between clinical and epidemiological diagnosis of asthma. Eur Respir J 1998; 11(3):599–605.

114. Toren K, Brisman J, Jarvholm B. Asthma and asthma-like symptoms in adults assessed by questionnaires. A literature review. Chest 1993; 104(2):600–608.

115. Glasgow N, Ponsonby AL, Yates R, McDonald T, Attewell R. Asthma screening as part of a routine school health assessment in the Australian Capital Territory. Med J Aust 2001; 174:384–388.

116. Jenkins MA, Clarke JR, Carlin JB, et al. Validation of questionnaire and bronchial hyperresponsiveness against respiratory physician assessment in the diagnosis of asthma. Int J Epidemiol 1996; 25(3):609–616.

117. Grassi M, Rezzani C, Biino G, Marinoni A. Asthma-like symptoms assessment through ECR11S screening questionnaire scoring. J Clin Epidemiol 2003; 56(3):238–247.

118. Hall CB, Wakefield D, Rowe TM, Carlisle PS, Cloutier MM. Diagnosing pediatric asthma: validating the Easy Breathing Survey. J Pediatr 2001; 139(2):267–272.

119. Remes S, Pekkanen J, Remes K, Salonen R, Korppi M. In search of childhood asthma: questionnaire, tests of bronchial hyperresponsiveness, and clinical evaluation. Thorax 2002; 57:120–126.

120. Kaur B, Anderson H, Austin J, et al. Prevalence of asthma symptoms, diagnosis, and treatment in 12–14 year old children across Great Britain (international study of asthma and allergies in childhood, ISAAC UK). Br Med J 1998; 316:118–124.

121. Grant EN, Daugherty SR, Moy JN, Nelson SG, Piorkowski JM, Weiss KB. Prevalence and burden of illness for asthma and related symptoms among kindergartners in Chicago public schools. Ann Allergy Asthma Immunol 1999; 83(2):113–120.

122. Gerald LB., Redden D, Turner-Henson A, et al. A multi-stage asthma screening procedure for elementary school children. J Asthma 2002; 39(1):29–36.

123. Ryu JH, Scanlon PD. Obstructive lung diseases: COPD, asthma, and many imitators. Mayo Clin Proc 2001; 76(11):1144–1153.

124. Sears MR, Jones DT, Holdaway MD, et al. Prevalence of bronchial reactivity to inhaled methacholine in New Zealand children. Thorax 1986; 41(4): 283–289.

125. Rijcken B, Schouten J, Weiss S, Speizer F, van der Lende R. The relationship of nonspecific bronchial responsiveness to respiratory symptoms in a random population sample. Am Rev Respir Dis 1987; 136:62–68.

126. Peat J, Britton W, Salome C, Woolcock A. Bronchial hyperresponsiveness in two populations of Australian schoolchildren. III. Effect of exposure to environmental allergens. Clin Allergy 1987; 17:291–300.

127. Woolcock A, Peat J, Salome C, et al. Prevalence of bronchial hyperresponsiveness and asthma in a rural adult population. Thorax 1987; 42:361–368.

128. Burney P, Chinn S, Britton J, Tattersfield A, Papacosta A. What symptoms predict the bronchial response to histamine? Evaluation in a community survey of the bronchial symptoms questionnaire (1984) of the International Union against Tuberculosis and Lung Disease. Int J Epidemiol 1989; 18: 165–173.

129. Toelle BG, Peat JK, Salome CM, Mellis CM, Woolcock AJ. Toward a definition of asthma for epidemiology. Am Rev Respir Dis 1992; 146:633–637.

130. Toelle B, Peat J, van den Berg R, Dermand J, Woolcock A. Comparison of three definitions of asthma: a longitudinal perspective. J Asthma 1997; 34:161–167.

131. Toelle BG, Xuan W, Peat JK, Marks GB. Childhood factors that predict asthma in young adulthood. Eur Respir J 2004; 23(1):66–70.

132. Shaw RA, Crane J, Pearce N, et al. Comparison of a video questionnaire with the 1UATLD written questionnaire for measuring asthma prevalence. Clin Exp Allergy 1992; 22(5):561–568.

133. Pattemore PK, Asher MI, Harrison AC, Mitchell EA, Rea HH, Stewart AW. The interrelationship among bronchial hyperresponsiveness, the diagnosis of asthma, and asthma symptoms. [sec comment]. Am Rev Respir Dis 1990; 142(3):549–554.

134. Enarson D, Vedal S, Schulzer M, Dybuncio A, Chan-Yeung M. Asthma, asthma-like symptoms, chronic bronchitis, and the degree of bronchial hyperresponsiveness in epidemiologic surveys. Am Rev Respir Dis 1987; 136:613–617.

135. Salome C, Peat J, Britton W, Woolcock A. Bronchial hyperresponsiveness in two populations of Australian schoolchildren. I. Relation to respiratory symptoms and diagnosed asthma. Clin Allergy 1987; 17:271–281.

136. Peat J, Toelle B, Gray E, et al. Prevalence and severity of childhood asthma and allergic sensitisation in seven climatic regions of New South Wales. Med J Aust 1995; 163:22–26.

137. Higgins B, Britton J, Chinn S, et al. The distribution of peak expiratory flow variability in a population sample. Am Rev Respir Dis 1989; 140:1368–1372.

138. Brand P, Duiverman E, Postma D, et al. Peak flow variation in childhood asthma: relationship to symptoms, atopy, airways obstruction and hyperresponsiveness. Eur Respir J 1997; 10:1242–1247.

139. Salome C, Roberts A, Brown N, Dermand J, Marks G, Woolcock A. Exhaled nitric oxide measurements in a population sample of young adults. Am J Resp Crit Care Med 1999; 159:911–916.

140. Mannino D, Homa D, Akinbami L, Moorman J, Gwynn C, Redd S. Surveillance for Asthma—United States, 1980–1999. In: CDC Surveillance Summaries: MMWR; 2002:1–13.

141. Beasley R, Pearce N, Crane J. International trends in asthma mortality. Ciba Foundation Symposium 1997; 206:140–150.

142. Rea H, Scragg R, Jackson R, Beaglehole R, Fenwick J, Sutherland D. A case-control study of deaths from asthma. Thorax 1986; 41:833–839.

143. Beasley R, Pearce N, Crane J, Burgess C. Beta-agonists: what is the evidence that their use increases the risk of asthma morbidity and mortality? J Allergy Clin Immunol 1999; 104(2 Pt 2):S18–S30

144. Stolley P, Schinnar R. Association between asthma mortality and isoproterenol aerosols: a review. Prev Med 1978; 7:519–538.

145. Jalaludin B, Smith M, Chey T, Orr N, Smith W, Leeder S. Risk factors for asthma deaths: a population-based, case-control study. Aust NZ J Public Health 1999; 23(6):595–600.

146. Smyth E, Wright S, Evans A, Sinnamon D, MacMahon J. Death from airways obstruction: accuracy of certification in Northern Ireland. Thorax 1996; 51:293–297.

147. Hunt L, Silverstein M, Reed C, O'Connell E, O'Fallon W, Yunginger J. Accuracy of the death certificate in a population-based study of asthmatic patients. JAMA 1993; 269:1947–1952.

148. Guite H, Burney P. Accuracy of recording of deaths from asthma in the UK: the false negative rate. Thorax 1996; 51:924–928.

149. Sidenius K, Munich E, Madsen F, Lange P, Viskum K, Soes-Petersen U. Accuracy of recorded asthma deaths in Denmark in a 12 months period in 1994–1995. Respir Med 2000; 94(4):373–377.

150. Jones K, Berrill W, Bromly C, Heudrick D. A confidential enquiry into certified asthma deaths in the North of England, 1994–1996: influence of co-morbidity and diagnostic inaccuracy. Respir Med 1999; 93:923–927.

151. Sears M, Rea H, de Boer G, et al. Accuracy of certification of deaths due to asthma. A national study. Am J Epidemiol 1986; 124:1004–1011.

152. Jorgensen IM, Bulow S, Jensen VB, Dahm TL, Prahl P, Juel K. Asthma mortality in Danish children and young adults, 1973–1994: epidemiology and validity of death certificates. Eur Respir J 2000; 15:844–848.

153. Reid D, Hendrick V, Aitken T, Berrill W, Stenton S, Hendrick D. Age-dependent inaccuracy of asthma death certification in Northern England, 1991–1992. Eur Respir J 1998; 12:1079–1083.

154. Stewart C, Nunn A. Are asthma mortality rates changing? Chest 1985; 79: 229–234

155. Australian Bureau of Statistics. Causes of death: Australia 2001.Cat. no. 3303.0. Canberra: ABS; 2002.
156. Baker DF, Marks GB, Poulos LM, Williamson M. Review of proposed National Health Priority Area asthma indicators and data sources. Report. Canberra: Australian Institute of Health and Welfare; 2004. Report No.: ACM2.
157. Woolcock A. Worldwide trends in asthma morbidity and mortality. Explanation of trends. Bull Int Union Tuberc Lung Dis 1991; 66:85–89.
158. Australian Bureau of Statistics. The health and welfare of Australia's Aboriginal and Torres Strait Islander peoples. Cat. no. 4704.0. Canberra: ABS; 2001.
159. Castro M, Schechtman K, Halstead J, Bloomberg G. Risk factors for asthma morbidity and mortality in a large metropolitan city. J Asthma 2001; 38(8):625–635.
160. Grant E, Lyttle C, Weiss K. The relation of socio-economic factors and racial/ethnic differences in US asthma mortality. Am J Public Health 2000; 90(12):1923–1925.
161. Tong S, Drake P. Hospital admission and mortality differentials of asthma between urban and rural populations in New South Wales. Aust J Rural Health 1999; 7(1):18–22.
162. Kozak L. Under reporting of race in the National Hospital Discharge Survey. Adv Data 1995; 265:1–12.
163. Marks G, Bumey P. Diseases of the respiratory system. In: Charhon J, Murphy M, eds. The Health of Adult Britain 1841–1994. Vol. 2. London: The Stationary Office, 1997:93–113.
164. Weiss K. Seasonal trends in US asthma hospitalizations and mortality. JAMA 1990; 263:2323–2328.
165. Diette GB, Krishnan JA, Dominici F, et al. Asthma in older patients: factors associated with hospitalization. Arch Intern Med 2002; 162(10):1123–1132.
166. Christakis D, Mell D, Koepsell T, Zimmerman F, Connell F. Association of lower continuity of care with greater risk of emergency department use and hospitalization in children. Pediatrics 2001; 103:524–529.
167. Boston Consulting Group. Report, on the cost of asthma in Australia. Victoria: National Asthma Campaign; 1992.
168. Phelan P, Bishop J, Baxter K, Duckett S. Hospitalisation of children under 15 years in Victoria. Aust Health Rev 1993; 16(2):148–159.
169. Ashton C, Del Junco D, Souchek J, Wray N, Mansyur C. The association between the quality of inpatient care and early readmission: a meta-analysis of the evidence. Med Care 1997; 35(10):1044–1059.
170. Russo M, McConnochie K, McBride J, Szilagyi P, Brooks A, Roghmann K. Increase in admission threshold explains stable asthma hospitalization rates. Pediatrics 1999; 104(3 Pt 1):454–462.
171. Abramson M, Matheson M, Wharton C, Sim M, Walters EH. Prevalence of respiratory symptoms related to chronic obstructive pulmonary disease and asthma among middle aged and older adults. Respirology 2002; 7(4):325–331.
172. Adams RJ, Smith BJ, Ruffin RE. Patient preferences for autonomy in decision making in asthma management. Thorax 2001; 56(2):126–132.

173. Blais L, Ernst P, Boivin J, Suissa S. Inhaled corticosteroids and the prevention of readmission to hospital for asthma. Am J Respir Crit Care Med 1998; 158:126–132.

174. Madge P, McColl J, Paton J. Impact of a nurse-led home management training programme in children admitted to hospital with acute asthma: a randomized controlled study. Thorax 1997; 52:223–228.

175. Mayo P, Richam J, Harris H. Results of a program to reduce admissions for adult asthma. Ann Intern Med 1990; 112:864–871.

176. Slack R, CE B. Readmission rates are associated with differences in the process of care in acute asthma. Quality in Health Care 1997; 6(4):194–198.

177. Sibbritt DW. Validation of a 28 day interval between discharge and readmission for emergency readmission rates. J Qual Clin Pract 1995; 15:211–220.

178. Brameld KJ, Holman CD. Estimation of excess risk of readmission to hospital after an index inpatient separation. Med Care 2003; 41(5):693–697.

179. Kendrick SW, Douglas MM, Gardner D, Hucker D. Best-link matching of Scottish health data sets. Methods Inf Med 1998; 37(1):64–68.

180. Australian Institute of Health and Welfare. Australian hospital statistics 2000–2001. AIHW cat. no. HSE 20. Canberra: AIHW; 2002.

181. Vollmer WM, Osborne ML, Buist AS, Uses and limitations of mortality and health care utilization statistics in asthma research. Am J Respir Crit Care Med 1994; 149(2 Pt 2):S79–S87; discussion S8–S90.

182. Osborne M, Vollmer W, Buist A. Diagnostic accuracy of asthma within a health maintenance organization. J Clin Epidemiol 1992; 45:403–411.

183. Gergen P, Mitchell H, Lynn H. Understanding the seasonal pattern of childhood asthma: results from the national cooperative innter-city asthma study (NCICAS). J Pediatr 2002; 141:631–636.

184. Fleming D, Cross K, Sunderland R, Ross M. Comparison of the seasonal patterns of asthma identified in general practitioner episodes, hospital admissions and deaths. Thorax 2000; 55:662–665.

185. Harju T, Tuuponen T, Keistinen T, Kivela S. Seasonal variations in hospital treatment periods and deaths among adult asthmatics. Eur Respir J 1998; 12:1362–1365.

186. van Rensen E, Straathof K, Veselic-Charvat M, Zwinderman A, Bel E, Sterk P. Effect of inhaled steroids on airway hyperresponsiveness, sputum eosinophils, and exhaled nitric oxide levels in patients with asthma. Thorax 1999; 54:403–408.

187. Waalkens H, Gerritsen J, Krouwels F, van Aalderen W, Knol K. Budesonide and terbutaline or terbutaline alone in children with mild asthma: effects on bronchial hyperresponsiveness and diurnal variation in peak flow. Thorax 1991; 46:499–503.

188. Ward C, Pais M, Bish R, et al. Airway inflammation, basement membrane thickening and bronchial hyperresponsiveness in asthma. Thorax 2002; 57(4):309–316.

189. Ind PW, Dal Negro R, Colman NC, Fletcher CP, Browning D, James MH. Addition of salmeterol to fluticasone propionate treatment in moderate-to-severe asthma. Respir Med 2003; 97(5):555–562.

190. Lalloo UG, Malolepszy J, Kozma D, et al. Budesonide and formoterol in a single inhaler improves asthma control compared with increasing the dose of corticosteroid in adults with mild-to-moderate asthma. Chest 2003; 123(5):1480–1487.

191. Malmstrom K, Rodriguez-Gomez G, Guerra J, et al. Oral montelukast, inhaled beclomethasone, and placebo for chronic asthma. A randomized, controlled trial. Montelukast/Beclomethasone Study Group. Ann Intern Med 1999; 130:487–495.

192. Ducharme FM. Anti-leukotrienes as add-on therapy to inhaled glucocorticoids in patients with asthma: systematic review of current evidence. Br Med J 2002; 324(7353):1545–1551.

193. Anis AH, Lynd LD, Wang XH, et al. Double trouble: impact of inappropriate use of asthma medication on the use of health care resources. CMAJ Can Med Assoc J 2001; 164(5):625–631.

194. Nestor A, Calhoun AC, Dickson M, Kalik CA. Cross-sectional analysis of the relationship between national guideline recommended asthma drug therapy and emergency/hospital use within a managed care population. Ann Allergy Asthma Immunol 1998; 81(4):327–330.

195. Gerdtham UG, Hertzman P, Jonsson B, Boman G. Impact of inhaled corticosteroids on acute asthma hospitalization in Sweden 1978 to 1991. Med Care 1996; 34(12):1188–1198.

196. Kuo A, Craig TJ. A retrospective study of risk factors for repeated admissions for asthma in a rural/suburban university hospital. Journal of the American Osteopathic Association 2001; 101(5 Suppl):S14–S17; quiz S517–8.

197. Suissa S, Ernst P, Kezouh A. Regular use of inhaled corticosteroids and the long term prevention of hospitalisation for asthma. Thorax 2002; 57(10): 880–884.

198. Lynd LD, Guh DP, Pare PD, Anis AH. Patterns of inhaled asthma medication use: a 3-year longitudinal analysis of prescription claims data from British Columbia, Canada. Chest 2002; 122(6):1973–1981.

199. Poluzzi E, Resi D, Zuccheri P, et al. Use of anti-asthmatic drugs in Italy: analysis of prescriptions in general practice in the light of guidelines for asthma treatment. Eur J Clin Pharmacol 2002; 5S(l):55–59.

200. Finkelstein JA, Lozano P, Farber HJ, Miroshnik I, Lieu TA. Underuse of controller medications among Medicaid-insured children with asthma. Arch Pediatr Adolesc Med 2002; 156(6):562–567.

201. Gaist D, Hallas J, Hansen NC, Gram LF. Are young adults with asthma treated sufficiently with inhaled steroids? A population-based study of prescription data from 1991 and 1994. Br J Clin Pharmacol 1996; 41(4):285–289.

202. Drake AJ, Howells RJ, Shield JP, Prendiville A, Ward PS, Crowne EC. Symptomatic adrenal insufficiency presenting with hypoglycaemia in children with asthma receiving high dose inhaled fluticasone propionate. Br Med J 2002; 324(7345):1081–1082.

203. Todd GR, Acerini CL, Ross-Russell R, Zahra S, Warner JT, McCance D. Survey of adrenal crisis associated with inhaled corticosteroids in the United Kingdom. Archives of Disease in Childhood 2002; 87(6):457–461.

204. Shelley M, Croft P, Chapman S, Pantin C. Is the ratio of inhaled corticosteroid to bronchodilator a good indicator of the quality of asthma prescribing? Cross sectional study linking prescribing data to data on admissions. Br Med J 1996; 313:1124–1126.
205. Jacobson GA, Peterson GM. Prescribing trends for anti-asthma drugs in Tasmania following the National Asthma Campaign. J Clin Pharm Ther 1996; 21(5):317–324.
206. McNiece R, Majeed A. Socioeconomic differences in general practice consultation rates in patients aged 65 and over: prospective cohort study. Br Med J 1999; 319(7201):26–28.
207. Saxena S, Majeed A, Jones M. Socioeconomic differences in childhood consultation rates in general practice in England and Wales: prospective cohort study. Br Med J 1999; 318:642–646.
208. Charles J, Valenti L, Britt H. GP visits by healthcare card holders. A secondary analysis of data from Bettering the Evaluation and Care of Health (BEACH), a national study of general practice activity in Australia. Aust Fam Physician 2003; 32(1–2):85–88, 94.
209. Gibson PG, Coughlan J, Wilson AJ, et al. Self-management education and regular practitioner review for adults with asthma (Cochrane Review). In: The Cochrane Libraiy, Issue 2 2002; Oxford: Update Software.
210. Fleming DM, Cross KW, Sunderland R, Ross AM. Comparison of the seasonal patterns of asthma identified in general practitioner episodes, hospital admissions, and deaths. Thorax 2000; 55(8):662–665.
211. Laurence C, Beilby J, Marley J, Newbury J, Wilkinson D, Symon B. Establishing a practice based primary care research network. The University Family Practice Network in South Australia. Aust Fam Physician 2001; 30(5): 508–512.
212. Hansell A, Hollowed J, McNiece R, Nichols T, Strachan D. Validity and interpretation of mortality, health service and survey data on COPD and asthma in England. Eur Respir J 2003; 21(2):279–286.
213. Britt H, Miller G, Knox S, Charles J, Valenti L, Henderson Jea. General Practice Activity in Australia 2001–02. Canberra: Australian Institute of Health and Welfare, 2002.
214. Stafford RS, Ma J, Finkelstein SN, Haver K, Cockburn I. National trends in asthma visits and asthma pharmacotherapy, 1978–2002. J Allergy Clin Immunol 2003; 111(4):729–735.
215. Pearson M, Goldacre M, Coles J, et al. Health Outcome Indicators: Asthma. Report of a working group to the Department of Health. Oxford: National Centre for Health Outcomes Development; 1999.
216. Marks G, Dunn S, Woolcock A. An evaluation of an asthma quality of life questionnaire as a measure of change in adults with asthma. J Clin Epidemiol 1993; 46:1103–1111.
217. Juniper E, Wisniewski M, Cox F, Emmett A, Nielsen K, O'Byrne P. Relationship between quality of life and clinical status in asthma: a factor analysis. Eur Respir J 2004; 23:287–291.
218. Guyatt G, Feeny D, Patrick D. Measuring health-related quality of life. Ann Intern Med 1993; 118:622–629.

219. Kirshner B, Guyatt G. A methodological framework for assessing health indices. J Chron Dis 1985; 38(1):27–36.
220. Bousquet J, Knani J, Dhivert H, et al. Quality of life in asthma: I. Internal consistency and validity of the SF-36 questionnaire. Am J Respir Crit Care Med 1994; 149:371–375.
221. Bradley C. Importance of differentiating health status from quality of life. Lancet 2001; 357:7–8.
222. Centre for Disease Control (CDC). Measuring healthy days–population assessment of health related quality of life. Atlanta, USA: U.S. Department of Health and Human services; 2000 November 2000.
223. Testa M, Simonson D. Assessment of quality-of-life outcomes. N Engl J Med 1996; 334(13):835–840.
224. McHorney C, Ware J, Raczek A. The MOS 36-item short-form health survey (SF-36): II. Psychometric and clinical tests of validity in measuring physical and mental constructs. Med Care 1993; 31:247–263.
225. Revicki D, Leidy N, Brennan-Diemer F, Sorensen S, Togias A. Integrating patients preferences into health outcome assessments. The multi-attribute Asthma Symptom Utility Index. Chest 1998; 114:998–1007.
226. Mishra G, Schofield MJ. Norms for the physical and mental health component summary scores of the SF-36 for young, middle-aged and older Australian women. Qual Life Res 1998; 7(3):215–220.
227. Ware J, Gandek B. Overview of the SF-36 Health survey and the International Quality of Life Assessment (IQOLA) Project. J Clin Epidemiol 1998; 51(11): 903–912.
228. Australian Centre for Asthma Monitoring. Measuring the impact of asthma on quality of life in the Australian population. Canberra: Australian Institute of Health and Welfare, 2004. AIHW Cat No. ACM 3.
229. Marks GB et al. Use of "preventer" medications and written asthma management plans among adults with asthma in NSW. MJA 2000; 173:407–410.

17

Role of Pharmacists in Asthma Monitoring

C. L. ARMOUR, B. SAINI, S. BOSNIC-ANTICEVICH, and I. KRASS

Faculty of Pharmacy, University of Sydney,
Sydney, Australia

Pharmacists in the Health Care System

The management of a chronic disease such as asthma involves the patient regularly visiting and communicating with several health care professionals within the health care system. It is assumed that each one of these health care professionals will in some way contribute to the management of the patient's disease state. The involvement of all members of the health care team in disease management can then have a positive effect on patient outcomes (1,2). In fact, a co-operative and co-ordinated approach to health care has been considered an essential requirement for the delivery of health care since the 1990s (3,4) and research has shown that highly successful interventions in chronic disease management involve the active participation of a variety of health care professionals (5).

One such profession critical to the improvement of health care is the pharmacist (6,7). In a systematic review of the literature from the Cochrane Database, Bero and colleagues defined the extended role of the pharmacist as encompassing a wide range of services such as home visits, screening for various diseases, and a health advisory role for minor self-limiting conditions. However, the potential role of the pharmacist in disease management is not limited to the services described in the review. In order to appreciate the vital role of the pharmacist in the health care team and in asthma management, the skills, knowledge, and trends in provision of health care by the pharmacist need to be considered.

Pharmacists and Chronic Diseases

It is well recognized that pharmacists provide ease of access to patients and are in a pivotal position to check if patients are using their medication appropriately, for example, in the case of asthma; to identify overuse of reliever medications, underuse of preventative medications, or incorrect inhalation device technique. They are the last health care professional the patient sees prior to administering their prescription or non-prescription medication. Hence it is not surprising that traditionally the role of the pharmacist primarily focused on the provision of counseling and education associated with use of medication. This is a critical role as appropriate use of prescription medication is critical to disease care (8).

Thus, the role of the pharmacist in appropriate medication use remains. However, over the years the role of the pharmacist has changed. The service that pharmacists are able to provide to patients has expanded beyond the distribution of and counseling about medications to the provision of clinical services and pharmaceutical care (9–14). This has resulted in a change in the way in which the profession of pharmacy sees its role in health care and within the health care team. The role of the pharmacist has expanded so that it does not only focus on medication use alone but rather on patient welfare (14) and overall disease management (15–17). In essence, this has meant that pharmacists have been able to build on their traditional role in order to provide a primary health care role.

Many studies have been conducted in the traditional areas of delivery of drug information, provision of counseling and monitoring of drug side effects. They have described the role of the pharmacist and have shown that as a result of pharmacist involvement, there is an increase in the quality use of medicines and a decrease in costs associated with medication use (7,18–20). With regard to asthma management, it was recognized by the National Asthma Education and Prevention Program Expert Panel Report released in 1995 that pharmacists have a role in educating patients about asthma medications, instructing patients about the proper use of inhaler medications, monitoring medication use and refill intervals to help identify patients with poorly controlled asthma, encouraging patients who are purchasing over the counter inhalers to seek medical care, helping patients monitor their lung function, and helping patients use written asthma self-management plans (21).

An element of the broader role of the pharmacist still associated with medication use is the medication review process, otherwise known as the performing of medication reviews, home medicines reviews, or domiciliary medication reviews. In fact, the process of medication review which involves the identification of drug/dosage discrepancies, such as drug dose above or below the recommended dose, incorrect dosage schedule for the drug, incorrect strength for the drug, missing information/no directions etc. as well as the identification of potential therapeutic problems such as drug–drug interactions, duplication of therapy, underutilization of drugs, contraindications to drug use, etc.(22) can be seen as a pharmacy service in itself. It has been shown that the impact of pharmacists performing medication reviews is positive both in terms of patient health outcomes and health care professional collaboration (23–25).

Current Issues with Asthma Management: Where Can the Pharmacist Help?

In Australia, asthma is one of the top 15 conditions contributing to the burden of disease and injury in the community as a whole (26). Various audits and surveys of asthma practices in Australia have documented that asthma is being sub-optimally managed (27), and have highlighted the issues which still remain for the care of people with asthma. This sub-optimal treatment is, in fact, a trend which is not only seen in Australia but all over the world (28). The issues associated with asthma management have been documented globally and highlight the need for asthma management interventions from all members of the health care professions. Broadly, the issues associated with sub-optimal asthma management practices fall into the following categories:

1. Patient-related issues.
2. Health professional-related issues.
3. Public health-related issues.

Patient-Related Issues

One major problem associated with the person with asthma is inappropriate medication use. Inappropriate use of medications can lead to sub-optimal control, morbidity (29), a higher risk for fatal and near fatal attacks, and result in significantly higher utilization of health care resources (29,30). Studies have demonstrated that inappropriate use of medications can be as high as 75% in adults (31) and 80% in children (29). The reasons for inappropriate medication taking by people with asthma has been related to a variety of different factors, including underuse of appropriate medication

(31,32), fear of side effects (33), patient dissatisfaction with asthma treatment (34), and poor adherence with medication regimens (31).

Another issue associated with the person with asthma and asthma management is their lack of adherence to self-management practices. It has been shown that asthma self-management, which should optimally be coupled with a written self-management plan and regular review, (35) can reduce asthma-related hospitalizations (36). Ideally with self-management comes responsibility for care of the disease and the need to be informed about optimal management for the disease. Lack of self-management by the person with asthma has been linked to preventable asthma deaths. In an investigational study of pediatric asthma deaths in Victoria, Australia, it was shown that the majority of the patients under 20 who had died could not be labeled as "high risk" patients, and that in 39% of cases the deaths were associated with preventable factors such as poor patient compliance with medications (in 53% of cases) and delay in seeking medical help (in 47% of cases) (37). Some studies have also investigated the lack of self-management by the person with asthma and have identified that many people with asthma
are either reticent to self-manage their asthma or may not have been given appropriate directions to do so (31). These studies highlight the need for all health care professionals to focus on asthma self-management for the person with asthma.

Health Professional-Related Issues

Whilst patient-related behavior may be a very important predictor of asthma outcomes, asthma management practices of health professionals must be considered if asthma management is to be optimized.

Data collected over five years indicate that although there is no difference in the rate of presentation of asthma, there has been a decrease in the number of people with asthma who undergo regular review with their general practitioner (38). This obviously identifies a significant problem in optimal asthma management as recommended in the national guidelines (39).

Further, studies have shown that there appears to be a mismatch between the perceptions of health care professionals and actual patient behavior. In a study designed to describe asthma management and morbidity in patients attending general practitioners in Australia, it was found that, over one-third of the patients had at least moderate asthma, two-thirds of the patients used reliever medication, about one-half used inhaled corticosteroids, 65% reported themselves to be mostly compliant, and 16% monitored their lung function with a peak flow meter. When the general practitioners were questioned on these issues, there was an obvious mismatch between GP and patient report on medication usage, with GPs overestimating preventative and reliever medication usage in their patients, as well as action plan (written self-management plan) usage (29). This mismatch is a non-obvious barrier to optimal asthma management.

In many cases, however, health care professionals may recognize that there are barriers to optimal asthma management and lack of time, lack of knowledge, and patient attitudes have commonly been reported as major barriers to improving asthma care.

Despite the barriers identified by health care professionals, studies investigating asthma management practices in Finland have suggested that health care professionals need to enhance their educational activities and collaboration in training people with asthma to self-monitor and to self-manage their asthma with medications (40). This could be through education and the use of written self-management plans.

Australian data indicate that although 52% of patients reported having a verbal action plan, only 9% of people with asthma and 11% of school children with asthma reported having a written asthma self-management plan (28,31). In Western Europe, although the reported written self-management plan ownership has been reported to be higher (61% in school children and 50% in adults with asthma), a suboptimal level of written self-management plan ownership is also evident (28).

Further, a lack of regular review by the health care professional may be a major contributor to sub-optimal asthma management practices. In Australia, it has been shown that asthma reviews are not as regular as they should be (38).

Public Health-Related Issues

In Australia, attempts have been made to co-ordinate public health and research directives, however, there may still be gaps between the person with asthma and the health professional expectations and health care service delivery. Poor communication between physicians, people with asthma, and other health care professionals (41) can widen this gap. There is a specific need for health care professionals to take on a more active collaborative role with regards to asthma management (42). A collaborative approach can result in enhanced exchange of information between health care professionals and this in turn can result in improvements in patient outcomes (43). In fact, the involvement of other health care professionals, who complement the physician in such areas as assessment, treatment management, seif-management, and follow-up, has been shown to improve adherence to management guidelines and patient satisfaction (5). The pharmacist is ideally placed to take on this challenge and there is evidence that this has been successful.

Current Trends in Pharmacy Management of Asthma

Pharmaceutical care is the determination of the drug needs for a given individual and a provision not only of the drugs required, but also the necessary services, before, during, and after treatment, to assure optimal, safe, and effective therapy. It includes a feedback mechanism as a means of facilitating continuity of care by those who provide it (44). It should involve the responsible provision of drug therapy for the purpose of achieving definite outcomes that improve a patient's quality of life (14).

Many large scale projects that involve pharmacists in the provision of pharmaceutical care have been instituted in the United States. Examples are the Institute of Pharmaceutical Care; the University of Minnesota that initiated Minnesota Pharmaceutical Care Project (45); and the Therapeutic Outcome Monitoring project initiated by the University of Florida (46). Individual pharmacists have also switched to the provision of pharmaceutical care in response to state-based health care reforms (47).

In most cases, provision of pharmaceutical care has led to improved patient outcomes, regardless of the disease modality targeted. Pharmacy interventions have been shown to increase the information given to patients about medications, promote more effective self-administration, and increase awareness about side effects (48). This is true for complex care situations, for example HIV clinics (49), cancer (50), congestive heart failure (51), and for routine chronic conditions like hypertension, dyslipidemia, asthma, anticoagulation, and peptic ulcers (52). Clinical, humanistic, and even economic outcomes have been shown to improve.

Pharmaceutical Care and Asthma

Many models of practice have been implemented to service patients with asthma and most of them have shown positive outcomes. Within pharmaceutical care, various models have been trialed, i.e., nationally driven (53,54), programs based on therapeutic outcome monitoring (55–57), programs based on patient empowerment (58), and programs based on a number of pharmaceutical elements (59,60). Some of the common features of all these programs include:

- Provision of continuity of care (61).
- Patient self-management and empowerment education (53).
- Clinic/appointment-based setting (62).
- Individualized patient education sessions (55–57).
- Physical collaboration (61–63).
- Long-term patient follow-up and monitoring (55–57,60,64).

A variety of positive outcomes have been demonstrated by pharmacy-based provision of specialized services for asthma including clinical benefits (58), for example, improved peak flow readings (57,60,64) and improved symptoms scores (55–57,65). Drug utilization has been shown to be optimized after specialist pharmacist interventions, for example, improved regimen profiles (53,55–57) and improved inhalation technique (66,67). Reduction in health care utilization has also been documented, i.e., decrease in number of hospitalizations (64), decreased loss in productivity (65). Decreases in emergency room and acute care visits also have been demonstrated (68). Humanistic outcomes also often change for the better after pharmacist provided asthma-related intervention and care provision (59,64,69,70). Improvement in self-efficacy and self-management skills has been shown in some programs (58,59), as has improvement in patient's asthma knowledge (53,55–57,59,65,69). Patients express satisfaction with care and have reported in some cases, to be willing to pay for asthma care services received by them from their pharmacists (60,71).

The design of various pharmacist asthma-related interventions has varied, and yet the results have been all positive in terms of clinical, humanistic, and economic outcomes (Table 1).

In some of these models, adherence to research protocols has not been adopted, and these programs have mostly been based on subjective evaluation or evaluation of process type indicators (61,63). In other cases, although a research protocol was adopted, the design selected was either a pre-test post-test design or a post-test design, which does not control for the possibility of a beneficial effect on patient's asthma-related outcomes resulting from sources other than the pharmacist intervention (57,58,71,72). In other cases, the intervention delivered was a very focused one and did not look at the overall management of asthma (78,79). In other cases, the pharmacist's interventions were based in the hospital setting, thus targeting only the severe population of asthma patients (65,68,77). In some cases, the outcomes measured concentrated on only a few aspects of better asthma control (75,79). Some of the pharmacy-based interventions were simply "one off" measures, such as conducting a "National Asthma Day," for example, the large nationally disseminated asthma programs carried out in Sweden (53,82). In most of the models, active collaboration between health care professionals was not sought.

Optimizing Pharmacy-based Interventions and Outcomes

Four studies have attempted to optimize their designed interventions for asthma. These are the TOM asthma project carried out in Denmark (55,56), and the pharmaceutical care programs carried out in Malta, U.S.A., and Germany (59,60,64). These four research projects were well designed;

Table 1 Review of Different Models of Pharmaceutical Care-Based Programs for Asthma

Model type	Research design	Place	Elements	Results	Reference
Asthma integrated management program—community pharmacy-based report of an ongoing program	Pre–Post-test design	Indiana, U.S.A.	Disease state management model (pediatric), patients referred from a HMO by contract, scheduled appointment with patients and carers, peak flow monitoring, patient education, patient follow up at 12 months after baseline	Improved quality of life, decreased hospital and acute care visits, contracted payment from the HMO for the asthma review for each patient	72
Community pharmacy based, patient focused interventions, 188 patients at three intervention pharmacies, 401 control patients	Parallel controlled group study	Virginia, U.S.A.	Patient education, follow-up, feedback and patient behavior modification interventions, patient follow-up for 16 months in a disease management model	Cost savings in the range of U.S. $144–293 per patient per month	73
Community pharmacy based and initiated by individual pharmacist	Not research driven	Indiana, U.S.A.	Pharmacy restructuring to have a waiting area, a health information center and a laboratory. Close collaboration with and referral from physicians, use of SOAP, electronic records, and contracts with MCOs, targets pediatric patients for asthma	Increased referrals from physicians, reimbursement in the range of $ 22.5–350 per patient	61

Community asthma management network program—community pharmacy-based 20 patients	Quasiexperimental, one group pre-test post-test design	Virginia, U.S.A.	Pharmacist training, patient empowerment through education, communication with other pharmacists and physicians, group education conducted by pharmacists, needs-based individual consultation, addressing problems and issues raised by patients, and patient follow-up at 6 months after intervention	Improved self-efficacy asthma knowledge and compliance with medications	58
Community pharmacy—12 community pharmacies, 11 general practices, and 103 patients	Post-test measures	Sussex, U.K.	Pharmacists were trained to identify patients for review, these pharmacists recruited patients, delivered and documented interventions and referred patients to the general practitioners, no follow-up	A large number of problems were addressed, 122 interventions were delivered across 58 patients	74
Community pharmacy—15 control, 16 intervention pharmacies, 500 patients, 236 control and 264 intervention patients	Experimental, parallel controlled design	Denmark	Controlled study. Pharmacist training, therapeutic outcome monitoring, MDI inhalation technique checking, patient education, peak flow monitoring and self-management principles, patient follow-up at 6 and 12 months after baseline	Study patient's asthma status improved more than control patients, as did days of sickness, quality of life and knowledge about asthma and inhaler techniques. There was a greater decrease in reliever usage, increase in symptom controller and preventer drug usage as compared to controls	55

(Continued)

Table 1 Review of Different Models of Pharmaceutical Care-Based Programs for Asthma (*Continued*)

Model type	Research design	Place	Elements	Results	Reference
Community pharmacy—5 community pharmacies, 110 patients	Two parallel group pre-test post-test design	South Africa	Peak flow and symptom monitoring, provision of individualized self-management plans, patient follow-up at 2 months after intervention	Adherence to self-management plans in the group who received peak flow monitoring counseling was achieved	75
Community pharmacy—48 pharmacies, 242 patients, 161 intervention and 81 control	Controlled intervention study	Germany	Pharmacist training to provide pharmaceutical care, inhalation technique correction, self-management, pharmacotherapy assessment, patient follow-up at 0,6, 12 months after baseline	Improvement of asthma severity, inhalation technique, quality of life and self-efficacy	59
Community pharmacy based, 172 patients with asthma recruited from 10 pharmacies	Post-test measures	Kentucky, U.S.A.	Asthma management initiated by community pharmacists, no patient follow-up in terms of clinical outcomes reported, the program consists of three monthly appointments with a trained pharmacist who conducted a needs assessment, provided information and interventions and helped set goals with patients	Satisfaction with and willingness to pay for pharmacist's time	71

Community pharmacy based, 11 intervention and 11 control pharmacies, 86 intervention and 66 control group patients	Prospective randomized controlled trial	Malta, Spain	Collaboration with specialists, pharmacist training, peak flow monitoring, patient education, patient follow-up at 0, 4, 8, 12 months after baseline	Positive impact on quality of life, inhaler technique and peak flows	64
Community pharmacies—consultations with patients, 4 community pharmacies, 28 intervention patients	Pre-test Post-test design	Finland	Pharmacist training, patient recruitment by physicians and pharmacists, therapeutic outcome monitoring method involving peak flow monitoring, self-management principles, a 1-year intervention with patient follow-up at baseline, and 4, 8, 12, and 24 months after baseline	Improved patient knowledge of and attitude towards asthma medications, improved asthma severity scores, improved regimens, patient satisfaction, resolution of patient problems	40,57,76
Community pharmacy-based pharmaceutical care program, 36 community drugstores, 1,113 patients with COPD and asthma	Randomized controlled trial	Indianapolis, U.S.A.	Provision of recent patient specific data, training, customized patient education materials, peak flow meters, monthly telephone interviews conducted by researchers, pharmacist delivered interventions and documented these at occasions when the patient came in for prescriptions, researchers completed follow-up interviews in person at baseline, 6 and 12 months and accessed documented data from pharmacists	At 12 months, patients in pharmaceutical care group had significantly higher peak flow rates when compared to usual care groups and patients receiving pharmaceutical care were more satisfied with their care.	60

(Continued)

Table 1 Review of Different Models of Pharmaceutical Care-Based Programs for Asthma (*Continued*)

Model type	Research design	Place	Elements	Results	Reference
Outpatient clinic-based care co-provided by pharmacist with a pulmonologist	Controlled group design	Ohio, U.S.A.	Comprehensive education program provided by pharmacists, patients followed 45 days after the education program was delivered	Increased likelihood of monitoring peak flows, increased satisfaction with care	65
Outpatient education delivered by hospital pharmacists, 29 patients	Pre-test– Post-test design	Hamamatsu, Japan	Pharmacist instruction to patients receiving inhaled corticosteroids,	Improvement in percentage of patients with correct device technique from 24% to 91%, increase in PEF values by 13%, compliance increased from 55% to 93%	77
Outpatient clinic setting—15 intervention subjects, 101 control patients	Controlled intervention study	Tokyo, Japan	Pharmaceutical care—optimization of therapy, patients followed up 24 months after baseline	ER visits and hospital admissions lower in the intervention group patients	68
Telepharmacy model, 15 intervention and 21 test patients	Experimental design	Arkansas, U.S.A.	Metered dose inhaler technique counseling via a telepharmacy model, targeting rural adolescents, patients followed up 2–4 weeks after the intervention	Improvement in counseling group in inhaler techniques	78
Electronic intervention model, 6 intervention patients	Pre-test– Post-test	Illinois, U.S.A.	Patient education, personalized pager messages, patients followed 30 days after the intervention	Increase in self-reported compliance	79

Program	Design	Location	Intervention	Outcomes	Ref
Emergency department based, co-pharmacist managed, physician directed program, 25 patients with asthma	Pre-test–Post-test measures	Florida, U.S.A.	Clinic-based small group education program, individualization of therapy, patients followed three times in a 12-month period	Reduction in the number of ER visits, total cost savings of U.S. $30,683 and $68,393	80
Education delivered by pharmacists to patients referred by the physician	Pre-test–Post-test design	France	Trained pharmacists delivered education to patients who were referred to them by physicians in the vicinity of the pharmacy, patients were followed up after 12 months	Fewer emergency consultations, increased use of preventative therapy, improved inhaler technique	81
Disease management-based care provided by chain of pharmacies–ProCare program, ongoing	Non research based	CVS Pharma-cies Inc., U.S.A.	Use of a clinical information management system linking physicians with pharmacists, analyzing prescribing patterns and drug utilization, automated dispensing allowing pharmacists to focus on the patient	Demonstrated cost effectiveness	63
National public health model, based in community pharmacies throughout Sweden, 900 pharmacies, 4.5 million patients	Post-test measures only	Sweden	Use of pharmacist and pharmacy staff education, distribution of free resources materials for pharmacists, conducting a "National Asthma Day"	Increased knowledge, awareness about medications	53
National public health model, based in community pharmacies throughout Canada, 4080 patients	Pre-test–Post-test	Canada	National Asthma Day, asthma control assessment, individualized education based on patient needs and telephone follow-up	Decreased frequency of day and nighttime symptoms, decreased use of reliever medication	82

consisting of a parallel control design in the case of the Danish and the German model (59), and a randomized controlled trial in the case of the American and Maltese model (64). In the case of the Danish model, clinical, humanistic, and economic evaluation of the project was carried out. In the case of the American, German, and the Maltese models, an economic evaluation was not conducted. All models used a variety of standard asthma outcome measures such as: asthma severity, use of reliever medications, frequency of symptoms, quality of life, asthma-related knowledge, medication device technique, self-reported adherence. Except for the American model, none of these models demonstrated remarkable differences in objective measures of lung function, nor was there any documentation of the provision of self-management guidelines such as written action plans, nor were interventions regarding lifestyle issues such as triggers documented. However the Danish, German, and Maltese models demonstrated a shift to more clinically appropriate medication regimens for asthma. Although the adherence to medications was measured based on self-report, none of the models investigated patient beliefs about their medications or documented problems that patients reported about using their medications. Publications arising out of these models do not indicate a concordance approach, issues identified were those that were addressed by the pharmacists, but patient priorities regarding their asthma were not documented or used in a collaborative setting between the patient and their provider. Thus, patient self-management was not a central theme despite evidence for its success. All the four models espoused the concept of adherence rather than the concordance model (83), that is based on collaborative goal setting between the patient and their health care provider. The American model serviced both asthma and COPD patients, and data for patients with asthma was not presented separately.

None of the four models adopted a standard set of national or international guidelines for the management of asthma. The needs of local practitioners were not generally taken into account in the American, German, or the Maltese models before starting the research (or at least this step was not documented).

Training provision for pharmacists was thus prescriptive and not needs based. Collaboration between the community pharmacists and GPs was established mainly for recruitment purposes, and there are no reports of collaboration being established between pharmacists and other health care professionals in the area where pharmacists delivered the interventions. Sustainability, in terms of patient's willingness to pay for such services was also not evaluated in any of the three models. Motivation of practitioners was another issue not addressed by any of the above service models and this in turn could imply lesser probability of the services being offered and the project being sustained after termination of the project tenure.

In terms of long-term or consistent and continued care for asthma, rather than treatment of asthma as a series of isolated episodes, monitoring of the disease process and feedback to the patient are essential. The cycle of needs analysis, targeted interventions, goal setting, and feedback are critical elements in changing patient behavior (Fig 1). Goal setting in collaboration between the health care professional and the patient involves a contract to which both agree. Using this approach, patients become more involved in the management of their own disease and in so doing change their behavior. Pharmacists are ideally placed to carry out these elements of the cycle (Fig 1) and in so doing contribute to collaborative care of asthma patients.

While many of the pharmaceutical care or disease management programs conducted by pharmacists have demonstrated improvement in clinical outcomes, self-management behavior such as uptake and use of action plans, adjustment in lifestyle factors, concordance with medication regimens or goal setting have not been evaluated. A recent study carried out in NSW, Australia used a controlled trial design to evaluate the impact of a pharmacy delivered service based on the National Asthma Guidelines (84,87). The training and service program used the structure of the six-step Asthma Management Plan (85). The six steps are:

1. assess asthma severity;
2. achieve best lung function;
3. maintain best lung function by avoiding trigger factors;
4. maintain best lung function by optimizing medication regimen;
5. develop a written action plan;
6. educate and review regularly.

While some steps have level one or two evidence for their effectiveness, other steps have been included based on evidence from other types of trials or studies (39).

The pharmacy asthma program involved a series of three visits over 6 months with the initial visit assessing individual patient needs, designing targeted interventions around the six step plan, showing how to monitor the disease process and setting collaborative goals for the next visit. At each follow-up visit, the goals were reviewed, the results of monitoring discussed, and new collaborative goals set for the subsequent visit. The monitoring undertaken by each patient was peak expiratory flow. Pharmacists provided feedback on the results of this self-monitoring and at each visit monitored the disease process. Specific factors that were monitored by the pharmacist included concordance with therapy, changes in lifestyle factors, changes in severity (based on symptoms and beta agonist use), and the number of new written asthma action plans. The cycle of care on which the program was based (Fig. 1) resulted in significant improvement in health outcomes for the intervention group compared to the control group. In addition, both economic and humanistic outcomes were improved following the program.

CYCLE OF MONITORING, REVIEW
AND FEEDBACK

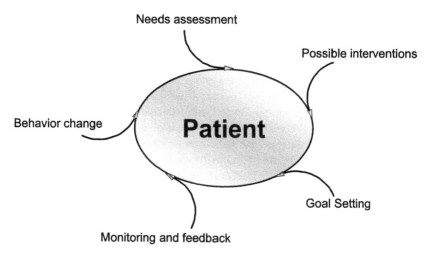

Figure 1   Cycle of care achieved in a pharmacy-based model.

When costs of asthma care were compared pre- and postservice, changes in severity of disease based on optimal management resulted in approximately a U.S.$ 1500 per patient saving for the health care system. Such savings cannot be ignored. More importantly, patients were happy with this approach and reported their satisfaction with the process and they wanted it to continue. Pharmacists also reported a high level of satisfaction with this new model of care. Studies such as these that highlight the contribution of health care professionals and how their role can be optimized for the benefit of the patient are needed on a national or international basis (Table 2).

While many of the models described above have implemented complex clinical service models, monitoring of patient outcomes is a role that can be explored as part of a complex or simple pharmacy model (Table 2). The impact of pharmacy interventions has been extremely positive and the opportunity to review behavior is unique to the community pharmacy setting.

Specific Monitoring of Asthma in the Pharmacy Setting

Monitoring is an important part of asthma management and is directed at the early detection of exacerbations and monitoring the day to day control of asthma (36).

Table 2 Brief Summary of Outcomes Monitored by Pharmacists

Outcomes	Description	Advantages	Disadvantages	References
Clinical Outcomes				
Symptom scores	Symptoms include nighttime or daytime wheeze, nighttime cough, increased mucous secretion, allergies scored on a scale of 0–10	Easy to use, easy to diarise, patients can relate to this measure	Some symptoms included in the score may not be meaningful to the patient, differentiation between score levels is subjectively decided by the patient	57,75,82,122
	Symptoms not defined but monitored as 'nighttime' or 'daytime' symptoms, activity levels	Easy to use and monitor, relatively easy to record	Simple definitions of symptoms often do not differentiate between different types of symptoms, the record is very subjective	74
	3-item symptom score—mild, moderate, severe	Easy to record	May be too simplistic and subjective	55
	Days of sickness	Quite easy to remember and record, can be corroborated by checking whether this coincides with a doctor visit, has both clinical and economic ramifications, patients may have been sick for a different reason, but felt stressed and record this as "asthma"	Depends on patients record	55,64

(Continued)

Table 2 Brief Summary of Outcomes Monitored by Pharmacists (*Continued*)

Outcomes	Description	Advantages	Disadvantages	References
Peak expiratory flow	Morning and evening peak flows, three peak flows recorded	Objective, can be done by patients at home, some patients feel in control by knowing what their lung function is	Tedious to record peak flows everyday, in acute asthma, peak flows may be hard to do and cause symptoms, peak flow is not the most accurate lung function measurement possible, it is also patient effort dependent	57,59,60, 64,75
	Peak flow of the day	Easy for patients—no daily records	This can only give a picture of lung function at one given time point and may not be meaningfully extrapolated	55,59
	The Jones Morbidity Index	Very simple to use, not time consuming, has been tried in GP settings	May be too simple and not differentiate between symptom types	89
	Forced expiratory volume in 1 sec	A more accurate measure than peak flow, easy to measure with a FEV_1 meter	FEV_1 meters may be more expensive than peak flow meters	59
Medication usage	Record of all medication being used by the patient	Easy to maintain in the pharmacy, all medication records can help with medication review	Recording of medications from dispensing history need not necessarily indicate usage	57
	Defined daily doses of medication	Needs daily recording by patients	A truer reflection of use as compared to just keeping a record of medications	55

Reliever medication used	No. of times reliever used in a particular period	Easy to record	prescribed or dispensed, depends on patient recording accuracy	74
			Depends on patient recall and recording accuracy, patients may be using relievers in order to feel "safe" rather than for symptoms	
Plasma theophylline concentration	Measured through blood sample analysis	Accurate profile of drug use and adherence	Invasive, not possible daily in the community pharmacy or home setting	68
Patient compliance	An important measure, simply can be judged through experience	Patients may be made aware of their own usage patterns when questioned	Very subjective to bias and patient recall, there is no good way to actually measure compliance simply by questioning.	64,74
Inhaler techniques	Observed by pharmacist	Easily demonstrated by patients, actual demonstration therefore correct	Patients often forget to bring their devices to the pharmacy to demonstrate, some patients may know how to use it correctly but may not be doing so everyday, some patients may dislike the feeling of being checked upon or corrected, the observation has to be done by a professional who is quite experienced in the	74,78

(Continued)

Table 2 Brief Summary of Outcomes Monitored by Pharmacists (*Continued*)

Outcomes	Description	Advantages	Disadvantages	References
			use of inhalation devices themselves	
	Inhaler techniques checked using a checklist	"	May be more accurate and repeatable to measure correctness of inhaler technique using a checklist	59,64
	Inhaler technique scored as number of errors per patient per device	"		56
Humanistic Outcomes				
Quality of Life	Global quality of life, SF-36	Easy to administer	Not asthma specific	56,59,60,64
	Asthma-related quality of life	Easy to administer, asthma specific	Does not uncover generic issues about the patients health	56
	Living with asthma questionnaire	"		59,64
Patient satisfaction	Interviews or questionnaires	Important from the patient's viewpoint, good feedback and constructive comments help shape future care provision	There are no validated instruments to measure patient satisfaction especially with pharmacy services for asthma	40,56,60,64
Self-efficacy	Questionnaire technique	Easy to administer	Dependent on the accuracy of patient answers	59
Economic Outomes				
	Days of sickness recorded by patient	Easy to record	May be misleading sometimes as patients may have two	56,59,64

		different illnesses, dependant on patient recall	
Hospital visits	Easy to record, an important indicator as it is a high cost event	Difficult in terms of sample size, as the hospitalization event is comparatively rare in people with mild to moderate asthma and thus very large sample sizes may be needed	56,64
Costs of medications	Relatively easy to record and find	The analysis may be confusing as in some cases medication costs are government subsidized or covered by private insurance, also costs relate to dispensed drugs and not the actual amount of drug used	55,122
Absenteeism from work or school	Easy to record	Some patients may be reluctant for this data to be recorded, and self-report may not be very accurate	56,64

Monitoring issues are determined by who will do the monitoring. This has implications for the type of data that can be collected, their validity and their accuracy. Some issues are outlined in Table 3.

The pharmacy setting is ideal for the purposes of regular review of a patient's asthma, as patients may see a pharmacist more frequently than other health care practitioners, in order to procure prescriptions, or buy over the counter products. As outlined in earlier sections, pharmacists have

Table 3 Monitoring Issues in Asthma

	Advantages	Disadvantages
Patient	Close, usually accurate, monitoring their own asthma can help palients self-manage	May not have the correct perception about themselves, may lose interest, and find it tedious. Data depends on self-report and may be biased.
Physician	Accurate, valid data, allows investigation of asthma control and reasons for poor control, allows physical examination and thorough spirometric testing	Time consuming and can only be done intermittently, some GPs may not have spirometric apparatus
Specialists	Accurate, valid data, asthma control and reasons for poor control may be assessed	Time consuming, can only be done intermittently
Pharmacists	Accurate, valid data. In addition to clinical data, data on quality of care, cost of care, medication usage, and patient satisfaction with care may be possible	Physical examination cannot be done, monitoring can be done more frequently than by a physician
Nurse educators	Accurate, valid data, asthma control can sometimes be assessed and spirometry can also be performed	Time consuming, can only be done intermittently
Family or carers	Carers may be more responsible than the patient themselves and are in a position to observe the patient closely	Data may be subjectively biased

begun to take up programs based around the pharmaceutical care or the disease management concept, both of which advocate monitoring.

Monitoring Outcomes (Table 2)

Currently trends in outcome measurement include three dimensions–economic, clinical, and humanistic outcomes (86). This has been given the acronym "the ECHO model." The ECHO model may provide a useful reference for the inclusion of criteria to be used as monitoring tools for the patient with asthma.

Clinical Outcomes

In asthma clinical outcomes may be focused on:

1. Symptoms— and their monitoring to assess control and severity.
2. Lung function—as an objective measure of disease severity.
3. Triggers and allergen response—to aid the identification of triggers and build an avoidance schedule.
4. Medication usage—as an indicator of control or severity, effectiveness of therapy, appropriateness of regimen and devices.
5. Adherence.
6. Ownership of action plans—built on various criteria such as symptoms and lung function.

Symptom-Based Outcomes– Severity and Control

Review of asthma symptoms by the pharmacist is a useful way in which current asthma severity or control can be assessed. There are several ways in which this can be done (Table 2).

One involves following the Australian National Asthma Council's Handbook on Asthma Management for health care professionals (2000) which has been used successfully in a Pharmacy setting (87). It classifies asthma severity into either mild, moderate, or severe, and uses a simple table that can be used by health professionals to score a patient's severity based on the frequency and intensity of symptoms, and limitations posed on the individual's daily activities.

The second involves the Jones Morbidity Index, which uses three simple questions, and has been validated for use in general practice settings and has also been tried in a community pharmacy setting to assess whether it can be used to identify people with poorly controlled asthma (88). Results showed that the Jones Morbidity Index was significantly associated with factors that imply sub-optimal asthma management (89). As the three questions only take a minute to administer, it may be considered a valuable tool for use by community pharmacists, such that patients with high morbidity levels can then be followed up by referral to a physician if need be, or by counseling patients to take necessary steps based on an action plan provided by their physicians.

Various other questionnaires have been validated for the assessment of either severity or control (90–92), and these can be adapted for use in a pharmacy setting.

Lung Function Tests

Although not currently practical to any great extent, pharmacists can become involved in spirometry measurements. Spirometry gives a very accurate snapshot of asthma severity and the degree of airways obstruction (93). A group of researchers are currently trialing the use of spirometric screening in community pharmacies (94); however, there are not many reports of spirometric testing through community pharmacies. This may become a method of monitoring asthma in the community pharmacy in the future, but specific training will be required.

Peak expiratory flow rates (maximal expiratory flow achieved during a forced expiration) are not quite as reliable as FEV_1 (95), yet peak flow meters are cheap, portable, and easy to use. It is important however to instruct patients on how to use and interpret peak flow meters and peak flow readings. Reddel et al. (1995) investigated various indices of peak flow and found that the best index, that correlated well with airway hyperresponsiveness, was the lowest morning pre-bronchodilator peak flow measured over a period (e.g., a week or a fortnight), expressed as a percentage of the recent best peak flow or the predicted best,

$$\text{Peak flow index} = \text{lowest morning peak flow/recent best best peak flow} \times 100$$

This can be a simple and useful measurement for patients. With continuing measurements of PEF, patients should be involved in the decision making about what action should be taken when changes occur. Pharmacists can provide feedback and encouragement for this self-management.

Monitoring Trigger Factors

Pharmacists can play an important role in identifying and advising about avoidance of trigger factors. Outcomes that can be possibly measured relative to trigger factors, would simply involve documenting whether the patient has made efforts to identify possible triggers, has sufficient knowledge about triggers and avoidance measures and has started taking measures to avoid or limit exposure to these triggers. Pharmacists can encourage patients to keep a symptoms diary and note occasions when symptoms are worse to detect a pattern. Pharmacists may also offer a visit to the patient's home to help identify possible triggers. Several useful approaches have been identified and validated for the assessment of occupational sensitizers as triggers and these can be adapted to the investigation of other triggers (96,97).

Monitoring Medication Outcomes

As mentioned previously, appropriate prescription medication use is critical to asthma care and the pharmacist's role is evident (8). Medication side effects are common in patients with asthma and lead to medication taking decisions that may often compromise asthma control (33). Patient dissatisfaction with asthma treatment has been associated with problems in belief in asthma medications (34). Thus, it is important to document the asthma medication profiles that patients have before and after interventions geared to optimize asthma therapy.

The use of computerized pharmacy records has very often served as a research tool to investigate asthma patterns. For example, a research initiative in California used a cohort of all 2344 adult Northern California members of a health maintenance organization hospitalized for asthma over a 2-year period. Computerized pharmacy data were used to ascertain asthma medications dispensed during the 3-, 6-, and 12-month intervals preceding hospitalization for asthma. It was found through multiple logistic regression analysis that high level inhaled β_2 agonist use was associated with a greater risk of intensive care unit (ICU) admission for asthma after controlling for asthma severity (98).

1. The Asthma Card was an initiative of the pharmacy profession to develop a method of monitoring purchases of over the counter inhaled bronchodilator medication. The Asthma Card was developed in response to ongoing concern about the overuse of bronchodilators.

2. In most states in Australia short-acting bronchodilators are available without a prescription. The Asthma Card is the size of a credit card and consists of a small four-sided folded card. One half has place for the patient details and the number of bronchodilators used. The other contains the six-step asthma management plan that is written on one side and an action plan to be filled out by the physician on the other side. All patients who purchase bronchodilator inhalers from a pharmacist without a prescription are required to possess an Asthma Card and produce it for review whilst purchasing the bronchodilator medication. In a survey conducted in Sydney in 1996 with 231 pharmacists, 53% of the pharmacists indicated that they had increased the number of referrals made by them to the physician regarding asthma reviews. The

majority of pharmacists reported the card to be a useful tool for initiating a counseling session (99). It was reported that of the 3677 patients referred by pharmacists to their doctor, 32% had a written action plan, 42% visited their physician regularly, and 695 used their bronchodilator inhaler more than three times a week.

Some of the measures that have been successfully used to monitor medication use in pharmacy intervention studies are:

- calculating changes in daily defined doses of drugs pre- and post intervention (70);
- monitoring asthma medication profiles using defined daily doses (70);
- monitoring serum concentrations of drugs like theophylline;
- documenting frequency of adverse drug reactions and side effects (100).

Adherence

In terms of monitoring medication outcomes, adherence to a drug regimen is a key factor. Adherence refers to the degree, to which a patient's medication use corresponds to the prescribed regimen. To assess and understand adherence behavior in asthma requires recognition of the diversity and complexity of medication taking behavior. In general, (101) non-adherence with prescribed medication can range from not filling prescriptions, taking incorrect doses, improper dosing intervals through to premature discontinuation of therapy. It is also useful to distinguish between *intentional* non-adherence (for example, if a patient does not believe that they have asthma and therefore chooses not to take the medication) and *unintentional* non-adherence (for example, forgetting to take a medication).

In asthma, the common non-adherent behaviors include over use of reliever medication especially during acute attacks, underuse of preventative medication, non-avoidance of triggers and not taking appropriate measures in an exacerbation, or even non-recognition of an exacerbation. Often, people with asthma exhibit an erratic pattern of medication use which alternates between fully adherent (usually when symptomatic) to underuse or non-adherent (when symptom-free). Another factor which can undermine the efficacy of treatment is lack of adherence to instructions for correct use of metered dose inhalers and use of spacers. Research suggests that poor technique is widespread (102).

Factors Associated with Adherence to Asthma Therapy

Factors shown to influence general adherence to therapy are summarized in Table 4. Broadly, they may be divided into patient, carer, disease, and therapy-related factors.

Table 4 Risk Factors for Non-Adherence

Patient factors	*Carer factors*
Cognitive impairment	Health beliefs of the carer/friends
Health beliefs	Lifestyle of carers/friends
Physical impairment	Prescriber–patient relationship
Lifestyle (occupation, schedules)	Information that carers/friends have
Health beliefs (perceived susceptibility, severity, barriers, and benefits)	about disease and therapy
Information and knowledge about disease and therapy	
Therapy factors	*Disease factors*
Multiple regimen	Asymptomatic nature
Multiple doses	Fluctuating severity
Lifestyle modification needed (trigger avoidance)	Effect of the disease on lifestyle
Difficult techniques (metered dose inhalers)	

Key influences on adherence behavior in asthma, however, center on patients' or carer's beliefs about asthma and its medications. Particular issues surrounding medications relate to the perceived need for medications and concerns about long-term use. The characteristics of the regimen itself are also related to adherence behavior, especially a regimen involving more than twice daily administration (102).

Strategies to Improve Adherence to Medication Regimens

In the case of chronic diseases such as asthma, research has clearly shown that successful interventions to support adherence need to be complex and multi-faceted and include a combination of counseling, education, more convenient care, self-monitoring, re-enforcement, reminders, and other forms of enhanced attention or supervision (103). Moreover, the combination of interventions selected need to target both systemic barriers such as irregular access to health care professionals as well as the individual needs of the patient. A targeted strategy should be used (Table 5).

The Pharmacist's Role in Supporting Adherence

Adherence support is considered to be one of the key roles that pharmacists can play. The pharmacist is likely to see patients on long-term treatment programs more regularly than their GP, and as is well known, adherence to medication regimens decreases over time. Hence, the pharmacist is well placed to offer ongoing monitoring and supervision. Given that the key non-adherent behaviors in asthma revolve around misconceptions about

Table 5 Adherence Support Strategies

Barrier	Strategy
Knowledge deficits	Tailor information to meet the needs of the patient
Health beliefs	Clarify misconceptions. Encourage partnership between patient and health care professional in treatment plan
Complex regimen	Simplify regimen Dosette
Forgetfulness	Select a reminder, or cue, such as a clock time, mealtime, or other ritual behavior that fits into the patient's lifestyle Use repeat refill reminders (telephone call, letter)
Adverse effects	Consider alternatives
Physical difficulties, e.g., co-ordination, eyesight	Large print, special devices
Lack of self-efficacy	Teaching and reinforcing skills for self-management

the role of medicines in asthma control, pharmacists as drug experts are well suited to educating patients about their disease and therapy.

Providing Adherence Support

Within the development of pharmaceutical care models for asthma in community pharmacy (40,55,56,59,60,64), many of the core features that have been incorporated correspond to well identified strategies for the delivery of adherence support to patients with chronic diseases (Table 5). For example individualised education aimed at improving the patient's understanding of their disease and the role that different therapies play in controlling asthma (40,55,56), and long term follow-up have been integral components of many of the programs reported in the literature (40,55,56,59,60,64).

Pharmacists have an important role to play in improving adherence to medication regimens in asthma. Through regular contact with the patient and use of medication records they can identify non-adherence, investigate its causes by careful questioning of the patient and provide targeted interventions based on individual patient assessment.

Inhalation Technique

The effectiveness of inhaler therapy depends not only on adherence but also on inhaler technique. Inhaler techniques can be assessed by using lung deposition studies (104), by subjective assessment, measuring improvements in lung function (FEV_1) (105), and by using a checklist of skill items (79,106). Of these, the most feasible in a community pharmacy setting would be observation using an inhaler technique checklist for all possible devices used by a patient.

Use of Written Asthma Action Plans

The use of written action plans allows self-management by patients, hence, a desired outcome of any asthma education intervention would be ownership of action plans by all participants. It has been suggested that self-monitoring of asthma by patients be coupled with a written action plan and regular medication review by a physician. In a systematic review of randomized controlled trials, self-management was shown to reduce the relative risk of hospitalization for asthma by 39% (107). Symptom-based self-monitoring and peak flow-based monitoring have similar benefits, and pharmacists can encourage the use of either depending on patient preference or a knowledge of the patient's perception levels. If patients are poor perceivers and remain asymptomatic despite a considerable fall in lung function, it may be better for the pharmacist to encourage peak flow-based self-monitoring.

Humanistic Outcomes

Quality of Life

Health care research outcomes should target outcomes that are important to patients (108). Patient assessed health outcomes can be:

1. *Health status:* this relates to patient's functional status and quality of life.
2. *Health utilities:* refers to patient's values for a particular state of health.
3. *Patient satisfaction.*

Pharmacists can share in the care of patients by monitoring quality of life. Among the quality of life measures for asthma, the most popular are those reported by Hyland, Juniper et al., and Marks et al. (109–111). Of these, the Marks quality of life questionnaire is the shortest with 20 items and has been demonstrated to be valid, reliable, and responsive (111). The Marks asthma quality of life questionnaire can be self-administered in the pharmacy or at home and uses an easy to score Likert Scale. Hence, it is both respondent and scorer friendly.

Perceived Control of Asthma

Psychological factors can play a role in asthma symptoms and may play a role in how individuals manage their asthma (112). Since self-management of asthma is part of most consensus guidelines, it becomes important to have an understanding of how much control patients perceive they have over their asthma. Pharmacist interventions have been shown to have a positive impact on the patient's perceived control of asthma (87). Reference 112a reported the development and validation of an 11-item questionnaire that measures perceived control of asthma. This questionnaire measures the three constructs of self-efficacy, learned helplessness, and locus of control. Although there are several scales to measure self-efficacy in asthma (113–115), there are no other instruments that specifically measure perceived control of asthma.

Knowledge

It has been proposed that knowledge is one of the factors that affects self-efficacy, attitudes, and behavior (115). Thus, it is relevant for pharmacists to measure asthma knowledge. Measurement of knowledge is also important as gaps in patient's knowledge can be identified and appropriate education designed. Many instruments to measure knowledge are available. One commonly used in Australian settings is the 31-item validated asthma knowledge questionnaire developed by researchers and clinicians at the University of Newcastle. This questionnaire has 31 true or false items and can be self-administered in the community pharmacy or at home (116).

Patient Satisfaction

Patient satisfaction is a concept that has been derived from the broader construct of customer satisfaction, and has been defined as a personal evaluation of health care services and providers (117). Usually qualitative methods can be used to assess patient satisfaction. No validated patient satisfaction instrument is available in the literature with respect to asthma care in the community pharmacy. However, several instruments measure generic satisfaction with pharmacy services. A University of California instrument has been validated, called the client satisfaction questionnaire. This questionnaire has eight items, and has been shown in many studies to perform very well and is reliable as a global measure of patient satisfaction (117). Willingness to pay for services also indicates levels of patient satisfaction, and has been a factor measured in many intervention studies including pharmacy-based asthma services (118–120).

Economic Outcomes

Disease management requires measurement of economic outcomes as well as clinical ones. The most commonly used economic outcome measures used in community pharmacy asthma-based interventions are reduction in hospitalizations, decreased days of sickness, decreased doctor visits (55). Hospitalization data may be a simple frequency of admission, relapse rate, rate of presentation at accident and emergency department, length of stay, etc. Of these, the number or rate of hospitalization is a measure that is simple, easy for patients to recall and used widely. Patient symptom diaries can be used to measure days of work lost or doctor visits.

Prescription databases have been used to generate cost center analyses. For example, four affiliated health maintenance organizations recruited a total of 25,614 asthmatics identified from a population of approximately 673,000 members in the health maintenance organization. Annual charges for asthma care were analyzed by age and gender. It was found that charges for acute care were inversely related to the dollars spent on pharmaceuticals. This study demonstrated the ability of a combined medical and pharmacy database to document the charges for care and possibly identify indicators of undertreated populations (121).

Conclusion

Pharmacists are an integral part of the health care system and are accessible to people with asthma on a daily basis. There are issues in the current management of asthma and pharmacists have specific skills which can address these issues. Pharmacy practice is changing from a traditional role restricted to the supply of medicines to the provision of ongoing care for the patient and the provision of services associated with medication use. Controlled trials have provided evidence of the value of these services. Monitoring the outcomes of interventions designed to improve asthma care has demonstrated clinical, humanistic, and economic benefits. Adherence to medication regimens is one area in which there is a definite need for intervention and in which pharmacists can have a significant impact. However, provision of continuity of care, empowering patients through education, monitoring with regular appointments and review are all areas in which pharmacy has had an impact and should continue to develop for the benefit of the person with asthma.

References

1. Litaker D, Mion L, Planavsky L, Kippes C, Mehta N, Frolkis J. Physician–nurse practitioner teams in chronic disease management: the impact on costs, clinical effectiveness, and patients' perception of care. J Interprof Care 2003; 17:223–237.
2. Stevenson K, Baker R, Farooqi A, Sorrie R, Khunti K. Features of primary health care teams associated with successful quality improvement of diabetes care: a qualitative study. Fam Pract 2001; 18:21–26.
3. Blumenthal D. Part 1: Quality of care—what is it? N Engl J Med 1996; 335:891–894.
4. Øvretveit J. Medical managers can make research-based management decisions. J Manag Med 1998; 12:391–397, 322.
5. Wagner EH. The role of patient care teams in chronic disease management. (comment). Br Med J 2000; 320:569–572.

6. Blais R, Gregoire JP, Rouleau R, Cartier A, Bouchard J, Boulet LP. Ambulatory use of inhaled β_2-agonists for the treatment of asthma in Quebec : a population-based utilization review. Chest 2001; 119:1316–1321.

7. Bero LA, Mays NB, Barjesteh K, Bond C. Expanding the roles of outpatient pharmacists: effects on health services utilisation, costs, and patient outcomes. Cochrane Database Syst Rev 2000.

8. Moyer P. Low hanging fruit. Manag Health 1995; Sept:S11–S12, S48.

9. Holland RW, Nimmo CM. Transitions, part 1: beyond pharmaceutical care. Am J Health Syst Pharm 1999; 56:1758–1764.

10. Holland RW, Nimmo CM. Transitions in pharmacy practice, part 2: who does what and why. Am J Health Syst Pharm 1999; 56:1981–1987.

11. Nimmo CM, Holland RW. Transitions in pharmacy practice, part 3: effecting change—the three-ring circus. Am J Health Syst Pharm 1999; 56: 2235–2241.

12. Holland RW, Nimmo CM. Transitions in pharmacy practice, part 4: can a leopard change its spots? Am J Health Syst Pharm 1999; 56:2458–2462.

13. Nimmo CM, Holland RW. Transitions in pharmacy practice, part 5: walking the tightrope of change. Am J Health Syst Pharm 2000; 57:64–72.

14. Hepler CD, Strand L. Opportunities and responsibilities in pharmaceutical care. Am J Hosp Pharm 1990; 447:533–543.

15. Giberson S, Cox T. Indian Health Service: leader in pharmaceutical care. US Pharm 2000; 25:HS20, HS25–HS26, HS31–HS32.

16. Brock PL. Disease state management clinics. ASHP Annual Meeting 2000; 57:PI–2.

17. Skledar SJ, Hess MM. Implementation of a drug-use and disease-state management program. Am J Health Syst Pharm 2000; 57:S23–S29.

18. Jones AN, Benzie JL, Serjeant CS, Swan GT. Activities of clinical pharmacists at ward level. Aust J Hosp Pharm 1984; 114:77–81.

19. Hatoum HT, Catizone C, Hutchinson RA, Purohit A. An eleven-year review of the pharmacy literature: documentation of the value and acceptance of the clinical pharmacy. Drug Intell Clin Pharm 1986; 20:33–48.

20. Wood J, Bell D. Evaluating pharmacist involvement in drug therapy decisions. Pharm J 1997; 259:342–345.

21. National Asthma Education and Prevention Program. The role of the pharmacist in improving asthma care. Am Pharm 1995; NS35:24–29.

22. Chen TF, Casson C, Krass I, Benrimoj S. Medication regimen review process. A guide for community pharmacy. Aust Pharm 1996; 15:681–686.

23. Chen TF, Crampton M, Krass I, Benrimoj SI. Collaboration between community pharmacists and GPs—the medication review process. J Soc Admin Pharm 2001; 16:145–156.

24. Chen TF, Crampton M, Krass I, Benrimoj SI. Collaboration between community pharmacists and GPs—the medication review process. J Soc Admin Pharm 1999; 16:145–156.

25. Krass I, Smith C. Impact of medication regimen reviews performed by community pharmacists for ambulatory patients with general medical practitioners. Int J Pharm Pract 2000; 8:111–120.

26. Mathers CD, Vos ET, Stevenson CE, Begg SJ. The Australian Burden of Disease Study: measuring the loss of health from diseases, injuries and risk factors. Med J Aust 2000; 172:592–596.

27. Matheson M, Wicking J, Raven J, Woods R, Thien F, Abramson M, Walters EH. Asthma management: how effective is it in the community? Int Med J 2002; 32:451–456.

28. Rabe KF, Vermiere PA, Sorino JB, Meier WC. Clinical management of asthma in 1999: The asthma Insights and Reality in Europe (AIRE) study. Eur Respir J 2000; 16:802–807.

29. Bauman A, Young L, Peat JK, Hunt J, Larkin P. Asthma under-recognition and under-treatment in an Australian community. Aust N Z J Med 1992; 22:36–40.

30. Anis AH, Lynd LD, Wang XH, King G, Spinelli JJ, Fitzgerald M, Bai T, Pare P. Double trouble: impact of inappropriate use of asthma medication on the use of health care resources. Can Med Assoc 2001; 164:625–631.

31. Campbell DA, McLennan G, Coates JR, Frith PA, Gluyas PA, Latimer KM, Luke CG, Martin AJ, Roder DM, Ruffin RE. A comparison of asthma deaths and near-fatal asthma attacks in South Australia. Eur Respir J 1994; 7:490–497.

32. Vermeire PA, Rabe KF, Soriano JB, Maier WC. Asthma control and differences in management practices across seven European countries. Respir Med 2002; 96:142–149.

33. White MV, Sander N. Asthma from the perspective of the patient. J Allergy Clin Immunol 1999; 103:S47–S52.

34. Markson LE, Vollmer WM, Fitterman L, O'Connor E, Narayanan S, Berger M, Buist AS. Insight into patient dissatisfaction with asthma treatment. Arch Intern Med 2001; 161:379–384.

35. Gibson PG, Powell H, Coughlan J, Wilson AJ, Abramson M, Haywood P, Bauman A, Hensley MJ, Walters EH. Self-management education and regular practitioner review for adults with asthma. Cochrane Database Syst Rev 2005:(CD001117).

36. Gibson PG. Monitoring the patient with asthma: an evidence based approach. J Allergy Clin Immunol 2000; 106:17–26.

37. Robertson CF, Rubinfeld AR, Bowes G. Pediatric asthma deaths in Victoria: the mild are at risk. Pediatr Pulmonol 1992; 13:95–100.

38. Britt H, Miller GC, Knox S. General Practice Activity in Australia 2000–2001 General Practice Series No.8. In: AIHW Cat No GEP 5. Canberra, ACT: Australian Institute of Health and Welfare, 2001.

39. National Asthma Council. Asthma Management Handbook. Melbourne, Victoria: National Asthma Council, 2002.

40. Narhi U, Airaksinen M, Enlund H. Do asthma patients receive sufficient information to monitor their disease—a nationwide survey in Finland. Pharm World Sci 2001; 23:242–245.

41. Davis P, Man P, Cave A, McBennett S, Cook D. Use of focus groups to assess the educational needs of the primary care physician for the management of asthma. Med Educ 2000; 34:987–993.

42. Le Gouldec N, Tahar A, Sonneville A. The physician–pharmacist team in education of patients. Allerg Immunol 2001; 33:383–387.
43. Osman LM, Abdalla Ml, Russell IT, Fiddes J, Friend JA, Legge JS, Douglas JG. Integrated care for asthma: matching care to the patient. Eur Respir J 1996; 9:444–448.
44. Brodie DC, Parish PA, Poston JW. Societal needs for drugs and drug related services. Am J Pharm Educ 1980; 44:276–278.
45. Meade V. Pharmaceutical care in a changing health care system. Am Pharm 1994; NS34:43–46.
46. Grainger-Rousseau TJ, Miralles MA, Hepler CD, Segal R, Doty RE, Joseph R. Therapeutic outcomes monitoring: application of pharmaceutical care guidelines to community pharmacy. J Am Pharm Assoc 1997; NS37:647–661.
47. Meade V. Adapting to provide pharmaceutical care. Am Pharm 1994; NS34:37–42.
48. Fischer LR, Scott LM, Boonstra DM. Pharmaceutical care for patients with chronic conditions. J Am Pharm Assoc 2000; 40:174–180.
49. Geletko SM, Poulakos MN. Pharmaceutical care in an HIV clinic. Am J Health Syst Pharm 2002; 59:709–713.
50. Augustine SC, Norenberg JP, Colcher DM, Vose JM, Tempero MA. Combination therapy for non-Hodgkin's lymphoma: an opportunity for pharmaceutical care in a specialty practice. J Am Pharm Assoc 2002; 42:93–100.
51. Varma S, McElnay JC, Hughes CM, Passmore AP, Varma M. Pharmaceutical care of patients with congestive heart failure: interventions and outcomes. Pharmacotherapy 1999; 19:860–869.
52. Dent LA, Stratton TP, Cochran GA. Establishing an on-site pharmacy in a community health centre to help indigent patient's access medications and to improve care. J Am Pharm Assoc 2002; 42:497–507.
53. Lisper B, Nilsson JL. The asthma year in Swedish pharmacies: a nationwide information and pharmaceutical care program for patients with asthma. Ann Pharmacother 1996; 30:455–460.
54. Haahtela T, Klaukka T, Koskela K, Erhola M, Laitinen LA. Asthma programme in Finland: a community problem needs community solutions. Thorax 2001; 10:806–814.
55. Herborg H, Soendergaard B, Froekjaer B, Fonnesbaek L, Jorgensen T, Hepler CD, Grainger-Rousseau TJ, Ersboell BK. Improving drug therapy for patients with asthma—part 1: patient outcomes. J Am Pharm Assoc 2001; 41: 539–550.
56. Herborg H, Soendergaard B, Jorgensen T, Fonnesbaek L, Hepler CD, Hoist H, Froekjaer B. Improving drug therapy for patients with asthma—part 2: use of antiasthma medications. J Am Pharm Assoc 2001; 41:551–559.
57. Narhi U, Airaksinen M, Tanskanen P, Erlund H. Therapeutic outcomes monitoring by community pharmacists for improving clinical outcomes in asthma. J Cfin Pharm Ther 2000; 25:177– 183.
58. Odedina FT, Leader AG, Venkataraman K, Cole R. Feasibility of a community asthma management network (CAMN) program: lessons learnt from and exploratory investigation. J Soc Admin Pharm 2000; 17:15–22.

59. Schulz M, Verheyen F, Muhlig S, Muller JM, Muhlbauer K, Knop-Schneick-ert E, Petermann F, Bergmann KC. Pharmaceutical care services for asthma: a controlled intervention study. J Clin Pharmacol 2001:41.

60. Weinberger M, Murray MD, Marrero DG, Brewer N, Lykens M, Harris LE, Seshadri R, Caffrey H, Roesner JF, Smith F, Newell AJ, Collins JC, McDonald CJ, Tierney WM. Effectiveness of pharmacist care for patients with reactive airways disease: a randomized controlled trial. J Am Med Assoc 2002; 288:1594–1602.

61. Sellers JA. Community pharmacy strives for continuity of care. Am J Health Syst Pharm 1998; 55:635–637.

62. McCallian DJ, Carlstedt BC, Rupp MT. Developing pharmaceutical care plans for desired outcomes. J Am Pharm Assoc 1996; NS36:270–279.

63. Frederick J. Staying on the cutting edge of pharmacy services. Drug Store News, New York, 1999.

64. Cordina M, McElnay JC, Hughes CM. Assessment of a community pharmacy based program for patients with asthma. Pharmacotherapy 2001; 21: 1196–1203.

65. Knoell DL, Pierson JF, Marsh CB, Allen JN, Pathak DS. Measurement of outcomes in adults receiving pharmaceutical care in a comprehensive asthma outpatient clinic. Pharmacotherapy 1998; 18:1365–1374.

66. Self T, Brooks JB, Lieberman P, Ryan MR. The value of demonstration and the role of the pharmacist in teaching the correct use of pressurized bronch-odilator. Can Med Assoc J 1998; 128:129–131.

67. Ekedahl A. Open-ended questions and show-and-tell way to improve pharma-cist counseling and patients' handling of their medicines. J Clin Pharm Ther 1996; 21:95–99.

68. Watanabe T, Ohta M, Murata M, Yamamoto T. Decrease in emergency room or urgent care visits due to management of bronchial asthma inpatients and outpatients with pharmaceutical services. J Clin Pharm Ther 1998; 23: 303–309.

69. Buchner DA, Butt LT, De Stefano A, Edgren B, Suarez A, Evans RM. Effects of an asthma management program on the asthmatic member: patient-centered results of a 2-year study in a managed care organization. Am J Manag Care 1998; 4:1288–1297.

70. Herborg H, Sondergaard B, Frokjaer B, Fonnesbaek L, Hepler C, et al. Phar-maceutical care value proved. Int Pharm J 1996; 10:167–168.

71. Blumenschein K, Johannesson M, Yokoyama KK, Freeman PR. Hypothetical versus real willingness to pay in the health care sector: results from a field experiment. J Health Econ 2001; 20:441–457.

72. Rupp MT, McCallian DJ, Sheth KK. Developing and marketing a community pharmacy-based asthma management program. J Am Pharm Assoc 1997; NS37:694–699.

73. Munroe WP, Kunz K, Dalmady-lsrael C, Potter L, Schonfield WH. Economic evaluation of pharmacist involvement in disease management in a community pharmacy setting. Clin Ther 1997; 19:113–123.

74. Cairns C, Eveleigh M. Community pharmacists contribution to managing patients with asthma. Asthma J 2000; 5:80–83.

75. Bheekie A, Syce JA, Weinberg EG. Peak expiratory flow rate and symptom self-monitoring of asthma initiated from community pharmacies. J Clin Pharm Ther 2001; 26:287–296.
76. Narhi U, Vainio K, Ahonen R, Airaksinen M, Enlund H. Detecting problems of patients with asthma in a community pharmacy—pilot study. J Soc Admin Pharm 1999; 16:127–133.
77. Matsumoto K, Nishikawa M, Hashimoto H, Hayakawa H, Chida K, Toyoshima M, Satoh A. Effect of pharmacist's instruction on the treatment of asthmatics with inhaled steroid. Arerugi 1998; 47:404–412.
78. Bynum A, Hopkins D, Thomas A, Copeland N, Irwin C. The effect of tele-pharmacy counseling on metered-dose inhaler technique among adolescents with asthma in rural Arkansas. Telemed J E Health 2001; 7:207–217.
79. Erickson SR, Ascione FJ, Kirking DM, Johnson CE. Use of a paging system to improve medication self-management in patients with asthma. J Am Pharm Assoc 1998; 38:767–769.
80. Pauley TR, Magee MJ, Cury JD. Pharmacist managed, physician directed asthma management program reduces emergency department visits. Ann Pharmacother 1995; 29:5–9.
81. Serrier P, Muller D, Sevin C, Mechin H, Chanal I. Evaluation of an educational program on asthma for pharmacists. Presse Med 2000; 29:1987–1991.
82. Diamond SA, Chapman KR. The impact of a nationally coordinated pharmacy-based asthma education intervention. Can Respir J 2001; 8:261–265.
83. Raynor DK, Thistlethwaite JE, Hart K, Knapp P. Are health professionals ready for the new philosophy of concordance in medicine taking? Int J Pharm Pract 2001; 9:81–84.
84. Saini B, Krass I, Armour C. Improvement in asthma management through a specialty pharmacy. Am J Respir Crit Care Med 2002; 165:A321.
85. Woolcock AJ, Rubinfeld AR, Seale P. Asthma management plan 1989. Med J Aust 1989; 151:650–653.
86. Kozma CM, Reeder CE, Schulz RM. Economic, clinical and humanistic outcomes: a planning model for pharmacoeconomic research. Clin Ther 1993; 15:1121–1132.
87. Saini B, Jogia R, Krass I, Armour C. Evaluation of a practice-based research design using an asthma care model. Int J Pharm Pract 2002; 10:177–184.
88. Jones KP, Bain DJ, Middleton M, Mullee MA. Correlates of asthma morbidity in primary care. Br Med J 1992; 304:361–364.
89. Nishiyama T, Chrystyn H. The Jones Morbidity Index as an aid or community pharmacists to identify poor asthma control during the dispensing process. Int J Pharm Pract 2003; 11:41–46.
90. Gibson PG, Wilson AJ. The use of continuous quality improvement methods to implement practice guidelines in asthma. J Quality Clin Pract 1996; 16:87–102.
91. Juniper EF, O'Byrne PM, Guyatt GH, Ferrie PJ, King DR. Development and validation of a questionnaire to measure asthma control. Eur Respir J 1999; 14:902–907.
92. Rosier MJ, Bishop J, Nolan T, Robertson CF, Carlin JB, Phelan PD. Measurement of functional severity of asthma control. Am J Respir Crit Care Med 1994; 149:1431–1441.

93. Enright PL, Lebowitz MD, Cockroft DW. Physiologic measures: pulmonary function tests. Am J Respir Crit Care Med 1994; 49:S9–S18.

94. Burton MA, Gissing P, Simpson M, Walker J, Archer M, Bowman S, Burton M. Spirometry screening in country pharmacies—A pilot study. Australian Asthma Conference, Fremantle, 9–12 Sept, 2001.

95. Giannini D, Paggiaro PL, Moscato G, Gherson G, Bacci E, Bancalari L, Dente FL, Di Franco A, Vagaggini B, Giuntini C. Comparison between peak expiratory flow and forced expiratory volume in one second (FEV1) during bronchoconstriction induced by different stimuli. J Asthma 1997; 34:105–111.

95a. Reddel HK, Salome CM, Peat JK, Woolcock AJ. Which index of peak expirations flow is most useful in the management of stable asthma. Am. J. Resp. Cri. Care Med 1995; 151(5):1320–1325.

96. Chan-Yeung M, Malo JL. Occupational asthma. N Engl J Med 1995; 333:107–112.

97. Malo JL. The case for confirming occupational asthma: why, how much, how far? Eur Respir J 1999; 13:477–478.

98. Eisner MD, Lieu TA, Chi F, Capra AM, Mendoza GR, Selby JV, Blanc PD. Beta agonists, inhaled steroids, and the risk of intensive care unit admission for asthma. Eur Respir J 2001; 17:233–240.

99. Comino EJ, Carroll P, Fonteyn P, Whicker S, Armour C, Bauman A, Dan E. The asthma card in NSW—the experience of community pharmacists. Aust Pharm 2000; 19:179–182.

100. Shane R, Gouveia WA. Developing a strategic plan for quality in pharmacy practice. Am J Health Syst Pharm 2000; 57:470–474.

101. Matsui D. Drug compliance in pediatrics: clinical and research issues. Pediatr Clin North Am 1997; 44:1–14.

102. Sabate E. Adherence to long-term therapies: evidence for action. Geneva, Switzerland: World Health Organisation, 2003.

103. Haynes RB, Montague P, Oliver T, McKibbon KA, Brouwers MC, Kanani R. Interventions for helping patients to follow prescriptions for medications. Cochrane Database Syst Rev. 2000:(CD000011).

104. Dolovich MB. Measuring total and regional lung deposition using inhaled radiotracers. Respir Med 2001; 14:S35–S44.

105. Cochrane MG, Mohan B, Downs KE, Mauskopf J, Ben-Joseph R. Inhaled corticosteroids for asthma therapy: patient compliance, devices and inhalation technique. Chest 2000; 117:542–550.

106. Manzella BA, Brooks CM, Richards JM Jr, Windsor RA, Soong S, Bailey WC. Assessing the use of metered dose inhalers by adults with asthma. J Asthma 1989; 26:223–230.

107. Gibson PG, Coughlan J, Wilson AJ, Abramson M, Bauman A, Hensley MJ, Walters EH. Self-management education and regular practitioner review for adults with asthma. Cochrane Database Syst Rev. 2000:(CD001117).

108. Richards JM, Hemstreet MP. Measures of life quality, role performance and functional status in asthma research. Am J Respir Crit Care Med 1994; 149:S31–S39.

109. Hyland ME. The living with asthma questionnaire. Respir Med 1991; 85(suppl B):13–16.

110. Juniper EF, Guyatt GH, Epstein PS, Ferrie PJ, Jaeschke R, Hiller TK. Evaluation of impairment of health related quality of life in asthma: development of a questionnaire for use in clinical trials. Thorax 1992; 47: 76–83.

111. Marks GB, Dunn SM, Woolcock AJ. A scale for the measurement of quality of life in asthma. J Clin Epidemiol 1992; 45:461–472.

112. Lehrer PM. Asthma and emotion, a review. J Asthma 1993; 30:5–21.

112a. Katz PP, Yelin EH, Smith S, Blanc PD. Perceived control of asthma: development and validation of a questionnaire. Am. J. Respir. Crit. Care Med 1997; 155:577–582.

113. Bailey WC, Wilson KB, Weiss RA, Windsor RA, Wolle JM. Measures for use in asthma clinical research. Am J Respir Crit Care Med 1994; 149:S2–S8.

114. Tobin DL, Wigal JK, Winder JA, Holroyd KA, Creer TL. The "Asthma Self-Efficacy Scale". Ann Allergy 1987; 59:273–277.

115. Wigal JK, Stout C, Brandon M, Winder JA, McConnaughy K, Creer TL, Kotses H. The Knowledge, Attitude, and Self-Efficacy Asthma Questionnaire. Chest 1993; 104:1144–1148.

116. Allen RM, Jones MP. The validity and reliability of an asthma knowledge questionnaire used in the evaluation of a group asthma education self-management program for adults with asthma. J Asthma 1998; 35:537–545.

117. Ware JE, Snyder MK, Wright RW, Davies AR. Defining and measuring patient satisfaction with medical care. Eval Program Plan 1983; 6:547–563.

118. Gore PR, Madhavan S. Consumers' willingness to pay for pharmacist counselling for non-prescriptin medicines. J Clin Pharm Ther 1994; 19:17–25.

119. Bala MV, Mauskopf JA, Wood LL. Willingness to pay as a measure of health belief. Pharmacoeconomics 1999; 15:9–18.

120. Barner JC, Mason HL, Murray MD. Assessment of asthma patients willingness to pay for and give time to and asthma self management program. Clin Ther 1999; 21:878–894.

121. Stempel DA, Hedblom EC, Durcanin-Robbins JF, Sturn L. Use of a pharmacy and medical claims database to document cost centers for 1993 annual asthma expenditures. Arch Fam Med 1996; 5:36–40.

122. Leone FT, Grana JR, McDermott P, MacPherson S, Hanchak NA, Fish JE. Pharmaceutically-based severity stratification of an asthmatic population. Respir Med 1999; 93:788–793.

18

Monitoring the Impact of Asthma Drug Therapy: Database Studies

PIERRE ERNST

Division of Clinical Epidemiology, Royal
Victoria Hospital, McGill University
Health Center,
Montreal, Canada

SAMY SUISSA[*]

Division of Clinical Epidemiology, Royal
Victoria Hospital, McGill University
Health Centre, and the Departments of
Epidemiology and Biostatistics and
Medicine, McGill University,
Montreal, Canada

Introduction

To bring a drug to market regulatory agencies require demonstration of benefit on a narrow range of outcomes and a lack of safety concerns. For asthma, the outcome of many randomized clinical trials has been a measure of flow such as FEV1 or PEF, as well as symptoms and use of rescue medications. More recently, measures of quality of life have been added to broaden the scope of benefits examined. These randomized clinical trials often do not have sufficient power or duration of follow-up to allow one to compare the rates of clinically important outcomes such as severe exacerbations requiring hospitalization, death, or long-term non-respiratory effects, for example, on growth or bone metabolism. Moreover, the selection criteria for clinical trials are quite strict. Subjects are usually required to be non-smokers, to have little or no co-morbid disease, and

---

[*] Samy Suissa is the recipient of a Distinguished Scientist award from the Canadian Institutes of Health Research.

to be compliant with therapy. Of course, once the medication is marketed, it is used by a broader range of subjects and often, not in the exact way intended. Once a drug is marketed, unexpected and severe adverse events are frequently detected by spontaneous reports of adverse events. Detection of adverse events will be less likely, however, if the adverse event is a worsening of the disease itself, for example, a worsening of asthma severity over time or an aggravation of the severity of asthma attacks.

In this chapter, we describe how observational studies using databases provide important information on the benefits and hazards of medications used to treat asthma, which extends considerably what can be learned from clinical trials. To do this, we will use, as examples, studies we have carried out and controversies we have been involved with over the last 15 fifteen years.

Advantages and Limitations of Database Studies

To be usable for research purposes, databases must meet certain minimum specifications. The diagnoses provided must have sufficient validity to permit accurate identification of subjects with the conditions and the outcomes under study. One must be also able to identify subjects without the condition or outcome of interest to serve as controls such that exposures to medications can be compared among those with and without the outcome examined. There must be a unique identifier that allows linkage between the conditions studied, for example, asthma hospitalization or fracture, and the drugs dispensed to the patient, since these two types of information are usually gathered separately and in different ways. Specialized software is required to make this link. There must be a link to vital statistics in order to ascertain deaths completely and to identify the cause of death. Finally, a guarantee of strict confidentiality is needed to assure that individual subjects and prescribers cannot be identified. The biggest advantage of databases is the large number of subjects for whom information is available and the resulting statistical power which cannot be matched by clinical trials. The major limitation is the lack of information on various confounding factors that may influence the relationship between the exposure of interest, usually a drug, and the outcome under study. This results from the fact that most databases were created to administer health programs and not to provide patient information for research purposes.

Our group has had most experience using the administrative databases of Saskatchewan Health. The province of Saskatchewan, Canada has had computerized databases for more than 35 years in order to administer various health programs that provide universal coverage to over 90% of the population. The only exceptions are those subjects whose health care falls under the responsibility of another level of government such as native

Indians. A health registration file contains dates of birth and gender as well as dates of coverage by the program. Termination of coverage is usually the result of death or emigration from the province. This contrasts with many databases in the United States where coverage often depends on employment such that there is considerable movement of patients in and out of the database. This creates selection bias since employment and health status may be linked. In Saskatchewan, a prescription drug database records medications dispensed since 1976. Medications must be on the provincial formulary, that is, they must have been accepted for reimbursement. This includes approximately 90% of all prescriptions. Newer drugs, however, may take some time to be accepted on the formulary, thus limiting there uptake by prescribers and patients, and thereby limiting the ability to study new medications quickly. The information is of high quality since it is used for the reimbursement of pharmacists and undergoes regular auditing.

The hospital services file records primary and secondary discharge diagnoses using four digit ICD-9 codes. Coding is carried out by health record librarians locally at each hospital. Access to medical records is restricted, however. The validity of these discharge diagnoses has been studied and has been found to be quite good at identifying patients with asthma or COPD, but not at distinguishing between the two (1). A physician services file provides information on claims for payment made by physicians and includes a diagnosis field (three digit ICD-9 codes) as well as procedure codes. The validity of these physician diagnoses has not been adequately studied. These different administrative files are linked by a unique identifier.

Causes of death are obtained from a federal agency thus allowing one to identify deaths occurring anywhere in Canada or deaths signaled to the government. Linkage to the Saskatchewan health services number, the unique identifier, is only available from 1992. Linkage of deaths to health information prior to 1992 requires probability matching based on age and gender.

The major strength of the Saskatchewan databases is the electronic linkage of the different sources of information through a unique identifier and the link to vital statistics information for a population as a whole, thus providing denominator information for the calculation of rates and a source for choosing control subjects. Furthermore, information is available for more than 90% of dispensed medications. This information is likely more valid than information on prescriptions only, since these may not be filled by the patient.

The limitations of these databases results from the small size of the population of Saskatchewan, approximately 1 million permanent residents. The study of rare outcomes, such as asthma deaths, is difficult. By including all subjects included in the prescription database since 1976, one can increase the sample size to approximately 2 million subjects. Moreover, information on confounding factors such as occupational and environmental exposures, exercise, smoking, and obesity is not available.

For studies of outcomes common to the elderly, such as osteoporotic fractures and cataracts, we have used the databases used to administer the health programs of the province of Quebec. All permanent residents aged 65 years or more, or approximately 850,000 subjects, receive universal health coverage including prescription drugs (2). A unique identifier allows reliable linkage to information on physician visits, hospitalisations and vital statistics (3,4). The additional limitation here is the lack of information on drugs dispensed prior to the age of 65 years.

A unique database which has frequently been used in pharmacoepidemiology is the General Practice Research Database or GPRD. It is the world's largest computerized database of anonymized patient information from general practice records and currently contains approximately 44 million patient years of recorded information (Carlos Martinez, personal communication). It takes advantage of the well-organized British system of health care where the General Practitioner is the gatekeeper for almost all of health care for the great majority of the population. It is currently collecting health information on 3 million active patients in the United Kingdom by having physicians enter clinical information in a standard fashion into a computerized database. Practices are required to record a minimum of 95% of prescriptions and other events resulting from encounters with patients. There is some variability in diagnostic terms so that for some patients, symptoms such as cough or dyspnea might be noted, while in other instances, a diagnosis such as asthma may be provided. The patient population it contains is broadly representative of the U.K. population as a whole (5). The advantage over other databases is the availability of information on the indication for a prescription, on various confounding factors noted by the physician or by the specialist physician in his reports to the General Practitioner, and on the occurrence of important medical events such as pregnancy. A potential major limitation is that information is available on prescribed rather than dispensed medications. Agreement between information obtained from the Prescription Pricing Authority based on dispensed medications appears good, however (5).

Adverse Effects of Inhaled β_2-Agonists

After their introduction in the 1970s, inhaled β_2-agonists were commonly used regularly, several times per day, for symptom control. In 1989, Sears et al. (6) published a study which put this practice into question. In a randomized trial, he found that asthma patients using fenoterol on a regular basis had poorer control of their asthma than subjects using the same medication, as needed, for symptom control. A reanalysis of this study emphasized the deleterious effect of regular fenoterol use on lung function and bronchial hyper-responsiveness to methacholine (7). A similar increase in bronchial responsiveness has also been shown with albuterol (8), though the clinical deterioration with regular use of albuterol was not apparent over 4 weeks (9) or quite subtle (10). The question of whether or not short-acting β_2-agonists should be used regularly or as needed has become less relevant with the introduction of long-acting β_2-agonists, such as salmeterol and formoterol, and the recommendation that the need for rescue or as-needed bronchodilator be used to judge asthma control and mark the need to modify maintenance therapy (11,12). Evidence, so far, suggests that, when used in conjunction with inhaled corticosteroids, these longer acting agents improve asthma control and reduce exacerbations (13,14). Use without concomitant inhaled corticosteroids, however, is associated with rapid and significant deterioration in asthma among adults (15,16) which likely results from lack of attention to the chronic inflammatory component of the disease (17,18) rather than to the minor effects of these agents on bronchial responsiveness (19).

Evidence on the safety of long-acting β_2-agonists in asthma from database studies is limited. Meie and Jick (20) using the GPRD database from the United Kingdom found less deaths among subjects prescribed salmeterol for the first time than similarly severe subjects with initial prescriptions for ipratropium bromide or theophylline. There were only 28 respiratory deaths identified with the short 16-week follow-up chosen and as such, none of the differences between groups were statistically significant. Furthermore, subjects receiving ipratropium and theophylline were more likely to have COPD rather than asthma and therefore a worse prognosis independent of the treatment prescribed. The risk of severe acute attacks of asthma in relation to the use of salmeterol was examined in a cohort of patients formed by using the health insurance claims records of a New England insurer (21). Subjects prescribed salmeterol were more severe as attested to by more frequent hospitalization and more intense use of asthma medications prior to receiving salmeterol. After adjusting for this greater severity subjects dispensed salmeterol had similar risk of emergency care, hospitalization and admission to an intensive care unit than patients dispensed sustained release theophylline.

Database studies have contributed very substantially to understanding the association between the occurrence of life-threatening or fatal attacks of asthma and the use of inhaled short-acting β_2-agonists. Concern about such an association was brought to the forefront by the publication of three case–control studies from New Zealand, the latter two carried out to address limitations of the prior study (22–24). Each of these studies reported a significant excess in mortality among asthma patients prescribed fenoterol as opposed to albuterol. All three studies were carried out by assembling a case series of asthma deaths and comparing their use of asthma drugs prior to death with asthmatic patients who had not died. The absence of a well-defined source population from which the case and control patients were derived left open the question of differences in determinants of selection into the study which may have rendered the two groups not comparable. Furthermore, information on which drugs were used by patients was based on notes in medical records at various times in the past, thus not necessarily reflecting drug use at the time of the critical event in the cases or the corresponding moment in the patients chosen for comparison.

The association between the occurrence of life-threatening or fatal attacks of asthma and the use of inhaled short-acting β_2-agonists was re-examined using the databases of Saskatchewan Health. A cohort of 12,301 subjects, aged 5–54 years, who had been dispensed a minimum of 10 prescription drugs was formed and the factors associated with a fatal or near fatal attacks of asthma were determined (25). Case patients and control subjects without a life-threatening attack of asthma were selected from the same source population, the cohort of 12,301 subjects, thus assuring that cases and controls were representative of this population. This nested case–control approach provides equivalent information to a cohort analysis but is simpler to perform. Such an approach to analysis also provides an anchor point, the date of the event or a corresponding date for the control patients, from which exposure to the medications under study can be examined. This allows one to select time windows of exposure most relevant to the disease mechanisms at hand; for example, exposure within the prior month if acute toxicity is hypothesized, or exposure in the last year, if a gradual worsening of asthma in relation to exposure is thought to be more pertinent. The nested case–control analysis found an excess of asthma deaths in relation to use of both fenoterol and albuterol during the prior 12 months, although the relationship was stronger with fenoterol (25). The complete information on prescriptions dispensed further allowed one to demonstrate a dose response relationship with risk of a life-threatening attack increasing with each canister prescribed in the prior 12 months. As expected, a full cohort analysis examining the determinants of asthma death found similar results but also permitted calculation of rates of death in the different treatment groups (26). Complete information on dispensed medications further allowed a refined analysis of exposure which identified a threshold dose at which risk of death increased. This analysis showed that risk increased only after the use of 1.4 canisters or more of inhaled short-acting β_2-agonists per month suggesting strongly that recommended doses were not associated with asthma deaths (26). A further refinement of the nested case–control analysis examined the pattern of use of inhaled short-acting β_2-agonists in the 12 months prior to the index event (fatal or near-fatal asthma) and found that increasing use of inhaled short-acting β_2-agonists as the date of the index event approached was much more strongly linked to the risk of fatal or near-fatal asthma than the actual number of canisters dispensed. This suggests that worsening of asthma control might be identified by the increasing need for rescue medication and life-threatening attacks potentially prevented (27).

Both the nested case–control and cohort analyses of the cohort of 12,301 asthmatic subjects found a higher risk of life-threatening asthma attacks with fenoterol as compared to the more commonly used albuterol. While much has been written about potential mechanisms for the greater toxicity of fenoterol (28,29), the most convincing explanation is channeling. The occurrence of channeling in relation to prescribing of fenoterol was first suggested in The Netherlands by Petri and Urquhart (30) using a pharmacy prescription database. They found that subjects dispensed fenoterol appeared to have more severe asthma as judged by concurrent use of other asthma medications including oral corticosteroids. According to the authors of the three New Zealand case–control studies, such channeling of fenoterol to patients with more severe asthma, although it did occur, did not explain their findings (31). In both the Dutch and New Zealand studies, use of asthma medications was measured at one point in time. The longitudinal data on drug exposure available in the Saskatchewan Health databases allowed us to examine the channeling phenomenon more accurately. While subjects whose initial prescription for an inhaled short-acting β_2-agonist was for albuterol or fenoterol did not appear to differ as to the severity of their asthma, subjects who switched from one inhaled short-acting β_2-agonist to another were more severe, and this greater severity was most marked for subjects who had switched from albuterol to fenoterol (32). Moreover, approximately 70% of new users of fenoterol were being switched from albuterol while only 9% of new users of albuterol had previously been dispensed fenoterol. It therefore appears that, at least in Saskatchewan, physicians were prescribing fenoterol to patients whose asthma was more severe and who were poorly controlled while taking albuterol. There was thus, confounding by indication, with fenoterol being preferentially prescribed to patients who were at higher risk for major asthma related adverse events. Such confounding remains the most likely explanation for the differences observed in the risk of life-threatening attacks of asthma among subjects dispensed albuterol and fenoterol.

In attempting to understand whether users of fenoterol and albuterol differed as to asthma severity and therefore differed in their baseline risk of experiencing fatal or near-fatal asthma independently of which inhaled short-acting β_2-agonist they received, the information available in most databases is limited. For example, there is no information on symptoms, provoking factors or lung function. This lack of information on important determinants of prognosis in asthma makes it likely that any association between asthma treatment and adverse outcomes might be related, at least in part, to residual confounding. In other words, any association found between treatment and outcome might be explained by unmeasured factors associated with the treatment prescribed and the outcome observed. It is therefore of interest, if possible, to supplement the information available in databases. We did this in Saskatchewan by examining hospital records and asking physicians to complete a questionnaire in the presence of the patient's office chart for the subjects included in the case–control analysis (33). We identified several factors associated with life-threatening asthma, such as previous loss of consciousness during an attack of asthma, attacks precipitated by food and severity of prior attacks. Adjustment for these clinical markers of severity did not account for the association between life-threatening asthma and use of inhaled short-acting β_2-agonists, however (34). This points to the limited information available in hospital and physician charts and residual confounding by severity, rather than to a causal relationship between the use of inhaled short-acting β_2-agonists and life-threatening asthma. For example, for only 21 of the cases of fatal and near-fatal asthma could evidence be found that spirometry had ever been done (34).

The benefits of obtaining good clinical information for control of confounding by severity was demonstrated in a study from New Zealand by Garrett et al. (35). Before adjusting for severity of asthma, they found an association between the use of fenoterol and life-threatening attacks of asthma. The strength of the association was attenuated after adjusting for prior hospitalization and oral corticosteroid use, but disappeared completely when using information on the severity of asthma recorded in a standardized manner during previous visits to the Emergency Department (35). Interestingly, they did find evidence that fenoterol had been preferentially prescribed to more severe patients in New Zealand. Recently, Lanes et al. (36) have re-examined the association between the use of asthma drugs and fatal asthma using the GPRD data in the United Kingdom. Once again, use of inhaled short-acting β_2-agonists, mostly albuterol, in excessive amounts, was the strongest predictor of asthma death with a relative risk of 51.6 (95% confidence interval, 7.9–345) among subjects prescribed 13 or more canisters in the past year. These data were collected from 1994 to 1998, several years after publication of the Saskatchewan studies, suggesting that physicians have yet to adopt excessive use of inhaled short-acting β_2-agonists as a marker of life-threatening asthma that requires prompt attention.

There have been several database studies which have examined non-asthma related adverse events associated with the use of β-agonists. There were 30 cardiac deaths among the 12,301 subjects in the Saskatchewan asthma cohort. There was an association between acute cardiac death and the use of oral or nebulized β-agonists as well as theophylline, but no increase in risk with the use of inhaled short-acting β_2-agonists delivered by metered dose inhaler (37). In contrast, Au et al. (38) reported an increase in the risk of myocardial infarction in new users of inhaled short-acting β_2-agonist delivered by metered dose inhaler. There was no dose response, however, and one must be concerned that the association might be due to protopathic bias; that is, β-agonists may have been prescribed for early signs of coronary ischemia (for example, shortness of breath and chest tightness) misinterpreted by the physician as signs of respiratory disease. If this were the case, the prescription would have resulted from early signs of acute coronary disease as opposed to having precipitated myocardial infarction. In a more recent study, a dose-related increase in acute coronary syndromes was found in patients who appeared more likely to have COPD rather than asthma based on age and smoking history (39).

Benefits of Inhaled Corticosteroids

In the original cohort of 12,301 subjects from Saskatchewan, the dispensing of 12 or more inhalers of inhaled corticosteroids, mostly low-dose beclomethasone, in the prior 12 months was associated with a profound reduction in the risk of fatal and near-fatal asthma (odds ratio 0.1, 95% confidence interval 0.02–0.6) (40). The conclusions that could be drawn were limited, however, by the small number of subjects among the 129 cases and 655 controls, only 37 subjects, who had actually been dispensed inhaled corticosteroids in such a sustained fashion. Of interest, subjects who were dispensed inhaled corticosteroids in a less sustained manner tended to have an increased risk of life-threatening asthma.

To better estimate the association between inhaled corticosteroids and asthma death, we formed a new cohort of patients from the databases of Saskatchewan Health. We identified 30,569 subjects, 5–44 years of age, who had been dispensed at least three prescriptions for an asthma drug in any one-year period from September 1995 through December 1991. These subjects were followed to the earliest of December 31st, 1997, age 55, death, or emigration from the province. All death certificates were examined and 66 deaths due to asthma were identified. A nested case–control analysis was performed such that these deaths were matched to all available controls who had been followed for a similar amount of time and had entered the cohort within 3 months of the case. Such matching assures that the cases and controls have a similar duration of disease and are therefore at similar points in the natural history of their condition and that the treatment occurred at similar calendar times. The latter is needed to account for time trends in the treatment of asthma. For example, over the last 20 years inhaled corticosteroids have been used in progressively milder cases of asthma. Since cases who died of asthma are likely to be more severe, matching of controls was also carried out for various predictors of life-threatening asthma such as hospitalization for asthma, use of excess amounts of inhaled short-acting β_2-agonists and dispensing of oral corticosteroids. As one might expect, despite such matching case patients still appeared to have more severe disease than controls. Such differences are adjusted for in the logistic regression analysis so that the independent association between inhaled corticosteroids and fatal asthma could be correctly evaluated. After the matching and the adjustment, there was a dose-related decrease in the risk of asthma death with increasing numbers of prescriptions dispensed for inhaled corticosteroids in the prior year (41). The death rate from asthma among users of inhaled corticosteroids was reduced by approximately half with the dispensing of six inhalers as compared to non-users of inhaled corticosteroids. Of note, subjects who discontinued use of inhaled corticosteroids were at a substantially increased risk of fatal asthma in the 3 months following such discontinuation (41) thus explaining the increase in risk of life-threatening asthma observed with unsustained use of inhaled corticosteroids observed in the original Saskatchewan cohort (40). Thus, use of a nested case-control approach allowed careful examination of the patterns of exposure to inhaled corticosteroids in relation to the time the adverse event occurred. The dose response and the increase in risk with discontinuation of therapy strongly suggest that the reduced asthma mortality is causally related to the sustained use of low-dose inhaled corticosteroids.

Using a similar approach among the same cohort of patients, we were able to examine the relationship between use of inhaled corticosteroids and the risk of myocardial infarction (42). Overall, the risk of myocardial infarction was reduced by almost half among subjects who had been dispensed inhaled corticosteroids in the prior year (rate ratio 0.56, 95% confidence interval 0.32–0.99). The protective effect increased by an estimated 12% with each extra canister of inhaled corticosteroids dispensed in the prior year and the protective effect was most marked among subjects with more severe asthma. The most likely explanation for these results is that poorly controlled asthma increases the risk of an acute coronary syndrome among subjects with underlying coronary heart disease.

There was some evidence available that, at least in adults, earlier treatment with inhaled corticosteroids might be more beneficial than treatment instituted later in the course of the disease (43,44). We were able to examine this question in the Saskatchewan Health databases by selecting a cohort of 13,563 subjects ages 5–44 years, who were initiating treatment with a controller therapy for asthma, in this case, either theophylline or inhaled corticosteroids. When inhaled corticosteroids or theophylline were initiated along with β-agonist bronchodilators, subjects dispensed inhaled corticosteroids were 40% less likely to have a first asthma-hospitalization. Inhaled corticosteroid users were 80% less likely to be hospitalized for asthma when this medication was used in preference to theophylline as first maintenance therapy after initial prescriptions of β-agonists (45).

We were also interested in the benefits of inhaled corticosteroids on hospitalization among subjects with more severe asthma. We therefore identified subjects hospitalized for asthma and examined the protective effects of inhaled corticosteroids on the risk of a rehospitalization for asthma (46). After the first 15 days from hospital discharge and for up to 6 months, the dispensing of inhaled corticosteroids was associated with a 40% reduction in the risk of a readmission to hospital for asthma (46). The benefit disappeared, however, after 6 months. The most likely explanation appeared to be that subjects continuing their use of inhaled corticosteroid beyond 6 months were more severe and therefore more likely to have a readmission for asthma. There was concern, however, that the benefits of inhaled corticosteroids on risk of hospitalization might wane over time. For this reason, we examined the effects of inhaled corticosteroids on asthma hospitalization after excluding from consideration the first year of asthma treatment (47). Use of inhaled corticosteroids after this first year was associated with a 31% reduction in the risk of an asthma admission to hospital and a 39% reduction in the risk of a readmission for asthma (47). Furthermore, the benefit was similar in the first 4 years of follow-up as in follow-up after these first 4 years, strongly suggesting that the benefits of inhaled corticosteroids did not wane over time.

Risks of Inhaled Corticosteroids

Fractures

Dose-related decreases in bone density in relation to the use of inhaled corticosteroids is well recognized (48,49). It is uncertain, however, whether this translates into an increase in the risk of fractures. Hubbard et al. (50) undertook a study of the relationship of inhaled corticosteroid use and hip fracture in the GPRD database in the United Kingdom. They identified 16,341 cases of hip fracture and matched these to almost 30,000 control subjects of similar age and gender chosen from the same practice as the case and with information available on prescribed medications over the same period of time. The mean age of subjects was 79 years and only 6% had a diagnosis of asthma or COPD recorded. Information on prescribed medication was only available for an average of 2.7 years. There was a dose-related increase in the rate of hip fracture, such that, at doses of inhaled beclomethasone or budesonide between 400 and 800 µg/day, there was an approximate 30% increase in risk of hip fracture (50). This association persisted when the analysis was restricted to subjects without a prescription for oral corticosteroids. Given the limited duration of prescribing information, however, subjects on higher doses of inhaled corticosteroids may have been more likely to have received oral corticosteroids prior to the time prescribing information was available. A recent study using the health care administrative databases of the province of Ontario did not find a link between the use of inhaled corticosteroids and fracture of the hip in elderly women (51). The power of the study was limited, however, with only 913 fractures observed. Furthermore, only rapid effects of inhaled corticosteroids were examined since subjects who had been dispensed these medications more than 365 days before the event were excluded.

To further examine the relationship between inhaled corticosteroids and fracture risk, we assembled a cohort of elderly subjects from the Quebec databases (52). Among subjects over the age of 65, we selected subjects who had been dispensed at least three prescriptions of drugs commonly used in the treatment of asthma and COPD on at least two different dates in any one-year period. We then selected cases with a first fracture of the hip or upper extremity after a minimum of 4 years of follow-up in order to assure that detailed information of sufficient duration on the use of oral and inhaled corticosteroids was available for all study subjects. We identified more than 9500 cases of fracture, 3326 hip fractures, and 6298 fractures of the upper extremity using hospital discharge codes. These cases were matched, on age only, to over 191,000 control subjects, actually control person moments (vide infra). Adjustment for differences in the severity of the underlying respiratory disease was made in the analysis by accounting for differences between cases and controls in the intensity of use of other respiratory drugs. Adjustment for comorbid conditions which might modify the risk of fracture was also done according to medications dispensed. Furthermore, the effect of inhaled corticosteroids was examined after adjusting for the cumulative exposure to oral corticosteroids in the prior 4 years. There was no association observed between inhaled corticosteroid use and fracture of the hip. For upper extremity fracture, there was a 12% increase in risk per 1000 µg increase in the mean daily dose of inhaled corticosteroids expressed as beclomethasone equivalents. Analyses were repeated among a sub-group with at least 8 years of information on corticosteroid use. Only the use of over 2000 µg of inhaled corticosteroids per day was associated with an increased risk of fracture of the hip or upper extremity (rate ratio 1.61, 95% confidence interval, 1.04–2.50). This means that 58 subjects (95% confidence interval, 24–1767 subjects) would have to be treated with such high daily doses to result in one extra fracture.

It therefore appears that, at doses commonly recommended, inhaled corticosteroids to not substantially increase the risk of osteoporotic fractures.

Cataracts and Glaucoma

The risk of cataracts with the use of inhaled corticosteroids has been the subject of several recent studies (53–56). Using the Quebec health databases, Garbe et al. (54) examined the risk of cataract extraction with the use of these drugs in subjects aged 70 years or greater. They found a threefold increase in risk with use of inhaled corticosteroids for more than 3 years. The risk was most evident among users of high doses, equivalent to more than 1 mg of beclomethasone per day (odds ratio 3.40, 95% confidence interval 1.49–7.76), while the risk at lower doses was equivocal and did not achieve statistical significance (odds ratio 1.63, 95% confidence interval 0.85–3.13). This increased risk of cataract extraction persisted even after excluding subjects who had been dispensed oral corticosteroids (54).

The association between the use of oral and inhaled corticosteroids and the risk of open angle glaucoma was also examined using the Quebec health databases. A dose-related increase in the occurrence of a diagnosis of ocular hypertension, open angle glaucoma, or treatment for these conditions, was found with the current use of oral corticosteroids (57). For inhaled corticosteroids, such a risk was only observed among subjects who had been dispensed high doses of inhaled corticosteroids, 1600 or more micrograms of beclomethasone or the equivalent, continuously for at least 3 months (58). The overall increases in risk of ocular hypertension or open angle glaucoma were small (odds ratios of less than 2) and these studies may be criticized for including many cases, almost half, that were quite mild since they did not undergo any treatment for their condition.

In examining the link between glaucoma and the use of corticosteroids, a nested case-control approach to the analysis of these cohort studies was again used. The choice of control subjects differed from the usual practice of choosing controls randomly from all subjects in the cohort, perhaps matching on several important determinants of risk such as age or comorbid conditions. Instead, control subjects were selected from among patients who were visiting an ophthalmologist. This was made necessary by the nature of the condition under study. Glaucoma may be asymptomatic for a prolonged period of time and usually requires a visit to an ophthalmologist for the diagnosis to be made and for treatment to be instituted. Therefore, selection of subjects as controls from the cohort as a whole will include subjects with the condition under study. This would reduce the strength of any association with use of medications. Furthermore, subjects dispensed corticosteroids may be more likely to be referred to an ophthalmologist if their physician is concerned about an association between corticosteroid treatment and eye disease. If controls are selected from the cohort as a whole, a false association between corticosteroid therapy and glaucoma will be created since a subject receiving corticosteroids will be more likely to be diagnosed. Selection of controls from among subjects visiting an ophthalmologist will prevent such a selection bias (59).

Asthma Prognosis

When patients initiate therapy for their asthma, the longer term prognosis is often unclear. To shed light on this question, we formed a cohort of patients from Saskatchewan, ages 5–44 years, who were initiating treatment for asthma as attested to by the absence of any prescriptions for asthma drugs dispensed in the prior 24 months (60). We classified patients according to intensity of asthma drug therapy over consecutive 12 month periods. Subjects whose initial drug therapy suggested their asthma was mild tended to remain mild as attested to by the absence of an increase in asthma treatment intensity over the subsequent 3–5 years. Subjects whose treatment intensity was appropriate for severe disease tended to become less severe with 61 % of subjects no longer being dispensed treatment appropriate for severe disease at 5 years. Such a waning in the intensity of treatment for asthma was more likely to occur among subjects less than 15 years old among whom 80% were no longer receiving therapy for severe disease at 5 years and a third were receiving therapy consistent with mild disease at 5 years. These results suggested that mild asthma tended to remain so, at least over an initial period of 5 years after the onset of therapy, and that severe disease on initial presentation tended to remit especially in children.

These conclusions, however, are based on accepting treatment intensity as a surrogate for asthma severity. We therefore examined the occurrence of other markers of asthma severity available in the Saskatchewan Health databases in relation to the groups defined by treatment intensity. Subjects dispensed treatment consistent with severe disease were 10 times as likely to be hospitalized for asthma than subjects dispensed therapy that suggested their asthma was mild (60). Thus, we felt that treatment intensity was a valid marker of asthma severity.

Methodological Issues in Observational Study Designs

Several non-experimental or observational epidemiologicai designs may be used to study the benefit and risk of asthma treatment using information recorded in databases. The particularity of these designs is that they address issues not considered in clinical trials, namely infrequent and severe asthma outcomes, longer term effects and, most importantly, they provide information in the real life context of asthma treatment. These designs include ecological, case–control, cohort, and nested case–control approaches. We describe the strengths and limitations of each of these approaches, with illustrations.

Ecological Designs

Ecological studies are epidemiologicai studies that correlate population-based geographical or secular trends in asthma outcomes with corresponding trends in a risk factor, notably the use of medications. In the first instance, several geographical regions (countries, states, counties, provinces, etc.) can be identified and rates of asthma outcomes and of medication use can be obtained for each. With the region as the unit of analysis, a correlation between the two rates can be estimated and used to indicate the association between the two. In the second instance, a single region is selected and rates of asthma outcomes and of medication use are obtained for several years (or other units of time) for that same region. Ecological studies in asthma have used the latter secular trend approach rather than a geographical approach.

Ecological studies can provide useful information on the potential population impact of a drug on major asthma outcomes. These studies are facilitated in countries where statistics on asthma outcomes such as morbidity and mortality are routinely collected in a consistent and exhaustive manner and are readily available. In addition, data on medication use should also be readily available. Most studies have used sales data from IMS to estimate rates of population drug use.

Studies based on the ecological design, however, have several limitations. First, ecological studies, in general, are inherently limited since they cannot link subjects who have the asthma outcome with their drug exposure on an individual basis. In fact, such a study design cannot even distinguish directionality, namely whether treatment precedes the outcome, since drug use and outcome rate are obtained at the same time point. Thus, while an increase in outcomes with increased use of a drug can be interpreted as the drug causing the outcome, the reverse is also possible with such a design. Furthermore, no individual information is available on confounding factors which might explain any association between the drug in question and the outcome. Therefore, such potential confounding cannot be controlled for in the analysis. Another issue in these studies is the limited information on drug use, particularly with respect to indication and age. For example, drug sales data on a bronchodilator do not provide this information by age groups that may be relevant if one is interested in asthma mortality in younger patients. Moreover, such information does not distinguish whether the drug was used for asthma or COPD.

The first use of the ecological design in monitoring asthma treatment was to examine the increase of asthma deaths observed in England and Wales in the 1960s, that coincided with the introduction of high dose formulations of isoproterenol, a non-selective β-agonist in use at the time (61,62). This same approach was used to "confirm" this relationship, by showing that asthma mortality did not increase in the United States, a country where this product was not available (63). Subsequently, a similar ecological evaluation in Australia did not find such a temporal relationship between isoproterenol use and asthma mortality in that country (64). Moreover, these studies have not used any quantitative analysis to assess the association between asthma deaths and bronchodilator sales, but have relied rather on a simple visual approach. This same visual approach was used more recently to relate the market share of fenoterol, a selective β_2-agonist, with asthma mortality in New Zealand between the mid-1970s to the late 1980s (65,66). Garrett et al. (67) concluded that the decrease in asthma mortality was most likely due to an increase in use of inhaled corticosteroids as reflected in sales of these medications in New Zealand as a whole. On the other hand, Pearce et al. (68) basing themselves on a visual assessment of sales and mortality information concluded that the impact of inhaled corticosteroids was minimal.

A major problem with most of these studies is that an analysis based simply on a visual inspection of data can be deceiving and the overall message may be changed by simply modifying the scale of the two factors under study (69,70). A better alternative is to fit the rates of asthma outcomes by Poisson or logistic regression models in order to estimate the effect of drug use on these outcomes. This approach was used to analyze the same New Zealand data, and showed that the rate of asthma mortality was reduced by 50% for each increase of one metered-dose inhaler of corticosteroids per asthmatic per month (71). This analysis also allowed one to control the effects of other antiasthma medications and strongly suggested that increasing inhaled corticosteroid use, rather than use of β-agonists, was the strongest factor in reducing the New Zealand asthma mortality epidemic. A more recent ecological study on asthma mortality in Japan, the first country to use a leukotriene receptor antagonist, also found an association between increasing anti-inflammatory medication use and a decrease in asthma mortality (72). This study was able to quantify the impact in various ways. First, it indicated that the stable yearly asthma death rate of around seven deaths per million before the introduction of leukotriene receptor antagonists in 1995 decreased by 23% (95% confidence interval 17–27%) thereafter, reaching 3.5 per million in 1999. In addition, the Poisson regression analysis showed that the rate ratio of asthma death was 0.96 (95% CI: 0.95–0.97) per one million 25-day treatment courses of inhaled corticosteroids and 0.80 (95% CI:0.76–0.83) for every one million 25-day treatment courses of leukotriene receptor antagonists, consumed per year in Japan.

Such epidemiological and statistical measures that allow one to quantify the impact of asthma medications on major outcomes in a population are essential to give credence to ecological studies in this field. The ecological design continues to be popular for monitoring outcomes in asthma in relation to drug use. In addition to the studies above, it has also been used to evaluate the impact of inhaled corticosteroids on asthma morbidity and mortality in several countries around the world, including the United Kingdom, New Zealand, Israel, Sweden, and Finland (67,73–77). Due to their important limitations, ecological studies are best used to generate hypotheses rather than for causal inference, in contrast to the more robust case–control and cohort study designs.

Case–Control Studies

The traditional case–control design, in contrast with the nested case–control design (see below), is not common in the evaluation of the impact of asthma drug therapy on major asthma outcomes, especially in studies using computerized databases. With this design, cases of major asthma outcomes such as asthma hospitalization or mortality are identified from a population and a control series of subjects who do not have this outcome at the same point in time are selected from the same population to estimate the association between drug therapy and the risk of this asthma outcome. The New Zealand case–control studies of asthma mortality were the first to address the effects of medications on this major outcome (22–24). Such field studies that collect information from patients, physicians, or medical charts are, however, the exception. The great majority employ existing health databases. For example, the GPRD was used to evaluate the impact of inhaled corticosteroids on the risk of hip fracture (50). The entire GPRD was used to identify 16,341 cases of hip fracture and a random sample of 29,889 subjects selected as controls. This design is attractive because of its efficiency in using only a sample of subjects to estimate an effect for an entire population. Such an approach, however, can be deceiving for specific diseases such as asthma because of the illusion of large sample sizes. Indeed, all cases of hip fracture selected within a population such as the GPRD suggests a very large sample size for the study, along with the very large number of controls. However, in assessing the effect of inhaled corticosteroids, a drug pertinent exclusively to the population of asthma or COPD patients, a large proportion of the cases and the controls are in fact irrelevant to the question at hand. Thus, for example, for the GPRD case–control study of hip fracture risk, only 878 of the 16,341 cases and 1335 of the 29,889 controls were subjects with asthma or COPD (50). With its 16,341 cases and 29,889 controls, the study appears at first more powerful than the Quebec study, based on 3326 cases of hip fracture and 66,237 controls selected from the asthma/COPD population (52). Consequently, the inference on the effect of inhaled corticosteroids is actually based on many fewer subjects than believed. This point is particularly relevant for studies that find no significantly increased risk, since, despite appearances, conclusions are based on fewer numbers of cases and controls with respiratory disease and thus lower power than expected. Furthermore, the estimate of effect may be biased if the outcome of interest, in this instance fractures, is also associated with the disease itself (asthma or COPD) and not only with the medications used to treat these conditions. In this case, the bias due to the association with the disease can only be eliminated by restricting the analyses to the population of patients who have the disease (52).

Cohort Studies

The majority of observational database studies that evaluate asthma drug therapy have used a cohort design. The distinguishing factor between the different cohorts is the definition of cohort entry or time zero. The Saskatchewan asthma cohorts have defined asthma as well as its onset by the dispensing of medications used to treat the condition. Patients were considered to have asthma as of the first time they received three prescriptions for an asthma medication, including bronchodilators, inhaled steroids, and other asthma drugs, on at least two different dates within a one-year period. The date of the third prescription defined the onset and diagnosis of asthma and patients were then followed from that point on for the occurrence of asthma outcomes. Such a definition is not entirely accurate for two reasons: subjects with asthma may be hospitalized as their initial presentation and medications for asthma are used for other conditions such as COPD. In an attempt to exclude patients with COPD, age criteria were used, including only patients to the age of 44, and also excluding oral corticosteroids as one of the defining drugs for asthma.

Alternatively, cohort entry may be defined by calendar time. For example, a cohort formed from a health maintenance organization in eastern Massachusetts defined cohort entry as October 1, 1991 (78,79). This cohort of 16,941 asthma patients was followed from this date or registration in the insurance plan to September 30, 1994. Such calendar time-based definitions of cohort entry will inherently define cohorts with patients who have varying durations of disease at time zero (cohort entry). Such a "prevalent" cohort, to be distinguished from an "incident" cohort defined by patients with new onset of asthma, are subject to serious biases when evaluating the association between drug use and asthma outcomes. Indeed, if the risk of the asthma outcome and of being dispensed the drug under study are both associated with the duration of asthma, such prevalent cohorts will produce biased estimates of this association unless the duration of the condition can somehow be adjusted for. A source of selection bias for such prevalent cohorts is that the treatment itself may change because of prior events that are not included in the period of observation. For example, if a patient was hospitalized for asthma in the past and, as a result, was prescribed inhaled corticosteroids, such a patient may be at increased risk of a further hospitalization and of being dispensed inhaled corticosteroids subsequently. For such studies to be valid, information on the history of asthma prior to cohort entry, which includes the duration of the disease and prior outcomes such as asthma hospitalizations as well as prior drug exposures are required for purpose of adjustment or for testing for effect modification. A frequent problem with computerized database studies is that these historical data on the duration and history of the disease before cohort entry are rarely available.

The third type of cohort defines cohort entry by a specific clinical event, such as hospitalization, emergency room visit, or a physician visit. Here again, these cohorts can be incident or prevalent if these cohort defining events are either the first one ever or rather the first to occur after a certain date. An example of this approach is a study from the Saskatchewan databases where patients were hospitalized for asthma for the first time and followed until readmission. The use of inhaled corticosteroids subsequent to the first hospitalization was evaluated with respect to the rate of readmission (46). A similar cohort definition was used with the Ontario database, although this cohort was based on elderly asthma patients and the asthma hospitalization defining cohort entry was not necessarily the first one to occur in their disease (80). The use of a physician visit or an emergency room visit was used as the cohort entry defining event in a recent study of the effectiveness of inhaled corticosteroids (81).

Immortal Time Bias in Cohort Studies

Irrespective of the type of cohort definition, the greatest challenge in cohort studies is in data analysis. Indeed, since asthma drug therapy, the exposure of interest, changes over time, data analysis must take this variability into account. However, such variability in exposure over time is not simple to incorporate in the analysis. Due to the complexity of such analyses, several of the studies mentioned above employed a time-fixed definition of exposure, by invoking the principle of intention-to-treat analysis. This principle, borrowed from randomized controlled trials, is based on the premise that subjects are exposed to the drug under study immediately at the start of follow-up. This information is unknown in database studies.

To imitate randomized controlled studies in the context of cohort studies, some authors have looked forward after cohort entry for the first prescription of the drug under study. In this way, a subject who was dispensed a prescription for such drug was considered exposed and subjects of who did not were considered unexposed. Different time periods of exposure assessment were used. For instance, in the context of COPD, a prescription for inhaled corticosteroids during the period of 90 days after cohort entry was used to define exposure (82). For asthma, periods of 1 year and 3 years were used to consider subjects exposed to inhaled corticosteroids in assessing their impact on mortality (80,83). This approach, however, leads to immortal time bias, a major source of distortion in the rate ratio estimate (84).

Immortal time bias arises from the introduction of immortal time in defining exposure by looking forward after cohort entry. Indeed, if an exposed subject was classified as such because they were observed to have been dispensed their first prescription for an inhaled corticosteroid 80 days after cohort entry, they necessarily had to be alive on day 80. Therefore, this 80-day period is immortal. While some exposed subjects will have very short immortal time periods (a day or two), others can have very long immortal periods. On the other hand, unexposed subjects do not have any immortal time, and in particular, the subjects who die soon after cohort entry, with too little time to receive the drug under study. Therefore, the exposed subjects will have a major survival advantage over their unexposed counterparts, because they are guaranteed to survive at least until their drug was dispensed.

This generation of immortal time in exposed subjects, but not in the unexposed subjects, causes an underestimation of the rate of the outcome among the exposed subjects. This underestimation results from the fact that the outcome rate in the exposed is actually composed of two rates. The first is the true rate, based on the person-time cumulated after the date of drug dispensing that defines exposure, while the second is that based on the person-time cumulated from cohort entry until the date of drug dispensing that defines exposure. The first rate will, therefore, be computed by dividing all outcome events in that group by the first rate person-time, while the second rate will, by definition, divide zero events by the second rate person-time. For example, the rate in the exposed

$$\text{Rate} = \text{deaths/total person} - \text{years} \tag{1}$$

is in fact

$$\text{Rate} = (0/\text{person-years pre-Rx}) + (\text{deaths/person-years after Rx}).$$

The zero component of the rate will necessarily bring down the exposed rate. Since thece is no such phenomenon in the unexposed group, the computation of the rate ratio will systematically produce a value lower than the true value because of the underestimation of the exposed rate. In particular, if the drug under study is altogether unrelated to the outcome, so that the true rate ratio is 1, this approach will produce rate ratios lower than 1, thus creating an appearance of effectiveness for the drug.

The immortal time in exposed subjects also causes an overestimation of the rate of the outcome among the unexposed subjects. This is because the zero component of the rate in the exposed group should in fact be classified in the unexposed group. Indeed, subjects are in fact unexposed to the drug under study between cohort entry until the date of drug dispensing that defines exposure. They only start to be exposed after the drug is dispensed. Thus, the zero rate should in fact be combined with the unexposed rate.

Immortal time bias is thus the result of simplistic yet improper exposure definitions and analyses that cause serious misclassification of exposure and outcome events. This situation is created by using an emulation of the randomized controlled trial to simplify the analysis of complex time-varying drug exposure data. However, such studies do not lend themselves to such simple paradigms. Instead, time-dependent methods for analyzing risks, such as the Cox proportional hazard models with time-dependent exposures or nested case–control designs, must be used to account for complex changes in drug exposure and confounders over time (84,85).

Nested Case–Control Studies

The complexity in data analysis is greater in the field of database studies because of the technical challenges presented by their large size. Indeed, the asthma cohort formed from the health maintenance organization in eastern Massachusetts included 742 asthma hospitalizations occurring during the 3 year follow-up period (78). With over 16,000 patients in the cohort, an analysis based on the Cox proportional hazards model with time-dependent exposure would require 742 risk sets (all patients in the cohort on the day of hospitalization) each containing approximately 16,000 observations with information on exposure and confounding factors measured at the point in time when the case occurred. Such an analysis would therefore require around 12 million observations, each with dozens of variables. Another example is the cohort study that included 6254 elderly asthma patients hospitalized for asthma in Ontario, Canada, of whom around 1500 either died or were readmitted for asthma (80). A proper time-dependent analysis would include in this case around 9 million observations, creating a serious technical challenge in statistical computing. As a result of this complexity, the temptation to analyze these cohorts with exposures that are assumed not to change over time is attractive which, as described above, can cause severe immortal time bias.

Rather than analyzing such cohort studies with proper but complex time-dependent techniques, methods based on sampling can produce practically the same results at greater efficiency. The nested case–control design, nested within the cohort, is precisely such an approach. It is based on using data on all the cases with the study outcome that occur during cohort follow-up. These represent the case series. A random sample of person-moments is then selected from all person-moments in the cohort to provide the control group for the nested case–control approach. For the cases, the index date, on which the timing of the exposure to the drug of interest is based, is simply the time at which the outcome occurred. For controls, the index date is a random person-moment during follow-up, or the same point in time of the corresponding case (86). Because of the highly variable nature of asthma drug exposure over time, it is important that person-moments are selected properly from all person-moments of follow-up for all members of the cohort. Thus, a subject may be selected more than once at different moments of their follow-up, and particularly person-moments preceding the index date of a case are valid control person-moments. For practical reasons and to conform with the Cox proportional hazards model, person-moments are usually selected from the risk set of each case. This approach involves identifying, for each case, all subjects who are at risk of the event at the time that the case occurred (the risk set) and controls are selected from this risk set. Part of the simplicity of this approach is that all subjects in a risk set are allocated the same index date as the set-defining case.

The advantage of this approach is the direct relationship between the Cox proportional hazard model with time-dependent exposure and the conditional logistic regression analysis that is used to analyze such nested case–control data. Thus, instead of using exposure data on all members of the risk set, as the Cox model would require, data on only a few subjects (usually 4 or 10 controls per case) are sufficient to provide a very efficient estimator of the rate ratio. Such ease of data analysis with the large size databases that are used in the field of asthma is crucial. As an example, with the cohort study of Donahue, if 10 controls per case were used for each of the 742 cases, the analysis would be based on 7420 observations instead of the 12 million observations necessary with the Cox model analysis.

In studying the effectiveness of treatment for asthma, one of the major problem is confounding by indication. The nested case–control approach becomes more useful, as it allows cases and controls to be matched on several measures of disease severity. Thus, the effect of a drug can be isolated, independently of the effects of the severity markers. Such a matched nested case–control study was used to evaluate the effectiveness of inhaled corticosteroids on asthma death (41). In that study, cases were identified from a cohort of over 30,000 asthma patients, from which 66 died of asthma. The Cox analysis would have required almost 2 million observations to be processed. For each case, however, the only members of the risk sets that were identified as controls were those with the same characteristics as the case, namely: prior hospitalization for asthma, oral corticosteroid use, number of canisters of β-agonists, use of theophylline, and nebulized β-agonists. Thus, cases and controls were similar on all these severity markers, except with respect to inhaled corticosteroids. As a result, the effect of inhaled corticosteroids could be assessed independently of potential confounding by severity.

Conclusion

Linked databases containing individualized information on important outcomes and on medications prescribed, or preferably dispensed, to patients provide important information on the safety and efficacy of medications used to treat asthma and other common conditions. Such information is not readily obtainable from randomized clinical trials or even meta-analyses of such trials. The information obtained relates directly to how medications are used in the real world clinical setting and therefore provide a more realistic estimate of the risks and benefits incurred when prescribing medications.

The analysis of these databases to obtain estimates of risk and benefit is not straightforward, however, and, thus far, insufficient attention has been given to the complexities involved and the biases that may result from a simplistic approach to these analyses. Careful attention to design, analysis, and interpretation of database studies is required if the valuable information which is obtainable from this source is not to be debased.

References

1. Rawson NS, Malcolm E. Validity of the recording of ischaemic heart disease and chronic obstructive pulmonary disease in the Saskatchewan health care datafiles. Stat Med 1995; 14(24):2627–2643.
2. Tamblyn R, Lavoie G, Petrella L, Monette J. The use of prescription claims databases in pharmacoepidemiological research: the accuracy and comprehensiveness of the prescription claims database in Quebec. J Clin Epidemiol 1995; 48(8):999–1009.
3. Wilchesky M, Tamblyn RM, Huang A. Validation of diagnostic codes in medical services claims data. Can J Clin Pharmacol 2001; 8:39.
4. Tamblyn R, Laprise R, Hanley JA, Abrahamowicz M, Scott S, Mayo N, et al. Adverse events associated with prescription drug cost-sharing among poor and elderly persons. J Am Med Assoc 2001; 285(4):421–429.
5. Walley T, Mantgani A. The UK General Practice Research Database (see comments). Lancet 1997; 350(9084):1097–1099.
6. Sears MR, Taylor DR, Print CG, Lake DC, Li QQ, Flannery EM, et al. Regular inhaled beta-agonist treatment in bronchial asthma (see comments). Lancet 1990; 336(8728):1391–1396.
7. Taylor DR, Sears MR, Herbison GP, Flannery EM, Print CG, Lake DC, et al. Regular inhaled beta agonist in asthma: effects on exacerbations and lung function (see comments). Thorax 1993; 48(2):134–138.
8. Drazen JM, Israel E, Boushey HA, Chinchilli VM, Fahy JV, Fish JE, et al. Comparison of regularly scheduled with as-needed use of albuterol in mild asthma. Asthma Clinical Research Network (see comments). N Engl J Med 1996; 335(12):841–847.
9. Chapman KR, Kesten S, Szalai JP. Regular vs as-needed inhaled salbutamol in asthma control. Lancet 1994; 343:1379–1382.
10. Taylor DR, Town Gl, Herbison GP, Boothman-Burrell D, Flannery EM, Hancox B, et al. Asthma control during long-term treatment with regular inhaled salbutamol and salmeterol. Thorax 1998; 53(9):744–752.

11. Boulet L-P, Becker A, Bérubé D, Beveridge R, Ernst P. Summary of recommendations from the asthma consensus report,1999. Can Med Assoc J 1999; 161(11 suppl):s1–s12.

12. National Asthma and Prevention Program. Guidelines for the diagnosis and management of asthma. Expert Panel Report 2. National Heart Lung and Blood Institute, editor. NIH Publication No. 97–4051, 1997.

13. Pauwels RA, Lofdahl CG, Postma DS, Tattersfield AE, O'Byrne P, Barnes, et al. Effect of inhaled formoterol and budesonide on exacerbations of asthma. Formoterol and Corticosteroids Establishing Therapy (FACET) International Study Group (see comments). N Engl J Med 1997; 337(20):1405–1411.

14. Matz J, Emmett A, Rickard K, Kalberg C. Addition of salmeterol to low-dose fluticasone versus higher-dose fluticasone: an analysis of asthma exacerbations. J Allergy Clin Immunol 2001; 107(5):783–789.

15. Lemanske RF Jr, Sorkness CA, Mauger EA, Lazarus SC, Boushey HA, Fahy JV, et al. Inhaled corticosteroid reduction and elimination in patients with persistent asthma receiving salmeterol: a randomized controlled trial. J Am Med Assoc 2001; 285(20):2594–2603.

16. Lazarus SC, Boushey HA, Fahy JV, Chinchilli VM, Lemanske RF Jr, Sorkness CA, et al. Long-acting beta2-agonist monotherapy vs continued therapy with inhaled corticosteroids in patients with persistent asthma: a randomized controlled trial. J Am Med Assoc 2001; 285(20):2583–2593.

17. Roberts JA, Bradding P, Britten KM, Walls AF, Wilson S, Gratziou C, et al. The long- acting beta2-agonist salmeterol xinafoate: effects on airway inflammation in asthma (see comments). Eur Respir J 1999; 14(2):275–282.

18. Mclvor RA, Pizzichini E, Turner MO, Hussack P, Hargreave FE, et al. Potential masking effects of salmeterol on airway inflammation in asthma. Am J Respir Crit Care Med 1998; 158(3):924–930.

19. Cockcroft DW, Swystun VA. Functional antagonism: tolerance produced by inhaled beta 2 agonists. Thorax 1996; 51(10):1051–1056.

20. Meier CR, Jick H. Drug use and pulmonary death rates in increasingly symptomatic asthma patients in the UK. Thorax 1997; 52(7):612–617.

21. Lanes SF, Lanza LL, Wentworth CE III. Risk of emergency care, hospitalization, and ICU stays for acute asthma among recipients of salmeterol. Am J Respir Crit Care Med 1998; 158(3):857–861.

22. Crane J, Pearce N, Flatt A, Jackson R, Ball M, Burgess C, et al. Prescribed fenoterol and death from asthma in New Zealand 1981–1983: case–control study. Lancet 1989; 1:917–922.

23. Pearce N, Grainger J, Atkinson M, Crane J, Burgess C, Culling C, et al. Case–control study of prescribed fenoterol and death from asthma in New Zealand, 1977–81 (see comments). Thorax 1990; 45(3):170–175.

24. Grainger J, Woodman K, Pearce N, Crane J, Burgess C, Keane A, et al. Prescribed fenoterol and death from asthma in New Zealand, 1981–7: a further case–control study. Thorax 1991; 46:105–111.

25. Spitzer WO, Suissa S, Ernst P, Horwitz Rl, Habbick B, Cockcroft D, et al. The use of beta-agonists and the risk of death and near death from asthma. N Engl J Med 1992; 326(8):501–506.

26. Suissa S, Ernst P, boivin JF, Horwitz RI, Habbick B, Cockroft D, et al. A cohort analysis of excess mortality in asthma and the use of inhaled beta-agonists. Am J Respir Crit Care Med 1994; 149(3 Pt 1):604–610.

27. Suissa S, Blais L, Ernst P. Patterns of increasing beta-agonist use and the risk of fatal or near-fatal asthma. Eur Respir J 1994; 7(9):1602–1609.

28. Taylor DR, Sears MR. Regular beta-adrenergic agonists. Evidence, not reassurance, is what is needed. Chest 1994; 106:552–559.

29. Sears MR, Taylor DR. The beta 2-agonist controversy. Observations, explanations and relationship to asthma epidemiology. Drug Saf 1994; 11(4):259–283.

30. Petri H, Urquhart J. Channeling bias in the interpretation of drug effects. Stat Med 1991; 10:577–581.

31. Beasley R, Burgess C, Pearce N, Woodman K, Crane J. Confounding by severity does not explain the association between fenoterol and asthma death. Clin Exp Allergy 1994; 24:660–668.

32. Blais L, Ernst P, Suissa S. Confounding by indication and channeling over time: the risks of beta-agonists. Am J Epidemiol 1996; 144:1161–1169.

33. Hemmelgarn B, Blais L, Collet J-P, Ernst P, Suissa S. Automated databases and the need for fieldwork in pharmacoepidemiology. Pharmacoepidemiol Drug Saf 1994; 3:275–282.

34. Ernst P, Habbick B, Suissa S, Hemmelgarn B, Cockcroft D, Buist AS, et al. Is the association between inhaled beta-agonist use and life-threatening asthma because of confounding by severity? (see comments). Am Rev Respir Dis 1993; 148(1):75–79.

35. Garrett JE, Lanes SF, Kolbe J, Rea HH. Risk of severe life threatening asthma and beta agonist type: an example of confounding by severity. Thorax 1996; 51(11):1093–1099.

36. Lanes SF, Rodriguez LAG, Huerta C. Respiratory medications and risk of asthma death. Thorax 2002; 57(8):683–686.

37. Suissa S, Hemmelgarn B, Blais L, Ernst P. Bronchodilators and acute cardiac death. Am J Respir Crit Care Med 1996; 154:1598–1602.

38. Au DH, Lemaitre RN, Curtis JR, Smith NL, Psaty BM. The risk of myocardial Infarction associated with inhaled beta-adrenoceptor agonists. Am J Respir Crit Care Med 2000; 161(3 Pt 1):827–830.

39. Au DH, Curtis JR, Every NR, McDonell MB, Finn SD. Association between inhaled beta-agonists and the risk of unstable angina and myocardial infarction. Chest 2002; 121(3):846–851.

40. Ernst P, Spitzer WO, Suissa S, Cockcroft D, Habbick B, Horwitz RI, et al. Risk of fatal and near-fatal asthma in relation to inhaled corticosteroid use. J Am Med Assoc 1992; 268(24):3462–3464.

41. Suissa S, Ernst P, Benayoun B, Baltzan M, Cai B. Low-dose inhaled corticosteroids and the prevention of death from asthma. N Engl J Med 2000; 343(5):332–336.

42. Suissa S, Assimes T, Ernst P. Inhaled short acting beta agonist use in COPD and the risk of acute myocardial infarction. Thorax 2003; 58(1):43–46.

43. Haahtela T, Jarvinen M, Kava T, Kiviranta K, Koskinen S, Lehtonen K, et al. Comparison of a beta 2-agonist, terbutaline, with an inhaled corticosteroid,

budesonide, in newly detected asthma (see comments). N Engl J Med 1991; 325(6):388–392.

44. Selroos O, Pietinalho A, Lofroos AB, Riska H. Effect of early vs late intervention with inhaled corticosteroids in asthma. Chest 1995; 108(5):1228–1234.

45. Blais L, Suissa S, boivin JF, Ernst P. First treatment with inhaled corticosteroids and the prevention of admissions to hospital for asthma (see comments). Thorax 1998; 53(12):1025–1029.

46. Blais L, Ernst P, boivin JF, Suissa S. Inhaled corticosteroids and the prevention of readmission to hospital for asthma. Am J Respir Crit Care Med 1998; 158(1): 126–132.

47. Suissa S, Ernst P, Kezouh A. Regular use of inhaled corticosteroids and the long term prevention of hospitalisation for asthma. Thorax 2002; 57(10):880–884.

48. Hanania NA, Chapman KR, Sturtridge WC, Szalai JP, Kesten S. Dose-related decrease in bone density among asthmatic patients treated with inhaled corticosteroids. J Allergy Clin Immunol 1995; 96(5 Pt 1):571–579.

49. Wong CA, Walsh LJ, Smith CJ, Wisniewski AF, Lewis SA, Hubbard R, et al. Inhaled corticosteroid use and bone-mineral density in patients with asthma (see comments). Lancet 2000; 355(9213):1399–1403.

50. Hubbard RB, Smith CJ, Smeeth L, Harrison TW, Tattersfield AE. Inhaled corticosteroids and hip fracture: a population-based case–control study. Am J Respir Crit Care Med 2002; 166(12 Pt 1):1563–1566.

51. Lau E, Mamdani M, Tu K. Inhaled or systemic corticosteroids and the risk of hospitalization for hip fracture among elderly women. Am J Med 2003; 114(2):142–145.

52. Suissa S, Baltzan M, Kremer R, Ernst P. Inhaled and nasal corticosteroid use and the risk of fracture. Am J Respir Crit Care Med 2004; 169(1):83–88.

53. Cumming RG, Mitchell P, Leeder SR. Use of inhaled corticosteroids and the risk of cataracts (see comments). N Engl J Med 1997; 337(1):8–14.

54. Garbe E, Suissa S, LeLorier J. Association of inhaled corticosteroid use with cataract extraction in elderly patients (published erratum appears in J Am Med Assoc 1998 Dec 2;280(21):1830). J Am Med Assoc 1998; 280(6):539–543.

55. Jick SS, Vasilakis-Scaramozza C, Maier WC. The risk of cataract among users of inhaled steroids. Epidemiology 2001; 12(2):229–234.

56. Smeeth L, Boults M, Hubbard R, Fletcher AE. A population based case–control study of cataract and inhaled corticosteroids. Br J Ophthalmol 2003; 87(10):1247–1251.

57. Garbe E, LeLorier J, Boivin JF, Suissa S. Risk of ocular hypertension or open-angle glaucoma in elderly patients on oral glucocorticoids. Lancet 1997; 350(9083):979–982.

58. Garbe E, LeLorier J, Boivin JF, Suissa S. Inhaled and nasal glucocorticoids and the risks of ocular hypertension or open-angle glaucoma. J Am Med Assoc 1997; 277(9):722–727.

59. Garbe E, Boivin JF, LeLorier J, Suissa S. Selection of controls in database case–control studies: glucocorticoids and the risk of glaucoma. J Clin Epidemiol 1998; 51(2):129–135.

60. Ernst P, Cai B, Blais L, Suissa S. The early course of newly diagnosed asthma. Am J Med 2002; 112(1):44–48.

61. Speizer FE, Doll R, Heaf P. Observations on recent increase in mortality from asthma. Br Med J 1968; 1(5588):335–339.

62. Inman WH, Adelstein AM. Rise and fall of asthma mortality in England and Wales in relation to use of pressurised aerosols. Lancet 1969; 2(615):279–285.

63. Stolley PD. Asthma mortality: why the United States was spared an epidemic of deaths due to asthma. Am Rev Respir Dis 1972; 105:883–890.

64. Gandevia B. Pressurized sympathomimetic aerosols and their lack of relationship to asthma mortality in Australia. Med J Aust 1973; 1(6):273–277.

65. Crane J, Burgess C, Pearce N, Beasley R, Jackson R. Asthma deaths in New Zealand. Brit Med J 1992; 304(6837):1307.

66. Suissa S, Ernst P, Spitzer WO. Asthma deaths in New Zealand. Brit Med J 1992; 305(6858):889–890.

67. Garrett J, Kolbe J, Richards G, Whitlock T, Rea H. Major reduction in asthma morbidity and continued reduction in asthma mortality in New Zealand: what lessons have been learned? Thorax 1995; 50(3):303–311.

68. Pearce N, Beasley R, Crane J, Burgess C, Jackson R. End of the New Zealand asthma mortality epidemic (see comments). Lancet 1995; 345(8941):41–44.

69. The Visual Display of Quantitative Information. Cheshire, CT: Graphics Press, 1983.

70. Cleveland CT, Diaconia P, McGill R. Variables on scatterpiots look more highly correlated when the scales are increased. Science (Wash) 1982; 216:1138–1141.

71. Suissa S, Ernst P. Optical illusions from visual data analysis: example of the New Zealand asthma mortality epidemic. J Clin Epidemiol 1997; 50(10): 1079–1088.

72. Suissa S, Ernst P. Use of anti-inflammatory therapy and asthma mortality in Japan. Eur Respir J 2003; 21(1):101–104.

73. Devoy MA, Fuller RW, Palmer JB. Asthma mortality and beta-agonists. Chest 1995; 108(6):1768.

74. Campbell MJ, Cogman GR, Holgate ST, Johnston SL. Age specific trends in asthma mortality in England and Wales, 1983–95: results of an observational study. Br Med J 1997; 314(7092):1439–1441.

75. Goldman M, Rachmiel M, Gendler L, Katz Y. Decrease in asthma mortality rate in Israel from 1991–1995: is it related to increased use of inhaled corticosteroids? J Allergy Clin Immunol 2000; 105(1 Pt 1):71–74.

76. Wennergren G, Kristjansson S, Strannegard IL. Decrease in hospitalization for treatment of childhood asthma with increased use of antiinflammatory treatment, despite an increase in prevalence of asthma. J Allergy Clin Immunol 1996; 97(3):742–748.

77. Haahtela T, Klaukka T. Societal and health care benefits of early use of inhaled steroids (editorial; comment). Thorax 1998; 53(12):1005–1006.

78. Donahue JG, Weiss ST, Livingston JM, Goetsch MA, Greineder DK, Platt R. Inhaled steroids and the risk of hospitalization for asthma. J Am Med Assoc 1997; 277(11):887–891.

79. Adams RJ, Fuhlbrigge AL, Finkelstein JA, Weiss ST. Intranasal steroids and the risk of emergency department visits for asthma. J Allergy Clin Immunol 2002; 109(4):636–642.

80. Sin DD, Tu JV. Inhaled corticosteroid therapy reduces the risk of rehospitalization and all-cause mortality in elderly asthmatics. Eur Respir J 2001; 17(3):380–385.
81. Smith M, Rascati KL, McWilliams BC. Inhaled anti-inflammatory pharmacotherapy and subsequent hospitalizations and emergency department visits among patients with asthma in the Texas Medicaid program. Ann Allergy Asthma Immunol 2004; 92(1):40–46.
82. Sin DD, Tu JV. Inhaled corticosteroids and the risk of mortality and readmission in elderly patients with chronic obstructive pulmonary disease. Am J Respir Crit Care Med 2001; 164(4):580–584.
83. Sin DD, Man SF. Low-dose inhaled corticosteroid therapy and risk of emergency department visits for asthma. Arch Intern Med 2002; 162(14): 1591–1595.
84. Suissa S. Effectiveness of inhaled corticosteroids in COPD: immortal time bias in observational studies. Am J Respir Crit Care Med 2003; 168:49–53.
85. Samet JM. Measuring the effectiveness of inhaled corticosteroids for COPD is not easy! Am J Respir Crit Care Med 2003; 168(1):1–2.
86. Suissa S. Novel approaches to pharmacoepidemiology study design and statistical analysis. In: Strom BL, ed. Pharmacoepidemiology. New York: John Wiley & Sons, Ltd., 2000:785–805.

Index